HORMONES
AND AGING

Edited by

Paola S. Timiras, M.D., Ph.D.
Department of Molecular and Cell Biology
University of California at Berkeley
Berkeley, California

Wilbur D. Quay, Ph.D.
Bio-Research Laboratory
New Bloomfield, Missouri

Antonia Vernadakis, Ph.D.
Department of Psychiatry and Pharmacology
University of Colorado Health Sciences Center
Denver, Colorado

CRC Press
Boca Raton   New York   London   Tokyo

Library of Congress Cataloging-in-Publication Data

Hormones and aging/edited by Paola S. Timiras, Wilbur B. Quay,
    Antonia Vernadakis.
        p.   cm.
    Includes bibliographical references and index.
    ISBN 0-8493-2446-7
    1. Endocrine glands—Aging.   2. Aging—Endocrine aspects.
    I. Timiras, Paola S.   II. Quay, Wilbur Brooks, 1927—1994.
    III. Vernadakis, Antonia, 1930—
    QP187.3.A34H67 1995
    612.4—dc20

                                                                    94-35653
                                                                    CIP

© 1995 by CRC Press, Inc.

No claim to original U.S. Government works
International Standard Book Number 0-8493-2446-7
Library of Congress Card Number 94-35653
Printed in the United States of America 1 2 3 4 5 6 7 8 9 0
Printed on acid-free paper

PREFACE

Chemical mediators have an important role in regulating the expression of the phenotype and in coordinating this expression in response to environmental demands. From the end of last century, the first time when these mediators, then called "internal secretions", were identified, they have been implicated as key factors in several functions indispensable for the survival of the individual (i.e., adaptation) and the continuation of the species (i.e., reproduction). Several current theories of aging consider the causative role of such mediators at the molecular, cellular, and organismic levels. Among the chemical mediators, hormones from the endocrine glands were the first to be identified and remain the best known; however, an increasing number of chemical substances from neurotransmitters to promoters or inhibitors of growth, to products of the immune system and to viral products, is continually being investigated for a better understanding of basic processes and the effectiveness of clinical interventions.

In 1982, we edited a first book on *Hormones in Development and Aging.* Ten years later, with Dr. W. B. Quay, we considered that sufficient progress had been made to justify another book on the topic of *Hormones and Aging,* hence the current publication. We are deeply sorry that Dr. Quay is no longer with us to rejoice in the final product of his earlier efforts, but we appreciate the three chapters he has contributed which are representative of his dual expertise in endocrinology and metabolism.

This book describes changes with aging in a wide spectrum of secretory functions: hormones from classical endocrine glands, hormone-like secretions and chemical mediators from diffuse cells within several systems, particularly the nervous and the immune systems. Changes in hormonal functions which occur in humans from young to old age under conditions of "normal" or "successful" aging focus on the menopause, changes in body composition and muscle mass, decline in metabolic rate, and alterations of oxidative metabolism. Pathological consequences of aging and associated hormonal changes discuss diabetes, osteoporosis, altered responses to stress, and cancer. The pathophysiology of these diseases is evaluated in the light of the most current, state-of-the-art biomedical advances, including molecular and genetic advances. Major preventive and therapeutic interventions are outlined, in particular the role of hormonal replacement therapy, growth promoting and cancer inhibitory substances, and influence of nutrition. Interactions of hormones with other systems, primarily the nervous and immune systems, have been implicated in the etiology of the aging process and are the basis of current neuroendocrine and immuno-endocrine theories of aging.

The book primarily considers humans but information is also provided by *in vivo* studies from uni- and pluricellular complex animal organisms as well as from cultured cells *in vitro.* Efforts were made to provide a concise review of a large variety of topics, integrating basic and clinical information. Contributors have been successful in providing a lucid and well-organized text, easily understandable to undergraduate and graduate students, as well as endocrinologists, gerontologists, and geriatricians.

In conclusion, the book represents a timely and useful contribution to a rapidly expanding field of chemical mediators and aging.

Paola S. Timiras
Antonia Vernadakis

REMEMBRANCE

Wilbur B. (Bill) Quay died Thursday, May 12, 1994, in New Bloomfield, Missouri, at the age of 67 years.

Bill was an extremely learned and scientifically prolific colleague. For all those who had the pleasure of knowing him, he would readily discuss almost any subject in science in considerable depth. Bill was a renaissance scholar who worked not only in the area of pineal biology, but also ornithology, population dynamics, and sebaceous glands, to name only a few. He was extremely well read and published widely on all of his interests; this work spanned fields from morphology, to circadian biology, to microbiology, to biochemistry and cellular biology.

Perhaps many of you did not personally know Bill Quay well. He was a thinker/loner and rarely engaged in social events. At meetings, rather than making "small talk", Bill would be in the nearby forests and streams communicating with the local fauna and flora; he never passed up an opportunity to inspect the natural environs around a meeting site.

I had the good fortune of knowing Bill Quay well as both a friend and scientist. I worked closely with him during the early days of pineal research and in conjunction with the *Journal of Pineal Research*; I discussed his personal and scientific life with him many times. I hope he considered me a good friend; it was a pleasure to have known him.

Bill published hundreds of papers in each of several different fields. He directed the training of eleven Ph.D. students and supervised twelve postdoctoral fellows. His broad perspective in biology and his wisdom for the field will be badly missed. I personally congratulate him on his many contributions but I know he would have accepted any accolade with reluctance. That was the nature of Bill Quay.

Bill, we all thank you for your many contributions and for your friendship. Thanks for enlightening our lives.

Russel J. Reiter
June, 1994

THE EDITORS

Dr. Paola S. Timiras is a Professor in the Department of Molecular and Cell Biology at the University of California at Berkeley (UCB). A native of Rome, Italy, Dr. Timiras is a graduate of the University of Grenoble, France (B.A.), the University of Rome (B.A., M.D., Summa cum Laude), and the University of Montréal, Quebec, Canada (Ph.D.).

Before joining the University of California in 1956, she was a faculty member of the University of Montréal (1950–1953) and the University of Utah (1953–1955). She chaired the Department of Physiology–Anatomy at the UCB from 1978 to 1984.

Her interest in development and aging has led her to participate in several related societies. She directed an innovative medical program (Health and Medical Science, 1973–1975) and a training program in developmental physiology and aging (1965–1976) at UCB. She was one of the founders and president (1978–1981) of the International Society of Developmental Neuroscience, as well as vice president and president of the International Society of Psychoneuroendocrinology (1974–1982). Her research on the neuroendocrinology of development and aging has resulted in the publication of more than 350 papers and several books.

Dr. Timiras is also a consultant for many government agencies concerned with biological research, and she is on the editorial boards of several journals. Her contributions to teaching and research have been recognized by several awards in the United States and abroad.

Dr. Timiras has recently edited *Physiological Basis of Aging and Geriatrics,* a comprehensive review of aging and geriatrics, published by CRC Press.

Dr. Antonia Vernadakis is a Professor in the Departments of Psychiatry and Pharmacology at the School of Medicine, University of Colorado, Denver. A native of Crete, Greece, she received her B.A., M.S., and Ph.D. degrees at the University of Utah in the Departments of Anatomy and Pharmacology. She was a Postdoctoral Fellow in the Department of Pharmacology, University of California, San Francisco (1961–1963). In 1964, she became a research faculty member of the Department of Physiology-Anatomy at Berkeley. In 1967, she joined the faculty of the School of Medicine of the University of Colorado and, in 1978, became a full professor.

Her main research interests are neuron-glia interactions during development and aging and, to this end, in 1986 she co-edited, with Sergey Fedoroff, three volumes on Astrocytes. She also contributed one of the first review articles in this field. She has been one of the first to explore the role of neuro-glia in the aging brain and has written several articles on the subject. Her research on regulatory mechanisms of development and aging has resulted into over 250 publications. In 1978, along with Ezio Giacobini, Dr. Vernadakis was the editor of the *International Journal of Developmental Neuroscience.*

Dr. Vernadakis was the first to initiate lectures in gerontological pharmacology as part of the medical pharmacology curriculum for second year medical students at the University of Colorado. She was also the first to establish an elective interdisciplinary course in gerontological pharmacology for graduate and postdoctoral students, again at the University's School of Medicine.

She has been the organizer of several conferences, workshops, and symposia and is considered one of the leaders of neurobiology.

CONTRIBUTORS

Jean-François Bach
Immulogie Clinique
INSERM U25
Hôpital Necker
Paris, France

Regina C. Casper
Department of Psychiatry and
  Behavioral Sciences
Stanford University School of Medicine
Stanford, California

Mireille Dardenne
Immulogie Clinique
CNRS URA 1461
Hôpital Necker
Paris, France

Elizabeth M. Dax
National HIV Reference Laboratory
Fairfield Hospital
Fairfield, Victoria, Australia

William C. Duckworth
University of Nebraska Medical Center
  and Veterans Administration
  Medical Center
Diabetes Section
Omaha, Nebraska

Gary L. Firestone
Department of Molecular and
  Cell Biology and
The Cancer Research Laboratory
University of California, Berkeley
Berkeley, California

Tamàs Fülöp, Jr.
Centre de Recherche en Gérontologie
  et Gériatrie
Hôpital d'Youville
Université de Sherbrooke,
  Faculté de Médecine
Sherbrooke, Quebec, Canada

Luis Goya
Instituto de Bioquímica
Facultad de Farmacia
Universidad Complutense
Madrid, Spain

Rodolfo Goya
INIBIOLP
Universidad National de la Plata
Facultad de Ciencias Medicas
La Plata, Argentina

Françoise Homo-Delarche
Immulogie Clinique
CNRS URA 1461
Hôpital Necker
Paris, France

Carol Hunter Winograd
Stanford University School of Medicine
Stanford, California and
Geriatric Research, Education, and
  Clinical Center
Palo Alto V.A. Medical Center
Palo Alto, California

James A. Joseph
United States Department of Agriculture
Agricultural Research Service
Human Nutrition Research Center
  on Aging
Tufts University
Boston, Massachusetts

Takashi Kachi
Department of Anatomy
School of Medicine
Hirosaki University
Hirosaki, Japan

Fran E. Kaiser
Division of Geriatric Medicine
St. Louis University Health Sciences
  Center and Geriatric Research,
  Education, and Clinical Center
Veterans Affairs Medical Center
Jefferson Barracks Division
St. Louis, Missouri

Anita C. Maiyar
Department of Molecular and Cell
  Biology and
The Cancer Research Laboratory
University of California, Berkeley
Berkeley, California

John E. Morley, M.B., B.Ch.
Division of Geriatric Medicine
St. Louis University Health Sciences Center
and Geriatric Research, Education,
and Clinical Center
St. Louis Veterans Administration Hospital
Jefferson Barracks Division
St. Louis, Missouri

Charles Y. C. Pak, M.D.
Center for Mineral Metabolism and
Clinical Research
Department of Internal Medicine
University of Texas Southwestern
Medical Center at Dallas
Dallas, Texas

A. M. Pascual-Leone
Instituto de Bioquímica
Facultad de Farmacia
Universidad Complutense
Madrid, Spain

Wilbur B. Quay*
Bio-Research Laboratory
New Bloomfield, Missouri

Ross A. Ramos
Department of Molecular and Cell Biology
and The Cancer Research Laboratory
University of California, Berkeley
Berkeley, California

Suresh I. S. Rattan, Ph.D., D.Sc.
Cellular Ageing Lab
Kemisk Institute
Aarhus Universitet
Aarhus-C, Denmark

Francisco Rivero
Instituto de Bioquímica
Facultad de Farmacia
Universidad Complutense
Madrid, Spain

Jacqueline Sentenac
Hopitaux de Gynecologie Chirugicale
School of Medicine
University of Bordeaux
Bordeaux, France

Paola S. Timiras, M.D., Ph.D.
Molecular and Cell Biology
University of California, Berkeley
Berkeley, California

Antonia Vernadakis
Departments of Psychiatry and
Pharmacology
University of Colorado Health
Sciences Center
Denver, Colorado

Rafael Villalobos-Molina
United States Department of
Agriculture
Agricultural Research Service
Human Nutrition Research Center at
Tufts University
Boston, Massachusetts
(Visiting Scientist
Seccion de Terapeutica Experimental
Departamento de Farmacologia y
Toxicologia
CINVESTAV-IPN
Mexico)

*Deceased

ACKNOWLEDGMENTS

The Editors are indebted to all contributors for their excellent chapters prepared within rather stringent deadlines. We are particularly grateful to those contributors (Drs. Dax, Duckworth, Homo-Delarche, Kachi, Kaiser, Joseph, Morley, Pak, Rattan, Vernadakis) and their associates who had prepared a chapter for an earlier (canceled) publication and have been willing to update their text for this edition. Special thanks go to Dr. L. L. Rosenberg for his substantive and constructive editoral criticisms of all chapters, and particularly for updating those of Dr. W. B. Quay. In this respect, we want also to thank Ms. Charlet Quay for making available to us all drawings and latest information for her husband's chapters.

We are grateful to Ana Duenas, who competently prepared the manuscript and dealt with the word processing and editing, and to Yuni Cho, who continued her word and guided the entire manuscript to its final completion. We would also like to thank bibliographic assistant, Ms. Anelia Popnikolova, and librarian, Ms. Ingrid Radkey, for their assistance with the bibliography.

CONTENTS

Part I: Introduction

Part II: Aging of the Endocrine Glands

Part III: Pathology and Hormonal Action in the Aged

Part IV: Molecular Regulatory Mechanisms

Part V: Conclusions and Perspectives

PART I

INTRODUCTION

1

Definitions, Evolution, and Theories

Paola S. Timiras

CONTENTS

I. INTRODUCTION

Hormones are molecules that are synthesized and secreted by specialized cells often localized in endocrine glands; they are released into the blood and exert biochemical effects on target

0-8493-2446-7/95/$0.00+$.50
© 1995 by CRC Press Inc.

cells at a distance from their site of origin. A more global definition of hormones includes, as well, substances secreted by cells and which act on targets situated in the immediate vicinity or nearby. The specificity of hormone action is determined by the presence of specific hormone receptors located either on the cell surface or intracellularly in the target cells. Cellular response is determined by the genetic programming of the particular cell, hence the same hormone has different actions on different cells.

Hormones classified in terms of chemical structure are listed in Table 1-1, and in terms of major actions in Table 1-2. While both structure and action will be discussed in detail throughout this book, the vital role of hormones should be underlined at the very onset together with the plurality of their actions affecting membrane permeability and transport, enzyme activation, and nuclear regulation. As a consequence of these multidimensional actions, hormones regulate growth and maturation during development, promote adaptation in adulthood, and many are indispensable for survival at all ages. Hormones regulate cellular and molecular functions directly as well as indirectly through other systems, i.e., by modulating neural and immune control.

In this chapter, definitions, demography, comparative aspects, and theories of aging are presented as a background to the aging of endocrine activity. All aspects of aging from molecular to organismic are influenced by hormones. Reciprocally, endocrine function may be modified during aging due to intrinsic alterations of the endocrine gland or cell, or to desynchronization of regulatory signals or to failure or impairment of target cell responses. The key role of hormones in growth and development is well demonstrated. A number of theories identify endocrine dysfunction as a cause of aging. They also imply that hormonal therapies are valid means to improve and prolong the lifespan.

The elderly comprise a growing proportion of the population in many nations; hence, the increased concern of the biomedical community in the problems of the aged and in understanding the aging process. More people live longer today than ever before and this trend is expected to continue in the next century. As people live longer, their later years are often marred by increasing disability and pathology. The pathology of aging has been extensively studied in terms of combating specific diseases associated with this high-risk group. In contrast, the biology of aging and its physiologic and psychosocial correlates have not been of dominant interest, partly because of the difficulty of distinguishing "normal" from "abnormal" aging as well as "successful" from "usual" aging.

Old age or senescence in humans has conventionally been accepted as that stage of the life cycle which starts around 65 years of age (often coinciding with retirement from the working force) and terminates with death. It is, however, extremely difficult to circumscribe the temporal boundaries in physiologic terms. Aging is commonly described as having its onset at some indeterminate point following maturity, in contrast to other periods of the life cycle in which the onset is clearly marked by specific physiologic events — such as menarche at puberty. Even body components age at different rates. These rates are themselves influenced by genetic and environmental factors. Aging has, so far, defied all attempts to establish objective landmarks that would precisely characterize its earlier stages.

II. DEFINITIONS OF AGING

It is impossible, at the present stage of our knowledge, to present an all-encompassing definition of aging — indeed, there are as many definitions as there are theories of aging. Maturity, connoting the achievement of optimal integrated function of all body systems, is used as a conceptual standard against which degrees of physiologic and pathologic deviation can be measured. In most biomedical textbooks, focus is on the mature organism — modeled in humans by the 70-k, 170-cm, 25-year-old man. During the years that follow maturity, physiologic change is far less rapid than during development and aging. In the absence of

TABLE 1-1 Selected Hormones Grouped by Structure

Peptides and proteins		Steroids	Amines
Glycoproteins	**Polypeptides**	**Steroids**	**Amines**
Follicle-stimulating hormone (FSH)	Adrenocorticotropic hormone (ACTH)	Aldosterone	Epinephrine
Human chorionic gonadotropin (hCG)	Angiotensin	Cortisol	Melatonin
Luteinizing hormone (LH)	Atrial natriuretic hormones	Estradiol	Norepinephrine
Thyroid-stimulating hormone (TSH)	Calcitonin	Progesterone	Thyroxine (T4)
	Cholecystokinin	Testosterone	Triiodothyronine (T3)
	Erythropoietin	Vitamin D	
	Gastrin		
	Glucagon		
	Gonadotropin-stimulating hormone (GnRH)		
	Growth hormone		
	Insulin		
	Insulin-like growth peptides (somatomedins)		
	Melanocyte-stimulating hormone (MSH)		
	Nerve growth factor		
	Oxytocin		
	Parathyroid hormone		
	Prolactin		
	Prolactin-inhibiting hormone (PIH)		
	Prolactin-releasing hormone (PRH)		
	Relaxin		
	Secretin		
	Somatostatin		
	TSH-stimulating hormone (TRH)		
	Vasopressin (ADH)		

TABLE 1-2 Selected Hormones Grouped by Function[a]

Membrane permeability and transport			Enzyme activation	Nuclear regulation
Glucose + amino acid	**Ions**	**H$_2$O and solutes**	**Enzyme activation**	**Nuclear regulation**
Insulin	Insulin	Aldosterone	Catecholamines	Steroids
TSH	Thyroid hormones	Vitamin D	Insulin	Thyroid hormones
Cholecystokinin	TSH	Glucocorticoids	Glucagon	Growth hormone
Glucagon		Parathyroid hormone	Calmodulin	Prolactin
Growth hormone		Gastrin	Steroids	Insulin
Thyroid hormones		Secretin		
Polypeptide tropic hormones				
Gonadal steroids				

[a] Some are involved in more than one function.

pathology, aging "is superimposed on maturity . . . imperceptibly."[1] Thus, the aging process can be viewed as an integral aspect of the continuous development of the organism: it has been defined as *the sum of all changes with the passage of time, eventually associated with functional impairment and reduced ability to maintain homeostasis* (Table 1-3).[2]

TABLE 1-3 Selected Definitions of Aging

Aging
  Stage of the lifespan
	• Sum of all changes occurring in an organism over time;
	  phase of normal life cycle

Aging (senescence)
  Deteriorative process
	• Sum of all changes occurring with time and leading to
	  functional impairment and death

Aging Cellular and molecular damage	• Changes with time in membranes, cytoplasm, and/or nucleus

A. Aging Characterized by Changes with the Passage of Time

Long before **gerontology** (the science that studies aging processes) became a field in its own right, aging phenomena were viewed, together with growth and development, as a continuum of physiologic events having their onset at fertilization and their termination at death (Table 1-4). Over the years, a definition was formulated that described the aging process as *the sum total of all changes that occur in the living organism with the passage of time.* The time frame for life is not yet clear. Psychologically, if not biologically, time flows faster and faster with age, as quoted by Whitrow:[3]

> For when I was a babe and wept and slept, Time crept;
> When I was a boy and laughed and talked, Time walked;
> Then when the years saw me a man, Time ran,
> But as I older grew, Time flew.

However, a "global" appreciation of the biologic history of the individual shows that chronologic and physiologic age rarely coincide because of the continuing interplay of genetic and environmental factors.[4] A more accurate picture of aging must recognize the decrement in physiologic competence that occurs at molecular, cellular, tissular, and organismic levels with advancing age. This decrement contributes to the progressively decreasing capacity of the organism to maintain its viability.

TABLE 1-4 Stages of the Lifespan

Stage	Duration
Prenatal	
Ovum	Fertilization through week 1
Embryo	Weeks 2–8
Fetus	Lunar months 3–10
Birth	
Postnatal	
Neonatal period	Newborn; birth through week 2
Infancy	3 Weeks until end of first year
Childhood	
Early	Years 2–6
Middle	Years 7–10
Later	Prepubertal: females 9–15 males 11–16
Adolescence	The 6 years following puberty
Adulthood	Between 20 and 65 years
Senescence[a]	From 65 years on
Death	

[a] Senescence is generally used interchangeably with aging. However, aging may be taken to refer to all changes observable throughout the lifespan, from birth to death, whereas senescence specifically circumscribes the later life period.

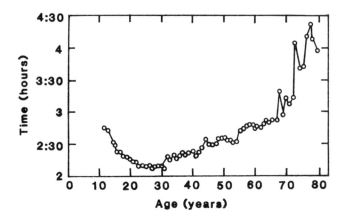

FIGURE 1-1   Age changes in world marathon records for men. Times first decrease from puberty to the minimum at approximately age 30. Thereafter, they increase progressively until about age 70 and then increase rapidly. (Redrawn from Comfort, A., *The Biology of Senescence,* 3rd ed., Elsevier, New York, 1979.)

B.   Aging, Homeostasis, and Stress

Alternatively, aging may be viewed as *the sum total of all changes that occur in a living organism with the passage of time and lead to functional impairment, increased pathology, and death.* Functional impairment is best manifested in a decreasing ability to maintain homeostasis and survive stress.

Homeostasis refers to the total ability of the organism to adjust and maintain the constancy of cells and molecules (i.e., the internal environment) in the face of changes in external conditions (generating stress). *Stress, in turn, may be defined as any environmental change that disrupts homeostasis.* The goal of homeostatic responses to stress is to provide the organism with the physiologic responses necessary to cope with environmental disruptive influences and to maintain the capacity for adaptation and survival. With aging, this homeostatic capability declines and the individual becomes more vulnerable to environmental challenges.[5] An illustrative example of the declining capability of the elderly in the performance of a demanding task (i.e., a stressful situation) is the increase of running time in a marathon race. Starting at about age 30, the time increases until it is about double at age 80 (Figure 1-1).[6] Maximum performance in this activity is dependent upon the excellent function of most, if not all, the major organ systems and, primarily, neuroendocrine interactions. These data are of particular interest because of the obvious selection for highly fit subsets of the population.

Under steady-state as well as stress conditions, the activity of several endocrines, most importantly the adrenal cortex, but also the gonads and the thyroid gland, must be synchronized by inputs from the hypothalamus and the pituitary and must be responsive to the needs of the many functions they regulate. With aging:

- Some of the efficiency of the hypothalamus-pituitary signals may be lost or altered,
- The secretory activity of the peripheral endocrines (e.g., adrenal cortex, thyroid, gonad) and the metabolism of their hormones may be altered, and
- The target on which the hormones act may be damaged.

All these perturbations may converge to induce a decline in homeostatic capability and a greater vulnerability to environmental challenges.

The linkage of stress and adrenocortical hormones and reproduction with aging and death is illustrated by the Pacific salmon and the Atlantic eel, which are prime examples of the inverse relationship between accumulation of damage, stress, and length of lifespan. Both fish age rapidly at the time of spawning and die shortly thereafter with all the signs (including adrenocortical hyperactivity) of exhaustion following stress (i.e., swimming upstream over rapids). However, if spawning and the associated stress is prevented, they will continue to live (albeit forfeiting reproduction) for several years.[7]

The compensatory attempts of the aging organism to adapt, such as the persistence of increased levels of adrenocortical hormones, may themselves be damaging (see Chapters 14 and 16). Chronic stress would lead to a progressive decline in efficiency of homeostasis, increase susceptibility to degenerative processes, induce disability and disease, and accelerate the probability of death.

C. Aging and Disease

It is difficult to isolate the effects of aging, alone, from those due to disease or to gradual degenerative changes that develop fully with the passage of time. For example, it may be questioned whether atheroma — the characteristic lesion of atherosclerosis — represents a degenerative process initiated early during development or an "actual" disease of the heart and arteries, and to what extent changes in the myocardium are due to age alone or are the consequence of cardiovascular pathology. Old age almost always seems to be "combined with or masked by morbid processes." Certainly, late life is a period of increasing and multiple pathology (Figure 1-2).[8] Death from "pure" old age is probably rare and certainly difficult to prove by objective evidence.

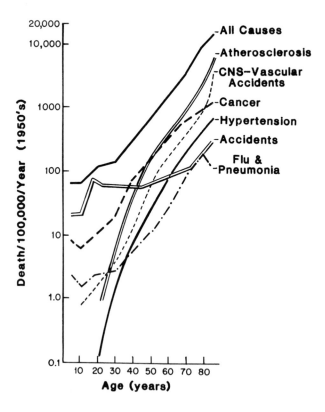

FIGURE 1-2 Some common causes of death by age in the United States. Atherosclerosis together with the accompanying vascular accidents of the central nervous system (CNS) and hypertension remain the major causes of death in the 1980s. (From Kohn, R. R., *Relations Between Normal Aging and Disease*, Johnson, H. A., Ed., Raven Press, New York, 1985.)

If aging is a disease, then the therapy of aging may be synonymous with treatment of disease. The latter is the scope of **geriatrics**, that branch of medicine which is concerned with the prevention and treatment of the diseases of old age. The usual clinical approach, fundamentally pragmatic, envisions no real chance of significantly influencing the overall aging process beyond removal or amelioration of disease. Carried to its extreme, this view defines aging as a disease on the argument that any deviation from the "ideal norm" embodied by the young adult, preferably the 25-year-old male, represents a condition of disease. (As defined in *Webster's Collegiate Dictionary*: "disease is an impairment of the normal state of the living animal or plant body that affects the performance of the vital functions".) Acceptance of aging as a disease because of its deviation from the adult norm would lead to the rather absurd parallel of youth as a disease — a view celebrated by the romantic poets, but hardly by biologists.

The difficulty of separating aging from disease is reflected by the lack of consensus in identifying and validating putative biological models and markers of intrinsic aging.[9,10] One marker that may meet some of the stringent criteria of validity — i.e., early onset and independence from intervening disease — is the rate at which lipofuscin pigments accumulate in the cytoplasm of certain cell types, including several endocrine cell types.[11]

A rigid view of "normal", tied as it is to the physiologic optimum of a specific age, is contrary to the dynamic nature of physiologic responses. For example, the reduced cellular availability of the hormone triiodothyronine in old individuals could be interpreted as a pathologic condition of thyroid hormone metabolism and nuclear binding with aging; it may just as well be a compensatory decline in the levels of the hormone in response to the decreased demands of older, less metabolically active cells.[12]

Treatment and eventual cure of many diseases may prolong life, but only by a few years. For example, if vascular diseases were cured overnight, the lifespan would be extended by only about 5 to 6 years. The spectacular advances in medicine in the last 90 years have been responsible, in large part, for the dramatic increase in the average lifespan, but further lengthening on this basis alone appears unlikely. With a better understanding of the basic mechanisms of the aging process per se, the etiopathology of the diseases of old age may be elucidated and further advances in rational treatment achieved.

Disease, by breaking down homeostatic defenses, can accelerate or induce aging. The more diseases encountered during the lifespan the greater the physiologic deterioration that accumulates, and the less the chance of survival at any age. Thus, childhood diseases are very important to health at all ages. Optimal development determines not only physical and mental well-being in adulthood but also quality of life in old age and length of the lifespan. Deleterious factors, though not lethal in themselves, may contribute to physiologic decline, predispose to functional losses or to specific diseases at a later age, and accelerate the time of death. Indeed, the logarithmic progression of the tendency to die with increasing age, described by epidemiologists from death rate curves, reflects both the decline in physiologic competence and the consequence of past and present diseases.

III. DEMOGRAPHY OF AGING

A. Life Expectancy and Lifespan

One of the most dramatic demographic changes witnessed in this century is the progressively greater number of people surviving to 65 years and older. Life expectancy at birth, that is, the number of years an individual in a given population is expected to live, was about 50 years at the turn of the century in the United States. A child born in 1992 can expect to live to 80 years of age and older, with women living 5 or more years than men (Figure 1-3). The extraordinary increase in the average lifespan (i.e., the average age reached by members of a

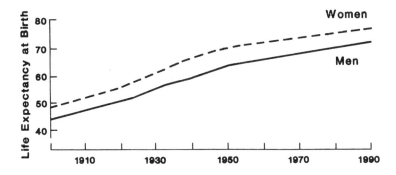

FIGURE 1-3 Increase in life expectancy in the United States between 1900 and 1990. This trend holds true also for developing countries' populations. Note the longer life expectancy for women.

population), unprecedented in history, has been ascribed to progress in the standard of living — particularly in sanitation, nutrition, and medicine.[13]

A direct consequence of the increase in the number of individuals reaching old age, with a relatively constant number of births, is the increased proportion of the elderly in the United States, Japan, and other economically developed countries. In 1910, 4% of our population was over 65 years of age; in 1980, 11%, and in 2030 it is predicted that 18% of the population will be 65 and older. Even more rapid is the increase in the population over 75 years of age (the so-called "old-old group"), increasing from 1% in 1910 to an expected 8% in 2030. Since 1985, the elderly over age 85, in percentage terms, are the most rapidly growing segment of our population (Figure 1-4). Impressive as these increases may appear they may underestimate future demographic changes.[14,15]

Historically, longevity was not a "problem" but a privilege. Most human deaths were premature: lives were cut short, usually by infectious diseases in infancy, childhood, and early maturity, that is, before old age. The question that demographers are expected to answer is how much larger, in both absolute and relative terms, will the population over 65 become in our demographic future? As the overall health status of the elderly improves and technology advances, "deceleration of aging may very well raise to 100 years the life expectancy of humans by the middle of next century, if not sooner."[16]

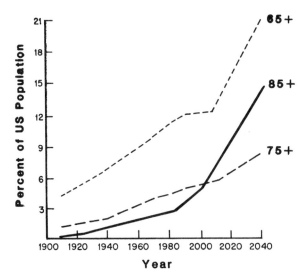

FIGURE 1-4 Age of United States population (in percent) from the year 1900 projected to the year 2040. The most rapidly increasing segment of the population is that of age 85 and older.

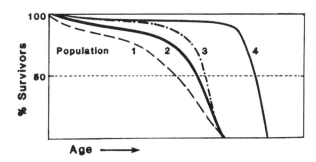

FIGURE 1-5 Survival curves measure age on the abscissa and the percentage of survivors (that is, that portion of the original population surviving) on the ordinate. The flatness of the curve indicates a high rate of survival, the 50% line represents the median age for survival; the tail indicates maximum lifespan (longevity). Curve 2 represents current survival. The relatively flat portion of Curve 2 indicates approximately 100% survival at early ages, but with increasing age the number of survivors decreases, as shown by the shoulder of the curve and the 50% population indicated by the dotted line; the tail of the curve indicates the maximum lifespan or maximum longevity of the population. Cumulative genetic or environmental hazards will shift the curve to the left as the number of survivors decreases (Curve 1). Improving genetic vigor and living conditions will increase the number of survivors and shift the curve to the right (Curve 3). Under both conditions, however, the maximum lifespan, that is, the length of life of the oldest members of a population, remains unchanged. In Curve 4, delayed onset of diseases of old age and increased maximum lifespan (rectangularization of the curve) is one of the goals of gerontologists, but is still today the most difficult one to achieve.

B. Survival Curves as Influenced by Genetic and Environmental Factors

Survival curves obtained from plots of life table survivorship are illustrated in Figure 1-5. Comparison of the four curves show that, at all ages, survivorship depends on both genetic and environmental factors: curves are shifted to the left (decreased survivorship) or to the right (increased survivorship) depending on the severity of genetic and environmental hazards or, vice versa, genetic vigor and improved conditions of life.

It is probably safe to state that most old individuals are affected by some disability or disease. In fact, it is the multiple pathology of old age (also referred to as co-morbidity) that impairs the quality of life in later years. However, some still very controversial observations suggest that changes in diet, physical and mental exercise, and daily routine may postpone the onset of disability and disease. This so-called "compression of morbidity" (i.e., shortening of time between the onset of disease and death) is already an ongoing process (according to some, but not all, epidemiologists) and is expected to lead to "rectangularization" of the survivorship curve (Figure 1-5) and to a healthier old age: declining function and increasing pathology would be banished to the very last months or weeks of life.[17,18]

C. Maximum Lifespan in Humans and Aging Worldwide

Among mammals, humans represent the longest-living species. Accurate records of human longevity (meaning length of life or long life) are difficult to collect due to recording errors or lack of recording and the well-known tendency of elderly individuals to exaggerate their age. Documented records have fixed the maximum lifespan (i.e., the greatest aged reached by any member of a species) in humans at 114 years, although a few of the partially documented records report a somewhat greater (up to 120 years) longevity.[6] Claims of extreme longevity (up to 130 years of age) abound in particular regions; often cited is the celebrated longevity of some inhabitants of the Caucasus, the high valleys of Ecuador, and the Karakoram Mountains.[19] Although there is no question that in these populations many subjects interviewed were very old, even centenarians, their exact ages and their proportion in the total population are questionable due to the lack of birth records.[20] While genetic isolation and separation from urban viruses and pollution, arduous work, and low calorie intake have been extolled as conducive to long life, any cause-to-effect relationship based on these populations' longevity is unwarranted.

More controversial is the question of whether the maximum lifespan for any animal species is fixed by absolute limits (established for humans at 70 years by Gompertz in 1825).[21] A common "prejudice" is that the human lifespan cannot be increased: the quality of life can be ameliorated and the number of individuals achieving a maximum possible lifespan can be increased, but the limits of life are biologically programmed and immutable. From an evolutionary perspective, the forces of natural selection become less important after the onset of reproduction; the individual would die from a number of causes which form the bases of the theories of aging. However, as will be discussed below, even the evolutionary perspective does not preclude the achievement of immortality; it implies that extension of human health and longevity depend not on "quick fixes" but on better understanding of the aging process and the continuing postponement of senescence. Accordingly, the human lifespan is not fixed; but, rather, it represents only a moving limit defined by the knowledge available to the successive generations of gerontologists.

Even in ancient times, when the usual lifespan lasted only two or three decades, some individuals lived to a very old age.[22] And even today in human populations with shorter average lifespans, a few individuals are capable of living as long a life as those from populations with a longer average lifespan (Figure 1-5). Indeed, individuals with unusually long lifespans have been found in populations living in rather hostile environments and under marginal economic conditions. It is well known that genetic make-up (perhaps genetic "vigor") is a determining component of longevity. Essentially, the best assurance towards a long life is the "choice" of parents who, themselves, lived long lives.

As indicated above, the standard of living, particularly in terms of sanitation and nutrition, is very important in human survival. In some developing countries, life expectancy, while still remaining well below that of economically advanced countries, has shown extraordinary progress since the 1950s. In India, for example, life expectancy which at the end of World War II ranged from 27 to 30 years, has now increased to 55 to 58 years.[23] The major concern of the public health policy in these countries continues to be the survival of the young during their early years (together with the reduction in the number of births) and the improvement of the health of the general population — two goals in which endocrine functions are directly implicated. As the proportion of the elderly in the population increases, this increasing number of individuals over 50 years will compete for medical and welfare benefits. This must be anticipated and addressed by government policy. The necessary strategies and interventions should include a better use of hormones.

IV. COMPARATIVE AND DIFFERENTIAL AGING

Senescence may be viewed as a manifestation of the process of adaptation. In evolutionary terms, the capacity to adapt has been solved by natural selection, that is by (1) the selection of inherited characteristics most favorable for survival and reproduction in a particular environment, and (2) the passage of the genes specifying these characteristics to the succeeding generations. In this sense, aging results from a decline of natural selection. Survival beyond the reproductive period would represent a luxury that few species could afford. Contrasting the immortality of the germ line with the mortality of somatic cells suggests that, at least in some species, limiting the individual lifespan may be a positively beneficial adaptation.

A gene that acted to insure a maximum number of offspring in youth but produces disease at later ages might be positively selected. "We grow old because to do otherwise would require . . . to invest resources in somatic maintenance . . . that are better spent on reproduction."[24]

**TABLE 1-5 Physiologic Correlation
with Longevity**

Index studied	Correlation
Body weight	Direct
Brain/body weight	Direct
Basal metabolic rate	Inverse
Stress	Inverse
Reproductive function	Inverse
Fecundity	Inverse
Length of growth period	Direct
Evolution	Uncertain

In other words, we age and die not because the damage (of wear and tear) is unrepairable, but rather because the cost of its repair is greater than the corresponding benefit, or it would be "cheaper to produce a 'disposable soma' than an eternally youthful one."[24,25]

However, in many species, and certainly in humans, longevity can theoretically be subject to positive selection based on criteria of fitness (e.g., optimal function) other than reproductive capacity. Some of the correlations between function and length of the lifespan are listed in Table 1-5 and discussed below.

A. Reproduction and Growth from an Evolutionary Perspective

In a general sense we think of fitness as health, strength, long life, and so forth, but in an evolutionary sense the meaning of fitness refers exclusively to the ability to successfully reproduce. Accordingly, senescence, as a decline in the force of natural selection, would begin with the onset of reproduction. "It is indeed remarkable that after a seemingly miraculous feat of morphogenesis, a complex metazoan should be unable to perform the much simpler task of merely maintaining what is already formed".[26] For an organism, to evolve increased longevity would require it to "reallocate reproductive energy . . . to postpone maturity, decrease litter size, increase offspring mortality, increase the time between litters, or some combinations of these."[27] Fecundity, measured by the number of young born per year of mature life, is inversely related to longevity — the shorter the lifespan the greater the fecundity (Table 1-5)

In experiments in which natural selection was used to create longer-lived stocks of fruit flies (*Drosophila melanogaster*), it was possible after about ten generations of selection for postponed senescence to create stocks with an increased mean and maximum lifespan.[28-31] Such stocks with postponed senescence exhibit depressed early fecundity. Other functions, however, such as the activity of the antioxidant enzyme superoxide dismutase, are enhanced, thereby denying the necessity to postulate a trade-off between early reproduction and senescence.

The duration of the period of growth before attaining reproductive maturity is directly related to the lifespan, the longer it takes an organism to reach maturity the longer the length of life. Duration of the growth period can be prolonged in experimental animals, primarily rodents. The onset of sexual maturation may be delayed by restricting food intake in terms of total calories or of some dietary components. With these dietary manipulations not only is the lifespan prolonged, but some specific functions such as reproduction and thermoregulation are maintained until an advanced age. Furthermore, the onset of aging-related pathology and its course are delayed and reduced.[32-34]

Currently, humans live well beyond their reproductive years — women some 40 years past the reproductive period. Longevity of a species beyond the reproductive years must be incidental to some earlier events, or the infertile individual must confer some advantage to

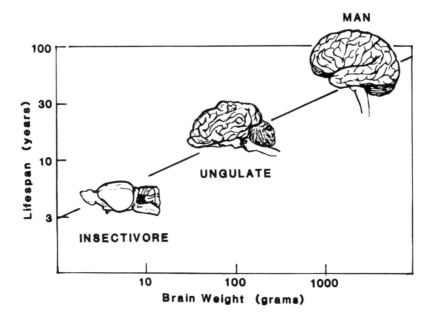

FIGURE 1-6 Relationship between lifespan and brain weight. Humans, with the longest lifespan among animals, have the heaviest brain relative to body weight.

those fertile. In our society this must be the case, for older members do contribute to the maintenance of the entire population structure and to the development and progress of society.

B. Brain Weight to Body Weight Ratio and Length of Lifespan

Comparison of several orders of placental mammals shows a highly significant relationship between lifespan and body weight — the larger the animal, the longer the lifespan. For example, the elephant may reach or exceed 70 years in captivity whereas the rat seldom lives more than 3 years. Many exceptions, however, qualify this generalization: humans may reach 114 years whereas other larger animals show a shorter potential longevity (horse, approximately 60 years; hippopotamus and rhinoceros, approximately 50 years; bear, 30 years; camel, 25 years). Among domestic animals cats generally live longer than dogs, although smaller in size.

An even more significant relationship exists between lifespan and brain weight: insectivores, with a smaller, simple brain have a shorter lifespan than ungulates. Humans, with the longest lifespan, have the heaviest brain in relation to body weight and also the most complicated brain structurally (Figure 1-6). The tentative explanation for this relationship is that the increase in size and complexity, especially of the cerebral cortex, provides for more precise homeostatic regulation and thus the greater chance for longer survival.[35] Such an interpretation seems well justified by the essential role that the nervous and endocrine systems play in regulating vital adjustments, especially responses to environmental demands.

The relationship of lifespan to brain size is a part of broader studies that attempt to identify the biologic constraints limiting how big a species' brain can be. Maternal metabolic rate and length of gestation have been suggested as important factors determining brain size.[36] Building bigger brains is reproductively expensive but has crucial consequences for a species' evolutionary ecology.[37] Some species live fast lives: they mature early, have large litters after a short gestation, and wean early; they also have small brains and short lifespans. By contrast, other species live long lives: they mature late, give birth to a single offspring after a long gestation, and wean late; they also have large brains and long lifespans.[38] In the first case, the potential reproductive output over a lifetime is large to accommodate the fluctuating availability of resources and is associated with high mortality. In the second case, building bigger brains demands a stable environment and leads to a slower but longer life.

C. Temperature, Basal Metabolism, and Length of Lifespan

Another physiologic parameter inversely related to the duration of life is the basal metabolic rate (also discussed in Chapter 5); the higher the metabolic rate, the shorter the lifespan.[39] The metabolic rate represents the amount of energy liberated per unit of time by the catabolism of food and physiologic processes in the body. The energy thus liberated appears as external work, heat, and stored energy; it is regulated by several factors among which the hormones, primarily thyroid hormones, play a key role. Conceivably, a higher metabolic rate would shorten the lifespan by accelerating the accumulation of nuclear errors (e.g., DNA damage) or of cellular damage (e.g., due to free radicals).

D. Selective Immortality

Senescence is assumed to occur in all vertebrates, hence its qualifications of being:

- Universal (i.e., occurring in all members of the same species),
- Intrinsic (i.e., independent from environmental factors),
- Progressive (i.e., occurring gradually and cumulatively), and
- Deleterious (i.e., leading to decreased function and to death).[40]

However, the evolutionary view does not preclude the achievement of immortality. When natural selection acts on lineages which reproduce asexually by symmetrical fission, then it will select for immortality, and immortality and reproduction coincide. This is the case for several unicellular organisms but not all: yeast and some ciliates which are also unicellular appear to undergo a well-defined senescence.

In some vertebrates, such as large fish and tortoises, the process of aging is so slow as to be almost undetectable. Similarly, in plants such as the bristlecone pine (*Pinus longaeva* D.K. Bailey), best known in the White Mountains of California, the rate of growth is very slow and the duration of life has been established at about 5,000 years. The bristlecone pine can survive in a region where faster developing plant forms cannot, and thus it stands alone in the harsh environment without having to share water and nutrients (Figure 1-7). At elevations above 9,500 feet the dry, cold, low-nutrient environment favors an extraordinarily slow growth rate, as well as a minimal rate of needle loss. The tree uses a strategy in which a portion of the bark and xylem are allowed to die when a supporting section of the tree's green crown is destroyed. During drought, fire, winds or other destructive bouts with nature, a portion of the wood is allowed to die, permitting the remaining photosynthetic crown to support a smaller quantity of live tissue and the tree to survive.

E. Usual Vs. Successful Aging

Comparative studies disclose differences in the rate of aging not only among plant and animal species but also in populations and individuals within the same species as well as in various functions within the same individual. In humans, physical appearance and behavior often belie biologic age and individuals are described as looking younger or older than their chronologic age: some 80-year-olds are as agile as 50-year-olds, whereas these, in turn, might act and look much older.

Within the same individual, both the rate and magnitude of the changes with aging vary depending on the cell, tissue, or organ considered. In certain functions (e.g., maintenance of the acid-base balance) regulation remains quite efficient until a late age — in others (e.g., eye accommodation), decrement appears at an early age.

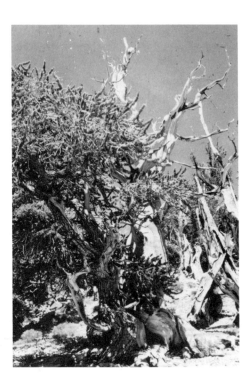

FIGURE 1-7 An ancient bristlecone pine specimen (4,000 years) from Schulman Grove, White Mountains, California.

Despite such individual and physiological heterogeneity, attempts have been made to establish a complete profile of the "average" older individual at progressive ages. Often, age-associated deficits and functional losses have been interpreted as age-determined. Lifestyle, habits, and psychological factors extrinsic to biologic aging actually may be major components of many age-associated declines.[41] Such factors, often underestimated, may be modifiable. This, then, offers a more immediate and encouraging basis for prevention and correction, or at least alleviation, of so-called age-related losses.

In an attempt to define normal aging, the focus is often on average aging and the great variability among the elderly is neglected. In an heterogeneous population of the elderly, among whom some age at a much slower rate than others, the aging process can be divided into:

- Usual aging, referring to the average physiologic decline, and
- Successful aging, referring to those individuals who have shown minimum functional decrements with aging.[42]

The distinction between usual, that is, average, and successful aging points to the importance of risk factors for age-associated diseases. Thus, age-linked increases in blood pressure, body weight, and serum cholesterol levels may be usual in the populations that have been most extensively studied. They are all risk factors for cardiovascular disease. These changes, which have been interpreted as age-intrinsic, are considered to be usual in prosperous, industrial countries, but are not or are much less so in developing but still prevalently pastoral and traditional agricultural societies.

It is at least a reasonable hypothesis, given such cross-cultural differences in human (and other) populations, that attributing change to age per se may often be exaggerated and that factors such as diet, exercise, drugs, and the psychosocial environment should not be underestimated or ignored as potential moderators of the aging process.

TABLE 1-6 Major Theories of Aging

Molecular Theories	
Somatic Mutation	Genetic mutations accumulate with increasing age; DNA repair may be inefficient, particularly for mitochondrial DNA damage/mutation
Error Catastrophe	Damage to mechanisms that synthesize proteins results in faulty proteins which accumulate to a level that causes catastrophic damage to cells, tissue, and organs; altered heat-shock proteins may contribute to alteration in protein disassembly and transport
Gene Regulation	Expression of proliferation promoting or inhibiting genes may lead to aging in yeasts, fruit flies, and nematodes
Cellular Theories	
Wear and Tear	Vital parts of cells and tissues may wear out; the faster the rate of living (i.e., metabolism) the shorter the lifespan
Free Radicals	Accumulated damage caused by oxygen radicals impairs membranes, DNA, and induces crosslinking
Crosslinking	Accumulation of crosslinked proteins damage cells and tissues, slowing down bodily processes
Systemic Theories	
Neuroendocrine	Biological clocks in the brain act through hormones to control the pace of growth, development, and aging
Immunologic	A programmed decline in immune system increases vulnerability to infectious diseases and incidence of auto-immune diseases leading to aging and death

V. THEORIES OF AGING

Theories of aging are numerous and most of them remain controversial. They may be categorized as molecular, cellular, and systemic (Table 1-6).

A. Molecular Theories and the Genetic Connection

These theories underline the importance of genetic control and assume that a genetic program or alterations of this program determines the various phases of the lifespan for each species. These theories and those concerning cellular aging are discussed in depth in Chapter 15; only a brief survey of some of the major theories is presented here.

1. Somatic Mutation and DNA Repair

The somatic mutation theory was originally formulated on the basis that irradiation shortens the lifespan in rodents. Genetic mutations due to ionizing radiation would cause cells to degenerate and die. Somatic mutations are no longer regarded as a probable cause of aging because (1) the rate at which they occur in the natural environment is too low to account for overall aging changes, and (2) DNA repair mechanisms may be sufficient to repair the damage. DNA repair mechanisms, however, may be insufficient when challenged by other toxic agents such as oxygen radicals or ultraviolet light acting on the cell for a long period of time. Failure to adequately repair DNA damage would lead to malfunction of genes, proteins, and cells and endanger function and survival. The ability to repair DNA damage by utilizing the various enzyme systems in the cell evolved for this purpose has been related to the length of the lifespan.[43]

Humans repair DNA faster and more efficiently than mice and other animals with a shorter lifespan. Defects in DNA repair have been detected in people with a familial genetic susceptibility to cancer (e.g., colon, breast cancer). The decline with aging in DNA repair processes would explain the increased incidence of cancer in older people.

DNA damage and repair follow different rates among organisms and cells in an individual organism. The most efficient repair occurs in germ cells; mitochondrial DNA is more susceptible to damage than nuclear DNA. Mitochondria represent organelles that are the principal cellular sites of metabolism and energy production and, as such, are more exposed to damaging oxygen radicals during metabolism (see below). Additionally, mitochondrial DNA lacks the protein coat that helps protect DNA in the nucleus from damage. Mitochondrial DNA damage (and eventually, mutations) increases with aging, and several diseases that appear in late life such as diabetes and degenerative neurologic (e.g., Parkinson's disease) and mental (e.g., Alzheimer's dementia) diseases have been traced to defects in mitochondria.[44,45]

2. Error Catastrophe and Heat Shock Proteins

Errors in the transmission of information through RNA to proteins would be responsible for aging.[46,47] Errors, such as the incorporation of the wrong molecules into messenger RNA (mRNA) during transcription, may change the triplet codons (three bases) in mRNA molecules. Accurate codon reading would not be possible (as in the codon restriction theory); rather, incorporation of the wrong amino acids into protein during translation may change the amino acid sequence. The initial error in proteins may be low, but would increase exponentially with the passage of time and lead to "error catastrophe" and cell death.[48]

While many reports contradict the occurrence of errors in proteins with aging,[49,50] other studies point to the possible role of specific proteins such as heat shock proteins.[51] These proteins are produced in cells exposed to various stresses (e.g., toxic substances, high temperatures). They may play a role in cell protein metabolism by helping the cells to disassemble and dispose of damaged proteins and to facilitate the transport of new proteins. Production of these proteins would decrease with aging.[51] The mechanisms by which heat shock proteins are formed and act are still unknown. Some experiments indicate that these proteins may be related to the adrenal cortical response to stress[52,53] and to alterations in brain proteins possibly involved in dementia.[54,55]

3. The Genetic Connection

Senescence may result from specific genes for longevity or death or from changes in the expression of genes after reproductive maturity has been achieved (see Chapter 15). Demonstration in the *Drosophila* that genes are linked to the lifespan (see above) has opened the way for further study of the genetic connection with longevity. Some of the genes found in yeasts, nematodes, and fruit flies promote longevity while others may shorten the lifespan. Only a few genes have been identified so far, but it is estimated that many more may be operative. Gene expression is the process through which the gene produces proteins: structural proteins that regulate cell morphology and enzyme proteins that regulate cell activity. Changes in gene expression may alter protein synthesis and thereby cause aging.

Certain genes trigger cell proliferation (e.g., the protooncogenes, *c-fos* or *ras,* genes); others interfere with cell proliferation.[56,57] In yeasts a gene, the longevity assurance gene LAG 1, promotes the number of cell divisions and, by inference, longevity.[58,59] In the nematode (*Caenorhabditis elegans*), mutation of a certain gene more than doubles the normal 3-week lifespan.[60,61]

Telomere length indicates how many divisions a cell has undergone and how many divisions remain before it becomes senescent. Telomeres are chromosome tails that have the same short sequence of DNA bases repeated thousands of times; they stabilize the chromosome during division, but with each cell division they lose a number of bases. While cancer cells divide indefinitely (are immortal?), normal somatic cells undergo only a limited number of cell divisions, during which they age and finally die.[62] Therefore the study of telomeres provides a model for studying the aging cell, its "programmed death", and the means to prevent or delay it.[63-66] Current studies connect the enzyme telomerase, present in cancer but not in normal cells, with the ability of preserving telomere length and insuring continuing cell division. The study of genes and telomeres that activate or inhibit cell proliferation represents an area in which aging research intersects not only with cancer research but, given the cell proliferative actions of several hormones, also with hormone research.

B. Cellular Theories

These theories relate to age-associated changes that occur in the structure and function of cells, particularly in response to environmental challenges. Again, for a more detailed discussion, the reader is referred to Chapter 15.

1. Wear and Tear and Rate of Living Theories

According to the wear and tear theory, living organisms are like machines, that is, with repeated use parts wear out, become defective, and the machinery ultimately fails to function.[39] However, organisms have mechanisms by which they can repair their damages whereas machines do not. The premise of this theory originates from the observation that environmental temperature may prolong (cold) or shorten (hot) the lifespan of some animals, perhaps by slowing down or accelerating wear and tear. As discussed earlier, the lifespans of different animal species are inversely proportional to the basal metabolic rate.[67] Within the same species, however, it is difficult to correlate individual differences in lifespan with the metabolic rate. The rate of living theory is a variation of the wear and tear theory and states that the greater the rate of basal metabolism, the faster the accumulation of free radical damage and, therefore, the shorter the lifespan.

2. Free Radical Theory

This theory postulates that free radical reactions (modified by genetic and environmental factors) are involved in aging and age-related disorders.[68-70] Reactions of free radicals — highly reactive chemical compounds — are ubiquitous in living organisms. Free radicals arise from both nonenzymatic and enzymatic reactions such as the reduction of O_2 to water or from exposure to ionizing radiation. Free radicals include O_2, HO-R (any organic radical), RO, and RO_2. Several enzymes (superoxide dismutase, catalase, glutathione peroxidase) and vitamins (E, C, carotenes) protect against oxidative attack. However, with aging this protection may be less effective, with the resulting peroxidation of lipids and aldehydes, and crosslinking of proteins and DNA.[71] Even these consequences may be repaired, but perhaps at a less efficient rate in old cells, thereby reducing or impairing function and increasing vulnerability to disease.

Support for the free radical theory comes from several observations such as the higher levels of the enzyme superoxide dismutase and of antioxidants in long-lived species, and the prolongation of average and maximum lifespan by the insertion of extra copies of the superoxide dismutase gene in fruit flies.

3. Crosslinking Theory

Many biologic molecules develop crosslinkages or bonds between identical or different molecules with the passage of time and these linkages may alter their physical and chemical properties.[72] In glucose crosslinking or glycosylation, glucose molecules attach themselves to proteins with consequent hardening of the tissues affected.[73] Sites of crosslinks involve the collagen, an extracellular fibrous protein which hardens with aging, as well as intracellular enzymes and nucleic acids.

Crosslinks have been related to a number of aging-associated diseases such as hardening of arteries (in atherosclerosis), cataracts, and diabetes. The link with diabetes is particularly important as this disease, associated with a shorter life expectancy, is often considered a model of accelerated aging (Chapters 10 and 11).

C. System Level Theories

The declining effectiveness of homeostatic adjustments with aging leads to failure of adaptation and survival. Adaptation, either to external environmental stimuli or internal signals such as hormones, depends upon control mechanisms regulated by nervous, endocrine, and immune systems. The activity of several endocrine glands such as the adrenals, gonads, and thyroid is controlled directly by the pituitary gland and indirectly by the signals (e.g., hormones, neurotransmitters) this gland receives from nervous centers, primarily the hypothalamus, as well as from signals (e.g., cytokines) from cells of the immune system. For proper adaptation, nervous, endocrine, and immune signals must be synchronized and responsive to the needs of the many functions they regulate. However, with aging, some of the efficiency of the hypothalamo-pituitary-immuno signals is lost or altered, and this results in decreased function and increased pathology of many organs and tissue systems.

The two major groups of theories under this category are the neuroendocrine and the immunologic. According to both, command cells would act as pacemakers that regulate a "biologic clock" or a genetically based program that governs development and aging. With the passage of time, the clock would deteriorate or cease to run. Likewise, the linkage to effector organs (e.g., muscle and glands) would cease. In either case, aging would be manifested through a slowing down or imbalance of a key organ or system such as the hypothalamus, pituitary, adrenal cortex, or thyroid gland for the neuroendocrine theories, and the thymus, lymph nodes, spleen or histocompatibility complex for the immune system. As these theories are central to the content of this book, they are discussed in the corresponding chapters.

D. Single Vs. Multiple Interdependent Theories

An overall view of the theories of aging shows that while it may be rationally satisfying to envision a single theory of aging, most gerontologists now would agree that a single theory cannot account for all the changes that take place with aging, especially in higher organisms such as humans. Our better understanding of the physiopathology of disease and the more efficient biotechnical tools at our disposal allow us to view aging from a new perspective involving many processes — interactive and interdependent — synchronized to determine good health and lifespan. Synchronization depends on environmental factors that have an impact on aging cells, tissues, and organs as well as on genetic control of the response to these factors.

REFERENCES

1. Lawton, A. H., The historical developments in the biological aspects of aging and the aged, *Gerontologist*, 5, 25, 1965.
2. Timiras, P. S., *Physiological Basis of Aging and Geriatrics*, 2nd ed., CRC Press, Boca Raton, FL, 1994.
3. Whitrow, G. J., *The Nature of Time*, Holt, Rinehart & Winston, New York, 1973, 43.
4. Finch, C. E., *Longevity, Senescence and the Genome*, University of Chicago Press, Chicago, IL, 1990.
5. Sapolsky, R. M., *Stress, the Aging Brain, and the Mechanisms of Neuron Death*, MIT Press, Cambridge, MA, 1992.
6. Comfort, A., *The Biology of Senescence*, 3rd ed., Elsevier, New York, 1979.
7. Robertson, O H. and Wexler, B. C., Histological changes in the organs and tissues of migrating and spawning Pacific Salmon, *Endocrinology*, 66, 222, 1960.
8. Kohn, R. R., Aging and age-related diseases: normal processes, in *Relations Between Normal Aging and Disease*, Johnson, H. A., Ed., Raven Press, New York, 1985, 1.
9. Finch, C. E., New models for new perspectives in the biology of senescence, *Neurobiol. Aging*, 12, 625, 1991.
10. Sprott, R. L., Development of animal models of aging at the National Institute of Aging, *Neurobiol. Aging*, 12, 635, 1991.
11. Martin, G. M., Cellular aging—postreplicative cells. A review (Part II), *Am. J. Pathol.*, 89, 513, 1977.

12. Timiras, P. S., Thyroid hormones and the developing brain, in *Handbook of Human Growth and Developmental Biology,* Vol. I, Part C, Meisami, E. and Timiras, P.S., Eds., CRC Press, Boca Raton, FL, 1988, 59.

13. Rabin, D. L., Waxing of the grey; waning of the green, in *Health in an Older Society,* Committee on an Aging Society, Institute of Medicine and National Research Council (America's aging), National Academy Press, Washington, D.C., 1985, 28.

14. Hoover, S. L. and Siegel, J. S., International demographic trends and perspectives on aging, *J. Cross-Cult. Gerontol.,* 1, 5, 1986.

15. Siegel, J. S. and Taeuber, C. M., Demographic perspectives on the long-lived society, *Daedalus,* 115, 77, 1986.

16. Brody, J. A., Brock, D. B., and Williams, T. F., Trends in the health of the elderly population, *Annu. Rev. Public Health,* 8, 211, 1987.

17. Fries, J. F., Aging, natural death, and the compression of morbidity, *N. Engl. J. Med.,* 303, 130, 1980.

18. Schneider, E. L. and Brody, J. A., Aging, natural death, and the compression of morbidity: another view, *N. Engl. J. Med.,* 309, 854, 1983.

19. Leaf, A., Long-lived populations: extreme old age, *J. Am. Geriatr. Soc.,* 30, 485, 1982.

20. Bennett, N. G. and Garson, L. K., Extraordinary longevity in the Soviet Union: fact or artifact?, *Gerontologist,* 26, 358, 1986.

21. Gompertz, B., On the nature and function expressive of the law of human mortality and on a new mode of determining life contingencies, *Phil. Trans. R. Soc. London,* 2, 513, 1825.

22. Kebric, R. B., Old age, the ancient military, and Alexander's army: positive examples for a graying America, *Gerontologist,* 28, 298, 1988.

23. *Directory and Yearbook,* Government of India, Official Publications, New Delhi, 1981.

24. Kirkwood, T. B. L., Immortality of the germ-line versus disposability of the soma, in *Evolution of Longevity in Animals, A Comparative Approach,* Woodhead, A D. and Thompson, K. H., Eds., Plenum Press, New York, 1987, 209.

25. Kirkwood, T. B. L. and Rose, M. R., Evolution of senescence: late survival sacrificed for reproduction, *Phil. Trans. R. Soc., Ser. B, London,* 332, 15, 1991.

26. Williams, G. C., Pleiotropy, natural selection, and the evolution of senescence, *Evolution,* 11, 398, 1957.

27. Guthrie, R. D., Senescence as an adaptive trait, *Perspect. Biol. Med.,* 12, 313, 1969.

28. Hutchinson, E. W. and Rose, M. R., Quantitative genetics of postponed aging in *Drosophila melanogaster.* I. Analysis of outbred populations, *Genetics,* 127, 719, 1991.

29. Rose, M. R., Vu, L. N., Park, S. U., and Graves, J. L., Jr., Selection on stress resistance increases longevity in *Drosophila melanogaster, Exp., Gerontol.,* 27, 241, 1992.

30. Rose, M. R., Nusbaum, T. J., and Fleming, J. E., *Drosophila* with postponed aging as a model for aging research, *Lab. Animal Science,* 42, 114, 1992.

31. Nusbaum, T. J., Graves, J. L., Jr., Mueller, L. D., and Rose, M. R., Fruit fly aging and mortality, *Science,* 260, 1567, 1993.

32. Segall, P. E. and Timiras, P. S., Patho-physiologic findings after chronic tryptophan deficiency in rats: a model for delayed growth and aging, *Mech. Ageing Dev.,* 5, 109, 1976.

33. Segall, P. E., Timiras, P. S., and Walton, J. R., Low tryptophan diets delay reproductive aging, *Mech. Ageing Dev.* , 23, 245, 1983.

34. Weindruch, R., Effect of caloric restriction on age-associated cancers, *Exp. Gerontol.,* 27, 575, 1992.

35. Sacher, G. A., Relation of lifespan to brain weight, and body weight, in *The Lifespan of Animals,* Wolstenholme, G. E. W. and O'Connor, M., Eds., Vol. 5, Little, Brown, Boston, 1959, 115.

36. Martin, R. D., *Human Brain Evolution in an Ecological Context,* American Museum of National History, (Fifty-second James Arthur Lecture on the evolution of the human brain, 1982), New York, 1983, 1.

37. Pagel, M. D. and Harvey, P. H., How mammals produce large-brained offspring, *Evolution,* 42, 948, 1988.

38. Partridge, L. and Harvey, P. H., The ecological context of life history evolution, *Science,* 241, 1449, 1988.

39. Sacher, G., Life table modification and life prolongation, in *Handbook of the Biology of Aging,* Finch, C. E. and Hayflick, L., Eds., Van Nostrand Reinhold, New York, 1977, 582.

40. Strehler, B. L., *Time, Cells, and Aging,* 2nd ed., Academic Press, New York, 1977.

41. House, J. S., Landis, K. R., and Umberson, D., Social relationship and health, *Science,* 241, 540, 1988.

42. Rowe, J. W. and Kahn, R. L., Human aging: usual and successful, *Science,* 237, 143, 1987.

43. Mullaart, E., Lohman, P. H., Berends, F., and Vijg, J., DNA damage metabolism and aging, *Mutation Res.,* 237, 189, 1990.

44. Wallace, D. C., Mitochondrial genetics: a paradigm for aging and degenerative diseases?, *Science,* 256, 628, 1992.

45. Wallace, D. C., Diseases of the mitochondrial DNA, *Annu. Rev. Biochem.,* 61, 1175, 1992.

46. Medvedev, Z. A., Repetition of molecular-genetic information as a possible factor in evolutionary changes of lifespan, *Exp. Gerontol.,* 7, 227, 1972.

47. Orgel, L. E., The maintenance of the accuracy of protein synthesis and its relevance to aging, *Proc. Natl. Acad. Sci., U.S.A.*, 49, 517, 1963.
48. Holliday, R. and Tarrant, G. M., Altered enzymes in aging human fibroblasts, *Nature*, 238, 26, 1972.
49. Fleming, J. E., Melnikoff, P. S., Latter, G. I., Chandra, D., and Bensch, K. G., Age dependent changes in the expression of *Drosophila* mitochondrial proteins, *Mech. Ageing Dev.*, 34, 63, 1986.
50. Stadtman, E. R., Starke-Reed, P. E., Oliver, C. N., Carney, J. M., and Floyd, R. A., Protein modification in aging, *Exs*, 62, 64, 1992.
51. Fargnoli, J., Kunisada, T., Fornace, A. J., Jr., Schneider, E. L., and Holbrook, N. J., Decreased expression of heat shock protein 70 mRNA and protein after heat treatment in cells of aged rats, *Proc. Natl. Acad. Sci., U.S.A.*, 87, 846, 1990.
52. Blake, M. J., Udelsman, R., Feulner, G. J., Norton, D. D., and Holbrook, N. J., Stress-induced heat shock protein 70 expression in adrenal cortex: an adrenocorticotropic hormone-sensitive, age-dependent response, *Proc. Natl. Acad. Sci., U.S.A.*, 88, 9873, 1991.
53. Blake, M. J., Buckley, D. J., and Buckley, A. R., Dopaminergic regulation of heat shock protein-70 expression in adrenal gland and aorta, *Endocrinology*, 132, 1063, 1993.
54. Cole, G. M. and Timiras, P. S., Aging-related pathology in human neuroblastoma and teratocarcinoma cell lines, in *Model Systems of Development and Aging of the Nervous System*, Vernadakis, A., Privat, A., Lauder, J. M., Timiras, P. S., and Giacobini, E., Eds., Martinius Nijhoff, Boston, MA, 1987, 453.
55. Blake, M. J., Nowak, T. S., Jr., and Holbrook, N. J., *In vivo* hyperthermia induces expression of HSP70 mRNA in brain regions controlling the neuroendrocine response to stress, *Brain Res.*, 8, 89, 1990.
56. Danner, D. B., The proliferation theory of rejuvenation, *Mech. Ageing Dev.*, 65, 85, 1992.
57. Goldstein, S., The biology of aging: looking to defuse the genetic time bomb, *Geriatrics*, 48, 76, 1993.
58. Jazwinski, S. M., Genes of youth: genetics of aging in Baker's yeast, *ASM News*, 59, 172, 1993.
59. Jazwinski, S. M., Chen, J. B., and Sun, J., A single gene change can extend yeast lifespan: the role of Ras in cellular senescence, *Adv. Exp. Med. Biol.*, 330, 45, 1993.
60. Johnson, T. E., Increased lifespan of age-1 mutants in *Caenorhabditis elegans* and lower Gompertz rate of aging, *Science*, 249, 908, 1990.
61. Johnson, T. E. and Lithgow, G. J., The search for the genetic basis of aging: the identification of gerontogenes in the nematode *Caenorhabditis elegans*, *J. Am. Geriatr. Soc.*, 40, 936, 1992.
62. Hayflick, L. and Moorehead, P. S., The serial cultivation of human diploid cell strains, *Exp. Cell. Res.*, 25, 585, 1961.
63. Harley, C. B., Futcher, A. B., and Greider, C. W., Telomeres shorten during ageing of human fibroblasts, *Nature*, 345, 458, 1990.
64. Harley, C. B., Telomere loss: mitotic clock or genetic time bomb?, *Mutation Res.*, 256, 271, 1991.
65. Levy, M. Z., Allsopp, R. C., Futcher, A. B., Greider, C. W. and Harley, C. B., Telomere end-replication problem and cell aging, *J. Mol. Biol.*, 225, 951, 1992.
66. Vaziri, H., Schachter, F., Uchida, I., Wei, L., Zhu, X., Effros, R., Cohen, D., and Harley, C. B., Loss of telomeric DNA during aging of normal and trisomy 21 human lymphocytes, *Am. J. Hum. Genet.*, 52, 661, 1993.
67. Sohal, R. S., Metabolic rate and lifespan, in *Cellular Ageing, Concepts, and Mechanisms, Part I: General Concepts*, Cutler, R. G., Ed., Interdisciplinary Topics in Gerontology, Vol. 9, Karger, Basel, 1976, 25.
68. Harman, D., Free radical theory of aging, *Mutation Res.*, 275, 257, 1992.
69. Harman, D., Role of free radicals in aging and disease, *Ann. N.Y. Acad. Sci.*, 673, 126, 1992.
70. Harman, D., Free radical involvement in aging. Pathophysiology and therapeutic implications, *Drugs and Aging*, 3, 60, 1993.
71. Ames, B. N., Shigenaga, M. K., and Hagen, T. M., Oxidants, antioxidants, and the degenerative diseases of aging, *Proc. Natl. Acad. Sci., U.S.A.*, 90, 7915, 1993.
72. Bjorksten, J., The crosslinkage theory of aging, *J. Am. Geriatr. Soc.*, 16, 408, 1968.
73. Cerami, A., Hypothesis. Glucose as a mediator of aging, *J. Am. Geriatr. Soc.*, 33, 626, 1985.

PART II

Aging

of the Endocrine Glands

2

Steroid-Secreting Endocrines: Adrenal, Ovary, Testis

Paola S. Timiras

CONTENTS

0-8493-2446-7/95/$0.00+$.50

25

I. INTRODUCTION

This and the following three chapters survey major structural, functional, and biochemical characteristics of the endocrine glands. Functional implications for normal aging of the entire organism and correlations to disease are drawn in subsequent chapters as indicated. A synopsis of the normal function of each gland in the mature individual provides the basis for comparison with the older individual. The simple classification used here is based on the chemical structure of hormones in anatomically well-defined endocrine organs. The four endocrine divisions represented include glands secreting steroids (Chapter 2), those secreting peptides or proteins (Chapter 3), those secreting amines (Chapter 4), and the contiguously located thyroid and parathyroid glands (Chapter 5). Other endocrine cells and their chemical mediators which are more diffusely or more complexly organized anatomically are discussed in Chapter 6.

II. ENDOCRINE GLANDS

Endocrine glands are organs that produce and secrete hormones. Hormones, however, are secreted not only by these glands but also by cells and groups of cells that are not segregated into anatomically discrete glands but are interspersed with other cells (Chapter 6). Major endocrine glands include the adrenals, gonads, pancreas, parathyroid, pituitary, and thyroid. The pineal (Chapter 4) and thymus (Chapter 20) have endocrine attributes but their activities are atypical of the classically considered endocrine glands. Endocrine and neural involvement in aging have led to the formulation of neuroendocrine theories of aging discussed throughout this book.

A. Assessment of Endocrine Function

In humans, evaluation of endocrine function relies primarily on clinical laboratory measurement of blood hormone levels under basal (resting or steady state) conditions. Such an evaluation is often incomplete and may lead to erroneous conclusions. One kind of circumstance giving rise to such difficulties results from the marked 24-hour rhythmic and briefer episodic fluctuations in outputs and levels of some of the hormones. An adequate endocrine evaluation focuses on several levels (Table 2-1):

  • At the endocrine gland, for regulation of hormone synthesis and release,
  • At the organism, for circulating hormone levels, hormone metabolism, and excretion,
  • At the target cell, for hormone receptor interaction and molecular events inside the cell.

Hormones regulate their own secretion and their actions on target cells by a number of feedback mechanisms which should also be measured. Feedback represents the return to the input of part of the output and are positive or negative. The net effect of a feedback, respectively, may be stimulatory or inhibitory on the endocrine cells of origin. One example of *positive feedback is the stimulatory action of ovarian estrogens on the release of hypothalamic and pituitary hormones.* Just prior to ovulation, the raising levels of estrogens:

- Increase the secretion of hypothalamic gonadotropin-releasing hormone (GnRH),
- Increase the sensitivity of the pituitary to this releasing hormone, and thus
- Increase the secretion (surge) of pituitary luteinizing hormone (LH) and the induction of ovulation.

A negative feedback inhibits secretion of the hormone. One example of *negative feedback is the reduction of both GnRH and LH release by the same estrogens, operative after ovulation.* Changes with aging may appear minor singly, but when compounded at several levels they may modify various attributes of the endocrine signal at the target cell as well as the ability of the target cell to respond normally.

TABLE 2-1 Hierarchical Level of Endocrine Activity

Level	Function
The gland	Synthesis and release of hormone
The feedback	Neural regulation; hormonal regulation, endocrine-endocrine interactions
The organism	Blood levels, metabolism and excretion (clearance)
The target	Hormone-receptor interaction(s); intracellular responses

B. Some Generic Endocrine Changes With Aging

Aging influences endocrine glands directly or indirectly through endogenous or exogenous factors.[1-7] Direct effects may manifest themselves as gland atrophy and weight loss, vascular changes, fibrosis, and tumors associated with alterations in hormone synthesis and release. Indirect effects may be due to changes in other endocrines and the nervous and immune systems, as well as in metabolism and body composition, and in cellular and molecular activities. Even more complex are the indirect effects of the complications of disease, medications, drugs, and the influence of diet and exercise (Table 2-2).

Some hormones act exclusively on one target; other hormones act on many cell types by diverse mechanisms. The same hormone may have different actions on different tissues. With aging, one of the many actions, or one of the many targets, may be selectively affected while other actions and targets are preserved.

Basal hormone levels may be maintained with age in humans and animals. One clear-cut exception is the fall in ovarian hormones following menopause. Regulation of hormone synthesis and release depends on neurotransmitters from neurons and cytokines from immune cells. These interact with an array of actions of other chemical mediators, including some other hormones. Alterations in one or several of these controls may significantly affect endocrine function. Secretory and clearance rates often decrease with aging, although it is not clear

TABLE 2-2 Contributors to Endocrine Aging

Endogenous	• Endocrine
	• Neural
	• Immune
	• Body composition
	• Target cells and molecules
	• Diseases
Exogenous	• Disease
	• Medications
	• Drugs, including smoking and alcohol
	• Diet
	• Exercise
	• Socioeconomic factors

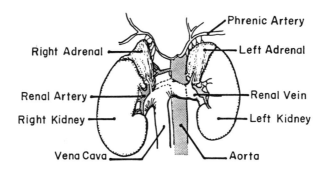

FIGURE 2-1 Diagram of the kidneys and adrenals.

whether the primary change involves secretion or clearance. The question remains to what extent is the capacity to maintain normal levels of plasma hormones preserved in old age?

The specificity of hormonal actions depends on a particular kind of receptor located on the cell membrane or intracellularly. The cellular response is determined by the genetic program within the nucleus of the target cell. With aging, receptor binding and intracellular responses tend to vary greatly, depending on the hormone and the target cell (Chapters 17 and 19).

III. THE ADRENAL CORTEX

The adrenals are paired glands embedded in fat tissue attached to the upper pole of the kidney (Figure 2-1). They are formed of an **outer cortex** and an **inner medulla**. The adrenal cortex secretes several steroid hormones: aldosterone, necessary to sustain life; cortisol, involved in carbohydrate and protein metabolism; and sex hormones, with minor androgenic effects (Figure 2-2).[8]

The adrenal medulla, a modified ganglion of the sympathetic nervous system, secretes epinephrine and norepinephrine with circulatory, nervous, and metabolic actions. Although not essential for life, these amines help the individual to deal with emergencies (Chapter 4).

A. Synopsis of Adrenocortical Function in the Adult

Hormones of the adrenal cortex are derivatives of cholesterol and are categorized chemically as steroids, hence the designation of adrenocorticosteroids or corticoids. Steroidogenesis comprises the steps in steroid biosynthesis from cholesterol and acetate to the final hormonal products. In both the adrenal cortex and the gonads the major reactions are summarized in Figure 2-3. On the basis of chemical structure and actions, adrenal steroids are distinguished as:

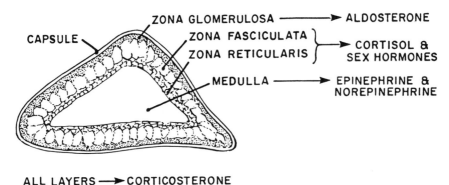

FIGURE 2-2 Diagram of a transverse section of an adrenal. Illustration of the three cortical zones, the medulla and their hormones.

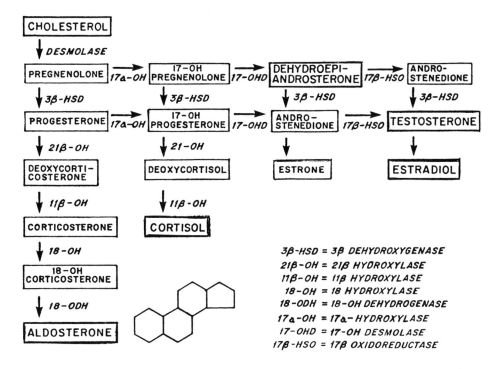

FIGURE 2-3 Synopsis of steroid hormones synthesis in the adrenal cortex. The major secretory products are emphasized by larger print and darker outline. Note the presence of sex hormones (progesterone, estradiol, and testosterone) also secreted by the ovary and testis.

- Glucocorticoids (pertaining to their actions on carbohydrate metabolism) such as cortisol and corticosterone (C_{21} steroids),
- Sex steroids (or adrenal androgens) such as dehydroepiandrosterone (DHEA) (C_{19} steroids). Both C_{21} and C_{19} hormones are secreted primarily from the two inner cortical zones, the zona fasciculata and the zona reticularis,
- Mineralocorticoids, in reference to their regulation of minerals or electrolytes in body fluids. They are secreted by the outer cortical cells, the zona glomerulosa. Aldosterone is the physiologically most effective C_{21} steroid insofar as mineralocorticoid activity and survival are concerned.

1. Glucocorticoids

Glucocorticoids (Figure 2-4) act on intermediary metabolism to increase amino acid uptake, protein synthesis, and gluconeogenesis (i.e., amino acid conversion to glucose) in liver, but to decrease amino acid uptake and protein synthesis in muscle. Decreased protein synthesis in connective tissue, bone, lymphatic tissue, and muscle are the general catabolic actions of these corticoids. They possess an anti-insulin effect as they raise blood sugar levels, and thus exacerbate diabetes mellitus. They also induce lipolysis and mobilize serum lipids and cholesterol.

In addition to these metabolic actions, glucocorticoids have anti-inflammatory activity when administered in superphysiologic doses. These inhibitory effects on inflammatory reactions form the basis for the frequent therapeutic use of these hormones as medications for a number of medical conditions (asthma, various types of allergies) and as effective immuno-suppressants to prevent rejection of transplanted organs. Effects are predominantly caused by the inhibition of expression of specific genes important in these processes. The mechanism of this negative gene regulation is not known, but it has been hypothesized that steroid receptors

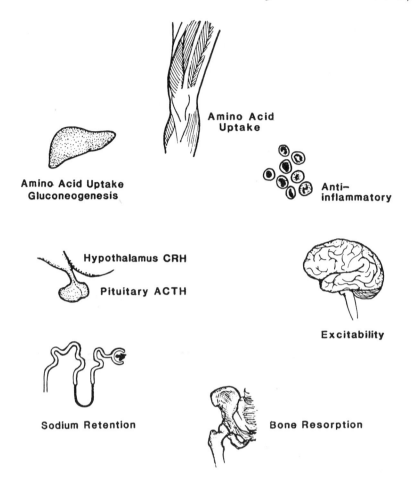

FIGURE 2-4 Some major targets of glucocorticoid action.

negatively regulate gene expression by interfering with the activity or binding of other important transcriptional factors.

Glucocorticoids have essentially excitatory effects on the nervous system, evidenced by the presence of hormone receptors on neurons and glia (Chapters 14 and 16), induction of neurotransmitter enzymes, EEG changes, and increased convulsiveness. Glucocorticoid toxicity to neurons of the hippocampus and its consequences on regulation of the hypothalamo-pituitary-adrenocortical axis are discussed in Chapter 14 and form the basis for the "glucocorticoid cascade hypothesis".

Other actions of glucocorticoids include: retention of sodium by renal tubules (but much less effectively than aldosterone), increased bone resorption and decreased bone production and altered calcium metabolism, maintenance of work capacity, increased stomach acid and pepsin secretion, and promotion of appetite. Despite the lipolytic effects, glucocorticoid excess increases fat deposition (in specific body areas). This paradox is explained by the effects of these hormones to increase appetite and to induce hyperglycemia.

2. Sex Steroids

Androgens are hormones that exert masculinizing effects, and promote protein synthesis (anabolism) and growth. Adrenal androgens, such as DHEA, are considerably less effective than androgens from the testis (e.g., testosterone). Some of the androgens are converted to

TABLE 2-3 Major Hormones Involved in
Glucocorticoid Regulation

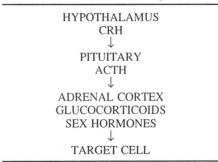

HYPOTHALAMUS
CRH
↓
PITUITARY
ACTH
↓
ADRENAL CORTEX
GLUCOCORTICOIDS
SEX HORMONES
↓
TARGET CELL

estrogens in the circulation and some estrogens are secreted by the adrenal, but their amount is apparently too small to be physiologically effective.

3. Corticotropin-Releasing Hormone (CRH) and Adrenocorticotropic Hormone (ACTH or Corticotropin)

Synthesis and release of glucocorticoids and adrenal androgens are regulated by hypothalamic CRH and pituitary ACTH (Table 2-3). Through their negative feedback on the hypothalamus and pituitary, glucocorticoids inhibit the secretion of both CRH and ACTH: the higher the levels of the circulating steroids, the lower the secretion of CRH and ACTH; the lower their levels, the higher CRH and ACTH release. Plasma ACTH and cortisol levels are not continuous, but are episodic with short-term fluctuation. They also follow a circadian rhythm with levels highest in the early morning and lowest in late evening. They are characteristically responsive to stress. Stress stimulates release of CRH which, in turn, stimulates release of ACTH and this promotes cortisol secretion.[9,10]

The feedback actions of corticoids have been categorized as resulting from changes in gene expression affecting metabolic and cellular events or in RNA and proteins synthesis with inhibition of CRH, ACTH, and ADH synthesis (for ADH, see Chapter 3). Sensitivity of adrenal cells and neurons to CRH and ACTH changes with stress and aging (Chapters 14 and 16).[11]

4. Mineralocorticoids

Aldosterone, the major mineralocorticoid, is indispensable for survival. Aldosterone increases sodium reabsorption from the renal tubular fluid, saliva, and gastric juice. In the kidney, it acts on the epithelium of the distal tubule and collecting duct where it facilitates the exchange of sodium for potassium and hydrogen ions. It may also increase potassium and decrease sodium in muscle and brain cells (Figure 2-5).

Secondary actions include:

- Maintenance of blood pressure (due to sodium-water retention and increased blood volume);
- Moderate potassium diuresis; and
- Increased urine acidity (sodium taken up is exchanged for potassium and hydrogen ions that are excreted).

5. Renin and Angiotensin II

Aldosterone secretion is regulated only partially by ACTH. The major regulator is angiotensin II, a potent vasopressive octapeptide formed in the body from angiotensin I which is liberated by the action of renin (an enzyme from the juxtaglomerular cells of the kidney) acting on a

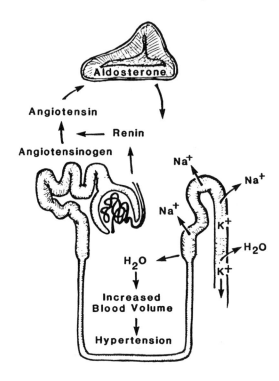

FIGURE 2-5 The renin-angiotensin-aldosterone system. Renin released from the juxtaglomerular apparatus in the kidney acts on circulating angiotensinogen — a protein from the liver — through a series of steps leading to angiotensin II, the most potent vasoconstrictor. Angiotensin II stimulates the adrenal cortex (the glomerulosa zone) to secrete aldosterone. The mineralocorticoid regulates sodium-potassium exchange in the distal renal tubule and collecting duct. Excess aldosterone may lead to increased sodium and water retention followed by increased blood volume, increased blood pressure, and eventually, hypertension.

circulating globulin, angiotensinogen (Figure 2-5). Changes in plasma Na+ (decrease) and K+ (increase) represent a third regulating mechanism of aldosterone secretion, although a weak one.

6. Corticoid Binding

Cortisol in the circulation is bound to a globulin called corticosteroid-binding globulin (CSBG) or transcortin and to a lesser degree to albumin. Other corticoids, including aldosterone, are similarly bound to circulating globulins and their bound form appears to be physiologically inactive. The active free cortisol and aldosterone diffuse across the plasma membrane into the target cell where they bind to specific receptor proteins in the cytoplasm. The resulting hormone-receptor complexes are activated and translocated to the nucleus where they bind to the DNA/chromatin complex. This stimulates the synthesis of heterogeneous RNA (hnRNA) which is processed into mature messenger RNA (mRNA). The mRNA is transported into the cytoplasm where it is translated into protein which causes the biological response.

7. Metabolism and Clearance

Corticoids are metabolized in the liver and their metabolites excreted in the urine (clearance). The rate of this hepatic metabolic inactivation is depressed in liver disease, during surgery and stress in the adult individual, and, as discussed below, with aging.

8. Diseases

Excess glucocorticoids, as in Cushing's disease, lead to abnormalities of intermediary metabolism; excess aldosterone, as in Conn's disease, leads to hypertension and electrolyte disturbances; adrenocortical insufficiency, involving both gluco- and mineralocorticoids, as in Addison's disease, leads to hypotension, shock, and death.

B. Changes With Aging Under Basal Conditions

1. Structural Changes

With aging, the adrenal cortex in humans and some animal species decreases in weight, except with the frequent occurrence of nodules (e.g., multifocal adenomas or localized hyperplastic changes, perhaps reactive to reduced blood supply). The adrenocortical cells (typical secretory cells, rich in mitochondria and endoplasmic reticulum, with lipid droplets indicating steroid hormone storage) undergo numerous changes:

- Accumulation of lipofuscin granules,[12] amyloid inclusions,[13] and lymphocytic infiltration,[14]
- Thickening of the supporting connective tissue shown by the thick capsule and the perivascular fibrous infiltrations, and
- Atherosclerotic involvement of adrenal vessels.

Despite these anatomic and histologic changes, basal plasma glucocorticoid levels do not differ significantly from maturity well into old age in humans[15-17] and other animals (cows, goats, dogs, monkeys)[18-21] although they may increase in some animals (rats) (Chapter 14). In contrast, DHEA[22] and aldosterone[23-26] levels decrease significantly in all animals studied, including humans.

Early studies in elderly (mostly hospitalized) individuals reported a reduced rate of secretion for all steroids and a slowed down steroidogenesis.[27-28] Reduced steroidogenesis with aging was ascribed to a reduced responsiveness, locally, of cortical cells to ACTH (due to loss of receptors, membrane alterations, and availability of precursors) or, more generally, to a reduced sensitivity of the hypothalmic-pituitary-adrenal (HPA) axis to feedback regulation. More recent studies in healthy men and women (volunteers from the community) show that levels of plasma cortisol and tests of adrenocortical function undergo little change with aging.[17]

2. Glucorticoids

With aging, glucocorticoids plasma levels remain normal in healthy ambulatory individuals. In some elderly the secretion rate is low, but it may be compensated by reduced clearance, that is, reduced metabolism and excretion (Figure 2-6). The reduced urinary excretion rate is no longer present when the urinary values are adjusted in relation to creatinine excretion, which is also decreased with aging.[7] If the glucocorticoid excretory rate is unchanged and circulating levels are normal despite reduced secretion, then compensation must depend on decreased metabolism. That this is the case is demonstrated by the decreased rate of cortisol removal from the circulation in individuals aged 60 years and older. This decline has been ascribed to a number of factors (decreased size, blood flow, enzyme activity) affecting the liver (the primary metabolizing organ).

In some male (but less so in female) rats levels of blood corticosterone (the major glucocorticoid in rats) increase with aging and high corticosterone levels after stress return more slowly to prestress values than in young or adult rats. This response to stress has been related to a failure of inhibitory inputs from the hippocampus to block CRH production in the hypothalamus (Chapter 14).

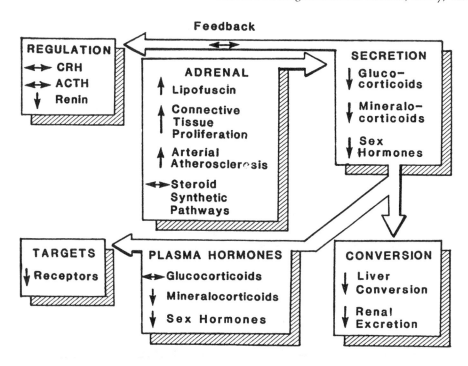

FIGURE 2-6 Diagram of age-related changes in corticosteroids in terms of regulation, biosynthesis, secretion, metabolism, and effects on targets. Under basal (steady state) conditions in the adrenal, steroid synthesis is unchanged. However, secretion of all hormones may be reduced. The feedback regulation of CRH and ACTH may not change but renin levels are reduced. Plasma levels of glucocorticoids remain unchanged despite low secretion, perhaps because of slower metabolism. For comparison with changes under stress conditions see Chapter 14. Plasma levels of mineralocorticoids and sex hormones are reduced. Reduced receptors impair target tissue response to all hormones.

3. Mineralocorticoids

Secretory rate and plasma levels of aldosterone are reduced by approximately 50% in elderly subjects despite a reduction in the metabolic clearance rate of the hormones.[8] The cause of this reduction probably lies in a reduced plasma renin activity.[23-26] That plasma electrolyte balance is maintained despite the drop in aldosterone output and levels may reflect hormonal (changes in ADH secretion, Chapter 3) and renal adjustments (changes in glomerular filtration). The decline in plasma renin activity has been ascribed to alterations in the sympathetic regulation of the juxtaglomerular apparatus in the kidney which secretes renin and, in aged rats, has been related to the general decline in adrenergic receptor activity.[29]

4. DHEA Changes and Replacement Therapy

The marked reduction in DHEA secretion and levels with aging has led to the speculation that reduction of this major androgen may be responsible for some of the aging decrements.[30] Therefore, replacement therapy with DHEA has been attempted in animals to induce anti-aging effects. Indeed, long-term DHEA administration reduces the incidence of mammary tumors, increases survival, and delays onset of immune dysfunction in mice.[31] With DHEA administration both body weight and food intake decrease, suggesting that the hormone, despite its minor anabolic action, might act in a manner similar to food restriction which also retards tumor development and immunologic senescence.

While the use of DHEA as an anti-aging agent in humans awaits adequate proof of its direct efficacy, historically, androgen deficiency has long been suggested as a cause of aging. The first association between endocrines and aging, as well as one of the primary secretory actions attributed to an organ (the testis) were drawn by the French physiologist C.E. Brown-Sequard, who extolled the anti-aging properties of testicular secretions (androgens).[32] Testicular transplants and administration of androgens as rejuvenating measures have been attempted repeatedly to delay or reverse aging, but with little success.

5. Changes in Adrenal Steroid Binding

As indicated above, hormone binding to specific intracellular receptors, activation of such hormone-receptor complexes, and the interaction of these complexes, at nuclear receptor sites are all events that mediate corticosteroid actions. In all target tissues at least two classes of corticosteroid receptors are present: type 1 (mineralocorticoids) and type 2 (glucocorticoids). These receptors differ in affinity and specificity for both naturally occurring and synthetic corticosteroids.[33] Specificity may be conferred by the presence in target tissues of some enzyme, such as is the case for aldosterone.[34]

Activation of steroid-receptor complexes leads to conformational changes which enable the complexes to interact with specific acceptor sites on chromatin and modulate gene expression. Receptor binding may depend upon various domains which confer specificity and coupling.[35] Modification of these domains as well as the number, and some physicochemical properties of receptors by extrinsic and intrinsic factors, may influence receptor response during development and aging.[36] For example, in rats, nuclear binding can be achieved *in vitro* by incubation of the hormone-receptor complex at a specific temperature and under high ionic conditions or by exposure to positively charged amino acid residues on the surface of the receptor molecule. Effects of temperature (25°C) and Ca^{2+} (20 mM at 0°C) vary with the age of the animal (from immature to mature) and with the organ considered. In cerebral hemispheres, kidney, liver, and skeletal muscle the number of receptors, but not their affinity, is reduced with age,[36] including old age.[37] Both heat and calcium activate the hormone-receptor complex at young and mature ages, but the magnitude of activation varies. In cerebral hemispheres, heat activation loses effectiveness as the animal matures, while the opposite occurs in liver; in both tissues Ca^{2+} activation is equally effective at all ages. In skeletal muscle and kidney, Ca^{2+} activation is less in older animals but heat activation is equally efficient.[38,39]

Hormones, like enzymes, may respond differentially depending on the cellular and molecular environmental conditions. Adaptive responses are also age related. An example of receptor adaptability taken from the immune system is the promotion of T-cells by such substances as interleukin-2 (IL-2). This promotion depends on activation of the antigen receptor and associated molecules.[40] The presence, in murine T cells, of a specific DHEA receptor, probably involved in the regulation of IL-2 production,[41] supports the suggestion of a physiologic role for DHEA in human immune responses[42] and provides the rationale for the administration of the hormone in old age (see above).

Many hormone receptors respond to binding by initiating a series of reactions including increased concentration of intracellular Ca^{2+} ions, phosphorylation, and rearrangement of membrane and intracellular proteins. Hormones may also occur in different forms and many consist of polypeptide dimers. The isomers may interact with the different domains of the same receptor to produce different actions.[43] At least some of the changes in hormonal actions with aging may best be ascribed to changes in target cells and molecules.

6. Responses to CRH, ACTH, and Stress

See discussion in Chapter 14.

IV. THE OVARY

A. Synopsis of Ovarian Function in the Adult

The ovary is the primary reproductive endocrine gland of the female. As does the testis, the corresponding primary endocrine gland in the male, the ovary produces both the germ cells (ova in the female and spermatozoa in the male) and sex hormones (primarily estrogens and progesterone in the female and testosterone in the male). The ovary is unique among endocrine glands because at a specific time of the lifespan (menopause in women) it ceases its gametogenic and hormonal functions.[44,45]

1. The Female Reproductive Tract

The major components of the female reproductive tract are the two ovaries (containing the female germ cells) and the *secondary female sex organs* which include two oviducts (or Fallopian tubes), the uterus, cervix, and vagina (Figure 2-7). Other structures, the breast (mammary gland) and the external genitalia (vulva), are also secondary sex organs. Development and function of these secondary sex organs depend on ovarian hormones. Also dependent on ovarian hormones are the *secondary sex characteristics* (hair distribution, voice pitch, adipose tissue distribution, stature, muscle and bone development, and so forth) which embody femininity.

The ovaries, located in the pelvic cavity, are small oval structures (in women, walnut-sized); they lie on either side of the uterus and are covered by the fimbriae, the fringed open end of the oviducts. These tubes, in which fertilization occurs, lead to the uterus. The uterus is a muscular organ that serves as a gestation sac for the developing embryo and fetus. The vagina is a slight curved muscular canal that serves as the receptive organ during intercourse and as the birth canal at parturition.

Estrogens are secreted from granulosa and thecal cells lining the ovarian follicles and by cells of the corpus luteum. The latter cells also produce progesterone and relaxin. Thecal cells also secrete androgens. Inhibin is another hormone secreted by both ovary and testis. In the testis it inhibits FSH secretion, but in the ovary its function is still uncertain. The hormone relaxin is secreted in the nonpregnant woman by the cells of the corpus luteum and, during pregnancy, by these cells and those of the placenta.

2. Major Hormones Involved in Ovarian Regulation

These hormones, all of which are affected by aging, are operative at different levels (Table 2-4):

- At the hypothalamus, the gonadotropin-releasing hormone (GnRH) is a polypeptide secreted into the portal blood vessels and carried to the anterior pituitary where it stimulates the synthesis and release of the two gonadotropins, the follicle stimulating hormone, FSH, and the luteinizing hormone, LH. Starting at puberty, GnRH secretion occurs cyclically and the cyclic secretion entrains the cyclicity of the reproductive function, (the menstrual cycle in humans). Other brain areas, particularly the limbic system, are involved in reproduction and in sexual behavior;
- At the anterior pituitary, the two glycoproteins, FSH and LH, are regulated by the hypothalamic GnRH and by the positive (stimulatory) or negative (inhibitory) feedbacks from the plasma ovarian hormones. FSH promotes the maturation of the follicle and secretion of estrogens. LH promotes the rupture of the follicle with the extrusion of the egg at ovulation. Both FSH and LH support the formation of the corpus luteum and its secretion of estrogens and progesterone;
- At the ovary, the major hormones, estrogen and progesterone, are steroids. Like the corticoids, they derive from cholesterol through a series of enzymatically catalyzed steps. The most biologically active of the estrogens, 17-β-estradiol, is followed by estrone and estriol in

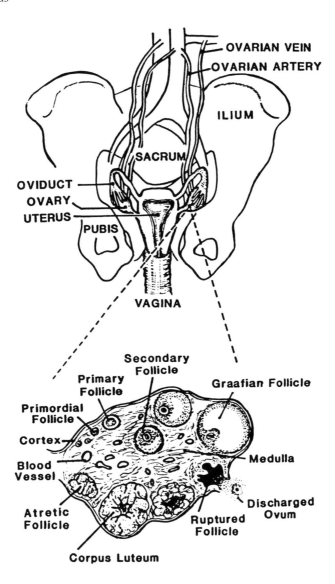

FIGURE 2-7 Diagram of the human female genital tract and ovary. Illustrated in the upper portion are the major female reproductive organs lying in the pelvic cavity. The lower portion shows an enlargement of the ovary with progressive stages of follicular development. The primordial follicle is present at birth, and eventually progresses through stages of primary, secondary, and mature (Graffian) follicle; this ruptures under the influence of an LH surge and releases the ovum at ovulation (approximately midway through the menstrual cycle), and thereafter forms the corpus luteum which (in the absence of pregnancy) undergoes atresia. Not all follicles complete maturation; those that do not mature undergo atresia (i.e., atretic follicles).

decreasing order of potency. Progesterone is secreted by the corpus luteum which also produces estrogens. Androgens, especially weak androgens such as DHEA, are synthesized in the ovary; this synthesis becomes significant in the postmenopausal woman when the feminizing actions of estrogens can no longer counteract the virilizing actions of androgens. Inhibin and relaxin are two polypeptides also secreted by the ovary but their role is primarily with pregnancy and, therefore, of little known import in aging.

• At the periphery, estrogens and progesterone follow the same mechanism of action as corticoids at the target cells. They bind to nuclear receptors and stimulate RNA and protein synthesis responsible for the many actions of these hormones.

TABLE 2-4 Major Hormones Involved in Ovarian Regulation

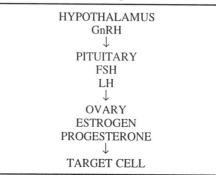

HYPOTHALAMUS
GnRH
↓
PITUITARY
FSH
LH
↓
OVARY
ESTROGEN
PROGESTERONE
↓
TARGET CELL

3. Cyclicity of the Hypothalamo-Pituitary-Ovarian Axis

As just described, functional dependence of the ovary on neuroendocrine inputs from the hypothalamus and pituitary has led to the concept of a unified system, or hypothalamo-pituitary-ovarian axis, which, in the females, regulates reproductive activity in a cyclic fashion.

This particular cyclicity in females, as opposed to the noncyclicity in males, depends on the organization of the central nervous system (CNS).[46] At the gross level, the morphology of the nervous system is quite similar in the two sexes; however, more detailed analysis reveals sexual dimorphism (i.e., existing in two different forms: female or male) in neuronal number, size, shape, biochemistry, and pattern of connectivity. Sexual dimorphism has been described in laboratory animals, particularly rodents, but it is present in the human CNS as well although its functional role and the extent to which it is hormonally (or genetically) determined are not yet known.

Cyclicity in females may underlie periodic preparations for fertilization and pregnancy with the corresponding cyclic endocrine and behavioral rhythms. Changes in cyclicity with aging may depend on changes in hypothalamic neurotransmitters.[47] Cyclicity involves all hormones active in the reproductive function; each cycle lasts a definite period of time varying with the animal species, for example, about 28 days for the menstrual cycle in women and 3 to 5 days for the estrous cycle in rats.

In each cycle, the sequence of events is similar and includes for the menstrual cycle, in brief:

- At the beginning of the cycle (the first day of menstruation) several follicles begin to grow but one only will continue to grow and ovulate. For the others, development is arrested and expulsion of the ovum never occurs, hence the term of "atresia" given to this arrest and "atresic" to these follicles (from the Greek: nonperforated). Atresic follicles involute: the ovum degenerates first, followed by detachment of granulosa cells, coagulation of follicular fluid, membrane thickening, and loss of secretory (mainly estrogens) activity. At the onset of this stage pituitary FSH and LH levels are low, but FSH levels are rising because the circulating levels of sex hormones are low and, therefore, the negative (inhibitory) feedback of these hormones on the release of pituitary gonadotropins and hypothalamic GnRH is reduced;
- Under FSH stimulation, with the maturation of the follicle, estrogen levels increase and, through a positive feedback on the hypothalamo-pituitary axis, stimulate the release of LH (the so-called LH surge) which triggers ovulation at about the 14th postmenstrual day;
- At ovulation, the ovum is expelled into the oviduct to be fertilized. The site of the ruptured follicle is transformed into the corpus luteum, which secretes abundant amounts of both estrogens and progesterone; and finally

- In the case of pregnancy, the corpus luteum continues to secrete estrogens and progesterone necessary for uterine implantation of the fertilized ovum. In the absence of fertilization, the corpus luteum degenerates and estrogens and progesterone levels fall. The hypertrophic and hyperhemic uterine mucosa is shed and menstruation occurs.

B. Major Actions of Ovarian Steroids

Major actions of estrogens (Table 2-5) include:

- Postnatal development and maintenance of female secondary sex organs and characteristics;
- Both positive and negative feedbacks regulating GnRH, FSH, and LH;
- Stimulation of RNA and protein synthesis;
- Sexual and maternal behavior.

For progesterone (progestins):

- Maintenance of pregnancy,
- Antiestrogenic action on uterine excitability;
- Negative feedback on LH secretion;
- Thermogenic (elevated body temperature) and natriuretic (increased urinary sodium excretion) actions (shared with the corticoids);
- Stimulation of RNA and protein synthesis.

TABLE 2-5 Major Actions of Ovarian Hormones

Estrogens	Progesterone
Postnatal development and maintenance of female secondary sex organs and characteristics	Maintenance of pregnancy, anti-estrogenic action on uterine excitability
($\pm$) Feedback regulating GnRH and FSH and LH	($-$) Feedback of GnRH and LH
Stimulation of RNA and protein synthesis	Thermogenic and natriuretic stimulation of RNA and protein synthesis

1. Metabolism and Clearance

Most of the estradiol in plasma is bound to gonadal steroid-binding globulin (GSBP), and to other proteins (albumin). Free estradiol is the active form of the hormone. Estrogens and progesterone are oxidized in the liver or converted to glucuronide and sulfate conjugates. Metabolites are excreted in the urine but some are secreted in the bile and reabsorbed into the blood stream.

Cessation of the ovarian function with aging, its consequences, and treatment of menopause are discussed in Chapters 7 and 8.

V. THE TESTIS

A. Synopsis of Testicular Function in the Adult

The aging of the testis differs from that of the ovary. It undergoes a slow and progressive decline rather than a complete cessation of function. Testicular function appears to continue indefinitely; a male climacteric or "andropause", the equivalent in men of the menopause, if it occurs at all, generally begins at age 60 years and older. The male climacteric may be associated with some clinical and emotional symptoms and with minimal endocrine alterations involving a moderate decline in testosterone and a minimal increase in gonadotropins.[48] Thus, the andropause differs endocrinologically from the menopause, but shares with it some of the changes in nonreproductive organs and functions (Chapter 9).

1.   The Male Reproductive System

The testis or male gonad represents the male primary sex organ (Figure 2-8). The two testes produce the germ cells, or sperm, and the major steroid male hormone testosterone as well as the hormone inhibin and amounts of estrogens depending on species. Other components of the male reproductive system depend for development and function on testosterone; they are the secondary sex organs. They include, extending in order anatomically from the testis, the epididymis and vas deferens — which serve for transport of sperm — and the seminal vesicles and prostate (with associated glands such as the Cowper's glands) for the production of seminal fluid. The widespread changes in secondary sex characteristics (hair distribution, body configuration, genital size, voice, and behavior) that develop at puberty depend for development and maintenance essentially on testicular androgens responsible for masculinity.

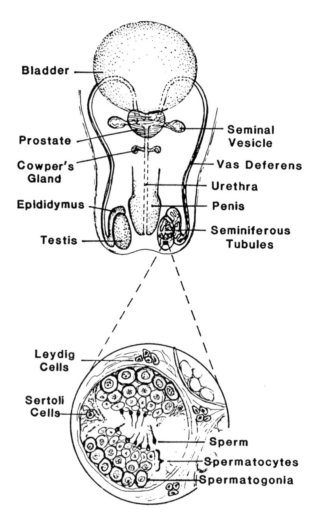

FIGURE 2-8 Diagram of the human male genital tract and testis. Illustrated in the upper portion are the major reproductive organs. The lower portion show an enlargement of the testis with a seminiferous tubule with Sertoli cells, spermatogonia, spermatocytes, and sperm. Also shown are Leydig cells in the intertubular spaces.

TABLE 2-6 Major Hormones Involved in
Testicular Regulation

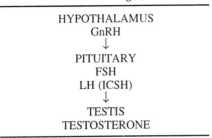

2. Major Hormones Involved in Testicular Regulation

As for the ovary, the hormones involved in male reproductive function are operative at several levels (Table 2-6); but unlike those of the ovary, they do not have a reproductive cycle. Rather, androgens have a 24-h rhythm, more marked in younger men than old. Regulatory controls include:

- At the hypothalamus, the secretion of polypeptide GnRH carried, as in females, through the portal vessels to the anterior pituitary to stimulate the synthesis and release of FSH and LH, similar to the corresponding hormones in the female.
- At the anterior pituitary, the synthesis and release of the two gonadotropins, FSH and LH (also called interstitial cell-stimulating hormone, ICSH). The gonadotropins are regulated by GnRH and through a negative feedback, by circulating levels of testosterone for LH and inhibin for FSH.
- At the testis, the major hormones are steroids: testosterone secreted by the interstitial cells of Leydig, and extremely small amounts of estradiol, probably secreted by both Leydig and Sertoli cells. Inhibin is secreted by the Sertoli cells situated at the base of the epithelium lining the seminiferous tubules where spermatozoa are formed. Inhibin secretion is stimulated by FSH; its levels inhibit FSH release from the pituitary and may also decrease GnRH.
- At the target cells, testosterone has the same mechanism of action as already described for other steroid hormones such as corticoids and ovarian hormones. It freely passes the plasma membrane and forms a cytoplasmic-activated steroid-receptor complex which is carried to the nucleus. The binding of the hormone to the nuclear acceptor sites results in the stimulation of protein and RNA synthesis to induce the characteristic masculinizing effects and growth-promoting actions of the hormone. In the prostate and several other tissues that are primary targets for testosterone, the hormone is converted to dehydrotestosterone (DHT). A small amount of testosterone is also converted to estrogens.

Androgens are also secreted by the adrenal cortex but they have little biological activity as compared with testosterone. Although their levels decline progressively with aging (see above), the contribution of this decline to reduced reproductive function with aging is minimal.

B. Major Actions of Testosterone

The major actions of testosterone have both organizing (i.e., inducing differentiation of the immature gonad into the testis) and metabolic importance (Table 2-7). The organizing actions are manifested prenatally, with the differentiation of the gonads and secondary sex organs in the male type. Organizing actions continue perinatally, with the differentiation of the hypo-thalamic control of gonadotropin release following the continuous patterns typical of the male. In the absence of androgens, differentiation of gonads and hypothalamus is of the female type. At puberty, testosterone regulates the development and maturation of the secondary sex

**TABLE 2-7 Major Actions of
Testosterone and
Dehydrotestosterone**

Prenatal
   Masculine differentiation of:
      Gonads
      Secondary sex organs
      Hypothalamus
Postnatal – Puberty
   Growth Stimulation
   Maturation of:
      Testis
      Male secondary sex organs
      Male sex behavior
Adult
Metabolic – Anabolic Behavior(s)

organs and sex characteristics. It also influences stature by first accelerating and then terminating body growth. In the adult, testosterone and its derivatives maintain the structure and function of secondary sex organs and male characteristics and behavior. Some of these actions are due directly to testosterone and others to its metabolite, dehydrotestosterone. Such is the case of the prostate where the active hormone is dehydrotestosterone (Chapter 9).

1. Metabolism and Clearance

Testosterone in plasma is bound primarily to a globulin called steroid hormone binding globulin (SHBG) and, to a much lesser extent, to other proteins. The remainder of testosterone is free and biologically active. A small amount of testosterone is converted to estrogens, but most of the circulating testosterone is metabolized in the liver and excreted in the urine.

    Aging of the testis and its consequences are discussed in Chapter 9.

REFERENCES

1. Gregerman, R. I. and Bierman, E. L., Aging and hormones, in *Textbook of Endocrinology,* 6th ed., Williams, R. H., Ed., W. B. Saunders, Philadelphia, 1981, 1192.
2. Korenman, S. G., *Endocrine Aspects of Aging,* Elsevier, New York, 1982.
3. Vernadakis, A. and Timiras, P. S., Eds., *Hormones in Development and Aging,* S. P. Medical & Scientific Books, New York, 1982.
4. Meites, J., *Neuroendocrinology of Aging,* Plenum Press, New York, 1983.
5. Everitt, A. and Meites, J., Aging and anti-aging effects of hormones, *J. Gerontol.,* 44, B139, 1989.
6. Green, M. F., The endocrine system, in *Principles and Practice of Geriatric Medicine,* 2nd ed., Pathy, M. S. J., Ed., John Wiley & Sons, New York, 1991, 1061.
7. Timiras, P. S., *Physiological Basis of Aging and Geriatrics,* 2nd ed., CRC Press, Boca Raton, FL, 1994.
8. Funder, J. W., Adrenal steroids: New answers, new questions, *Science,* 237, 236, 1987.
9. Dallman, M. F., Stress update: Adaptation of the hypothalamic-pituitary-adrenal axis to chronic stress, *TEM,* 4, 62, 1993.
10. De Kloet, E. R., Corticosteroids, stress, and aging, *Ann. N. Y. Acad. Sci.,* 663, 357, 1992.
11. Roberts, N. A., Barton, R. N., and Horan, M. A., Ageing and the sensitivity of the adrenal gland to physiological doses of ACTH in man, *J. Endocrinol.,* 126, 507, 1990.
12. Sohal, R. S., Ed., *Age Pigments,* Elsevier/North-Holland, New York, 1981.
13. Eriksson, L. and Westermark, P., Age-related accumulation of amyloid inclusions in adrenal cortical cells, *Am. J. Pathol.,* 136, 461, 1990.
14. Hayashi, Y., Hiyoshi, T., Takemura, T., Kurashima, C., and Hirokawa, K., Focal lymphocytic infiltration in the adrenal cortex of the elderly: immunohistological analysis of infiltrating lymphocytes, *Clin. Exp. Immunol.,* 77, 101, 1989.

15. Jensen, H. K. and Blichert-Toft, M., Serum corticotrophin, plasma cortisol and urinary excretion of 17-ketogenic steroids in the elderly (age group: 66-94 years), *Acta Endocrinol.*, 66, 25, 1971.

16. Waltman, C., Blackman, M. R., Chrousos, G. P., Riemann, C., and Harman, S. M., Spontaneous and glucocorticoid-inhibited adrenocorticotropic hormone and cortisol secretion are similar in healthy young and old men, *J. Clin. Endocrinol. Metab.*, 73, 495, 1991.

17. Barton, R. N., Horan, M. A., Weijers, J. W., Sakkee, A. N., Roberts, N. A., and van Bezooijen, C. F., Cortisol production rate and the urinary excretion of 17-hydroxycorticosteroids, free cortisol, and 6 beta-hydroxycortisol in healthy elderly men and women, *J. Gerontol.*, 48, M213, 1993.

18. Bowman, R .E. and Wolf, R. C., Plasma 17-hydroxycorticosteroid response to ACTH in *M. mulatta*: dose, age, weight, and sex, *Proc. Soc. Exp. Biol. Med.*, 130, 61, 1969.

19. Riegle, G. D. and Nellor, J. E., Changes in adrenocortical function during aging in cattle, *J. Gerontol.*, 22, 83, 1967.

20. Riegle, G. D., Przekop, F., and Nellor, J. E., Changes in adrenocortical responsiveness to ACTH infusion in aging goats, *J. Gerontol.*, 23, 187, 1968.

21. Rothuizen, J., Reul, J. M., Rijnberk, A., Mol, J. A., and de Kloet, E. R., Aging and the hypothalamus-pituitary-adrenocortical axis, with special reference to the dog, *Acta Endocrinol.*, 125(Suppl. 1), 73, 1991.

22. Orentreich, N., Brind, J. L., Rizer, R. L., and Vogelman, J. H., Age changes and sex differences in serum dehydroepiandrosterone sulfate concentrations throughout adulthood, *J. Clin. Endocrinol. Metab.*, 59, 551, 1984.

23. Noth, R. H., Lassman, M. N., Tan, S. Y., Fernandez-Cruz, A., Jr., and Mulrow, P. J., Age and the renin-aldosterone system, *Arch. Intern. Med.*, 137, 1414, 1977.

24. Hallengren, B., Elmstahl, S., Galvard, H., Jerntorp, P., Manhem, P., Pessah-Rasmussen, H., and Stavenow, L., Eighty-year-old men have elevated plasma concentrations of catecholamines but decreased plasma renin activity and aldosterone as compared to young men, *Aging*, 4, 341, 1992.

25. Luft, F. C., Fineberg, N. S., and Weinberger, M H., The influence of age on renal function and renin and aldosterone responses to sodium-volume expansion and contraction in normotensive and mildly hypertensive humans, *Am. J. Hypertension*, 5, 520, 1992.

26. Bauer, J. H., Age-related changes in the renin-aldosterone system. Physiological effects and clinical implications, *Drugs and Aging*, 3, 238, 1993.

27. Romanoff, L. P., Morris, C. W., Welch, P., Rodrigues, R. M., and Pincus, G., The metabolism of cortisol-4-C^{14} in young and elderly men. I. Secretion rate of cortisol and daily secretion of tetrahydrocortisol, (allotetrahydrocortisol), tetrahydrocortisone, and cortolone (20α and 20β), *J. Clin. Endocrinol. Metab.*, 21, 1413, 1961.

28. West, C. D., Brown, H., Simons, E. L., Carter, D. B., Kumagai, L. F., and Englert, E., Jr., Adrenocortical function and cortisol metabolism in old age, *J. Clin. Endocrinol. Metab.*, 21, 1197, 1961.

29. Roth, G. S., Mechanisms of altered hormone-neurotransmitter action during aging: from receptors to calcium mobilization, *Annu. Rev. Gerontol. Geriatr.*, 10, 132, 1990.

30. Meikle, A. W., Daynes, R. A., and Araneo, B. A., Adrenal androgen secretion and biologic effects, *Endocrinol. Metabol. Clin. N. Am.*, 20, 381, 1991.

31. Araneo, B. A., Woods, M. L., and Daynes, R. A., Reversal of the immunoscenecent phenotype by dehydroepiandrosterone: hormone treatment provides an adjuvant effect on the immunization of aged mice with recombinant hepatitis B surface antigen, *J. Inf. Dis.*, 167, 830, 1993.

32. Timiras, P. S., Neuroendocrinology of aging: retrospective, current, and prospective views, in *Neuroendocrinology of Aging*, Meites, J., Ed., Plenum Press, New York, 1983, 5.

33. Meyer, J. S., Biochemical effects of corticosteroids on neural tissues, *Physiol. Rev.*, 65, 946, 1985.

34. Funder, J. W., Pearce, P. T., Smith, R., and Smith, A. I., Mineralocorticoid action: target tissue specificity is enzyme, not receptor, mediated, *Science*, 242, 583, 1988.

35. Kobilka, B. K., Kobilka, T. S., Daniel, K., Regan, J. W., Caron, M. G., and Lefkowitz, R. J., Chimeric α2-ß2-adrenergic receptors: delineation of domains involved in effector coupling and ligand binding specificity, *Science*, 240, 1310, 1988.

36. Sharma, R. and Timiras, P. S., Glucocorticoid receptors, stress and aging, in *Regulation of Neuroendocrine Aging*, Everitt, A. V. and Walton, J. R., Eds., Karger, Basel, 1988, 98.

37. Roth, G. S., Age-related changes in specific glucocorticoid binding by steroid-responsive tissues of rats, *Endocrinology*, 94, 82, 1974.

38. Sharma, R. and Timiras, P. S., Regulatory changes in glucocorticoid receptors in the skeletal muscle of immature and mature male rats, *Mech. Ageing Dev.*, 37, 249, 1987.

39. Sharma, R. and Timiras, P. S., Regulation of glucocorticoid receptors in the kidneys of immature and mature male rats, *J. Intern. Biochem.*, 20, 141, 1988.

40. Shaw, J. P., Utz, P. J., Durand, D. B., Toole, J. J., Emmel, E. A., and Crabtree, G. R., Identification of a putative regulator of early T-cell activation genes, *Science*, 241, 202, 1988.

41. Meikle, A. W., Dorchuck, R. W., Araneo, B. A., Stringham., J. D., Evans, T. G., Spruance, S. L., and Daynes, R. A., The presence of a dehydroepiandrosterone-specific receptor binding complex in murine T cells, *J. Steroid Biochem. Mol. Biol.,* 42, 293, 1992.

42. Suzuki, T., Suzuki, N., Daynes, R. A., and Engleman, E. G., Dehydroepiandrosterone enhances IL2 production and cytotoxic effector function of human T cell, *Clin. Immunol. Immunopathol.,* 61, 202, 1991.

43. Hart, C. E., Forstrom, J. W., Kelly, J. D., Seifert, R. A., Smith, R. A., Ross, R., Murray, M. J., and Bowen-Pope, D. F., Two classes of PDGF receptor recognize different isoforms of PDGF, *Science,* 240, 1529, 1988.

44. Kawagoe, S., The aging process of the reproductive organs: an overview, *Horm. Res.,* 39(Suppl. 1), 3, 1993.

45. Meldrum, D. R., Female reproductive aging — ovarian and uterine factors, *Fertility and Sterility,* 59, 1, 1993.

46. Fishman, R. B. and Breedlove, S. M., Sexual dimorphism in the developing nervous system, in *Handbook of Human Growth and Developmental Biology,* Vol. I, Part C, Meisami, E. and Timiras, P. S., Eds., CRC Press, Boca Raton, FL, 1988, 45.

47. Wise, P. M., Weiland, N. G., Scarbrough, K., Larson, G. H., and Lloyd, J. M., Contribution of changing rhythmicity of hypothalamic neurotransmitter function to female reproductive aging, *Ann. N.Y. Acad. Sci.,* 592, 31, 1990.

48. Johnson, L., Evaluation of the human testis and its age-related dysfunction, *Progr. Clin. Biol. Res.,* 302, 35, 1989.

3

Protein- and Peptide-Secreting Endocrines

Paola S. Timiras

CONTENTS

I. INTRODUCTION

Included in this category are the pituitary (or hypophysis), a typical endocrine gland; the pancreas, a gland with both endocrine and exocrine secretions; and the hypothalamus, a brain area with hormone-secreting neurons.

The pituitary, ovoid in shape, lies at the base of the skull within a recess (sella turcica) in the sphenoid bone. It is comprised of an anterior lobe (or adenohypophysis), an intermediate lobe (rudimentary in humans and a few other mammalian species), and a posterior lobe (neurohypophysis). It is surrounded by membranes (or meninges) covering the brain. These form a diaphragm separating the gland from the cerebrospinal fluid and the blood-brain barrier. It is suspended from the hypothalamus by a stalk which, through an opening in the diaphragm, carries the portal hypophysial blood vessels from the median eminence of the hypothalamus to the anterior lobe. The stalk also carries the nerve projections from the hypothalamic neurons to the posterior pituitary.[1] Pituitary hormones are proteins and peptides.

Peptide hormones are major secretions of the hypothalamus. Part of the anterior diencephalon, the hypothalamus is an important neural center for the regulation of visceral (autonomic) functions (e.g., sleep, hunger, thirst, temperature). It also secretes hormones which are transported through neural connections to the posterior pituitary and through vascular connections to the anterior pituitary. The concept of neuroendocrinology has emerged from the neural and vascular link between the hypothalamus and the pituitary, that is, between a designated brain region and an endocrine gland. Neuroendocrinological research has demonstrated that the brain regulates the secretion of endocrine glands and that hormones, in turn, act on the central nervous system (CNS) to modify brain function.[2] With aging, dysfunction could arise in this neuroendocrine articulation as well as within the individual endocrines.

Cells within the "satiety and feeding center" of the hypothalamus are sensitive to the level of glucose utilization. Likewise, cells in the pancreas secrete hormones which are sensitive to glucose and regulate its uptake into cells. Pancreatic cells secrete four peptide hormones with important functions in the regulation of the intermediary metabolism of carbohydrates, proteins, and fats.

II. HYPOTHALAMIC PEPTIDES AND HYPOPHYSIOTROPIC HORMONES

Once known primarily as the "head ganglion of the autonomic system", the hypothalamus is recognized also as the source of numerous hormones, neurotransmitters, and other biologically active substances. Peptides can be secreted by both neurons and gland cells. For example, somatostatin, when secreted by neurons (in the hypothalamus), acts as a neurotransmitter. When secreted by gland cells (in the pancreas) it acts as a hormone and as a paracrine mediator, affecting activities of other nearby endocrine cells.

Of the following nine major hypothalamic hormones (Table 3-1), two, usually designated as posterior pituitary hormones, are carried (by axonal transport) to the posterior pituitary: vasopressin (also called antidiuretic hormone, ADH) and oxytocin. Seven hypophysiotropic hormones are carried (by the portal vessels) to the anterior pituitary: corticotropin-releasing hormone (CRH), thyrotropin-releasing hormone (TRH), growth-hormone-releasing hormone (GRH), growth-hormone-inhibiting hormone (GIH, also called somatostatin or somatotropin release inhibitory factor SRIF), luteinizing-hormone releasing hormone (LHRH) (also called gonadotropin-releasing hormone, GnRH, in the presumed absence of a specific follicule-stimulating releasing hormone), prolactin-releasing hormone (PRH), and prolactin-inhibiting hormone (PIH).

Hypothalamic peptides are part of a large family of neuropeptides distributed within and without the CNS and often abundant in the hypothalamus.[3,4] These neuropeptides include:

- Hypothalamic/posterior pituitary and hypophysiotropic hormones;
- Pituitary hormones synthesized also in various brain areas or carried to the brain by the circulation;
- Opioid peptides, derivatives, with ACTH and MSH, of the precursor molecules pro-opiomelanocortin and pro-dynorphin.

TABLE 3-1 Major Hypothalamic Hormones

Hormone	Structure	Primary function
Posterior Pituitary Hormones		
Arginine-vasopressin or antidiuretic hormone, ADH	9-Amino-acid peptide with disulfide linkage	Promotes water retention in the kidney by ↑ permeability of renal collecting duct cells
Oxytocin	9-Amino-acid peptide with disulfide linkage	↑Smooth muscle contraction, milk release, and uterine contraction during labor
Hypophysiotropic Hormones		
Thyrotropin-releasing hormone (TRH)	3-Amino-acid peptide	↑Pituitary TSH
Corticotropin-releasing hormone (CRH)	41-Amino-acid peptide	↑Pituitary ACTH
Luteinizing hormone releasing hormone (LHRH) or gonadotropin-inhibiting hormone (GnRH)	10-Amino-acid peptide	↑Pituitary LH (or ICSH) and FSH
Somatostatin or growth hormone-releasing hormone (GIH)	14-Amino-acid peptide with disulfide linkage	↓Pituitary GH
Growth-hormone-releasing hormone (GRH)	44-Amino-Acid peptide	↑Pituitary GH
Prolactin-inhibiting hormone (PIH)	Amine (dopamine)	↓Prolactin
Prolactin-releasing hormone (PRH)	??	↑Prolactin

Other neuropeptides, to be discussed in Chapter 6, are

- Blood-borne gastrointestinal peptides (e.g., substance P, VIP, CCK) located in the stomach, intestinal walls, and CNS; and
- Peptides distributed in CNS and other tissues (e.g., neurotensin, angiotensin II, atrial natriuretic factors).

A. Vasopressin (ADH) and Oxytocin in the Adult

1. Synthesis and Transport

These hormones are nona (amine) peptides; they are

- Synthesized as large precursor hormones in the cell bodies of neurons of the supraoptic and paraventricular nuclei of the hypothalamus,
- Packaged there along with processing enzymes into membrane-bound granules,
- The granules are transported within the neuronal axons to the posterior pituitary lobe, and
- Stored there in the nerve endings.

Processing of the prohormones to the hormonal forms occurs during axonal transport. Pre-pro-pressophysin contains a leader sequence of 19 amino acids, signal peptide (cleaved within the cysternae of the neuronal endoplasmic reticulum as synthesis of the precussor occurs), followed by the amino acid sequence of vasopressin (arginine vasopressin in humans), then the sequence of vasopressin neurophysin (Neurophysin II), followed by a glycopeptide. Pre-pro-oxyphysin contains the amino acid sequence of oxytocin and oxytocin neurophysin (Neurophysin I) but lacks the glycopeptide. The products of the processing reactions, including the nonapeptide hormones contained within the granules in the nerve endings, are released to the blood from the posterior lobe by the process of exocytosis when appropriate stimuli impinge on the hypothalamic neurons.

These hormones are also found in the endings of neurons that project to the brain stem and spinal cord, a location that may explain their involvement in cardiovascular control. They

TABLE 3-2 Major Actions of Vasopressin

Target organ	Action
Kidney, collecting duct	↑ Water and urea permeability
Arterioles	Vasoconstriction
Brain	Behavioral effects: memory enhancer
Anterior pituitary	↑ ACTH release

appear to be synthesized also in the adrenal cortex and gonads where they (at least vasopressin) may act as inhibitors of steroid biosynthesis. The evidence for extrahypothalamic and extrapituitary vasopressin secretory neurons and their projections, although incomplete and often inferential, suggests that the hormone may also fill a neurotransmitter role. Certainly, behavioral effects involving memory and learning have been ascribed to vasopressin and its analogs, and these may be specifically affected with aging.

2. Major Actions

The major physiologic actions of vasopressin (Table 3-2) are to promote:

- Retention of water by the kidney, hence its alternate name, antidiuretic hormone (ADH);
- Increased permeability of the renal collecting ducts so that water is filtered from the incipient urine into the hypertonic interstitium of the renal pyramids; and
- Concentration of the urine and reduction of its volume.

Other important actions of vasopressin include:

- Stimulation of aldosterone synthesis, thereby contributing to water reabsorption in the renal distal tubule,
- Release of ACTH from the anterior pituitary,[5,6] probably by activation of Ca^{2+} channels and the consequent rise in intracellular Ca^{2+},[7]
- Vasoconstriction, by its stimulatory action on the smooth muscle of the arterioles, and
- In large (supraphysiologic) doses it elevates blood pressure, thereby playing a role in blood pressure homeostasis and possibly in the etiology of some forms of hypertension.

Actions of oxytocin include:

- Activation of smooth muscle contraction, particularly that of the uterus (as in the uterine contractions during labor at delivery),
- Promotion of milk ejection at suckling, by inducing contraction of the myoepithelial cells lining the ducts of the mammary gland,
- Increased motility of the oviducts to facilitate sperm transport,
- In addition to its direct action on muscle, stimulation of the formation of prostaglandins — a group of cyclic unsaturated fatty acids with many functions, including stimulation of smooth muscle contractions.

3. Receptors and Factors Regulating Secretions

The action of both hormones is mediated by the binding to receptors. Those so far identified for vasopressin include:

- V_1 receptors found in brain and muscle for vasoconstrictor action; they increase phosphatidylinositol metabolism and cytoplasmic Ca^{2+};
- V_1 receptors also found in the liver for increased glycogenolysis and gluconeogenesis;

- V_2 receptors found in kidney for the antidiuretic action that act on adenylate cyclase to increase intracellular cyclic AMP; and
- Possibly V_3 receptors situated in the anterior pituitary for the stimulation of ACTH release, especially under stress conditions.

TABLE 3-3 Selected Stimuli Effecting Vasopressin Secretion

↑Vasopressin secretion	↓Vasopressin secretion
↑Plasma osmotic pressure	↓Plasma osmotic pressure
↓Extracellular fluid volume	↑Extracellular fluid volume
Pain, emotion, stress, drugs (nicotine)	Drugs (alcohol)

Oxytocin may bind to two kinds of receptors; one which subserves smooth muscle contraction and one relaxation. Receptors in the uterus may not only mediate control of muscle activity but also synthesis of prostaglandins. Binding of oxytocin to plasma membrane receptors increases markedly in the uterus at the end of pregnancy and in the mammary gland during lactation due to up-regulation of receptors under the influence of high estrogen levels.

Vasopressin secretion is regulated by a variety of stimuli summarized in Table 3-3, including changes in:

- Osmolality of extracellular fluid acting on osmoreceptor cells in the brain, and
- Blood volume and pressure acting on other specific receptors in the heart and great blood vessels.

Several drugs affect ADH secretion, among which alcohol has a significant depressant action. Glucocorticoids participate in the regulation of vasopressin mRNA expression in a subset of neurons of the paraventricular nucleus in adult animals. This regulation illustrates the potential of the adult genome to be influenced by hormones and synaptic signals.[8]

Absence or low levels of ADH or failure of the kidney to respond to adequate circulating levels of ADH results in the loss of large volumes of very dilute urine, a condition called *diabetes insipidus* (in contrast to *diabetes mellitus*, due to insulin deficiency). Excessive water loss is associated with both cellular and extracellular dehydration and, in an attempt to compensate for the loss of fluid, with polydipsia (increased thirst and fluid intake). High plasma concentrations of ADH are found in some conditions (e.g., trauma, pain, anxiety, and particularly nausea which will lead to vomiting), and diseases (e.g., ADH-secreting tumors) leading to a variety of osmoregulatory defects characteristic of the "syndrome of inappropriate secretion of ADH" (SIADH).

Oxytocin secretion is stimulated by reflexes initiated by mechanical stimuli associated with dilation of the cervix and contraction of the uterine muscle at parturition and by stimulation of the nipple by suckling during lactation. Drugs such as alcohol and stressful conditions depress oxytocin secretion.

Despite oxytocin role in parturition, normal deliveries have been reported in women with diabetes insipidus due to hypothalamic tumors and, presumably, with destruction of the oxytocin-secreting cells. The complex neuroendocrine regulation of parturition is not yet fully understood. This is not the case for lactation, where the presence of oxytocin in women is indispensable for contraction of the myoepithelial cells and milk ejection.

B. Vasopressin (ADH) and Oxytocin Changes With Aging

While several hypopthalamic nuclei show significant age-related changes with cell loss, accumulation of lipofuscin, and degenerative changes, the paraventricular and supraoptic nuclei are spared relatively.[9-11] When these changes do occur in aged rats, they include:

- Decreased nuclear volume, perhaps indicative of reduced functional activity;
- Depletion of neurosecretory material, especially in very old rats;
- Altered axoplasmic transport, with axonal fibers appearing varicose and dilated;
- Accumulation of lipofuscin;
- Presence of vacuoles, primarily in oxytocin-secreting neurons;
- Decreased neuronal activity (depletion of hormones, decrease in nuclear size) along with reduced axonal transport (varicose axonal fibers), consistent with the reported decreased stores of hormones in the posterior pituitary;
- Depleted stores, correlated with depressed neurohypophysial function in old rats and a high incidence of mild diabetes insipidus.

Perhaps, in an attempt to compensate for the declining functional capacity, some cells may be overactivated during aging, and these activated cells may eventually degenerate. Degenerating cells can be seen in selected hypothalamic nuclei as well as in extrahypothalamic brain areas containing or innervating vasopressin neurons. Because of the progressive nature of the process, cells in different stages of activation will alternate with cells undergoing destruction. The diverse aging patterns of these secretory cells may account for the controversial observation of low, high, or unchanged hormonal levels.[11] A decrease in hypothalamic cell size and number in elderly individuals affected by Alzheimer's dementia has been associated with reduced circulating levels of vasopressin but unchanged levels of oxytocin.[10,12,13]

1. ADH and Water Balance

Oxytocin secretion and its regulation are essentially associated with the reproductive years.[14,15] With aging, most of the changes involve alterations in ADH and its role in salt and water balance. A commonly agreed-upon finding in both the human and rat is that the ability of the kidney to concentrate urine is diminished with aging.[16] Impairment may occur at one of two levels (or a combination of the two):

- At the neurohypophysis where the ability to secrete ADH is impaired.
- At the kidney where renal responsiveness to ADH action is impaired.

The decline in renal efficiency with aging is well documented and ascribable to a variety of hormonal and extrahormonal factors.[16] Conversely, the possibility of a decline in ADH synthesis, secretion, or effectiveness has yielded conflicting data, still in need of further clarification. Thus, the redistribution of water from intracellular to extracellular sites, characteristic of old age, has been ascribed to a decline in ADH levels in humans and rats.[17] Perhaps more important than ADH levels in the pituitary and in blood is the ADH response to appropriate stimuli and its effectiveness on target cells in the renal collecting duct.

Aging may alter responses to ADH not only in the kidney but also in the brain. Brain osmoreceptors are specifically stimulated by increased osmolality of extracellular fluid as well as decreased extracellular volume of body fluids and decreased blood pressure. With aging, the sensitivity of this hypothalamic "osmostat" appears to be increased. The osmostat set-point would be the same in old and young people, but more ADH would be secreted in the elderly for a given stimulus.[18-22]

Both stimulation and inhibition of ADH secretion induce altered responses with increasing age.[23] Administration of alcohol (ethanol), known to depress ADH secretion, reduces ADH levels for as long as 120 minutes in young individuals. In old individuals, ADH levels are lowered almost immediately after alcohol ingestion but increase by 120 minutes, perhaps a sign of compensatory hypersecretion. In the young individual, low ADH levels are associated with the expected diuresis (or increased water clearance). In old individuals ADH inhibition occurs early after alcohol administration and then disappears; concomitantly, diuresis does not occur or is only minimal (Figure 3-1).

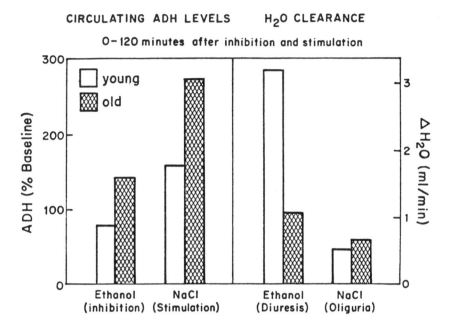

FIGURE 3-1 Age-related changes in ADH (vasopressin) effects on water balance. On the left, ADH responses in young and old individuals to ethanol and NaCl challenges; on the right, H₂O excretion in response to the same challenges.

As for inhibition, stimulation of ADH secretion (by injection of hypertonic sodium chloride) induces different responses in the elderly compared to the young. In response to the same osmotic challenge, ADH levels increase more in old subjects than in young, but in the former, the increased ADH levels are not accompanied by the expected increase in water retention observed in the young. In the elderly such reduction may occur primarily in those individuals with concomitant renal infections or hypertension and would not necessarily be associated with normal aging.[24,25]

In response to a standardized dose of ADH, the ability of the tubules to perform osmotic work and increase water retention and urine concentration is reduced in old rats.[26,27] Aged rats show decreased responsiveness of the collecting duct cells to ADH as the most likely cause for the impairment of urine-concentrating ability. Reduced secretion and levels of ADH may only be minimal and not play an important role in this impairment.

In conclusion, ADH alterations with aging reported to vary from nonexistent to severe appear to include:

- Depletion of pituitary hormone stores and perhaps reduced blood levels of the hormone under specific stimuli;
- Disturbances of axonal transport of the hormones;
- Degeneration of specific neuronal populations with persistance of others;
- Decreased sensitivity of target renal cells to ADH, and
- Defects in processing of precursors (a little-studied but definite possibility).

Other manifestations of possible ADH alterations with aging are represented by changes in the daily timing of urine voiding. In the elderly, "nocturia", that is, waking up at night to void, is a frequent if not universal phenomenon which has been referred to hypothalamic dysfunction.

2. ADH and Memory

There have been claims that this peptide acts on the CNS to facilitate memory consolidation and retrieval processes and to a lesser extent arousal and attention, as well as to modulate rewarded behavior and dependence on drugs of abuse.[28-30] These effects may be mediated by vasopressin actions on turnover of neurotransmitters, primarily monoamines but also acetylcholine.[31] Administration of vasopressin and some of its analogs to old rats, mice, and monkeys significantly improves some tests of behavior and memory performance in some animals, but in no case is the improvement great enough to restore the performance characteristic of young animals.[32] Without vasopressin and related peptides there is still learning and memory, but these are enhanced in the presence of such compounds. In the elderly, vasopressin ameliorates long-term memory and attention between the ages of 50 to 65 but has a less specific effect at later ages. Results from clinical tests of vasopressin therapy for senile dementia have been equivocal and the utility of this therapy remains questionable.

C. Hypophysiotropic Hormones in the Adult

These seven hormones induce release (five hormones) or inhibition of release (two hormones) of the hormones from the anterior pituitary, and derive their names from these activities (Table 3-1). While the two previously discussed hypothalamic hormones, vasopressin and oxytocin, reach the posterior lobe of the pituitary via neuronal axons, the hypophysiotropic hormones are carried directly (before entering the general blood circulation) to the anterior lobe of the pituitary by the specialized portal-hypophysial vessels. Within the hypothalamus are clusters of neurons comprising hypothalamic nuclei which secrete the various hormones. This is the case, described earlier, for the paraventricular and supraoptic nuclei which secrete vasopressin and oxytocin. The localization of the neurons which secrete the hypophysiotropic hormones is less circumscribed and there is considerable overlap in the secretion of the various hormones.

1. Major Actions of Hypophysiotropic Hormones

TRH stimulates the pituitary to secrete not only TSH but also prolactin (the functional significance of the latter secretion is uncertain). TRH widespread distribution within the CNS and its presence in the pancreas and gastrointestinal tract support a great range of actions in addition to release of anterior lobe TSH, including general arousal, activation of brain electrical activity, hypermotility, muscle tremor, and many other actions suggestive of involvement with several neurotransmitter systems.[33]

CRH stimulates the secretion of the adrenocorticotropic hormone, ACTH, as well as beta-lipotropin — both derived from a larger precursor molecule called pro-opiomelanocortin. The location of the secretory neurons in the anterior portion of the paraventricular nuclei may explain the interrelations with vasopressin.[34]

GnRH may stimulate the secretion of both luteinizing hormone, LH, and follicle-stimulating hormone, FSH, for it has not been possible to purify FSHRH from LHRH. Therefore, there is a good probability that only luteinizing hormone-releasing hormone LHRH (or more generically, gonadotropin-releasing hormone GnRH) affects pituitary release of both gonadotropins.[35]

Somatostatin inhibits not only GH but also TSH secretion (the functional significance of the latter is uncertain). Its wide distribution through the brain, pancreas, and intestine is associated with diverse modes of chemical mediation, including neurotransmission and endocrine and paracrine secretions (Chapter 6).

GRH and *PRH* are relatively newly characterized hormones and PRH appears, in fact, to be the neurotransmitter dopamine. With aging, dopaminergic neurons may undergo changes in number and dopamine content or remain unchanged, depending on the species, sex, and stress.[36,37]

Behavioral effects. One of the reasons for the interest in these hormones is their influence on behavior. While the data regarding this influence are still fragmentary, general concepts are being formulated that promise direct applicability to normal and abnormal human behavior.[38,39] The mechanisms and pathways by which these hormones operate have been classified in a number of often overlapping categories. One single peptide may regulate a variety of behaviors, such as TRH inhibition of food intake, lordosis, and sympathetic responses (lordosis is a curvature of the vertebral column which is assumed by female rats when receptive to males). Peptides also act at several CNS locations (e.g., LHRH can facilitate lordosis when infused in a variety of CNS loci) or, in fact, different peptides may act on the same structure to produce the same action (but probably by different mechanisms, e.g., lordosis may be facilitated by LHRH, prolactin, and substance P and inhibited by CRH and beta-endorphin).

Neurotransmitter effects. Brain peptides can interact or have close functional association, or may even coexist with neurotransmitters.[40-42] The peptides, in producing a specific behavior, serve as neurotransmitters at each CNS synapse along the neural pathway that regulates that specific behavior. This is the case in the behavioral examples cited. Neuropeptides can also synergize or antagonize neurotransmitter actions. For example, TRH can modulate serotonin release and/or directly stimulate serotonin receptors.[43]

Interrelation with steroid hormones. Many behaviors, including some indicated above, are regulated jointly by peptide and steroid hormones (e.g., lordosis is modulated by LHRH and estrogens and inhibited by CRH and opioids; LHRH, PRL, and oxytocin exert their respective actions only in the presence of estrogen).[39] The dependence of neuropeptides on this so-called "permissive" action of steroids has been ascribed to the steroid induction of proteins, including receptor proteins and the metabolic substrates necessary to maintain behavior.[39]

D. Changes With Aging in Hypophysiotropic Hormones

The many actions of the hypophysiotropic peptides testify to their wide range of effects. It is perhaps because of this very diversity and complexity that little is known of how they are affected by aging processes and how they can influence these processes. Neither the hypophysiotropic peptides nor the hypophysial hormones can be discussed in isolation, but must be considered as part of a system or axis. Illustrative of this interconnection are the hypothalamo-pituitary-adrenocortical, or hypothalamo-pituitary-thyroid, or hypothalamo-pituitary-gonad systems. Changes with aging usually involve the entire system, even though not all systems are equally affected. Therefore, the aging changes in such systems are more adequately discussed with the peripheral endocrine (adrenal cortex, Chapters 2 and 14; thyroid, Chapter 5; gonads, Chapters 7, 8, and 9).

TRH shows small differences in immunoreactivity between young and old rats.[44] This contrasts with TSH, which demonstrates an altered distribution of immunoreactive forms with aging.[45] In patients with Alzheimer-type dementia (occurring most frequently in elderly individuals), TRH concentration is decreased in the cerebrospinal fluid; in rats, TRH levels are lower in the hypothalamus but not in the cerebral cortex of old compared to young.[44] Whether these relatively minor changes play a role in the regulatory action of the hormone on such functions as thermoregulation, eating and drinking behavior, or pain perception and cognition, all of which are impaired with aging, remains to be investigated.

Somatostatin. In rats, age-related changes in this hormone have been reported in the caudal hypothalamus and median eminence or in the corpus striatum by some, and negated by others.[46] In the elderly, a significant correlation was not found between age and somatostatin in several brain areas. However, in patients with Alzheimer's disease, somatostatin levels were decreased in seven (e.g., hippocampus, parts of the frontal, parietal and occipital cortex) of eight brain regions that also exhibited acetylcholine deficits[47-50] and in the cerebrospinal fluid.[51] Somatostatin levels are also decreased in the cerebrospinal fluid and some cortical areas of patients with Parkinson's disease[52] but increased in basal ganglia in Huntington's disease (although levels are low in the cerebrospinal fluid).[53]

LHRH (GnRH) secretion is decreased in the aged rat[46] as well as is its content in the hypothalamus, its pulsatile release, and the pituitary responsiveness to its action.[54-56] LHRH-containing neurons themselves may not deteriorate with aging but the observed changes in LHRH may rather result from altered function of neurotransmitter (e.g., reduced norepinephrine) or opioid (e.g., higher opiate antagonism) systems important in LHRH regulation.[54]

In the human male direct data are not available, but using a pharmacologic stimulus to LHRH secretion (i.e., the drug clomiphene) no difference was observed between young and old men in the pulsatile LH release.[57] Thus, the rat model may not be appropriate for studying the CNS components of reproductive aging in the human male. Even in the rat, several environmental factors (e.g., housing, nutrition, stress) rather than aging, per se, may be responsible for the observed changes.[46]

E. Pro-Opiomelanocortin, Related Peptides, and Changes With Aging

Pro-opiomelanocortin (POMC) is a large precursor protein found in the anterior and intermediate lobes of the pituitary, in the brain, lungs, gastrointestinal tract, and placenta. It contains beta-endorphin, a 31-amino acid polypeptide, and other shorter endorphins. It also produces beta-lipotropin (BLPH), ACTH, and γ-MSH — the latter hormones are secreted by the pituitary. Despite the frequency of alterations with aging in the regional distribution of POMC-derived peptides, understanding and interpretations of these alterations remain incomplete.

Opioid peptides represent endogenous ligands that bind morphine receptors. They are comprised of closely related penta (five) peptides called enkephalins, endorphins, and dynorphins. They are synthesized from a larger precursor molecule, pro-enkephalin, pro-opiomelanocortin (discussed here), and pro-dynorphin. They all bind to opioid receptors present in brain tissue in different subtypes, but differing in their distribution in the brain and elsewhere (e.g., the gastrointestinal tract). They appear to act as synaptic transmitters, particularly to mediate pain sensations.

Post-translational processing of POMC involves (Figure 3-2):

- Cleavage of the c-terminal β-lipoprotein (beta-LPH) sequence from the parent molecule;
- Cleavage of ACTH from the 16-kDa N-terminal peptide;
- Cleavage of ACTH to form several intermediary products leading to the formation of α-melanocyte-stimulating hormone (α-MSH); and
- Splitting of β-LPH to form the β-endorphin sequence.

Although all of these steps have not been investigated with aging, those which have, show significant changes. α-MSH concentration and content are decreased with aging in the hypothalamus, preoptic area, and thalamus of female rats. Similarly, ACTH content and concentration decrease with aging in both male and female rats.[58] Its immunoreactive profiles and molecular weights likewise change with age and the brain region.[59] Concentration and content of β-LPH follow the same decreasing pattern as those of α-MSH and ACTH. In humans, cerebrospinal fluid β-endorphin decreases with increasing age and with both Huntington's and Alzheimer's disease according to some investigators[59] but not to others.[60]

Experimental protocols most often tend to compare a single age in young animals with a single age in old animals, thereby skipping all intermediate ages and failing to provide a comprehensive profile of developmental and aging changes. Therefore, it remains unclear whether the reported decline in old animals is due to senescence or occurs earlier during

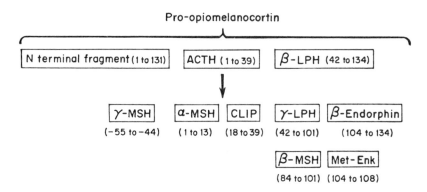

FIGURE 3-2 The biologically active hormones divided from pro-opiomelanocortin. Figures in parentheses represent the amino acid sequence in the respective polypeptide fragments and are numbered from ACTH. To the left they are represented by a minus designation.

maturation. Changes in β-endorphin immunoreactivity in various brain regions of rats occur primarily in early adulthood rather than at advanced age[46] and may be due to a changed cell population, especially to the increased number of astrocytes and to the glial hypertrophy which occurs with brain maturation.

In addition to changes in content and concentration, modification in structure and biological activity of these neural peptides may account for a loss of antigenicity and, thereby, failure of detection. Polypeptide hormones are found in various forms and this polymorphism changes with aging.[45,46] Likewise, enzymatic and receptor changes do occur with aging and involve abnormal processing of the various hormones from the precursor protein[61] or changes in receptor number and affinity.[62]

III. ANTERIOR AND INTERMEDIATE PITUITARY HORMONES

The pituitary gland regulates through tropic protein hormones several peripheral endocrines (adrenal cortex, thyroid, gonads) and, through the secretion of prolactin and growth hormone, other target tissues. The six established hormones secreted by the anterior pituitary are (Figure 3-3).

- Adrenocorticotropic hormone (ACTH),
- Follicle-stimulating hormone (FSH),
- Luteinizing hormone (LH),
- Thyroid-stimulating hormone (TSH, thyrotropin),
- Prolactin (PRL), and
- Growth hormone (GH).

ACTH, PRL, and GH are polypeptides and TSH, LH, and FSH are glycoproteins. PRL acts on the mammary gland; GH acts on soft and bone tissues and on the liver (for the production of local growth factors). The other four hormones stimulate the secretion of other endocrine glands. In addition, the anterior lobe also contains the above-described β-LPH. The regulation of target endocrine secretion depends on positive and negative feedbacks between the peripheral gland and the pituitary/hypothalamus through the circulating hormones. Further adjustments are controlled by the hypophysiotropic hormones through hypothalamo-pituitary feedbacks (Figure 3-3).

The intermediate lobe, partially mixed into and often indistinguishable from anterior lobe tissue in humans, contains the α and β melano-stimulating hormones (α- and β-MSHS, also referred to as melanotropin or intermedin). Both anterior and intermediate lobes contain

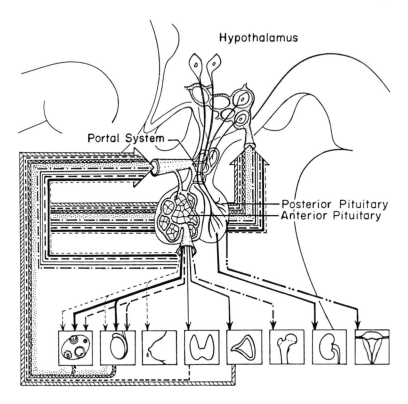

FIGURE 3-3 Diagram of the hypothalamus, pituitary, and peripheral target endocrines showing the complexity of
hormones, targets, and feedbacks. Hypophysioptropic hormones from the hypothalamus reach the
anterior pituitary through the portal vessels and stimulate the synthesis and release of various
hormones that act on target organs. From left to right they are:

    Ovary: prolactin, PL (- - -), luteinizing hormone, LH (█████), follicle-stimulating hormone, FSH (– – –);
    Testes: primarily interstitial-cell-stimulating hormone ISCH (similar to LH and to a lesser extent
    PL and FSH;
    Mammary gland: PL; thyroid gland: thyroid-stimulating hormone, TSH (━━━);
    Adrenal cortex: adrenocorticotropic hormone ACTH (———);
    Long bones: growth hormone GH (-•-•-).
    From the posterior pituitary, continuing from left to right:
    Kidney: antidiuretic hormone or vasopressin, ADH (▬▬)
    Smooth muscle, uterus: oxytocin (—••—••—).
    The hormones secreted by the peripheral endocrines [sex (: : : :) and adrenocortical (\\\\\\) steroids
    and thyroid hormones (- - - -)] feedback to stimulate or inhibit secretion from the anterior pituitary
    or hypothalamus. Likewise, tropic hormones from the pituitary can feedback and regulate hormone
    secretion by the hypothalamus. In this manner, short and long feedback loops are established.

pro-opiomelanocortin and β-endorphin. The posterior lobe stores and secretes the two above-
described peptides, vasopressin or (ADH) and oxytocin.

    ACTH, TSH, LH, and FSH are discussed with the corresponding endocrine which they
regulate (see Chapters 2, 5, and 7 to 9). This section briefly surveys the aging changes in the
anterior pituitary as a whole followed by a discussion of the aging changes involving GH,
PRL, and MSH.

A. Aging Changes in the Anterior Pituitary

The human anterior pituitary is made up of interlacing cell cords and an extensive network of
fenestrated capillaries. The cells contain granules of stored hormone that are extruded by
exocytosis. Cells are classified on the basis of their staining reactions into agranular

chromophobes and granular chromophils (acidophils: secreting GH and PRL; and basophils: secreting TSH, FSH, and LH).

Relatively few studies have explored systematically the changes with aging of the many important functions of the anterior pituitary; major changes include:

- Great individual variability within and among species;
- Differential alterations in secretion from maximal to unaltered; and
- Possible modification of age-related changes and effects on the lifespan produced by hypophysectomy (i.e., surgical ablation of the gland) in rats.

The selective rather than global nature of these changes and their importance for survival has led to the formulation of a number of neuroendocrine theories of aging based on the hypothesis that disorganization or desynchronization of hypothalamo-pituitary signals may cause, or at least be closely involved in, aging processes (Chapter 21).

1. Structural Changes

The anterior pituitary reaches its maximum size in middle age and then gradually becomes atrophic and fibrotic in old age. Histologically, cells undergo characteristic aging changes (e.g., accumulation of lipofuscin, increased connective tissue, vacuolation). However, the number of the specific cells that secrete the different hormones is not markedly altered except for the gonadotropes (secreting LH and FSH). While gonadotropin levels are increased, gonadotropes are lost in postmenopausal women and show changes (e.g., vacuolation) similar to those observed after castration in experimental animals (Chapter 7). In male rats, gonadotropes undergo a reduction in number and size but remain capable of keeping appropriate basal levels of LH and FSH.[63] Hyperplastic areas and, often symptomless, small tumors (adenomas), particularly prolactinomas (i.e., formed of PRL-secreting cells) commonly occur in old individuals.[64] Despite the progressive decrease in pituitary weight with aging (except with the presence of a tumor), tests of endocrine function based on hormone release in response to a specific stimulus or drug do not reveal any significant impairment of pituitary tropic hormone reserve.

The concept that pituitary and adrenocortical hormones may induce or accelerate aging was first suggested by clinical studies showing premature aging in patients with Cushing's syndrome. Studies in rats have reported an anti-aging action of hypophysectomy (surgical removal of the hypophysis) and have likened this action to the life-prolonging effects of undernutrition.[65]

B. Growth Hormone

In humans, GH, although immunologically highly specific, resembles in structure PRL and the placental hormone somatomammotropin (or placental lactogen, PL) and may have derived from the same common single hormone. In the young, GH promotes growth directly by stimulating the development of bone and tissues. It also acts indirectly by stimulating the liver and perhaps other tissues to produce local growth factors such as somatomedins, also called insulin-like growth factors IGFs I and II (Chapter 6). These growth factors are polypeptides responsible (mainly IGF I) for most of the (postnatal) growth effects of GH, especially on the skeleton. While GH is found in higher levels in infants and children than adults, its continuing presence in the pituitary and blood after cessation of whole-body growth maintains muscle mass, cartilage, and bone.

1. GH Promotes Muscle Mass and Function in the Elderly

Aging is associated, in very general terms, with decreased protein synthesis, lean body mass, and bone formation as well as increased adiposity — hence the potential involvement of GH

TABLE 3-4 Selected Factors Affecting GH
and PRL Secretion in the Adult

Factor	GH	PRL
Exercise	↑	↑
Sleep	↑	↑
Stress	↑	↑
Hypoglycemia and starvation	↓	—
Hyperglycemia	↓	—
Elevated FFA+	↓	—
Elevated AA++	↑	—
Obesity	↓	—
Pregnancy and nursing	—	↑
Dopamine		
Agonists	↑	↓
Antagonists	↓	↑

Note: FAA + = free fatty acids; AA ++ = free amino
acids.

because of its anabolic (i.e., promoting protein synthesis) and metabolic actions. Although acidophils (which include GH-secreting cells) may be lost in some elderly individuals, generally, the number of GH cells, the pituitary content of GH, and the basal plasma levels of the hormone and its clearance remain essentially unchanged into old age. Some studies, however, have reported a depressed GH secretory response to stress, surgical trauma, exercise, and arginine treatment — a response that is contrary to that found in the adult (Table 3-4).[66,67] In rats, GH basal levels appear decreased with age. Obesity is known to suppress GH levels in young individuals and the increased obesity often present in the elderly may contribute to the decreased GH levels,[68] although not all reports agree.[69]

GH secretion in humans undergoes a nocturnal peak during the first four hours of sleep, coinciding with stages 3 and 4 of slow-wave sleep; these are the stages most affected in aging.[70] Studies in older humans report a decrease in sleep-related GH secretion although the relation of GH changes with sleep remains as controversial as that with obesity. Whether this decrease is due to a decline in the releasing hormone GRH or to an increase in the inhibiting hormone somatostatin is not known. Other conditions such as metabolic alterations (e.g., hypoglycemia and fasting, increase in the amino acid arginine), increased catecholaminergic stimuli (e.g., administration of dopaminergic agonists or antagonists), and stress may represent factors responsible for GH changes with aging.

The declining release with advancing age of growth hormone (GH) from the pituitary may contribute to the decrease in lean body mass and the increase in mass of adipose tissue that occur in old age. The causes of the aging-related decline in muscle mass and strength are not clear; current data are insufficient to determine whether this decline is due solely to aging or also to other factors such as disuse (i.e., lack of practice of one or several functions), decreased motivation (for muscular activity and mobility), or disease. Irrespective of the causes, impaired physical function due to decline in muscle and bone strength is one of the main risk factors in falls, fractures, and loss of independence in the elderly.

In a study of healthy old men aged 61 to 81 years, some individuals were found to exhibit low IGF-I blood levels; they were injected with biosynthetic human GH for six months. During six months after the treatment, these men showed a 9% increase in lean body mass, a 15% decrease in adipose tissue, and a 2% increase in density of some (but not all) bones.[71]

While encouraging and supportive of the beneficial effects of GH in improving muscle mass and strength in adult and older individuals, these results should be considered as preliminary. GH and growth factors have a variety of actions in addition to those on muscle and adipose tissues. Several of these actions may lead to conditions reminiscent of acromegaly (a clinical condition caused by high GH levels in adults). Complications of GH treatment in the elderly include alterations of carbohydrate metabolism, hyperinsulinemia, glucose intolerance, and diabetes mellitus; in the musculoskeletal system it causes arthritis and athralgia; and in the cardiovascular system hypertension, edema, and congestive heart failure.

Other aspects of this treatment that remain to be elucidated are[72,73] the effects of long-term treatment of GH on muscle function (strength, motility) and quality of life; when (at which age) should the treatment begin; what is the minimal effective dose; and what are the treatment costs?

Further studies should be performed before adopting the use of GH treatment for the elderly. Declines in muscle strength are not inevitable. Elderly persons respond well to increased levels of physical activity (exercise and training) to restore, maintain, and enhance their physical strength and function. A number of hormones — androgens, estrogens, insulin, and thyroid hormones, in addition to GH — may improve muscle mass and strength either directly by their anabolic actions or indirectly by stimulation of IGFs release.[74]

C. Prolactin

The primary known action of prolactin (or lactogen or PRL), a protein synthesized and secreted from the cells (lactotropes) of the anterior pituitary, is to stimulate lactation during the postpartum period (Table 3-4). Milk secretion from the mammary glands involves increased productions of mRNA and of casein and lactalbumin, two major milk components. PRL is high during pregnancy and in the fetus and newborn infant, but its levels are quite low in the pituitary and blood at any other period of life; the possible function (if any) of PRL in males is unknown.

Metabolic actions of PRL may occasionally mimic those of GH, including a diabetogenic one. Administration of (ovine) PRL to GH-deficient patients results in positive nitrogen balance, lipolysis, and limited skeletal growth. In several species, but not in humans, PRL regulates osmolality by influencing salt and water metabolism. The hypothalamic control of PRL release, unlike that of other pituitary hormones, is predominantly inhibitory and is carried through the action of the neurotransmitter dopamine. Stimulatory factors include, in addition to a number of other hormones (e.g., TRH, PRH), metabolic conditions, stress, and drugs, as summarized in Table 3-4.

As with GH, PRL secretion is episodic and peaks in the early morning hours. This sleep-associated augmentation of PRL release is not part of a circadian rhythm but is strictly related to the sleeping period, regardless of when it occurs during the day.

1.   Changes With Aging

PRL pituitary content and circulating blood levels are significantly increased in aged men and women and experimental animals (rodents). This increase has been related to an age-associated reduction of hypothalamic dopamine, the inhibiting regulator. In the absence or low levels of dopamine, the hypothalamus shows a reduced capacity to send inhibitory signals to the anterior pituitary to block PRL synthesis and release. However, other factors (hormones) may also intervene. Immunocytochemical studies in aged subjects (past 80 years of age) reported numerous and well-developed PRL-containing cells in the pituitary in both sexes, but relatively low blood levels in women and high levels in men;[75] the low levels in women have been attributed to the lack of estrogens after menopause as estrogen stimulates PRL release.[76]

Differences in day-night levels associated with sleeping are somewhat dampened with aging. The declining rhythmicity of PRL as well as GH and adrenal and thyroid hormones and the clear-cut cessation of ovarian cyclicity may all underline the progressive failure of chronobiologic regulations with aging.

The high PRL levels in the elderly may, in some instances, be related to the high incidence of PRL-secreting pituitary tumors (e.g., chromophobe adenomas, prolactinomas).[77] Early manifestations of the tumors are gonadal dysfunction and impotence which are often over-looked because of the age of the patient and will not be diagnosed until later with the appearance of headache, visual impairment, and hypothyroidism.

D. Melanocyte-Stimulating Hormones (MSH)

While these hormones control skin coloration (through the pigment melanin) in fish, reptiles, and amphibians, their action in mammals is still unkown. Melanocytes synthesize melanin which is then transferred to skin cells and hair follicles and accounts for the pigmentation of hair and skin. Treatment with MSHs accelerates melanin synthesis and causes readily detect-able darkening of the skin in humans in 24 hours.

The number of melanocytes decreases with aging by approximately 8 to 20% per decade after the age of 30 in areas of the skin both exposed and unexposed to the sun. This reduction leads to irregular pigmentation, especially in sun-exposed areas (hence the "age spots" frequently seen on the back of the hands), and to the inability to tan as deeply as when younger. Other studies negate or at least minimize this reduction in melanocytes with aging.[78] Whether the reduction in melanocyte number is associated with a progressive decrease in MSH brain levels remains to be investigated.

In addition to their role in mediating pigmentation, MSHs share important functions with the other peptides of the POMC family: they may affect instinctive behavior, brain electrical activity, learning, memory, and attention.[79] As these functions are markedly impaired in old individuals, it appeared logical to implicate MSH decrements in these functional losses and suggest administration of the hormone for rehabilitation. So far, the promise for rehabilitation has not been fulfilled and even the implication of the hormone in the cognitive deficits of the elderly remains uncertain.

IV. PANCREAS

In a relatively high percentage of the elderly, 65 years of age and older, the ability to maintain glucose homeostasis, particularly after a glucose challenge, is impaired (lowered "glucose tolerence") (Chapters 10 and 11). Several factors may combine to alter glucose metabolism in the elderly. These include:

- Genetic predisposition,
- Diet,
- Exercise,
- Body composition (particularly fat content),
- Hormone levels,
- Medications and drugs, and
- Presence of disease.

The pancreas is formed of two functionally different parts:

- The exocrine pancreas, which is part of the gastrointestinal tract and, through the secretion of digestive enzymes, contributes to the processing of foods; and
- The endocrine pancreas, which is the source of the four hormones which directly (insulin and glucagon) and indirectly (somatostatin and possibly pancreatic polypeptide) modulate ab-sorption and storage of glucose.

A. Structure and Endocrine Function

The pancreas lies inferior to the stomach, in a bend of the duodenum. The hundreds of thousands of small endocrine cell clusters, the islets of Langerhans (with at least four cell

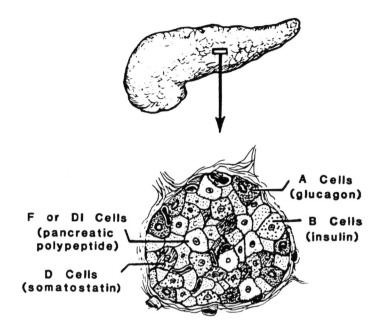

FIGURE 3-4 Diagram indicating the various cells and secretory products contained in a pancreatic islet.

types), are scattered within the glandular tissue of the exocrine portion and comprise approximately only 1% of the pancreatic mass (Figure 3-4). While insulin is secreted only by the islet cells, the other hormones are also secreted by the mucosa of the gastrointestinal tract (Chapter 6 and 10) and somatostatin is also found in the brain (see above).

B. Biochemistry of Insulin

Insulin is synthesized in the cells as part of a larger precursor, pre-pro-insulin, which includes a 23-amino-acid signal sequence attached to pro-insulin; this signal sequence is cleaved from the pro-insulin as the nascent protein enters the cysternae of the endoplasmic reticulum. Kallikrein, an enzyme present in the islets, then aids in the conversion of pro-insulin to insulin. In this conversion, a so-called C-peptide chain is removed from the pro-insulin molecule, producing the disulfide-connected A and B chains of insulin. In the circulation, insulin is degraded within 5 minutes in the liver and kidneys. C-peptide and kallikrein are also present in the circulation, having been secreted with the insulin.

C. Major Actions of Insulin

At the target cells, insulin binds with specific membrane receptors forming an insulin-receptor complex, which triggers several simultaneous actions that, most importantly, promote the entrance of glucose into the cell (by facilitated transport) in muscle, adipose tissue, and connective tissue (Table 3-5).

   In the liver, insulin facilitates glycogen deposition and decreases glucose output, with a net increase in glucose uptake; it induces (through key glycolytic enzymes) or represses (through gluconeogenic enzymes) the synthesis of many enzymes, but whether this is a direct or indirect action is not known. Other noninsulin-dependent cells for glucose transport include red blood cells, B-cells of the pancreas, and mucosal cells of the gastrointestinal tract.

   The receptor complex enters the target cell by endocytosis, where it is cleaved in the lysosomes and the receptor is recycled. High circulating levels of insulin reduce the number of receptors (down-regulation), and low levels of insulin increase the number and/or affinity

TABLE 3-5 Major Actions of Insulin and Glucagon

Insulin	Glucagon
Reduces blood glucose by facilitating glucose transport through certain cell membranes	Raises blood sugar
Promotes glycogen formation and storage	Stimulates glycogen release from stores and metabolism
Slows gluconeogenesis	Promotes gluconeogenesis
Regulates lipogenesis	Stimulates fat metabolism
Promotes protein synthesis and growth	Promotes injury repair

of receptors (up-regulation). The number of receptors per cell is decreased in obesity and acromegaly, and receptor affinity is reduced by excess glucocorticoids. The insulin internalized with the receptor is either destroyed or, perhaps, directly mediates some cellular actions.

Paracrine (local) functions of insulin include inhibition of glucagon secretion by neighboring A-cells. Somatostatin, released from the D-cells in response to most of the same stimuli that induce insulin release, also acts to reduce glucagon secretion. Pancreatic polypeptide, secreted by F-cells and, possibly, intestinal cells, may affect gastrointestinal secretion, also by a paracrine effect.

D. Function and Biochemistry of Glucagon

Glucagon, from the pancreatic A-cells as well as intestinal cells, derives, like insulin, from a larger polypeptide precursor (pro-glucagon) and is degraded in the liver. The A-cells also produce a peptide with some glucagon activity called glicentin. Major actions of glucagon are listed in Table 3-5.

Changes with aging in the endocrine pancreas and its hormones are discussed in Chapters 6, 10, and 11.

REFERENCES

1. Pelletier, G., Anatomy of the hypothalamic-pituitary axis, *Methods Achiev. Exp. Pathol.*, 14, 1, 1991.
2. Swaab, D. F., Hofman, M. A., Lucassen, P. J., Purba, J. S., Raadsheer, F. C., and Van de Nes, J. A., Functional neuroanatomy and neuropathology of the human hypothalamus, *Anat. Embryol.*, 187, 317, 1993.
3. Palkovits, M., Distribution of neuropeptides in brain. A review of biochemical and immunohistochemical studies, in *Peptide Hormones: Effects and Mechanisms of Actions*, Vol. 1, Negro-Vilar, A. and Conn, P. M., Eds., CRC Press, Boca Raton, FL, 1988, 3.
4. Meister, B., Gene expression and chemical diversity in hypothalamic neurosecretory neurons, *Mol. Neurobiol.*, 7, 87, 1993.
5. Rivier, C. and Vale, W., Modulation of stress-induced ACTH release by corticotropin-releasing factor, catecholamines and vasopressin, *Nature (London)*, 305, 325, 1983.
6. Raff, H., Interactions between neurohypophysial hormones and the ACTH-adrenocortical axis, *Ann. N.Y. Acad. Sci.*, 689, 411, 1993.
7. Mollard, P., Vacher, P., Rogawski, M. A., and Dufy, B., Vasopressin enhances a calcium current in human ACTH-secreting pituitary adenoma cells, *FASEB J.*, 2, 2907, 1988.
8. Baldino, F., Jr., O'Kane, T. M., Fitzpatrick-McElligott, S., and Wolfson, B., Coordinate hormonal and synaptic regulation of vasopressin messenger RNA, *Science,* 241, 978, 1988.
9. Choy, V. J., Altered polypeptide hormones and aging, in *Altered Proteins and Aging*, Adelman, R. C. and Roth, G. S., Eds., CRC Press, Boca Raton, FL, 1983, 135.
10. Fliers, E., Swaab, D. F., Pool, C. W., and Verwer, R. W. H., The vasopressin and oxytocin neurons in the human supraoptic and paraventricular nucleus; changes with aging and in senile dementia, *Brain Res.*, 342, 45, 1985.
11. Zbuzek, V. and Zbuzek, V. K., Vasopressin and aging, in *Regulation of Neuroendocrine Aging,* Everitt, A. V. and Walton, J. R., Eds., Karger, Basel, 1988, 125.

12. Rossor, M. N., Iversen, L. L., Mountjoy, C. Q., Roth, M., Hawthorn, J., Ang, V. Y., and Jenkins, J. S., Arginine vasopressin and choline acetyltransferase in brains of patients with Alzheimer type senile dementia, *Lancet*, 2, 1367, 1980.

13. Goudsmit, E., Neijmeijer-Leloux, A., and Swaab, D. F., The human hypothalamo-neurohypophyseal system in relation to development, aging and Alzheimer's disease, *Prog. Brain Res.*, 93, 237, 1992.

14. Melis, M. R., Stancampiano, R., Fratta, W., and Argiolas, A., Oxytocin concentration changes in different rat brain areas but not in plasma during aging, *Neurobiol. Aging*, 13, 783, 1992.

15. Wierda, M., Goudsmit, E., Van der Woude, P. F., Purba, J. S., Hofman, M. A., Bogte, H., and Swaab, D. F., Oxytocin cell number in the human paraventricular nucleus remains constant with aging and in Alzheimer's disease, *Neurobiol. Aging*, 12, 511, 1991.

16. Timiras, M. L., The kidney, the lower urinary tract, the prostate and body fluids, in *Physiological Basis of Aging and Geriatrics*, CRC Press, Boca Raton, FL, 1994.

17. Miller, M., Influence of aging on vasopressin secretion and water regulation, in *Vasopressin,* Schrier, R., Ed., Raven Press, New York, 1985, 249.

18. Reppert, S. M., Circadian rhythm of cerebrospinal fluid vasopressin. Characterization and physiology, in *Vasopressin,* Schrier, R., Ed., Raven Press, New York, 1985, 455.

19. Silverman, W. F., Aravich, P. A., Sladek, J. R., Jr., and Sladek, C. D., Physiological and biochemical indices of neurohypophyseal function in the aging Fisher rat, *Neuroendocrinology*, 52, 181, 1990.

20. Davies, I., Davidson, Y. S., Goddard, C., Moser, B., Faragher, E. B., Morris, J., and Wilkinson, A., The ageing hypothalamo-neurohypophysial system. An analysis of the neurohypophysis in normal hydration, osmotic loading and rehydration, *Mech. Ageing Dev.*, 51, 157, 1990.

21. Terwel, D., ten Haaf, J. A., Markerink, M., and Jolles, J., Changes in plasma vasopressin concentration and plasma osmolality in relation to age and time of day in the male Wistar rat, *Acta Edocrinol.*, 126, 357, 1992.

22. Duggan, J., Kilfeather, S., Lightman, S. L., and O'Malley, K., The association of age with plasma arginine vasopressin and plasma osmolality, *Age Ageing*, 22, 332, 1993.

23. Helderman, J. H., Vestal, R. E., Rowe, J. W., Tobin, J. D., Andres, R., and Robertson, G. L., The response of arginine vasopressin to intravenous ethanol and hypertonic saline in man: the impact of aging, *J. Gerontol.*, 33, 39, 1978.

24. Phillips, P. A., Rolls, B. J., Ledingham, J. G., Forsling, M. L., Morton, J. J., Crowe, M. J., and Wollner, L., Reduced thirst after water deprivation in healthy elderly men, *N. Engl. J. Med.*, 311, 753, 1984.

25. Phillips, P. A., Bretherton, M., Risvanis, J., Casley, D., Johnston, C., and Gray, L., Effects of drinking on thirst and vasopressin in dehydrated elderly men, *Am. J. Physiol.*, 264, R877, 1993.

26. Bengele, H. H., Mathias, R .S., Perkins, J. H., and Alexander, E. A., Urinary concentrating defect in the aged rat, *Am. J. Physiol.*, 240, F147, 1981.

27. Geelen, G. and Corman, B., Relationship between vasopressin and renal concentrating ability in aging rats, *Am. J. Physiol.*, 262, R826, 1992.

28. De Wied, D., Joels, M., Burbach, J. P. H., De Jong, W., De Kloet, E. R., Gaffori, O. W. J., Urban, I. J. A., Van Ree, J. M., Van Wimersma, Greidanus, T. B., Veldhuis, H. D., Versteeg, D. H. G., and Wiegant, V. M., Vasopressin effects on the central nervous sytem, in *Peptide Hormones: Effects and Mechanisms of Action*, Vol. 1, Negro-Vilar, A. and Conn, P. M., Eds., CRC Press, Boca Raton, FL, 1988, 97.

29. Thompson, G., Rodent models of learning and memory in aging research, in *Experimental and Clinical Interventions in Aging*, Walker, R. F. and Cooper, R. L., Eds., Marcel Dekker, New York, 1983, 261.

30. Bartus, R.T., Dean, R. L., and Beer, B., Neuropeptide effects on memory in aged monkeys, *Neurobiol. Aging*, 3, 61, 1982.

31. Dean, R. L., III, Loullis, C. C., and Bartus, R. T., Drug effects in an animal model of memory deficits in the aged. Implications for future clinical trials, in *Experimental and Clinical Interventions in Aging*, Walker, R. F. and Cooper, R. L., Eds., Marcel Dekker, New York, 1983, 279.

32. Legros, J. J., Gilot, P., Timsit-Berthier, M., and Bruwier, M. W. M., Vasopressin and memory during aging in the human, in *Experimental and Clinical Interventions in Aging*, Walker, R. F. and Cooper, R. L., Eds., Marcel Dekker, New York, 1983, 317.

33. Kalivas, P. W. and Prange, A. J., Central and peripheral actions of thyrotropin-releasing hormone, in *Peptide Hormones: Effects and Mechanisms of Action*, Vol. I, Negro-Vilar, A. and Conn, P. M., CRC Press, Boca Raton, FL, 1988, 165.

34. Taylor, A. L. and Fishman, L. M., Corticotropin-releasing hormone, in *Peptide Hormones: Effects and Mechanisms of Action*, Vol. I, Negro-Vilar, A. and Conn, P. M., Eds., CRC Press, Boca Raton, FL, 1988, 35.

35. Jinnah, H. A. and Conn, P. M., GnRH action at the pituitary. Basic research and clinical applications, in *Peptide Hormones: Effects and Mechanisms of Action*, Vol. I, Negro-Vilar, A. and Conn, P. M., CRC Press, Boca Raton, FL, 1988, 119.

36. Moore, K. E. , Demarest, K. T., and Lookingland, K. J., Stress, prolactin and hypothalamic dopaminergic neurons, *Neuropharmacology*, 26, 801, 1987.

37. Amoroso S., Di Renzo, G. F., Maurano, F., Maida, P., Taglialatela, M., and Annunziato, L., Lack of evidence for an impairment of tuberoinfundibolar dopaminergic neurons in aged male rats of the Sprague-Dawley strain, *Exp. Aging Res.*, 13, 85, 1987.

38. Swaab, D. F., Neuropeptides. Their distribution and function in the brain, *Prog. Brain Res.*, 55, 97, 1982.

39. Kow, L. M. and Pfaff, D. W., Behavioral effects of neuropeptides. Some conceptual considerations, in *Peptide Hormones: Effects and Mechanisms of Action*, Vol. I, Negro-Vilar, A. and Conn, P. M., Eds., CRC Press, Boca Raton, FL, 1988, 141.

40. Chan-Palay, V. and Palay, S. L., *Coexistence of Neuroactive Substances in Neurons,* John Wiley & Sons, New York, 1984

41. Wang, R.Y., White, F. J., and Voigt, M. M., Cholecystokinin, dopamine and schizophrenia, *Trends Pharmacol. Sci.*, 5, 436, 1984.

42. Anthony, E. L. and Bruhn, T. O., Do some traditional hypophysiotropic hormones play nontraditional roles in the neurohypophysis? Implications of immunocytochemical studies, *Ann. N.Y. Acad. Sci.*, 689, 469, 1993.

43. Barbeau, H. and Bedard, P., Similar motor effects of 5-HT and TRH in rats following chronic spinal transection and 5,7-dihydroxytryptamine injection, *Neuropharmacology,* 20, 477, 1981.

44. Pekary, A. E., Carlson, H. E., Yamada, T., Sharp, B., Walfish, P. G., and Hershman, J. M., Thyrotropin-releasing hormone levels decrease in hypothalamus of aging rats, *Neurobiol. Aging*, 5, 221, 1984.

45. Choy, V. J., Klemme, W. R., and Timiras, P. S., Variant forms of immunoreactive thyrotropin in aged rats, *Mech. Ageing Dev.*, 19, 273, 1982.

46. Dorsa, D. M. and Wilkinson, C. W., Regulation of neuropeptides in aging, in *Peptide Hormones: Effects and Mechanisms of Action*, Vol. I, Negro-Vilar, A. and Conn, P. M., Eds., CRC Press, Boca Raton, FL, 1988, 69.

47. Davies, P., Katzman, R., and Terry, R. D., Reduced somatostatin-like immunoreactivity in cerebral cortex from cases of Alzheimer's disease and Alzheimer senile dementia, *Nature* (London), 288, 279, 1980.

48. Davies, P. and Terry, R. D., Cortical somatostatin-like immunoreactivity in cases of Alzheimer's disease and senile dementia of the Alzheimer type, *Neurobiol. Aging*, 2, 9, 1981.

49. Ferrier, I. N., Cross, A. J., Johnson, J. A., Roberts, G. W., Crow, T. J., Corsellis, J. A., Lee, Y. C., O'Shaughnessy, D., Adrian, T. E., McGregor, G. P., Baracese-Hamilton, A. J., and Bloom, S. R., Neuropeptides in Alzheimer type dementia, *J. Neurol. Sci.*, 62, 159, 1983.

50. Serby, M., Richardson, S. B., Twente, S., Siekierski, J., Corwin, J., and Rotrosen, J., CSF somatostatin in Alzheimer's disease, *Neurobiol. Aging*, 5, 187, 1984.

51. Raskind, M. A., Peskind, E. R., Lampe, T. H., Risse, S. C., Taborsky, G. J., Jr., and Dorsa, D., Cerebrospinal fluid vasopressin, oxytocin, somatostatin, and β-endorphin in Alzheimer's disease, *Arch. Gen. Psychiatry*, 43, 382, 1986.

52. Dupont, E., Christensen, S. E., Hansen, A. P., de Fine Olivarius, B., and Orskov, H., Low cerebrospinal fluid somatostatin in Parkinson disease: an irreversible abnormality, *Neurology,* 32, 312, 1982.

53. Manberg, P. J., Nemeroff, C. B., Bissette, G., Widerlov, E., Youngblood, W. W., Kizer, J. S., and Prange, A. J., Jr., Neuropeptides in CSF and post-mortem brain tissue of normal controls, schizophrenics and Huntington's choreics, *Prog. Neuro-Psychopharmacol. Biol. Psychiatry*, 9, 97, 1985.

54. Steger, R. W., DePaolo, L. V., and Shepherd A. M., Effects of advancing age on hypothalamic neurotransmitter content and on basal and norepinephrine-stimulated LHRH release, *Neurobiol. Aging*, 6, 113, 1985.

55. Cocchi, D., Age-related alterations in gonadotropin, adrenocorticotropin and growth hormone secretion, *Aging*, 4, 103, 1992.

56. Sadow, T. F. and Rubin, R.T., Effects of hypothalamic peptides on the aging brain, *Psychoneuroendocrinology,* 17, 293, 1992.

57. Bremner, W. J., Tenover, J. S., and Matsumoto, A. M., Episodic luteinizing hormone secretion in normal men, in *The Episodic Secretion of Hormones,* Crowley, W. F., Jr. and Hofler, J. G., Eds., John Wiley & Sons, New York, 1987, 235.

58. Gambert, S. R., Garthwaite, T. L., Pontzer, C. H., and Hagen,T. C., Age-related changes in central nervous system β-endorphin and ACTH, *Neuroendocrinology*, 31, 252, 1980.

59. Facchinetti, F., Petraglia, F., Nappi, G., Martignoni, E., Antoni, G., Parrini, D., and Genazzani A. R., Different patterns of central and peripheral β-EP, β-LP and ACTH throughout life, *Peptides*, 4, 469, 1983.

60. Kaiya, H., Tanaka, T., Takeuchi, K., Morita, K., Adachi, S., Shirakawa, H., Ueki, H., and Namba, M., Decreased level of β-endorphin-like immunoreactivity in cerebrospinal fluid of patients with senile dementia of Alzheimer type, *Life Sci.*, 33, 1039, 1983.

61. O'Donohue, T. L., Handelmann, G. E., Miller, R. L., and Jacobowitz, D. M., N-acetylation regulates the behavioral activity of α-melanotropin in a multineurotransmitter neuron, *Science,* 215, 1125, 1982.

62. Gruenewald, D. A. and Matsumoto, A. M., Age-related decrease in pro opiomelanocortin gene expression in the arcuate nucleus of the male rat brain, *Neurobiol. Aging,* 12, 113, 1991.

63. Console, G. M., Gomez Dumm, C. L. A., and Goya, R. G., Immunohistochemical and radioimmunological study of pituitary gonadotrophs during aging in male rats, *Mech. Ageing Dev.*, 73, 87, 1994.

64. Walton, J. R. and Everitt, A. V., Hypothalamic-pituitary function in aging men, in *Regulation of Neuroendocrine Aging,* Everitt, A. V. and Walton, J. R., Eds., Karger, Basel, 1988, 21.

65. Everitt, A.V., Seedsman, N. J., and Jones, F., The effects of hypophysectomy and continuous food restriction begun at ages 70 and 400 days, on collagen aging, proteinuria, incidence of pathology and longevity in the male rat, *Mech. Ageing Dev.,* 12, 161, 1980.

66. Sonntag, W. E., Steger, R. W., Forman, L. J., and Meites J., Decreased pulsatile release of growth hormone in old male rats, *Endocrinology,* 107, 1875, 1980.

67. Rudman, D., Growth hormone, body composition, and aging, *J. Am. Geriatr. Soc.,* 33, 800, 1985.

68. Rudman, D., Kutner, M. H., Rogers, C. M., Lubin, M. F., Fleming, G. A., and Bain, R. P., Impaired growth hormone secretion in the adult population: relation to age and adiposity, *J. Clin. Invest.,* 67, 1361, 1981.

69. Elahi, D., Muller, D. C., Tzankoff, S. P., Andres, R., and Tobin, J. D., Effect of age and obesity on fasting levels of glucose, insulin, glucagon, and growth hormone in man, *J. Gerontol.,* 37, 385, 1982.

70. Prinz, P. N., Weitzman, E. D., Cunningham, G. R., and Karacan, I., Plasma growth hormone during sleep in young and aged men, *J. Gerontol.,* 38, 519, 1983.

71. Rudman, D., Feller, A. G., Nagraj, H. S., Gergans, G, A., Lalitha, P. Y., Goldberg, A. F., Schlenker, R. A., Cohn, L., Rudman, I. W., and Mattson, D. E., Effects of human growth hormone in men over 60 years old, *N. Engl. J. Med.,* 323, 1, 1990.

72. Vance, M.L., Growth hormone for the elderly?, *N. Engl. J. Med.,* 323, 52, 1990.

73. Kaplan, S. L., The newer uses of growth hormone in adults, *Adv. Intern. Med.,* 38, 287, 1993.

74. Joseph, J. A. and Roth, G. S., Hormonal regulation of motor behavior in senescence, *J. Gerontol.,* 48, 51, 1993.

75. Everitt, A.V., The hypothalamic-pituitary control of ageing and age-related pathology, *Exp. Gerontol.,* 8, 265, 1973.

76. Rossmanith, W. G., Szilagyi, A., and Scherbaum, W. A., Episodic thyrotropin (TSH) and prolactin (PRL) secretion during aging in postmenopausal women, *Horm. Metab. Res.,* 24, 185, 1992.

77. Kovacs, K., Ryan, N., Horvath, E., Singer, W., and Ezrin, C., Pituitary adenomas in old age, *J. Gerontol.,* 35, 16, 1980.

78. Marks, R., Skin disorders, in *Principles and Practice of Geriatric Medicine,* 2nd ed., Pathy, M. S. J., Ed., John Wiley & Sons, New York, 1991, 1011.

79. Beckwith, B. E. and Kastin, A. J., Central action of melanocyte-stimulating hormone (MSH), in *Peptide Hormones: Effects and Mechanisms of Actions,* Vol. I, Negro-Vilar, A. and Conn, P. M., Eds., CRC Press, Boca Raton, FL, 1988, 195.

4

Amine-Secreting Endocrines

Wilbur B. Quay and Takashi Kachi

CONTENTS

I. INTRODUCTION

Biogenic amines — small molecules made in the body from single amino acids — are the subject of this chapter. Biosynthesis endows the resulting compound with special and increased biological activities as compared to the amino acid precursor. These activities depend upon the existence of specific receptor molecules such as those in the plasma membrane of target or effector cells. Union of biogenic amine molecules with their receptors initiates a chain of chemical events within the target cells. The overall result is a series of changes in rates of some cellular activities. Biogenic amines serve a number of roles as hormones, neurotransmitters, neuromodulators, tissue humors, and others.

Two chemical classes of biogenic amine act as hormones, the catecholamines and indolamines. The catecholamines, primarily epinephrine (adrenalin, E) and to a lesser extent, norepinephrine (noradrenalin, NE) play multiple roles in humans and other animals, depending on the species and circumstances (Figures 4-1 and 4-2). They are secreted into the bloodstream by the chromaffin cells of the adrenal medulla, and have diverse actions as hormones on effector cells throughout the body. NE actions as a chemical mediator occur primarily within the nervous system, and here as a neurotransmitter rather than as a hormone, although some neurally released NE does find its way into the bloodstream.

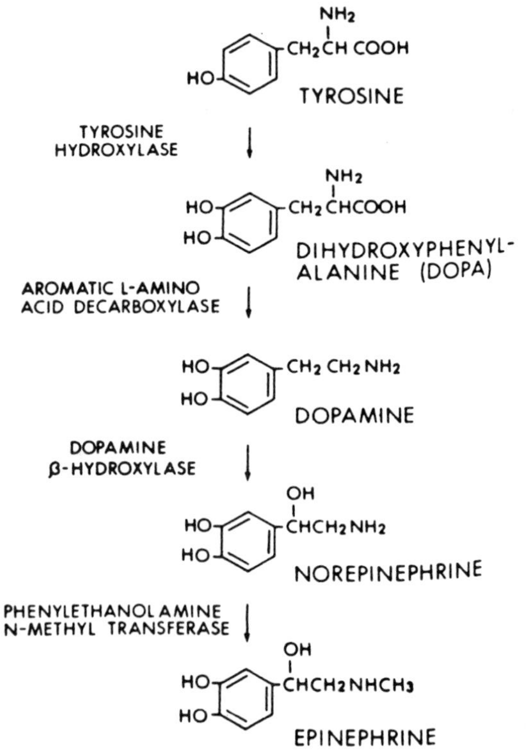

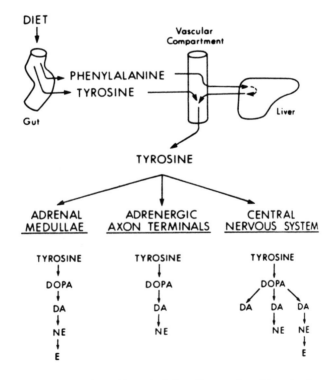

FIGURE 4-1 Major catecholamines and their biosynthesis. (From Cryer, P., *Endocrinology and Metabolism, 2nd ed.,* McGraw-Hill, New York, 1987, 651, with permission.)

FIGURE 4-2 Primary sites of catecholamine biosynthesis from dietary amino acids, and major end products in those sites. (From Cryer, P., *Endocrinology and Metabolism, 2nd ed.,* McGraw-Hill, New York, 1987, 651, with permission.)

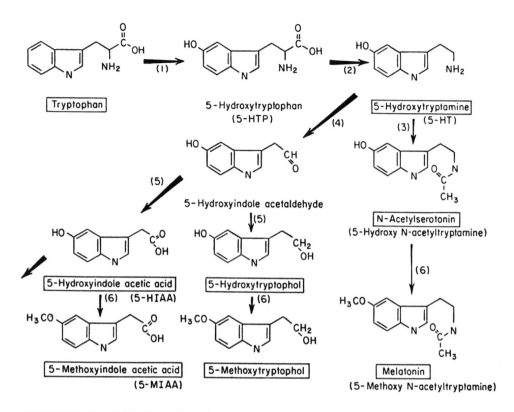

FIGURE 4-3 Pineal indolamines and their biosynthetic pathways. Heavier arrows signify major pathways; compounds within rectangles are measurable within pineal tissue. Enzymic steps: (1) tryptophan hydroxylase, (2) aromatic L-amino acid decarboxylase, (3) *N*-acetyltransferase, (4) monoamine oxidase, (5) aldehyde dehydrogenase, and (6) hydroxyindole-*O*-methyltransferase. (From Quay, W. B., *Pineal Chemistry in Cellular and Physiological Mechanisms,* Charles C Thomas, Springfield, IL, 1974, with permission.)

Indolamines, compared with catecholamines show a parallel range of biosynthetic steps, metabolic actions, specificity of anatomical and subcellular localization, modes of activity, and functional relationships (Figure 4-3). Melatonin (5-methoxy-*N*-acetyl-tryptamine, M) is synthesized in the pineal gland, secreted directly into the blood, and has widespread hormonal actions, primarily based upon its transport via the bloodstream.

A. Relationship Between Adrenal Medulla and Pineal Gland

The adrenal medulla and pineal gland share similar characteristics. Endocrine cells of both, embryologically, have a neuroectodermal origin — the adrenomedullary ones from neural crest cells, and the endocrine pinealocytes from neuron-like precursors in the roof of the diencephalon of the brain. Adrenomedullary endocrine cells are also called chromaffin cells due to the distinctive reaction of their catecholamines with chromates or chromic acid.[1] Chromaffin cells can be considered as postganglionic sympathetic neurons that have lost their axons and, instead of releasing catecholamines as neurotransmitters, secrete them directly to the blood where these catecholamines circulate and have hormonal function (Figure 4-2). Pinealocytes, the specialized endocrine cells of the pineal gland, have evolutionary precursors some of which in lower vertebrates are photosensory as well as endocrine in function, and have neuronal characteristics as well.[2-4]

Major control of the activities of both glands is imposed by sympathetic innervations — the pineal by postganglionic neurons of the paired superior cervical sympathetic ganglia, and the adrenal medulla by sympathetic preganglionic fibers in the greater splanchnic nerves. Both adrenomedullary and pineal cells are also affected by steroid and peptide hormones, and interact with these and other chemical mediators.

Although the endocrine cells of both gland, normally have relatively little ability to divide or regenerate in adult humans or other mammals, they remain present and active in appreciable numbers throughout life. Age changes in both systems show great individual variation and, when detectable, are largely related to subtle decrements in rates and magnitudes of responses, and in sharpness of timing of phase relationships.

II. ADRENAL MEDULLA AND CATECHOLAMINES

A. Catecholamines

Epinephrine (E), although not as widespread as norepinephrine (NE), is found in many different cells of the body in addition to the adrenal medulla.[5] Although nonadrenal occurrence of E is due mostly to uptake from the blood of E secreted from the adrenal medulla, a small amount is synthesized within the brain for an intrinsic, presumably neurotransmitter, role there.[6,7] Adrenalectomy does not lead to complete loss of E from the urine.[8] A very small amount of regulated E secretion occurs from scattered clusters of extra-adrenal chromaffin cells. However, physiologically effective blood levels of E depend primarily upon the adrenomedullary source, especially in adults.[9]

Human adrenal medullae can release NE into the circulation, along with large amounts of E.[10,11] This occurs for example in normal humans during heavy exercise.[9] NE plasma levels reflect release by the sympathochromaffin system as a whole, whereas E plasma levels mirror the anatomically more restricted releases by the adrenal medulla. Major physiologic and pathophysiologic correlates of plasma levels of these two hormonal amines in humans are compared in Figures 4-4 and 4-5. The greater involvement of E as compared to NE in metabolic functions is exemplified here by its greater responsiveness to hypoglycemia, ketoacidosis, and cardiac infarction.

E increases heart rate and cardiac output, but blood pressure may not be increased significantly. Blood flow in some organs is increased as much as 100%. The cardiovascular system is sensitive to very low concentrations of E; even 1 part in 1.4 billion parts of fluid medium is sufficient to accelerate a denervated mammalian heart. The marked effects of E on metabolism include:

- Increased O_2 consumption, and
- Increased basal metabolic rate.

Its hyperglycemic action is mediated by:

- Mobilization of hepatic carbohydrate stores (through activation of phosphorylase, and thereby, acceleration of the first step in the breakdown of glycogen to glucose);
- Promotion of conversion of muscle glycogen to lactic acid, from which in turn the liver can make new carbohydrate; and
- Stimulation of hypophyseal release of ACTH, which stimulates adrenocortical secretion of glucocorticoids which, in turn, stimulate gluconeogenesis.

These E actions while true on the main, represent an oversimplification of many indirect, direct, and counterbalancing effects of E on metabolism and plasma glucose level and the multiple interactions with the endocrine pancreas. These complex and multifactor neuroendocrine and target interactions make it difficult and deceptive to attribute particular changes during aging to single isolated factors (Chapter 10).

Biologic actions of catecholamines depend on their interactions with cellular receptors. Whereas steroid and thyroid hormones bind with intracellular receptors, catecholamines (also acetylcholine and the peptide hormones) react initially with plasma membrane receptors at the external surface of the target cell. Catecholamine (adrenergic) receptors are of two major

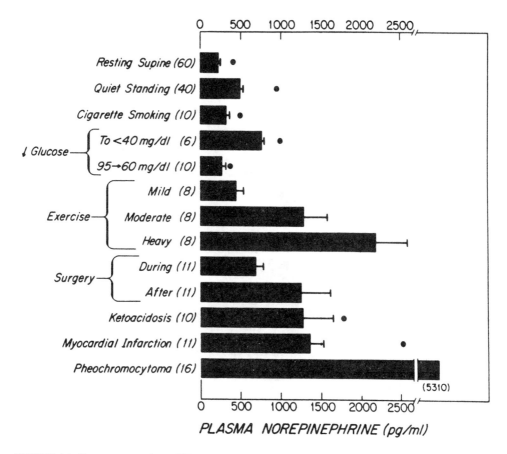

FIGURE 4-4 Human venous plasma NE concentrations in various physiologic and pathophysiologic states. Horizontal bars and lines represent means and standard errors, respectively, the dots are the highest observed values. Numbers of subjects studied are noted within parentheses. (From Cryer, P., *Endocrinology and Metabolism, 2nd ed.,* McGraw-Hill, New York, 1987, 651, with permission.)

types, α- and β-adrenergic receptors (adrenoceptors) with several subtypes, among which α1 and α2, and correspondingly, β1 and β2 adrenergic receptors are the best known.

Recognition and classification of adrenergic receptors was based initially on the differential biologic potency of the members of an array of agonist amines (e.g., methoxamine and clonidine for α1 and α2 receptors, and prenalterol and terbutaline for β1 and β2 receptors, respectively). Currently, the use of antagonists facilitates appropriate classification of the receptors (e.g., phentolamine and yohimbine for α1 and α2 receptors, and propanolol and butoxamine for β1 and β2 receptors, respectively). It should be realized that adrenergic receptor type and subtype activity, or specificity, is not absolute. NE and E are mixed agonists. They can interact with either α- or β-receptors. Other compounds, chiefly some drugs, generally have greater but not absolute receptor specificity. The response(s) of a target cell or tissue depend(s) upon the types and subtypes of adrenergic receptors that are present and the relative number of each.

Adrenergic receptors are in a dynamic state with respect to sensitivity to their agonists and their number per cell. Desensitization of β-receptors can occur after their phosphorylation, catalyzed by a receptor kinase which leads to uncoupling of the receptor from its postreceptor apparatus. This probably constitutes the basis of tolerance to amine-type drugs and to tachyphylaxis (i.e., decreasing responses that follow consecutive injections made at short intervals). Internalization of the receptors by their cells, perhaps, after phosphorylation, can decrease the number of plasma membrane receptors and the rates of receptor protein synthesis;

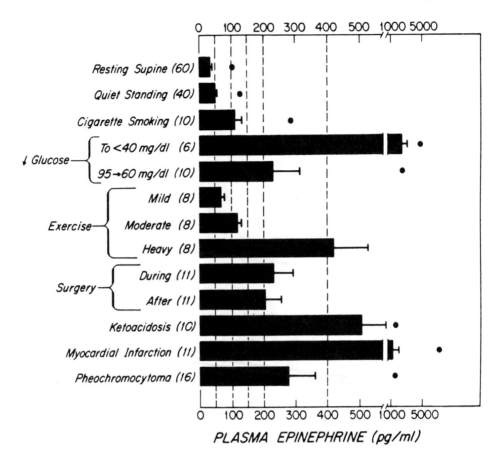

FIGURE 4-5 Human venous plasma E concentrations in various physiologic and pathophysiologic states. Explanations as in Figure 4-4. (From Cryer, P., *Endocrinology and Metabolism, 2nd ed.,* McGraw-Hill, New York, 1987, 651, with permission.)

both of these processes may play a role in the desensitization process. "Down-regulation" (desensitization) of receptors usually occurs in response to increased catecholamine levels and "up-regulation" (increased sensitization) to decreased levels. Rapid changes in receptor affinity for agonists can also contribute to changes in sensitivity of target cells to the catecholamines. Heterologous regulation or modulation of adrenergic receptors can occur too; for example, thyroid hormones and some steroids, which are not adrenergic receptor agonists or antagonists, can affect adrenergic receptors. This is one of a number of ways in which different hormonal systems can interact during adaptive and homeostatic responses, as well as during aging.

B. Adrenomedullary Characteristics

As the name suggests, the paired adrenal (suprarenal) glands lie close to the kidneys. In humans and other mammals the adrenal has a central core, or medulla, composed primarily of two major kinds of catecholamine-secreting (chromaffin) cells.[12] E is the major secretory product of one group and NE of the other. The methylation of NE to form E occurs in the more abundant E cells catalyzed by the enzyme PNMT (phenylethanolamine-*N*-methyltransferase) (Figure 4-1). The activity of this enzyme is maintained by the high concentrations of glucocorticoids (100 times higher than in systemic arterial blood) in the blood drainage of the adrenal cortices which constitutes the principal vascular supply of the medulla. Cortisol also stimulates the activities of tyrosine hydroxylase and dopamine β-hydroxylase, two enzymes

TABLE 4-1 Relative Number of Molecules of Various Compounds in a Single Adrenomedullary Chromaffin Granule

Constituents	Granule site or fraction	
	Membrane	Cytosol
Catecholamines		3,000,000
Nucleotides		930,000
Calcium		90,000
Ascorbic Acid		120,000
Peptides:		
Chromogranin A		5,000
Chromogranin B		80
Enkephalin-containing peptides		4,000
Free enkephalins (+ hexa-, hepta-, and octapeptides)		260
Neuropeptide Y		428
Dynorphin		9
Neurotensin		0.8
Substance P		0.4
Dopamine β-hydroxylase	210	140
Cytochrome b_{561}	1750	

Note: Bovine chromaffin granules were used.

Modified from Winkler, H., Apps, D. K., and Fisher-Colbrie, R., *Neuroscience*, 18, 261, 1986.

involved in the biosynthesis of the catecholamines. Thus, stimuli that signal the secretion of ACTH mobilize both cortisol and epinephrine.

The two major kinds of adrenomedullary endocrine cells are usually named A-cells (for epinephrine- or adrenaline-secreting cells) and NA-cells (for norepinephrine or noradrenaline-secreting). A third kind of adrenomedullary chromaffin cells with relatively small secretory chromaffin granules, so-called small-granule chromaffin (SGC) cells, are viewed as intermediates between typical chromaffin cells (A- and NA-cells) and sympathetic postganglionic neurons. Like the latter, they send out two or more long, axon-like processes, receive a rich innervation, and contain small synaptic-type vesicles in addition to the dense-cored secretory granules of a neurosecretory type.[13]

The major endocrine or chromaffin cells of the adrenal medulla store their catecholamine hormones in specialized cytoplasmic organelles, the chromaffin granules.[14] Part of the enzymatic apparatus for catecholamine biosynthesis is also located in these granules, which resemble the large dense-core vesicles of sympathetic neurons in their terminals, particularly in their biochemical composition.[15] Although catecholamines are quantitatively important compounds of chromaffin granules, many other kinds of molecules are also present (Table 4-1).[16] Still others continue to be found, and there are species and granule subtype differences in the occurrences and relative abundance of some of the chemical constituents.[17-20] Many of the greatest compositional differences occur in the granule peptide constituents. In humans, the A-cell's granules and Golgi complex are rich in glycoproteins, unlike these structures in NA-cells.[12] Possible functional significance of these differences and of the variety of components of the granules remain to be elucidated.

When chromaffin cells secrete, chromaffin granules discharge their soluble contents to the cell exterior by "exocytosis", a process involving fusion of the granule membrane with the cellular plasma membrane. The molecular mechanism linking a chemical stimulus, such as provided by the neurotransmitter acetylcholine, with the secretory or exocytotic event has been termed "stimulus-secretion coupling". It has many variants and interpretations, but that of the adrenomedullary chromaffin cells continues to be the most studied model.[21-23]

Adrenomedullary chromaffin cells and the nerve endings upon them show distinctive ultrastructural changes depending on functional activity and daily 24-h cycle. In the laboratory rat, where this has been best studied, some of these 24-h adrenomedullary changes are modified by removal of the pineal gland.[24,25] The study of the effects of pinealectomy reveals the close physiologic interrelations between the two amine-secreting glands and shows how some of the changes in the pinealectomized rat resemble those in the aged animal.[25]

C. Changes With Aging

Age changes in the sympathetic nervous system are perhaps better known than those in its major endocrine derivative, the adrenal medulla.[26] Even so, many of the aging-related functional changes in the sympathetic system are reflected in the adrenal medulla. Aging in the adrenomedullary and catecholaminergic endocrine system has been viewed from two perspectives:

- Changes in the adrenal medulla
- Changes in the responsiveness of target cells to adrenomedullary hormones

1. Changes With Aging in the Adrenal Medulla

In laboratory rats the adrenomedullary content of collagenous fibers[26] and the tendency for cell hyperplasia and hypertrophy[27-29] increase with older age, whereas rough endoplasmic reticulum decreases.[29] The adrenal medulla in elderly individuals shows a reduced nerve supply and structural alterations in its nerve fibers, although these changes are highly variable among the individuals studied. Scantiness of innervation does not increase proportionately with age, nor do changes in the nerve fibers become more noticeable with aging.[30] Perhaps these alterations in the human adrenal medulla are more related to diseases suffered during life than to any intrinsic aging process.[30]

Secretory activity of the adrenal medulla has been relatively little studied in older subjects. Reports on the possible relationships of age with plasma levels and urinary excretion of catecholamines in humans and laboratory mammals under basal conditions are contradictory. Estimates of catecholamine output from adult to senile subjects indicate no change with aging, or reduction in absolute and averaged circadian amplitude, or even increases with age.[31-34] This increase in humans was greater following standing and isometric exercise. In at least some studies, the elderly appear to have well-preserved sympatheticoadrenal function.[31] A decrease in peripheral clearance[35] or no change has been noticed.[36] In the interpretation of catecholamine plasma levels, failure to distinguish between adrenomedullary release and peripheral clearance of the hormone may be responsible for some of the current contradictions.

2. Changes in Responsiveness of Target Cells to Adrenomedullary Hormones

Aging-associated changes in responsiveness to adrenomedullary hormones are often difficult, if not impossible, to tease out from the complex neuroendocrine interactions (Chapter 20). Reported elevations of plasma and urinary catecholamines in the aged after various stimuli have been interpreted as representing compensatory reactions to the apparently increasing refractoriness of aged target cells to catecholamines, but even in young individuals, stimuli of different kinds often are not equally efficient in increasing plasma NE levels. As for glucocorticoid responses to stress, in the elderly the time necessary for return to baseline levels tends to be relatively prolonged (Chapter 14). Differential responsiveness is sometimes shown in comparisons of the output of the two major catecholamines. While plasma NE in the elderly is elevated during a mental stress test, plasma E is not. This can be interpreted as either lessening of PNMT activity or hyperactivity of the overall sympathetic system rather than of the adrenal medulla;[37] indeed, sympathetic nerve activity appears to increase with age.[38]

Target cells exhibit either an increased refractoriness or a decreased sensitivity to the catecholamines resulting from alterations in transport or binding. Clinical and experimental observations results either support the idea of:

1. Diminished responsiveness by some targets in some cases, or
2. No decrease, or
3. Increased responsiveness.

Decreased responsiveness with aging in humans and rodents is illustrated by:

1. Diminished efficiency of hemodynamic and cardiovascular responses to postural changes and to exercise (although some opposite cardiovascular effects may also be seen as in hypertension);
2. Slower dark adaptation of pupillary diameter; and
3. Impaired ability to respond to footshock, perhaps contributing to the increasing forgetfulness of senescent animals.[39]

E is one of the chemical mediators that, in some species, participates in the experimental production of atherosclerosis.[40] The locations of experimental lesions in the media of the arterial wall, however, do not correspond to the most frequent intimal site of the arterial lesions in the aging human.

Human subjects having behavioral patterns characterized by "aggressiveness, ambition, drive, competitiveness and a profound sense of time urgency" have higher daytime excretion of catecholamines, particularly NE. They characteristically also have raised serum lipid levels, shortened coagulation time, and higher incidence of coronary heart disease.[41,42] Excess catecholamines also alter lipid dynamics in animals and worsen the severity of atherosclerosis in animals fed excess cholesterol. They may influence lipid peroxides with the consequent increase in free radical production and aging-related diseases as well as extend or initiate myocardial damage directly or indirectly.[43]

3. Primary Disorders of the Adrenal Medulla

These primary disorders are few at all ages. The catecholamine-secreting tumor, pheochromocytoma, arising from chromaffin tissue including most often that of the adrenal medulla, is quite rare. Recognizable adrenomedullary deficiency conditions are almost unknown.[38] In spite of this, and especially in relation to the critical functional importance of changing responsiveness with age, drugs, and other factors, clinicians must remain acutely aware of the adrenal medulla's many functions (and extent of quantitative individual variation) during adaptation and diverse kinds of stress (Chapter 14). We owe early recognition and conceptual consolidation of the importance of this system in adaptation and stress to Walter Cannon[44] and Hans Selye.[45]

III. PINEAL GLAND AND INDOLAMINES

A. Indolamines

The amino acid tryptophan is the physiologic precursor of indolamine chemical mediators within the body (Figure 4-3). Of these, only melatonin (M) fits, so far, hormonal criteria in humans and other vertebrates. Other indolamines related to melatonin may also have hormonal actions, at least in some species.[2,3] These as well as melatonin are released into the blood by the pineal gland (Figure 4-2). The dependence of blood melatonin upon pineal presence has been demonstrated. Other tissues perhaps contribute to blood levels of M in some species and under some circumstances.[46-48]

Serotonin (5-hydroxytryptamine, or 5-HT) is not only an indolamine biosynthetic precursor of M (Figure 4-2), but it is also a widespread chemical mediator in its own right, with an ubiquity and versatility resembling NE. Both 5-HT and NE serve as important neurotransmitters in central and peripheral nervous systems. Both are cytoplasmic coinhabitants with a number of different peptide chemical mediators in aminergic and peptidergic endocrine cells. In blood, serotonin is almost completely bound to platelets. When released, as for example during some kinds of shock, it can have profound effects on several cells and processes affecting permeability and other functionally important characteristics, especially in and around smaller peripheral blood vessels. Such released, or "free", 5-HT is quickly cleared from the blood during circulation through the lungs. Blood levels of total 5-HT depend upon stores released by the gastrointestinal mucosa, rather than by the pineal or any other of the endocrine organs.[3]

B. Pineal Characteristics

The median and solitary pineal organ of humans and most other mammals is an extension of the brain. Its cell and tissue composition resembles that of the roof of the diencephalon, from which it is derived evolutionarily and embryologically. About 80% of its cells are pinealocytes, unique to the pineal and specialized for synthesis and secretion of melatonin, and probably for other as yet obscure activities and roles.[49] Among the endocrine pinealocytes at least, many have evolved from physiologically active photoreceptor cells in the ancestral pineal complex of lower vertebrates.[2-4] Even though direct and active photoreception seems to be greatly diminished or lost in humans and other mammals, there remains a strong physiologic heritage with adaptive and rhythmic mechanisms closely linked with environmental illumination. These and related considerations have led to the current concept that the pineal is a unique photoneuroendocrine organ.[2,4]

The pineal has a great diversity of functions among species of vertebrates. A common denominator is the mediation and modulation of some biorhythms.[2,50] This has been determined in most detail in relation to near-24-h (circadian) and seasonal or annual (circannual) rhythms. The most extensive experimental demonstration of this relationship has been with the photoperiodic timing of seasonal reproduction in some species.[51] Although a cause and effect relationship has not been demonstrated between human melatonin and pituitary-ovarian hormone levels, there is an inverse seasonal relationship between pineal and ovarian secretion in human populations at high latitudes.[52]

Pineal endocrine release of small amounts of M into the circulation affects the physiologic timing and phase relationships of a number, but probably not all, of the body's critically time-dependent activities. Despite the presence of specific binding sites for M in several peripheral tissues, including the spleen and the adrenal glands,[53] much of the action of this hormone is through receptors on target cells within the brain, probably within the hypothalamus. Pineal release of the M "trigger" is generally centered or concentrated during the usual hours of darkness, whether the animal is diurnal, nocturnal, or crepuscular. The amplitude (peak to valley dimension) of the pineal's M and related biochemical rhythms, and their great sensitivity to brief light exposure (mediated via retina, brain, and sympathetic innervation) are unique features.[54] These are giving us an excellent "window" on pineal mechanisms and their changes in health, disease, and aging.

C. Changes With Age

Human pineal weight decreases from mid to late adulthood, and may increase to a peak weight around the seventh decade of life to decline again gradually during the eighth and ninth decades (Table 4-2).[4,55] Great individual variation in pineal weight, and notably also in other of the pineal's quantitative features, should prompt caution in assuming that trends in a few arbitrarily chosen samples are necessarily attributable to all or most populations.

TABLE 4-2 Human Pineal Weight in Relation to Decade of Life

Age (years)	0–10	11–20	21–30	31–40	41–50	51–60	61–70	71–80	81–90
Absolute Weight (mg)									
Males	77	113	127	127	151	132	152	148	121
Females	70	83	106	148	160	133	164	155	156
Pineal/Brain Weight x 10^{-3}									
Males	9.25	11.75	10.20	10.54	8.71	10.12	8.57	8.64	10.57
Females	8.92	14.41	11.97	8.62	7.77	9.30	7.49	7.89	7.62

Note: Total number of specimens = 585.

Modified from von Eyl, O. and Gusek, W., *Verh. Dtsch. Ges. Path.,* 59, 400, 1975.

The aging-related pineal characteristic that has received the most attention is the occurrence of concretions within pineal tissue. Occurrence, tissue compartmental association, and relative number and size of these structures vary considerably among individual humans, and different mammalian species.[56] Indeed, some people, even in their ninth to tenth decades, have little if any pineal calcification with few changes in pinealocyte number and structure.[3,4,57-61] Since important pineal enzyme activities are not negatively affected by aging in human subjects, with or without pineal concretions, the latter do not appear to signify major involutional changes with age.[62,63] This contrasts with what often was assumed by early pathologists. Spectrometric assays of the calcium content of 1731 human pineals reveal great individual variation, without a strict age dependency.[64]

Pineal chemical constituents of diverse kinds may change quantitatively in older age.[3,4] Few of these so far have been linked metabolically or causally to pineal endocrine function or hormonal (M) output. For example, in the distal and middle portions of the pineal gland of aged mice, cavities, probably caused by degenerating parenchymal elements, are associated with reduced light responsiveness of pinealocyte glycogen, a primary energy source; likewise, cavities are often seen in elderly humans but their functional significance remains unknown.[65,66] By far the most clearly functionally relevant pineal constituent according to current information is M itself. Blood levels of M in humans and laboratory mammals determined by RIA decrease during old age.[46,51,67-72] The contradictory results from earlier studies could perhaps be ascribed to other conditions associated with altered M levels rather than advanced age per se.[70-72] Thus, M concentrations are apparently lower in human subjects with idiopathic pain syndromes, a subset of the pathologically depressed, and with dementia of the Alzheimer type as well as in the visually impaired.[73-78] Both bright and dim light can suppress nighttime M level in humans,[54] whereas some kinds of stress do not appear to affect M levels.[78]

There are several reasons for believing that the more recently demonstrated examples of decreased M in the aged are in fact age-related and not artifacts of pharmacological agents,[67,69,79,80] nor due simply to one or more of the other factors noted above:

1. *Melatonin levels are decreased during both night and day in elderly humans* (Figure 4-6, Table 4-3) and old rats (Figure 4-7).[68] The net effect is a dampening of the amplitude of the daily M rhythm.[75,81] It remains to be ascertained whether this is sufficient to compromise the hormone effectiveness in adjusting phase relations of biorhythms. Changes in M levels in the elderly are more marked than those in testosterone and LH, in direction, timing and magnitude (Table 4-4) although circadian rhythms in M and testosterone persist (Table 4-5).[81]

2. The daily M rhythm of the pineal and some related responses depend to a major extent upon the sympathetic innervation and β-receptors on the pinealocytes. *Innervation and receptors on the pinealocytes are reduced in number in old age,*[82,83] a reduction often associated with abnormal swelling of sympathetic nerve axons.[84]

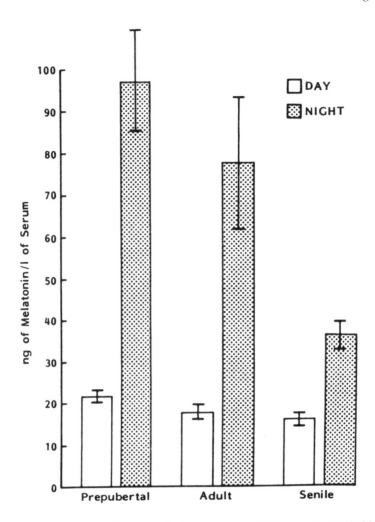

FIGURE 4-6 Plasma concentrations of melatonin in three age groups of Chinese males. Vertical bars represent means ± standard errors of six to nine samples. Analysis of variance indicated significant difference in time ($F = 50.03$; df = 1/39; $p < 0.05$) and age effect ($F = 6.95$; df = 1/39; $p < 0.05$). (From Pang, S., *Pineal Res. Rev.*, 3, 115, 1985, with permission.)

TABLE 4-3 Decrease With Age in Human Summer Nighttime Urinary 6-Hydroxymelatonin

	Age (years)			
	20–39	40–59	60–79	80+
Sex:				
Male	12.1 ± 5.1 (10)	11.1 ± 7.1 (7)	6.3 ± 2.7 (8)	6.2 ± 4.4 (5)
Female	11.4 ± 5.1 (10)	6.0 ± 3.2 (8)	5.1 ± 3.5 (7)	5.8 ± 3.3 (5)
Total	11.7 ± 5.0 (20)	8.4 ± 5.8 (15)	5.7 ± 3.0 (15)	6.0 ± 3.7 (10)

Note: 6-Hydroxymelatonin is in humans the major urinary metabolite of melatonin; it was measured here by a highly specific and sensitive gas chromatographic-negative ionization mass spectrometric method. Data are means [μg/17-h urine collection] ± standard deviations (number of subjects). Subjects (Oregon, U.S.A., uncontrolled in light exposure, sleep, activity, and diet) collected urine at home for three consecutive nights (5 p.m. and 10 a.m. the next morning) around the time of the summer solstice.

Extracted from Sack, R. L., Lewy, A. J., Erb, D. L., Vollmer, W. M., and Singer, C. M., *J. Pineal Res.*, 3, 379, 1986.

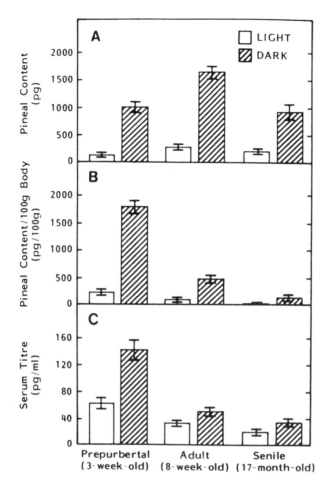

FIGURE 4-7 Age-related changes in rat pineal and serum contents of melatonin. Levels of melatonin are compared also at mid-light and mid-dark in the daily light-dark cycle. Each bar represents the mean ± standard error of six to nine samples. (From Pang, S., *Pineal Res. Rev.,* 3, 115, 1985, with permission.)

3. Observations of *reduced rhythm amplitude and sensitivity in circadian systems in the elderly* are consistent with evidence for decreased M levels with aging in humans and other animals.[85-89]

There are multiple effects of aging upon the distinctive circadian physiologic rhythms of humans and other animals.[86-89] In humans the age distribution of internal desynchronization is skewed toward older age.[90] This and other findings suggest that the ability to maintain appropriate phase relations and sensitivity among circadian physiological rhythms frequently deteriorates with advanced age.[89,90] An example is illustrated by laboratory rats with a slower rate of phase shifting at older age. The time required for phase shift of circadian activity (wheel-running) rhythm in old rats is longer in pinealectomized rats than in controls.[91] Pineal presence in the controls appears to stabilize the phase shift rate throughout life.[50] Another example system is the rat circadian rhythm in serum corticosterone. In this case too, aging and pinealectomy each result in increased morning corticosterone levels with decreased day-night differences.[91] In rats raised and maintained on a food (calories) restricted diet, M levels and amplitude of M rhythmicity are preserved and lifespan significantly prolonged.[79] From these results, it can be hypothesized that M, as a hormonal circadian mediator or modulator, is important in regulating or fine-tuning the phase relations of some circadian rhythms; in older

TABLE 4-4 Serum Levels of Melatonin (M), Free Testosterone (T_f), Total Testosterone (T_Σ) and LH in Elderly (E, N = 9, Age Range 69–80 Years) and Young Adult Men (A, N = 14, Age Range 26–36 Years)

Time:		08:00	12:00	16:00	20:00	24:00	04:00
M (pg/ml)	E	51.7 ± 15.1	47.9 ± 13.1	53.3 ± 12.7	51.6 ± 10.6	49.6 ± 15.9	58.5 ± 12.1
	A	43.7 ± 11.4	32.5 ± 9.3	49.2 ± 11.8	58.0 ± 17.9	103.0 ± 33.2	106.0 ± 37.9
T_f (ng/ml)	E	[a]7.5 ± 1.8	7.9 ± 4.5	8.6 ± 2.8	7.1 ± 2.9	7.3 ± 3.1	7.7 ± 2.8
	A	11.2 ± 2.3	9.1 ± 2.8	7.7 ± 2.0	7.3 ± 2.6	7.9 ± 2.3	9.3 ± 2.6
T_Σ (ng/ml)	E	[a]424 ± 150	437 ± 203	497 ± 156	414 ± 223	461 ± 224	422 ± 122
	A	650 ± 141	516 ± 168	447 ± 147	402 ± 123	481 ± 113	574 ± 136
LH (mIU/ml)	E	[a]12.1 ± 2.1					
	A	7.4 ± 1.2					

Notes: Subjects were nonobese without apparent liver, kidney, metabolic, or endocrine disease; studied during the winter (Italy); and without endocrine-altering drugs during the preceding three months. They were exposed daily to a fixed photoperiod schedule (light:dark = 14:10) starting at least two weeks before venous blood samples were taken at 4-hour intervals as shown. Data are ± standard deviation.

[a] $p < 0.05$ (Student-Fisher t) E vs. A group.

Modified from Carani, C., Baldini, A., Morabito, F., Resentini, M., Diazzi, G., Sarti, G., Del Rio, G., and Zini, D., *Fundamentals and Clinics in Pineal Research,* Trentini, G. P., DeGaetani, C., and Pévet, P., Eds., Raven Press, New York, 1987.

TABLE 4-5 Population Cosinor Summary: Study of the Circadian Rhythms of Serum Melatonin (M), Free Testosterone (T_f), and Total Testosterone (T_Σ) in Elderly (E) and Young Adult (A) Men

Rhythm Characteristics:		Mesor (±SD)	Mean	Amplitude Range (95% C.L.)		Mean Acrophase	*p*
M	E	51.7 ± 11.9	2.08	0.12 →	6.70	3.21	NS
	A	63.9 ± 16.3	37.40	23.00 →	51.80	1.27	<0.05
T_f	E	7.8 ± 1.8	0.24	0.61 →	1.45	11.83	NS
	A	8.6 ± 2.0	1.76	1.00 →	2.53	7.79	<0.05
T_Σ	E	445 ± 147	18.80	38.60 → 107.00		17.78	NS
	A	512 ± 119	108.00	59.40 → 157.00		6.90	<0.05

Notes: Subjects and original data as in Table 4-4. Mesor and amplitude of M are expressed as pg/ml; those of T_f and T_Σ as ng/100 ml; $p < 0.05$ (Student-Fisher t) E vs. A group. Additional abbreviations: C.L. = confidence limits; NS = not statistically significant; p = probability of nonrhythmic; SD = standard deviation.

Modified from Carani, C., Baldini, A., Morabito, F., Resentini, M., Diazzi, G., Sarti, G., Del Rio, G., and Zini, D., *Fundamentals and Clinics in Pineal Research,* Trentini, G. P., DeGaetani, C., and Pévet, P., Eds.,

age with lessening of M levels and amplitude of M rhythmicity, the orderliness and inter-relations of other circadian physiologic rhythms are disturbed. The importance of this kind of biologic orchestration for longevity has been questioned repeatedly, but its testing has been limited largely to insects. These die sooner in disruptive temporal conditions, such as repeated forced phase shifts, or longer-term maintenance in light-dark cycles with period lengths different from 24 hours.[92,93]

Reduced activity of the aging pineal gland has been also implicated in the progressive impairment with aging of immunomodulatory, metabolic, oncostatic, and autonomic functions.[94-100] Thus, improvement in pineal function, and particularly, normalization of M levels, may ameliorate these M-dependent functions and contribute to longevity.[99] Free radical production with aging (see Chapters 1 and 15) and its association with M is of particular interest when considering pineal function in relation to aging. M is an extremely efficient scavenger of the most toxic of the oxygen radicals, i.e., the hydroxyl radical.[98,101] As such, it normally protects cells and organs from degeneration associated with aging.[102,103] Because of its ability to so effectively scavenge the hydroxyl radical, decreasing melatonin levels, which are a usual consequence of age,[104] have been implicated in being either causative or contributory to a variety of age-related diseases[98,103,105] as well as to aging itself.[102,104-106] Furthermore, M administration to aging mice significantly prolongs their survival and maintains them in better health into advanced age.[99] In sum, the pineal gland, via its hormone melatonin, may be a major player in the processes of aging and senescence.[98,103,105,106]

REFERENCES

1. Boyd, J., Origin, development and distribution of chromaffin cells, in *Adrenergic Mechanisms,* (Ciba Foundation Symposium), Vane, J., Wolstenholme, G., and O'Connor, M., Eds., Little, Brown, Boston, 1960, 63.
2. Binkley, S., *The Pineal: Endocrine and Nonendocrine Function,* Prentice-Hall, Englewood Cliffs, NJ, 1988.
3. Quay, W. B., *Pineal Chemistry in Cellular and Physiological Mechanisms,* Charles C Thomas, Springfield, IL, 1974.
4. Vollrath, L., *The Pineal Organ,* Springer-Verlag, Berlin, 1981.
5. von Euler, U., *Noradrenaline. Chemistry, Physiology, Pharmacology and Clinical Aspects,* Charles C Thomas, Springfield, IL, 1956.
6. Axelrod, J., Following the trail of epinephrine from the periphery to the brain, in *Epinephrine in the Central Nervous System,* Stolk, J. M., U'Prichard, D. C., and Fuxe, K., Eds., Oxford University Press, Oxford, 1988, 3.
7. von Euler, U., Synthesis, uptake and storage of catecholamines in adrenergic nerves. The effects of drugs, in *Catecholamines,* Blaschko, H. and Muscholl, E., Eds., Springer-Verlag, Berlin, 1972, 186.
8. von Euler, U., Franksson, C., and Hellstrom, J., Adrenaline and noradrenaline output in urine after unilateral and bilateral adrenalectomy, *Acta Physiol. Scand.,* 31, 1, 1954.
9. Shah, S., Tse, T., Clutter, W., and Cryer, P., The human sympathochromaffin system, *Am. J. Physiol.,* 247, E380, 1984.
10. Brown, M. J., Jenner, D. A., Allison, D. J., and Dollery, C. T., Variations in individual organ release of noradrenaline measured by an improved radioenzymatic technique; limitations of peripheral venous measurements in the assessment of sympathetic nervous activity, *Clin. Sci.,* 61, 585, 1981.
11. Planz, G., Planz, R., Persigehl, M., Bundschu, H. D., and Heintz, R., Adrenaline and noradrenaline concentration in blood of suprarenal and renal vein of man with normal blood pressure and with essential hypertension, *Klin. Wochenschr.,* 56, 1109, 1978.
12. Benchimol, S. and Cantin, M., Ultrastructural cytochemistry of the human adrenal medulla, *Histochemistry,* 54, 9, 1977.
13. Kobayashi, S., Adrenal medulla: chromaffin cells as paraneurons, *Arch. Histol. Jpn.,* 40(Suppl.), 61, 1977.
14. Blaschko, H. and Welch, A. D., Localization of adrenaline in cytoplasmic particles of the bovine adrenal medulla, *N.-S. Arch. Exp. Path. Pharmak.,* 219, 17, 1953.
15. Lagercrantz, H., Isolation and characterization of sympathetic nerve trunk vesicles, *Acta Physiol. Scand.,* 366(Suppl.), 7, 1971.
16. Winkler, H., Apps, D. K., and Fisher-Colbrie, R., The molecular function of adrenal chromaffin granules: established facts and unresolved topics, *Neuroscience,* 18, 261, 1986.
17. Bjartell, A., Ekman, R., Sundler, F., and Widerlov, E., Delta-sleep-inducing peptide-like immunoreactivity in pituitary ACTH/MSH and adrenal-medullary cells, *Ann. New York Acad. Sci.,* 512, 476, 1987.
18. Bruhn, T., Engeland, W. C., Anthony, E. L., Gann, D.S., and Jackson, I. M., Corticotropin-releasing factor in the adrenal medulla, *Ann. New York Acad. Sci.* 512, 115, 1987.
19. Morel, G., Chabot, J. G., Garcia-Caballero, T., Gossard, F., Dihl, F., Belles-Isles, M., and Heisler, S., Synthesis, internalization, and localization of atrial natriuretic peptide in rat adrenal medulla, *Endocrinology,* 123, 149, 1988.

20. Schultzberg, M., Andersson, C., Unden, A., Troye-Blomberg, M., Svenson, S. B., and Bartfai, T., Interleukin-1 in adrenal chromaffin cells, *Neuroscience,* 30, 805, 1989.

21. Douglas, W., Stimulus-secretion coupling: the concept and clues from chromaffin and other cells, *Brit. J. Pharmacol.,* 34, 453, 1968.

22. Ohara-Imaizumi, M. and Kumakura, K., Receptor desensitization and the transient nature of the secretory response of adrenal chromaffin cells, *Neurosci. Lett.,* 70, 250, 1986.

23. Suchard, S. J., Corcoran, J. J., Pressman, B. C., and Rubin, R. W., Evidence for secretory granule membrane recycling in cultured adrenal chromaffin cells, *Cell Biol. Int. Reports,* 5, 953, 1981.

24. Kachi, T., Pineal actions on the autonomic system, *Pineal Res. Rev.,* 5, 217, 1987.

25. Kachi, T., Takahashi, G., Banerji, T. K., and Quay, W. B., Rough endoplasmic reticulum in the adrenaline and noradrenaline cells of the adrenal medulla: effects of intracranial surgery and pinealectomy, *J. Pineal Res.,* 12, 89, 1992.

26. Cryer, P., Diseases of the sympathochromaffin system, in *Endocrinology and Metabolism,* 2nd ed., Felig, P., Baxter, J., Broadus, A., and Frohman, L., Eds., McGraw-Hill, New York, 1987, 651.

27. Dribben, I. S. and Wolfe, J. M., Structural changes in the connective tissue of the adrenal glands of female rats associated with advancing age, *Anat. Rec.,* 98, 557, 1947.

28. Andrew, W., *Cellular Changes with Age,* Charles C Thomas, Springfield, IL, 1952.

29. Coupland, R. E. and Tomlinson, A., The development and maturation of adrenal medullary chromaffin cells of the rat in vivo: a descriptive and quantitative study, *Int. J. Dev. Neurosci.,* 7, 419, 1989.

30. Botar, G., *The Autonomic Nervous System. An Introduction to its Physiological and Pathological Histology,* Akademiai Kiado, Budapest, 1966.

31. Fisher, R., The urinary excretion of 4-hydroxy-3-methoxy mandelic acid in the elderly, *Gerontologia Clinica,* 13, 257, 1971.

32. Herbeuval, R., Masse, G., Cuny, G., and Guerci, O., L'excretion des catecholamines dans l'hypertension des viellards, *Rev. Franc. Gerontol.,* 9, 75, 1963.

33. Karki, N., The urinary excretion of noradrenaline and adrenaline in different age groups, its diurnal variation and the effect of muscular work on it, *Acta Physiol. Scand.,* 39(Suppl. 132), 1, 1956.

34. Tumer, N., Hale, C., Lawler, J., and Strong, R., Modulation of tyrosine hydroxylase gene expression in the rat adrenal by exercise: effects of age, *Mol. Brain Res.,* 14, 51, 1992.

35. Esler, M., Skews, H., Leonard, P., Jackman, G., Bobik, A., and Korner, P., Age-dependence of noradrenaline kinetics in normal subjects, *Clin. Sci.,* 60, 217, 1981.

36. Rubin, P. C., Scott, P. J., Mclean, K., and Reid, J. L., Noradrenaline release and clearance in relation to age and blood pressure in man, *Eur. J. Clin. Invest.,* 12, 121, 1982.

37. Barnes, R. F., Raskind, M., Gumbrecht, G., and Halter, J. B., The effects of age on the plasma catecholamine response to mental stress in man, *J. Clin. Endocrinol. Metab.,* 54, 64, 1982.

38. Davies, I. and Sever, P., Adrenoceptor function, in *Autonomic Failure, A Textbook of Clinic Disorders of the Autonomic Nervous System,* 2nd ed., Bannister, R., Ed., Oxford University Press, Oxford, 1988, 348.

39. Martinez, J. L., Jr., Schulteis, G., Janak, P. H., and Weinberger, S. B., Behavioral assessment of forgetting in aged rodents and its relationship to peripheral sympathetic function, *Neurobiol. Aging,* 9, 697, 1988.

40. Oester, Y. T., Adrenal medullary hormones and arteriosclerosis, *Ann. New York Acad. Sci.,* 72, 885, 1959.

41. Rosenman, R. H., Emotional factors in coronary heart disease, *Postgrad. Med.,* 42, 165, 1967.

42. Friedman, M., St. George, S., Byers, S. O., and Rosenman, R. H., Excretion of catecholamines, 17-ketosteroids, 17-hydroxycorticoids and 5-hydroxyindole in men exhibiting a particular behavior pattern (A) associated with high incidence of clinical coronary artery disease, *J. Clin. Invest.,* 39, 758, 1960.

43. Yagi, K., Role of peroxidases in aging and age-related diseases, in *New Trends in Biological Chemistry,* Ozawa, T., Ed., Springer-Verlag, Berlin, 1991, 207.

44. Cannon, W., *Bodily Changes in Pain, Hunger, Fear and Rage. An Account of Recent Researches into the Function of Emotional Excitement,* D. Appleton, New York, 1915.

45. Selye, H., *The Physiology and Pathology of Exposure to Stress, A Treatise Based on the Concepts of the General-Adapation-Syndrome and the Diseases of Adaptation,* Acta, Montreal, Canada, 1950.

46. Brown, G. M., Young, S. N., Gauthier, S., Tsui, H., and Grota, L. J., Melatonin in cerebrospinal fluid in daytime; its origin and variation with age, *Life Sci.,* 25, 929, 1979.

47. Pang, S., Brown, G. M., Grota, L. J., Chambers, J. W., and Rodman, R. L., Determination of N-acetylserotonin and melatonin activities in the pineal gland, retina, harderian gland, brain and serum of rats and chickens, *Neuroendocrinology,* 23, 1, 1977.

48. Ralph, C., Melatonin production by extrapineal tissues, in *Melatonin: Current Status and Perspectives,* Birau, N. and Schloot, W., Eds., Pergamon Press, New York, 1981, 35.

49. Quay, W. B., Pineal function in mammals: a reconsideration, *Pineal Res. Rev.,* 2, 87, 1984.

50. Quay, W. B., Pineal homeostatic regulation of shifts in the circadian activity rhythm during maturation and aging, *Trans. New York Acad. Sci.,* 34, 239, 1972.

51. Reiter, R. J., Johnson, L. Y., Steger, R. W., Richardson, B. A., and Petterborg, L. J., Pineal biosynthetic activity and neuroendocrine physiology in the aging hamster and gerbil, *Peptides,* 1 (Suppl. 1), 69, 1980.

52. Kauppila, A., Kivela, A., Pakarinen, A., and Vakkuri, O., Inverse seasonal relationship between melatonin and ovarian activity in humans in a region with a strong seasonal contrast in luminosity, *J. Clin. Endocrinol. Metab.,* 65, 823, 1987.

53. Stankov, B., Fraschini, F., and Reiter, R. J., The melatonin receptor: distribution, biochemistry and pharmacology, in *Melatonin: Biosynthesis, Physiological Effects and Clinical Applications,* Yu, H.-S. and Reiter, R. J., Eds., CRC Press, Boca Raton, FL, 1993, 155.

54. Bojkowski, C., Aldhous, M., English, J., Franey, C., Poulton, A. L., Skene, D. J., and Arendt, J., Suppression of nocturnal plasma melatonin and 6-sulphatoxymelatonin by bright and dim light in man, *Horm. Metabol. Res.,* 19, 437, 1987.

55. von Eyl, O. and Gusek, W., Zur Frage von Altersveränderungen der Zirbeldrüse beim Menschen, *Verh. Dtsch. Ges. Path.,* 59, 400, 1975.

56. Welsh, M., Pineal calcification: structural and functional aspects, *Pineal Res. Rev.,* 3, 41, 1985.

57. Arieti, S., The pineal gland in old age, *J. Neuropathol. Exp. Neurol.,* 13, 482, 1954.

58. Tapp, E. and Huxley, M., The weight and degree of calcification of the pineal gland, *J. Path.,* 105, 31, 1971.

59. Tapp, E. and Huxley, M., The histological appearance of the human pineal gland from puberty to old age, *J. Path.,* 108, 137, 1972.

60. Wildi, E. and Frauchiger, E., Modifications histologiques de l'epiphyse humaine pendant l'enfance, l'age adulte et le viellissement, *Progr. Brain Res.,* 10, 218, 1965.

61. Trentini, G. P., De Gaetani, C., Criscuolo, M., Migaldi, M., and Ferrari, G., Pineal calcification in different physiopathological conditions in humans, in *Fundamentals and Clinics in Pineal Research,* Trentini, G. P., De Gaetani, C., and Pévet, P., Eds., Raven Press, New York, 1987, 291.

62. Otani, T., Gyorkey, F., and Farrell, G., Enzymes of the human pineal body, *J. Clin. Endocrinol. Metab.,* 28, 349, 1968.

63. Wurtman, R., Axelrod, J., and Barchas, J., Age and enzyme activity in the human pineal, *J. Clin. Endocrinol. Metab.,* 24, 299, 1964.

64. Trentini, G., De Gaetani, C., Pierini, G., Criscuolo, M., Vidyasagar, R., and Fabbri, F., Some aspects of human pineal pathology, *Adv. Pineal Res.,* 1, 219, 1986.

65. Kachi, T., Fujita, M., Kanda, M., Hamada, K., Ueno, T., Takei, H., Yahara, O., Tanii, H., Ishibashi, H., Terasawa, K., Takatori, T., Hikichi, T., and Yoshida, A., Static and dynamic morphological studies of human pineal gland in neoplastic and systemic neurodegenerative disease cases and medico-legal autopsy cases, *Adv. Pineal Res.,* 3, 277, 1989.

66. Kachi, T., Matsushima, S., and Ito, T., Postnatal observations on the diurnal rhythm and the light-responsiveness in the pineal glycogen content in mice, *Anat. Rec.,* 183, 39, 1975.

67. Beck-Friis, J., von Rosen, D., Kjellman, B., Ljunggren, J., and Wetterberg, L., Melatonin in relation to body measures, sex, age, season and the use of drugs in patients with major affective disorders and healthy subjects, *Psychoneuroendocrinology,* 9, 261, 1984.

68. Pang, S., Melatonin concentrations in blood and pineal gland, *Pineal Res. Rev.,* 3, 115, 1985.

69. Touitou, Y., Bogdan, A., Claustrat, B., and Touitou, C., Drugs affecting melatonin secretion in man, in *Fundamentals and Clinics in Pineal Research,* Trentini, G. P., De Gaetani, C., and Pévet, P., Eds., Raven Press, New York, 1987, 349.

70. Sack, R. L., Lewy, A. J., Erb, D. L., Vollmer, W. M., and Singer, C. M., Human melatonin production decreases with age, *J. Pineal Res.,* 3, 379, 1986.

71. Waldhauser, F. and Trinchard-Lugan, I., Age-related alterations of human serum melatonin, in *Fundamentals and Clinics in Pineal Research,* Trentini, G. P., De Gaetani, C., and Pévet, P., Eds., Raven Press, New York, 1987, 369.

72. Vaughan, G., Melatonin in humans, *Pineal Res. Rev.,* 2, 141, 1984.

73. Almay, B. G., von Knorring, L., and Wetterberg, L., Melatonin in serum and urine in patients with idiopathic pain syndromes, *Psychiatry Res.,* 22, 179, 1987.

74. Beck-Friis, J., Kjellman, B. F., Aperia, B., Unden, F., von Rosen, D., Ljunggren, J., and Wetterberg, L., Serum melatonin in relation to clinical variables in patients with major depressive disorders and a hypothesis of a low melatonin syndrome, *Acta Psychiatrica Scandinavica,* 71, 319, 1985.

75. Skene, D. J., Vivien-Roels, B., Sparks, D. L., Hunsaker, J. C., Pévet, P., Ravid, D., and Swaab, D. F., Daily variation in the concentration of melatonin and 5-methoxytryptophol in the human pineal gland: effect of age and Alzheimer's disease, *Brain Res.,* 528, 170, 1990.

76. Boyce, P. M., 6-Sulphatoxy melatonin in melancholia, *Am. J. Psychiatry,* 142, 125, 1985.

77. Smith, J. A., O'Hara, J., and Schiff, A. A., Altered diurnal serum melatonin rhythm in blind men, *Lancet,* 2[8252], 933, 1981.

78. Vaughan, G. M., McDonald, S. D., Jordan, R. M., Allen, J. P., Bohmfalk, G. L., Abou-Samra, M., and Story, J. L., Melatonin concentration in human blood and cerebrospinal fluid: relationship to stress, *Clin. Endocrinol. Metab.,* 47, 220, 1978.

79. Reiter, R. J., The ageing pineal gland and its physiological consequences, *Bioessays,* 14, 169, 1992.

80. Surrall, K., Smith, J., Bird, H., Okala, B., Othman, H., and Padwick, D., Effect of ibuprofen and indomethacin on human plasma melatonin, *J. Pharm. Pharmacol.,* 39, 840, 1987.

81. Carani, C., Baldini, A., Morabito, F., Resentini, M., Diazzi, G., Sarti, G., Del Rio, G., and Zini, D., Further studies on the circadian rhythms of serum melatonin and testosterone in elderly men, in *Fundamentals and Clinics in Pineal Research,* Trentini, G. P., De Gaetani, C., and Pévet, P., Eds., Raven Press, New York, 1987, 377.

82. Greenberg, L. H. and Weiss, B., Beta-Adrenergic receptors in aged rat brain: reduced number and capacity of pineals to develop supersensitivity, *Science,* 201, 61, 1978.

83. Reuss, S., Spies, C., Schröder, H., and Vollrath, L., The aged pineal gland: reduction in pinealocyte number and adrenergic innervation in male rats, *Exp. Gerontol.,* 25, 183, 1990.

84. Jengeleski, C. A., Powers, R. E., O'Connor, D. T., and Price, D. L., Noradrenergic innervation of human pineal gland: abnormalities in ageing and Alzheimer's disease, *Brain Res.,* 481, 378, 1989.

85. Bremner, W. J., Vitiello, M. V., and Prinz, P. N., Loss of circadian rhythmicity in blood testosterone levels with aging in normal men, *J. Clin. Endocrinol. Metab.,* 56, 1278, 1983.

86. Feinberg, I., Changes in sleep cycle patterns with age, *J. Psychiatr. Res.,* 10, 283, 1975.

87. Weitzman, E. D., Moline, M. L., Czeisler, C. A., and Zimmerman, J. C., Chronobiology of aging: temperature, sleep-wake rhythms and entrainment, *Neurobiol. Aging,* 3, 299, 1982.

88. Wever, R., The meaning of circadian rhythmicity with regard to aging, *Verh. Dtsch. Ges. Pathol.,* 59, 160, 1975.

89. Halberg, F. and Nelson, W., Chronobiologic optimization of aging, in *Aging and Biological Rhythms,* Samis, H. V., Jr. and Capobianco, S., Eds., Plenum Press, New York, 1978, 5.

90. Samis, H. V., Jr., Aging: The loss of temporal organization, *Perspectives in Biology and Medicine,* 12, 95, 1968.

91. Oxenkrug, G., McIntyre, I., and Gershon, S., Effects of pinealectomy and aging on the serum corticosterone circadian rhythm in rats, *J. Pineal Res.,* 1, 181, 1984.

92. Ehret, C., Groh, K., and Meinert, J., Circadian dyschronism and chronotypic ecophilia as factors in aging and longevity, in *Aging and Biological Rhythms,* Samis, H. V., Jr. and Capobianco, S., Eds., Plenum Press, New York, 1978, 185.

93. Davis, F. C., Ontogeny of circadian rhythms, in *Handbook of Behavioral Neurobiology, Vol. 4, Biological rhythms,* Aschoff, J., Ed., Plenum Press, New York, 1981, 257.

94. Blask, D. E., Melatonin in oncology, in *Melatonin: Biosynthesis, Physiological Effects and Clinical Applications,* Yu, H.-S. and Reiter, R. J., Eds., CRC Press, Boca Raton, FL, 1993, 447.

95. Carneiro, R. C., Pereira, E. P., Cipolla-Nero, J., and Markus, R. P., Age-related changes in melatonin modulation of sympathetic neurotransmission, *J. Phamacol. Exp. Therap.,* 266, 1536, 1993.

96. Maestroni, G. J., Conti, A., and Pierpaoli, W., Pineal melatonin, its fundamental immunoregulatory role in aging and cancer, *Ann. N. Y. Acad. Sci.,* 521, 140, 1988.

97. Maestroni, G. J. and Conti, A., Melatonin in relation to the immune system, in *Melatonin: Biosynthesis, Physiological Effects and Clinical Applications,* Yu, H.-S. and Reiter, R. J., Eds., CRC Press, Boca Raton, FL, 1993, 289.

98. Poeggeler, B., Reiter, R. J., Tan, D. X., Chen, L. D., and Manchester, L. C., Melatonin, hydroxyl radical-mediated oxidative damage and aging: a hypothesis, *J. Pineal Res.,* 14, 151, 1993.

99. Pierpaoli, W., Dall'Ara, A., Pedrinis, E., and Regelson, W., The pineal control of aging: the effects of melatonin and pineal grafting on the survival of older mice, *Ann. N. Y. Acad. Sci.,* 621, 291, 1991.

100. Reiter, R. J., Pineal gland, cellular proliferation and neoplastic growth: an historical account, in *The Pineal Gland and Cancer,* Gupta, D., Attanasio, A., and Reiter, R. J., Eds., Brain Research Promotion, Tübingen and London, 1988, 41.

101. Reiter, R. J., Poeggeler, B., Tan, D. X., Chen, L. D., Manchester, L. C., and Guerrero, J. M., Antioxidant capacity of melatonin: A novel action not requiring a receptor, *Neuroendocrinol Lett.,* 15, 103, 1993.

102. Reiter, R. J., Tan, D. X., Poeggeler, B., Menendez-Pelaez, A., Chen, L. D., and Saarela, S., Melatonin as a free radical scavenger: implications for aging and age-related diseases, *Ann. N.Y. Acad. Sci.,* 719, 1, 1994.

103. Reiter, R. J., Poeggeler, B., Chen, L. D., Abe, M., Hara, M., Orhii, P. B., Attia, A. M., and Barlow-Walden, L. R., Melatonin as a free radical scavenger: theoretical implications for neurodegenerative disorders in the aged, *Acta Gerontol.,* 44, 92, 1994.

104. Reiter, R. J., The aging pineal gland and its physiological consequences. *BioEssays,* 14, 169, 1992.

105. Tan, D. X., Reiter, R. J., Chen, L. D., Poeggeler, B., Manchester, L. C., and Barlow-Walden, L. R., Both physiological and pharmacological levels of melatonin reduce DNA adduct formation induced by the carcinogen safrole, *Carcinogenesis,* 15, 215, 1994.

106. Reiter, R. J., Tan, D. X., Poeggeler, B., Chen, L. D., and Menendez-Pelaez, A., Melatonin, free radicals and cancer initiation, in *Advances in Pineal Research,* Vol. 7, Maestroni, G. J. M., Conti, A., and Reiter, R. J., Eds., John Libbey, London, 1994, 211.

5

Hormones of the Thyroid and Parathyroid Glands

Paola S. Timiras

CONTENTS

I. INTRODUCTION

In attempting to group hormones for easier association of their actions and changes with aging, the thyroid and parathyroid hormones are presented together in this chapter. These hormones, thyroxine and triiodothyronine from the thyroid gland and parathyroid hormone from the

0-8493-2446-7/95/$0.00+$.50
© 1995 by CRC Press Inc.

TABLE 5-1 Major Actions of Thyroid Hormones

Calorigenic
Metabolic (BMR)
Maturational (Brain)
Behavioral

parathyroid glands, while structurally and functionally not similar, are secreted by neighboring cells. The parathyroid glands are embedded in the posterior poles of the thyroid gland which also contains cells producing another hormone, calcitonin. The great significance of thyroid and parathyroid hormones lies in their widespread actions in the regulation of basal (thyroid hormones) and calcium (parahormone, calcitonin) metabolism. Therefore, changes with aging in these hormones will necessarily have broad general effects on lifespan and survival.

II. THYROID HORMONES

Thyroxine (T4) and triiodothyronine (T3) have for years sparked the interest of investigators seeking the causes of aging. Discovery of the importance of the thyroid gland for general health, identification of the major functions of thyroid hormones (Table 5-1) and, once they had been identified, the successful use of synthetic hormones in hypothyroid (myxedematous) patients for replacement therapy, have generated considerable interest in their possible role in aging.

During development, the thyroid gland is necessary for whole-body and organ growth and for maturation of the central nervous system (CNS): in children, hypothyroidism is associated with dwarfism and severe mental retardation (cretinism). In adulthood, T3 regulates tissue oxygen consumption (hence its effects on the basal metabolic rate) and influences behavior. Although the thyroid gland is not essential for life, hypothyroidism is associated with lower resistance to cold, and mental and physical slowing, and hyperthyroidism induces metabolic and behavioral alterations which impair well-being and endanger survival.

In humans, certain signs of aging resemble those of thyroid insufficiency or hypothyroidism. Hypothyroid individuals may develop a number of signs:

- Reduced metabolic rate,
- Hyperlipidemia,
- Accelerated atherosclerosis,
- Early aging of skin and hair,
- Slow reflexes, and
- Slow mental performance.

These could be interpreted as "precocious senescence". All signs can be ameliorated or eliminated by the administration of thyroid hormones. Given the importance of these hormones in normal development, it may be argued that they may also control the rate/site of aging.

As early as the turn of this 20th century, investigators optimistically attempted rejuvenation or prolongation of life through hormone administration.[1] Thyroid hormone administration to some animals (rats, mice) shortens lifespan[2] while thyroid insufficiency lengthens it.[3] In others animals (fowl), thyroid hormones may induce an apparent dramatic rejuvenation.[4] In humans, alterations of the thyroid state do not seem to alter the lifespan.

The ability to maintain a normal thyroid (euthyroid) state continues during aging despite a number of changes in various aspects of thyroid hormone production, secretion, and actions.

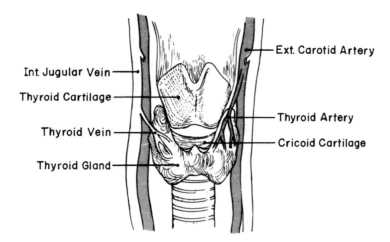

FIGURE 5-1 Diagrammatic location and structure of the thyroid gland. The thyroid gland and cricoid cartilages and the major blood vessels are included. Four parathyroid glands are imbedded in the superior and inferior poles of the thyroid gland. Calcitonin-secreting C-cells are dispersed throughout the thyroid gland. (Drawing by S. Oklund).

Nevertheless, as with most endocrines, normal thyroid function in the elderly is marginal and may be threatened by repeated challenges and stress; the resulting abnormal (dysthyroid) state may impair overall physiologic competence and lead to disease and aging.

A. Structure and Function of the Hypothalamo-Pituitary-Thyroid Axis

The thyroid gland, located in the region of the lower larynx and upper trachea, is composed of two lobes united by a narrow bridge or isthmus. It is one of the most vascularized endocrines (Figure 5-1). Vascularity, size, and microscopic structures vary with the levels of the pituitary tropic hormone, thyroid-stimulating hormone (thyrotropin or TSH), nutrition, temperature, sex, and age.

The follicle is the functional unit of the thyroid gland. Follicles are roughly spherical and consist of a single layer of epithelial cells supported on a basement membrane; the cells surround a central cavity or lumen filled with colloid. The colloid is a proteinaceous material containing an iodinated protein, thyroglobulin, necessary for the production of T3 and T4 (Figure 5-2). Thyroid gland control extends from the brain to the target organs (Table 5-2) through a series of integrated actions that include:

- At the hypothalamus: secretion of the tripeptide thyrotropin-releasing hormone (TRH) into the portal vessels and its transport to the anterior pituitary where it stimulates the release of TSH. TRH is present in many brain areas where it has extra-endocrine actions (Chapter 3).
- At the anterior pituitary: the release of TSH may be inhibited by thyroid hormones (negative feedback) or stimulated by TRH or low T3 and T4 levels. TSH is a glycoprotein and its major function is to stimulate the thyroid gland to produce its hormones. In the absence of TSH (as in hypophysectomy), the thyroid gland fails to grow, follicular cells become atrophic with enlarged colloid centers, and hormone synthesis and secretion are impaired.
- At the thyroid gland, the two major hormones secreted are T4 and T3. A third hormone, reverse T3 or rT3 (wherein iodination of the tyrosine ring is reversed) is present in the blood in small amounts and has little biological activity.

Stimulation of TSH receptors on thyroid cells activates intracellular cAMP and cell membrane changes responsible for TSH actions. TSH stimulates hormonogenesis which consists of:

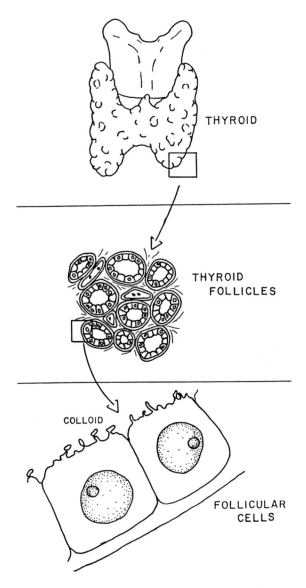

FIGURE 5-2 Diagrammatic representation of the thyroid gland and its microscopic structure. Top: thyroid gland; Center: thyroid follicles, the cells of which surround a central colloid-filled cavity; Bottom: thyroid cells with microvilli projecting into the central colloid. (Drawing by S. Oklund).

- Synthesis of thyroglobulin by the follicular cells;
- Secretion of thyroglobulin from follicular cells to lumen;
- Iodination of tyrosine residues of thyroglobulin at the luminal surface of follicular cells;
- Coupling of iodinated tyrosil residues to form iodinated thyronil residues, primarily T4 and, in lesser amount, T3 (both iodine-containing derivatives of the amino acid tyrosine);
- Retrieval of the iodinated thyroglobulin from lumen to cells;
- Secretion of T3 and T4 from the basal ends of follicular cells to the blood; and
- At the target tissues, T3, derived primarily from deiodination of T4, represents the most biologically active hormone.

Circulating T3 and T4 exist both free and protein-bound. They interact with receptors localized in membrane, mitochondria, cytoplasm, and nucleus of responsive cells. T3 and T4

TABLE 5-2 Spectrum of Thyroid Hormone Regulation Along the
Hypothalamo-Pituitary-Thyroid Axis

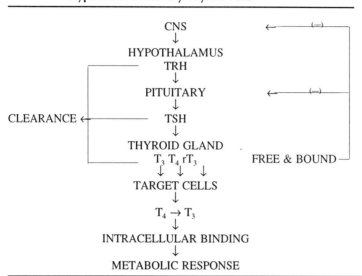

are deiodinated and deaminated in the tissues, conjugated in the liver, and excreted in the bile, feces, and urine.

B. Structural Changes in the Thyroid Gland With Aging

Characteristic of aging is a progressive decrease in gland size from maturity on, although in some cases the thyroid remains unchanged or may even enlarge due to the presence of nodules.[5,6] An increase may also be caused by mild endemic goiter (hypothyroidism due to iodine deficiency), but the incidence of this condition is higher at young ages.[7]

While the general shape of the gland is constant, several histological changes take place with aging and may lead to reduced function.[8,9] These include:

- Distension of follicles;
- Discoloration of colloid;
- Flattening of the follicular epithelium suggestive of reduced secretory activity;
- Fewer mitoses suggestive of reduced cell turnover;
- Increased fibrosis of interstitial connective tissue and parenchyma; and
- Vascular changes of atherosclerotic nature suggestive of decreased transport between cells, blood, and follicles.

The presence of nodules is another characteristic of the thyroid gland in some old individuals. Nodules consist of localized tissue proliferation with overlapping areas of cell involution and are frequently found in hyperthyroid elderly. The prevalence of micronodules and clinically palpable nodules, however, has been reported both to increase and to decrease with aging (Figure 5-3).[5-7] The prevalence of multinodular goiter may be as high as 70% in women over 60 years of age and might be associated with increased antithyroid antibodies (as manifested in the autoimmune diseases of the thyroid gland, discussed below). The much lower prevalence of goiter and nodules in men than in women does not vary significantly with age. Evaluation of thyroid nodules in elderly patients shows that, although more frequent, they are more benign (i.e., less likely to progress to carcinoma) than in young individuals. Nevertheless, occult thyroid cancer has been reported in 4 to 8% of patients with nodular goiter, irrespective of age.[10]

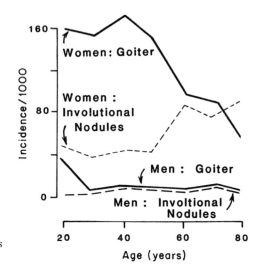

FIGURE 5-3 Incidence of thyroid goiter and nodules with age in men and women.

C. Changes in Blood Thyroid Hormone Levels

Of the two major thyroid hormones, T3 is biologically more active than T4 although T4 is the principal hormone secreted by the thyroid gland. Circulating T3 is derived primarily (about 80%) from deiodination of plasma T4 in the liver and kidney and not directly by secretion from the thyroid gland. The greater affinity of T3 for nuclear receptors as compared to T4 is the major reason for the greater T3 biological activity. Several proteins (globulin, albumin) bind to the circulating hormones and only the very small amounts of "free" (not protein-bound) hormones are the determinants of thyroid hormone activity. The protein-bound hormone comprises a large store which can dissociate to release the effective free hormone.

Changes with aging in thyroid hormone levels are controversial due to the variability of responses to various stimuli and diseases (Figure 5-4).[11-16] Total and free T4 levels may be unchanged, slightly decreased, or increased depending on age, sex, and general health.[17,18] In euthyroid healthy geriatric individuals, serum T4 levels declined by 15 to 20% in some individuals but increased by a similar percentage in others, irrespective of body weight, diagnosis, drug treatment, or age (ranging from 69 to 95 years). In most studies, T4 levels do not change with advancing age even when thyroid secretion may have decreased, in some cases, by as much as 50%.[19] A slowed hepatic (and tissue) metabolism and reduced renal excretion of the hormones may compensate — as in the case of glucocorticoids — for the reduced secretion. As for T4, the levels of the binding proteins (especially globulin) in serum have been reported unchanged, decreased, or increased with aging. However, the ratio of bound to free hormone, particularly in the absence of debilitating diseases, remains constant into old age.

While rT3 levels remain unchanged or may be slightly increased into old age, T3 blood levels are significantly reduced, but this reduction is often limited to individuals suffering from undernutrition and disease — frequent correlates of old age. Decreased T3 blood levels may reflect:

- Impaired T4 to T3 conversion in tissues;[20]
- Increased T3 degradation, metabolism, and excretion;
- Decreased T3 secretion from the thyroid gland due either to failure of TSH stimulation or primary, intrinsic alteration of the gland.

Current data do not permit distinguishing among these mechanisms nor do they exclude the possibility of a combination of all of them.[21-23]

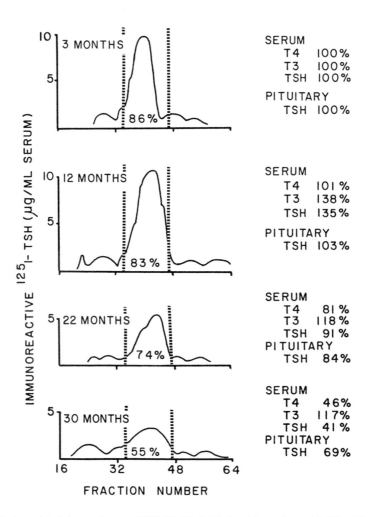

FIGURE 5-4 Age-related changes in serum TSH, T4, T3, in T4 thyroid secretion and in T4 to T3 conversion in tissues of humans. Changes from adult (50 years of age) to old age (85 years) are indicated by direction (+ or -) and the range by the hatching.

In summary, in healthy humans, old age is associated with

- Lower circulating T3 levels than at younger ages but generally within the normal (lower) range,
- Simultaneously decreased secretion and metabolic clearance of T4 with resulting essentially normal levels,
- Decreased peripheral conversion of T4 to T3, and
- Elevated TSH levels in 10% of the elderly, associated with an increase in antithyroid antibodies and present even in the absence of manifestations of hypothyroidism.

With respect to laboratory animals, not only are there differences with humans but also inter- and intraspecies differences.

D. Changes in the Hypothalamo-Pituitary-Thyroid Axis

Basal TSH levels are elevated in some relatively healthy persons over the age of 60, more so in women than in men, and often with normal T3 and T4 levels.[21-23] Whether such relatively

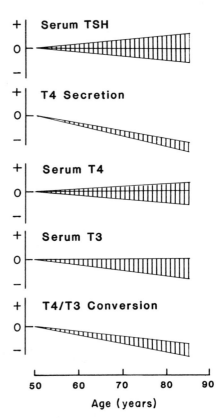

FIGURE 5-5 Changes with age (3 to 30 months) in TSH immunoreactivity in male Fisher-344 rats. Left: changes in TSH fractionation profile at progressive ages. Serum TSH was radioimmunoassayed to obtain the illustrated profiles. The amount of immunoreactive TSH in each fraction was corrected for the original serum volume and for the recovery from the affinity column so that the four plots are directly comparable. The percentages are relative to the total TSH recovered. Right: serum T4, T3, and TSH and pituitary TSH values measured at the same corresponding ages, taking three months as 100%. (Redrawn from Choy, V. J., Klemme, W. R., and Timiras, P. S., *Mech. Ageing Dev.*, 19, 273, 1982).

high TSH levels are a sign of mild hypothyroidism associated with old age or of alterations in the negative feedback of thyroid hormones on TSH has not been clarified in humans.

In the rat, both quantitative and qualitative TSH changes have been demonstrated.[24] The TSH glycoprotein is present in several forms, differing in molecular weight and immunoreactivity. In old rats, the major TSH form, which is also biologically the most active, decreases progressively while concomitantly the proportions of low- and high-molecular weight forms increase (Figure 5-5). The biologic significance of this age-related increase in TSH polymorphism remains speculative. Polymorphism is not limited exclusively to TSH but occurs in the other glycoprotein hormones of the pituitary, FSH and LH. In these gonadotropins the proportion of polymorphic forms also increases with age.[25]

In old rats, with the increased TSH levels and polymorphism, the typical circadian cyclicity of blood hormone levels is abolished. The functional significance of TSH rhythmicity is still obscure; however, the loss of specific pulsatile signals may suggest a progressive failure with aging of fine tuning of thyroid function. Additionally, in some rat strains low levels of T3 and/ or T4 occur together with normal or reduced TSH levels rather than the elevated TSH levels expected under these conditions (due to negative feedback on the pituitary). Impairment of thyroid hormone-pituitary negative feedback has been interpreted as a major factor in the alterations of the thyroid state with aging.

TSH levels are modulated not only by the circulating levels of T3 and T4 but also by the stimulatory effect of TRH on the synthesis and release of the hormone from the pituitary. The TRH test (based on TRH administration and subsequent measurement of circulating TSH and thyroid hormones), a sensitive tool in the diagnosis of the disorders of the hypothalamo-pituitary axis, shows an intact TSH responsiveness into old age. This is particularly well proven in women but less certain in men in whom the response is extremely variable.[26,27] Changes in extrahypothalamic TRH with advancing age have been discussed in Chapter 3.

E. Changes in Thyroid Hormone Receptors

The relative adequacy of the pituitary-thyroid axis into old age contrasts with the apparent symptoms of an altered thyroid state in the elderly. One possible explanation for this contrast is that age-related alterations occur essentially at the peripheral level,[28] primarily within the target cell and involve, to a lesser extent, the hypothalamo-pituitary-thyroid axis. Cellular actions are mediated through the binding of the hormone to specific cell molecules, the first-line being T3 receptors.

Thyroid hormone receptors, primarily for T3, have been identified in the nucleus, mito-chondria, plasma membrane, and cytosol.[29] The biologic actions of the hormone occur through nuclear binding and stimulation of protein synthesis.[30] *In vitro* studies of T3 nuclear binding in rat liver and brain show that the receptor number remains unchanged with aging. This absence of changes in receptor number occurs even though low circulating T4 levels *in vivo* might have forecast an upward regulation (indeed, the number of receptors seems to be inversely related to the circulating hormone levels — increasing when the levels are low and decreasing when they are high). The inability of tissues from old animals to adjust the receptor number upwards in response to low hormone levels suggests fundamental alterations in peripheral (cellular) hormone utilization.

In vivo, the major source of intracellular T3 is local conversion from T4. In the pituitary, the principal negative feedback at the thyrotrope is probably T4 taken from the blood and converted *in situ* to T3. *In vivo* administration of radiolabeled T4 results in lowered cytoplas-mic free T4 and T3 values in the brains of old as compared to adult rats and in high bound T4 values.[31] Furthermore, the amount of T3 derived intracellularly from conversion of T4 is reduced in the old animals, and nuclear binding of T3 is also reduced. These data indicate a reduction with aging of intracellular T3 production (from T4). At the same time, plasma T4 levels decrease with aging in these (Long-Evans strain) rats due to reduced thyroid secretion and this, combined with the reduced intracellular conversion, would result in markedly reduced availability of T3 for nuclear binding and, therefore, reduced T3 actions (Figure 5-6).

An alternative explanation for the decreased peripheral effectiveness of T3 actions is the presence of an antithyroid factor. One such factor of pituitary origin and secreted in progres-sively higher levels with advancing age was postulated some years ago,[32] but so far has not been isolated and the derived hypothesis is no longer plausible.

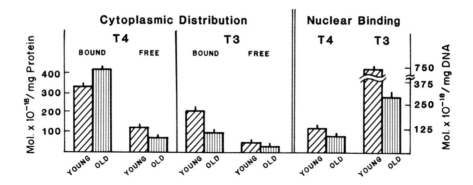

FIGURE 5-6 Changes with age in T3 and T4 cytoplasmic distribution and nuclear binding in cerebral hemispheres of rats. Cerebral bound T4 increases and free T4 decreases in 24-month-old as compared to 2-month-old Long-Evans male rats. Lower levels in older animals suggest depressed T4 deiodination with aging. The depressed free cytoplasmic T4 and T3 levels are also reflected in decreased nuclear binding of these hormones, particularly of T3. Similar results were also reported in the liver. (Redrawn from Margarity, M., Valcana, T., and Timiras, P. S., *Mech. Ageing Dev.*, 29, 191, 1985.)

III. PHYSIOPATHOLOGIC CORRELATES OF AGING-INDUCED THYROID HORMONE ALTERATIONS

Of the major actions of thyroid hormones listed in Table 5-1, those directing growth and development cease once adulthood has been reached. In some instances, still controversial, thyroid hormones appear to promote growth of adult tissues, even those such as the nervous tissue that reach maturity early in life.[33] A facilitatory action of these hormones has been reported in the recovery of spinal cord and peripheral nerve injuries in humans and other animals and in the induction of adrenergic enzymes in the adrenal medulla *in vitro*,[34] perhaps through the stimulatory action of T3 on the synthesis of nerve growth factor (NGF).[35] Catch-up whole-body growth and rehabilitation of some behaviors, induced by thyroid deficiency at an early age, have been described in adult rats after return to the normal thyroid state.[36,37]

Other actions of the thyroid hormones extant at all ages, but particularly important in old age, involve the cardiovascular system. Because of their complexity they will be mentioned here only briefly despite their relevance to aging and lifespan:

- Cholesterol levels are increased (and cholesterol metabolism is slowed down) in hypothyroidism, which, therefore, becomes a risk factor in atherosclerosis;
- Cardiac output depends indirectly on the thyroid state due to the stimulatory interaction of thyroid hormones and catecholamines on cardiac rate and strength of contraction;[11]
- Peripheral vascular resistance is decreased in hyperthyroidism due to increased cutaneous vasodilation.

Significant for the mental and neurologic state of the elderly are the behavioral changes which accompany alterations in the thyroid state.[38] Rapid mentation, increased irritability, restlessness, tachycardia, and sweating are frequent in hyperthyroid adults, and the opposite symptoms (slow mentation, slow responsiveness, apathy, fatigue, dry skin) in the hypothyroid; in the elderly, the mental state of hyperthyroid and hypothyroid individuals often are similar and characterized by severe depression (e.g., "apathetic thyrotoxicosis") and in some cases, dementia. These behavioral disturbances are probably mediated through neurotransmitter effects and not through changes in oxygen consumption which is unaffected by thyroid hormones in the adult and aged brain.[39]

A. Basal Metabolic Rate

T3 regulation of metabolic processes is manifested by its action on the basal metabolic rate (BMR), that is, the rate at which oxygen is consumed and carbon dioxide produced under conditions of physiologic and mental rest. BMR is customarily measured in terms of kilocalories per unit of time and body surface and has a value of approximately 39 to 40 kcal/m^2 of body surface/hour for a healthy (euthyroid) male weighing 80 kg and aged 20 to 30 years.

With age, from adolescence to old age, BMR decreases progressively in both men and women — in the latter, values are always slightly lower than in men — from 46 kcal in men and 43 kcal in women at 14 to 16 years of age, to 35 and 33 kcal, respectively, at 70 to 80 years of age. The cause for this progressive decrease is not known.[40] It may be associated at least in part with the age-related decline in T3 activity at the target cells, even though this decline is only slight and does not occur in all elderly.

The decrease in BMR with aging has also been ascribed to a progressive preponderance of adipose body mass (metabolically less active) at the expense of the diminishing lean body mass (metabolically more active). The metabolically active tissues and cells (such as muscle) would decrease with aging, as shown by an age-related decline in total body (or specific organ or tissue) potassium (the major intracellular electrolyte) and an increase in urinary excretion of creatine, a product of muscle metabolism. However, these very metabolic alterations could also result from changing hormone levels and cellular demands.

B.   Reduced Cell Demand or Reduced Hormone Secretion?

As in the case of the adrenal and the adrenal steroids (Chapters 2 and 14) and the pancreas and insulin (Chapters 10 and 11), both peripheral metabolism of thyroid hormones and tissue demands for these hormones may be altered with aging: T4 and corticosteroid turnover rates decline and resistance to insulin increases with aging. The most common explanation for the decline in thyroid hormone demand is the loss or reduction of metabolically active (lean) tissue mass. However, this explanation is not without flaws: endocrine changes usually occur early in life and precede body composition changes; such changes do not affect all individuals equally, and even when they occur, they may be secondary to endocrine changes.

Rather, altered responses to hormones may be due to a general decrease in protein synthesis and impaired target cell function (Chapters 17 and 19). Thyroid hormones necessary for growth and development when energy requirements are high, may become detrimental when the only energy needed is for homeostasis. A selective impairment of the general metabolic actions of thyroid hormones may occur with cessation of growth and subsequent aging, without a concomitant loss of catabolic effects. Injections of high doses of T4 are tolerated quite well in young animals: the animals respond with increased appetite and more rapid growth. The same doses injected in adult animals result in muscle wasting and body weight loss. These and other findings have led to the suggestions that there is an homeostatic wisdom in the arrangement whereby conversion of T4 to T3 is inhibited when metabolism is already hyperactive.[41] From this perspective the decline in thyroid hormone metabolism in old animals would reflect a need for protection against the catabolic actions of these hormones.[42] Therefore, the reduced intracellular availability of T3 for nuclear binding, and the consequent effects on protein synthesis, may represent an adaptive beneficial response to the decreased metabolic needs of the aged individual.

C.   Calorigenesis and Thermoregulation

T3 stimulates oxygen consumption in almost all tissues except adult brain, testis, uterus, spleen, lymph nodes, and anterior pituitary. The subsequent increased cellular metabolic rate leads to increased heat production or calorigenesis.

The thermogenetic effects of T3 depend on the initial metabolic rate and catecholamine interactions: the higher the levels of catecholamines and the lower the BMR at the time of T3 administration, the greater the calorigenic effect. With aging, thermoregulation is progressively impaired due to alterations in thyroid hormone function and in other metabolic and neural adjustments. Thermoregulation depends on the balance between heat production (stimulated by muscular contraction, food assimilation, and metabolic hormones) and heat loss (induced by conduction and radiation through skin, mucosae, sweat, respiration, urination, and defecation). In homeothermic (warm-blooded) animals, including humans, this balance is preserved by reflex and hormone responses integrated in the hypothalamus for the purpose of maintaining body temperature within a narrow range in spite of wide fluctuations of environmental temperature. With aging, alterations occur at several levels of thermoregulation:

- In peripheral temperature sensation as part of the sensory decline associated with old age;
- In the hypothalamus as part of autonomic and neuroendocrine decline; and
- In the higher cerebrocortical centers, with deficient perception and integration of the multiple inputs that are essential to determine adaptive effectiveness.

Inadequate thermoregulation with aging leads to the higher mortality of the elderly during "heat" or "cold waves" and may be attributed not only to physiologic decrements but often to economic (poor diet, clothing, housing) and emotional and mental (depression, dementia) impairments.

In rodents, when old rats are immersed in cold water body temperature falls lower and takes longer to return to normal than in younger animals.[43] This decreased thermoregulatory competence associated with aging can be delayed by modification of the aging process. Dietary restriction (by administration of a low tryptophan diet), initiated at weaning and continued for one year and followed by a normal diet, induces significant extension of thermoregulatory responses. The fall in body temperature is less severe and the return to normal is faster in old rats placed on the restricted regimen during their first year of life. This persistence of efficient thermoregulation in old animals represents one manifestation of the beneficial effects of dietary restriction on aging processes in rodents.

Responses to heat are also impaired with aging, as illustrated by a slower and delayed onset of sweating in the elderly. Fever response, the most universal hallmark of disease, is reduced as well. Fever depends on a "resetting" of the hypothalamic thermostat in response to a variety of agents (e.g., bacteria-induced interleukin-1; prostaglandins). Hypothalamic resetting is dampened in old humans and other animals.[44]

D. Cholesterol Metabolism

Serum cholesterol levels rise with aging in a number of animals including humans despite a fall in hepatic cholesterol synthesis, indicating altered cellular metabolism and turnover with consequent implications for the pathogenesis of atherosclerosis. The similarity of these changes to those seen in hypothyroidism has prompted several attempts to treat hyperlipidemia with thyroid hormones and their analogs.[45,46] Thyroidectomy in rats and other mammals reduces cholesterol turnover and elevates serum levels while exercise increases thyroid hormone levels and reduces cholesterol. In humans, a hyperbolic fall in serum cholesterol occurs with increasing T3 levels and, conversely, declining serum T3 levels are associated with decreased turnover of low-density lipoproteins and consequent cholesterol increase in both hypothyroid and aged individuals. The significance of altered lipoprotein metabolism in the development of atherosclerosis suggests that early attempts by investigators to relate declining thyroid function with factors predisposing to atherosclerotic lesions may not be entirely without foundation.

E. TSH Antibodies and Thyroid Autoimmune Diseases

The frequency of antithyroid antibodies primarily directed to TSH receptors on thyroid cells increases with age, reaching 20% after the age of 70 in women.[12,47] This may be due to the decline in the self-recognition ability of the immune system (Chapter 20) as well as the increased TSH polymorphism.

The incidence of the two probable autoimmune diseases of the thyroid — Graves' disease or toxic diffuse goiter and Hashimoto's disease or chronic lymphocytic thyroiditis — increases with age. Some of the characteristics of both diseases are summarized in Table 5-3. Although the events that trigger these diseases are not known, the immune system is strongly implicated.[12] These diseases may represent the extremes of a continuum of signs and symptoms resulting from a deranged immune system with hyperthyroidism at one end and hypothyroidism at the other. Antibodies against TSH receptors or components of the thyroid cell are present in both disorders, although in different proportions. TSH receptor antibodies compete with TSH at the receptor site on the thyroid cell and may either stimulate T4 and T3 secretion (Graves's) or block access to TSH and reduce hormone secretion (Hashimoto's).

Other antithyroid antibodies are those directed against thyroglobulin, the thyroid cell protein precursor of T4 and T3, antibodies against microsomal and nuclear components, and antibodies against T3 and T4 . The presence of these antibodies and the frequent invasion of the thyroid tissue by lymphocytes contribute to thyroid destruction.

TABLE 5-3 Immune System: Autoimmune Diseases of the Thyroid

Characteristics	Graves' Disease (Toxic Diffuse Goiter)	Hashimoto's Thyroiditis (Chronic Lymphocytic Thyroiditis)
Thyroid Status	Hyperthyroid	Hypothyroid
TSH	- Generally undetectable	- Normal to vastly elevated
T4, T3 (serum)	- Above normal	- Below normal
TSH-Receptor	Incidence - 80%	Incidence - 10%
Antibodies (ABs)	- ABs compete with TSH action at receptor site - Hence loss of TSH control over thyroid function	- Some ABs in this class block TSH action
Autoantibodies Against thyroglobulin, T3, T4, Thyroid microsomal and nuclear components	- Generally present	- Generally present
Lymphocytic Invasion	- Limited	- Marked (development of germinal center plasma cells)
Female:Male Ratio	- As high as 10:1	- As high as 10:1

IV. ABNORMAL THYROID STATES IN THE ELDERLY

The frequency of an altered thyroid state increases with advancing age.[13-16,48-50] Hypothyroidism has been identified in 2 to 4% of a population of geriatric patients and hyperthyroidism (more common among women) in 7 to 12%.[47] This age-related increase is often masked by the atypical manifestations in the elderly of an altered thyroid state. Thus, although modalities for treatment of thyroid disease are readily available and straightforward, the subtleties of diagnosis in the elderly often provide a challenge for the clinician. In the elderly, signs and symptoms of thyroid disease may be minimal, are frequently atypical, and are commonly assumed to be an inevitable consequence of aging or of other more common diseases of old age.[22,23,48-51]

A. Hyperthyroidism

Thyroid hormone excess or hyperthyroidism is caused by toxic (i.e., hypersecreting) *nodular goiter*; its prevalence is higher in older individuals while in younger individuals toxic *diffuse goiter* (e.g., Graves' disease) is prevalent. The majority of hyperthyroid patients over the age of 60 presents with clinical features of cardiovascular (or other age-associated) disease, hence the term of "masked hyperthyroidism" (Table 5-4). In general, most of the hyperkinetic features (related to catecholamine synergism) are minimal or absent in elderly patients

TABLE 5-4 Common Signs and Symptoms of Hyperthyroidism in the Elderly

Cardiovascular abnormalities
    Congestive heart failure
    Atrial fibrillation
    Angina
    Pulmonary edema
Tremor
Nervousness
Weakness
Weight loss and anorexia
Palpable goiter (possible ?)
Exophthalmos (possible ?)
Thyroid nodules

TABLE 5-5 Characteristics of Apathetic Hyperthyroidism

Blunted affect, i.e., withdrawal behavior with apathy and depression
Absence of hyperkinetic motor activity
Slowed mentation
Proximal weakness
Diarrhea
Edema of the lower extremity
Droopy eyelids
Cardiovascular abnormalities

whereas the signs related to tissue catabolism are prominent. In contrast to younger patients, the presenting symptom in the elderly is usually referable to a single organ system and the more widespread clinical features become apparent only on closer examination.

In one study, 79% of the elderly subjects had cardiovascular abnormalities; 67% had symptoms of congestive heart failure, 39% were in atrial fibrillation, 20% had symptoms of angina, and 8% presented pulmonary edema. Typical signs and symptoms such as tremor, nervousness, muscular weakness, depression, eye manifestations (e.g., exophthalmos and lid retraction) and weight loss are either absent or are ignored as they are common in the elderly. Since thyroid nodules are common in the elderly, it is difficult to raise suspicion of significant thyroid disease solely on the basis of their presence.

"Apathetic hyperthyroidism" is another term coined to designate a thyroid disease in the elderly. This condition, with several symptoms resembling those of hypothyroidism, is characterized by blunted affect (i.e., withdrawal behavior with depression and apathy), absence of hyperkinetic motor activity, slowed mentation, weakness, diarrhea, edema of the lower extremities, droopy eyelids, and cardiovascular abnormalities (Table 5-5). Untreated, this condition may insidiously decline into coma and death, but can be satisfactorily reversed with appropriate therapy.

Laboratory tests of hyperthyroidism or serum T3 and T4 determinations and a radionuclide thyroid scan can help differentiate Graves' disease from toxic nodular goiter. Treatment includes oral antithyroid medication (e.g., with the goitrogen propylthiouracil, which inhibits thyroid hormonogenesis) and radioactive (with radioactive iodine) or surgical ablation (thyroidectomy) of the gland.

B. Hypothyroidism

Thyroid hormone deficiency (hypothyroidism) may be congenital or caused by iodine deficiency or excess (as in the coastal goiter seen in Japan), by the ingestion of goitrogens which inhibit hormonogenesis (particularly when iodine intake is marginal), autoimmune disease, or excessive treatment of hyperthyroidism. Just as masked hyperthyroidism exists in the elderly so does "masked hypothyroidism" (Table 5-6). Typical symptoms of hypothyroidism such as fatigue, weakness, constipation, dry skin, hair loss, mental confusion, depression, and cold intolerance may be attributed to old age rather than thyroid deficiency. In addition, the insidious onset and slow progression of hypothyroidism makes it more difficult to diagnose. Laboratory diagnosis of hypothyroidism is best made by measuring plasma TSH levels, which are elevated, rather than measuring T4 or T3 levels which may remain apparently normal in mild cases. As with hyperthyroidism, the major signs involve the cardiovascular system and include dyspnea (a sensation of shortness of breath) in over half of the patients, chest pains in one quarter, and enlarged heart and bradycardia (slow cardiac rate) in most. Other frequent symptoms include anorexia (poor appetite), muscular weakness, mild anemia, depression (often severe), and joint pain.

TABLE 5-6 Common Signs and Symptoms of Hypothyroidism
in Elderly Patients that are Frequently Missed

Cardiovascular
Dyspnea
Chest pain
Enlarged heart
Bradycardia
Anorexia and constipation
Muscular weakness
Mild anemia
Depression
Cold intolerance
Joint pain

Treatment of hypothyroidism consists of appropriate replacement therapy primarily with T4, keeping in mind the necessity of administering the elderly lower doses than younger patients with the same degree of thyroid deficiency.

C. Screening for Thyroid Function

Given the difficulties of differential diagnosis of thyroid disease in the elderly, the role of laboratory screening becomes very important.[17,18,51-53] It has been argued that screening of the thyroid function in an healthy ambulatory geriatric population is not worthwhile. However, certain guidelines can be established for selection of those cases in which such screening is necessary. Patients over 60 years of age should have laboratory screening for thyroid disease under the following conditions: admission to acute-care hospital, nursing home, or psychiatric ward, dementia or altered mental status, and tachyarrhythmia, including atrial fibrillation.

Thyroid disease states, although potentially difficult to diagnose clinically in the elderly, can be detected if the possibility is entertained. The relative ease and success of treatment (once the risk of greater susceptibility of the elderly to thyroid hormone is taken into account)[53] makes such detection well worth while.

D. Thyroid Status and Longevity

Support for a role of thyroid hormones in the regulation of lifespan can be drawn from several lines of evidence such as the commonality of receptor genes among hormones (thyroid and some steroid hormones) involved in adaptation (hence, influencing the lifespan), experiments on longevity in rats under different thyroid states, and the possibility that thyroid hormones act as a signal for regulation of growth and development as well as aging.

The thyroid hormone receptor has been identified with multiple c-erbA genes in human chromosomes 3 and 17 and has been characterized as the cellular homolog of the v-erbA oncogen product.[54] Thus, the thyroid receptor belongs to the same gene family as the receptor for cortisol and estradiol, the three receptors forming a "superfamily" of regulatory genes. This commonality is also suggested by the transcriptional synergism of glucocorticoids and T3. The kinship of the thyroid hormone receptor with the steroid hormone receptors indicate that these molecules may all be part of regulatory proteins that have arisen over evolutionary time to match the increasing developmental and physiological needs of the more complex organism. The multiplicity of c-erbA genes in humans also predicts the existence of multiple receptors, and indeed, structurally different forms of T3 receptors have been characterized in the adult rat brain.[55,56] It seems likely that several genetic loci, encoding specific functional molecules, underlie the existence of a family of thyroid receptors that coordinately regulate overlapping networks of genes to control developmental (in the young) as well as metabolic and behavioral (in the adult) functions.[30] Aging may be the consequence of a genetic program geared to regulate development and aging or may result from the interruption and loss of the genetic program.[57]

The lower circulating T3 in the elderly and T4 in the aged rat, and the reduced conversion of T4 to T3 in target tissues, may be interpreted as beneficial compensations for the catabolic actions of thyroid hormones; they would represent a certain "homeostatic wisdom" reflecting the changing metabolic needs of the organism. That this may be the case is corroborated by studies in which rats made hypothyroid neonatally outlived the corresponding controls (with an average lifespan of 30 months) by about 4 months for males and 1 month for females.[3] The higher levels of T3 and T4 in males than females may explain these sex differences and the shorter lifespan of males; in females, hormonal influences may only slightly add to their already longer life. The life-extending effects of hypothyroidism resemble those found after removal of the pituitary gland.[58] They also resemble effects of dietary restriction, for the body and organ weights of hypothyroid rats are significantly reduced as compared to freely fed rats and growth inhibition may act as an anti-aging factor.[59] When thyroid hormone levels are increased (by exogenous T4 administration) for one or two years from an early age, the average lifespan is significantly shortened in the treated rats, but remains unchanged if the treatment is started in senescence. Thus, the life-shortening effects of excess thyroid hormones may not be due to the direct action of the hormones to initiate or promote old age diseases, the direct cause of death — rather, high thyroid hormone levels may accelerate the aging process by hastening the timetable of development. Thyroid hormones are seen as pacemakers capable of signaling not only certain key events during development (e.g., metamorphosis of tadpoles into frogs) but also signaling the aging process.

V. THYRO-PARATHYROID HORMONES

In humans, the four parathyroid glands embedded in the thyroid gland secrete the parathyroid hormone (PTH). The so-called C-cells, dispersed throughout the thyroid gland, the parathyroids, and the thymus (as well as identified in several other tissues) secrete another hormone, calcitonin (CT). Both PTH and CT are polypeptides; they play a significant role in the maintenance of calcium homeostasis, particularly with respect to bone. While PTH is the major hormone involved in calcium metabolism, thyroid hormones, as well, appear to act directly on bone resorption, formation, and remodeling.[60] Thyroid hormones may activate the rate of bone turnover, thereby allowing for faster bone repair and minimizing bone loss,[61] perhaps by influencing gut absorption of calcium, PTH, CT, and vitamin D.[21,62,63] States of thyroid hormone excess and deficiency are associated with alterations in bone integrity as evidenced by enzymatic, radiologic, and clinical signs and these signs can be normalized by the appropriate therapy.[64]

A. Bone Modeling and Remodeling

Both cortical (outer, more compact) and trabecular (inner, more porous) portions of bone consist of an organic matrix, collagen, and a solid, inorganic mineral phase of calcium and phosphorus. Availability of calcium for deposition into the matrix depends upon the balance of gains from intestinal absorption and excretory losses through the feces, urine, and sweat. Even in the normal state and at a young age, bone mineral content is not static, but represents a major supply source of calcium circulating through a continuous remodeling process (Chapter 13).

Bone remodeling processes involve several steps. "Modeling" refers to the initial growth of bones, as in the rapid elongation seen at adolescence. Bone "remodeling" occurs by a combination of resorption and new bone formation and represents the mechanism by which old bone is renewed. It occurs throughout life in the so-called Harvesian periosteal and endosteal envelopes and is defined by a set sequence of events. Cells are activated to become osteoclasts which then destroy and reabsorb bone. Osteoblasts, capable of generating new bone invade the area of resorption and deposit new bone. The sequence operates through the coupling of osteoclast and osteoblast functions into bone multicellular remodeling units.[61]

Rates of new bone formation and reabsorptive remodeling are equal and bone mass remains constant. Starting in young adulthood (25 to 30 years) bone mass is progressively lost with a negative net mineral balance: calcium loss by excretion exceeds dietary intake/absorption and bone resorption exceeds bone formation. Under these conditions bone mass is reduced, leading to osteoporosis and a high incidence of bone fractures (Chapter 13). This reduction depends on multiple factors:

- Genetic factors;
- Negative calcium balance due to decreased intestinal absorption;
- Defective renal adaptation to low calcium intake;
- Decreased lean body mass and mobility consequent to joint and muscle dysfunction and reduced weight-bearing;
- Decreased levels of vitamin D (due to reduced sun exposure) of the often immobilized, homebound elderly;
- Alterations in PTH, T3, and CT secretion and metabolism;
- Several drugs (steroids, anticonvulsants, alcohol); and
- Smoking.

B. PTH, CT, and Vitamin D Actions

The major action of PTH is to maintain normal levels of blood calcium. In response to hypocalcemia, PTH raises the concentration of plasma calcium by:

- Increasing renal calcium reabsorption;
- Mobilizing calcium from bones by stimulating the activity of osteoclasts, vitamin D being required for this action to take place;
- In the presence of adequate amounts of vitamin D, stimulating the absorption of calcium in the small intestine; and
- Lowering levels of plasma inorganic phosphate by inhibiting renal reabsorption of phosphate.

Calcitonin is secreted not only in response to calcium levels but also to gastrointestinal hormones such as glucagon. When administered in high (pharmacologic) doses, it lowers plasma calcium and phosphate levels by inhibiting bone resorption. However, it remains controversial whether the hormone plays an important physiological role in normal calcium metabolism.[65] CT would protect against the excess bone resorption that might otherwise be seen during times of high demand of calcium, such as pregnancy, lactation, and accelerated growth.[66] CT may augment renal clearance of calcium and phosphorus, thereby reducing their blood levels, but it does not appear to affect intestinal calcium absorption. It has also some minor action on water and electrolytes and decreases gastric acid secretion.

Vitamin D (as vitamin D_2, ergocalciferol, and vitamin D_3, cholecalciferol) is also considered a hormone regulator of calcium metabolism.[67] It reaches the body in two ways, by dietary ingestion and, under the influence of ultraviolet radiation (sunlight), by synthesis in the skin. It is hydroxylated in the liver to form 25-hydroxyvitamin D, and is further hydroxylated in the kidneys to form 1,25-dihydroxyvitamin D. It promotes calcium absorption from the small intestine; its deficiency leads to bone abnormalities (e.g., rickets, osteomalacia).

C. Changes With Aging

Structural changes with aging in the parathyroids and C-cells of humans and laboratory animals are few (e.g., presence of degenerating cells containing colloid and mitochondria showing bizarre patterns),[68] although in old rats the ratio of C-cells to thyroid cells appears to increase.

The study of immunoassayable PTH shows divergent results. PTH levels would decline after 60 years of age in white men but not in white women, with variable effects depending on race, or would increase with aging.[69,70] This increase in PTH levels may not be physiologically important as it may involve biologically inactive (but immunologically active) fragments of the molecule or may depend on impaired renal function.[71] Explanation for the increased PTH may be sought at the peripheral level (decreased metabolism and excretion), or at the endocrine gland itself (altered synthesis).[69,72,73] Both PTH and CT derive from the cleavage of preprohormones by proteases; with aging the cleavage of the precursor hormones may be altered, resulting in the secretion of less biologically active preprohormones rather than the adult biologically active hormone. Another interpretation relates PTH changes with aging to alterations in vitamin D. Vitamin D receptors have been identified in parathyroid cells and vitamin D metabolites reduce the synthesis of pre-pro-PTH mRNA.[74] When vitamin D levels are lowered, as occurs in the elderly,[75] synthesis, secretion, and circulating levels of PTH increase.[69] Such a provocative role for vitamin D in mediating an age-related increase in serum PTH is possible, but to date such a hypothesis remains to be substantiated.

Little is known of the changes, if any, with aging in CT, and their consequences. A decrease in CT has been reported in humans and is greater in men than women. However, *in vitro* studies show an increased immunoassayable CT in thyroid glands from old rats as compared to adult.[77] Since CT decreases bone resorption, its potential usefulness, eventually in association with the administration of thyroxine in the therapy of age-related demineralization and osteoporosis, has been explored but without beneficial results.[77]

D. Role of Calcium and Changes With Aging

Calcium has many actions indispensable for maintenance and regulation of vital functions (Table 5-7). The primary emphasis here has been on the role of calcium in bone. Other vital functions are summarized in Table 5-7. Several of these actions are altered with aging (Table 5-8). The consequences of these age-related changes may reflect or may depend on PTH and CT levels.[78-80] This interrelationship should be the basis of further studies as it has wide implications for cellular activities.

TABLE 5-7 Phenomena That May Be Regulated by Changes in Intracellular Calcium

Phenomena	Examples of regulation
Cell movement	Muscle contraction
	Ciliate and flagellate movement
	Chemotaxis
Cell excitability	Muscle action potential
	Myocardial action potential
	Response of the eye and other photoreceptors to light
Cell secretion	Neurotransmitter, hormone exocrine secretions
Phagocytosis	Engulfment of particles or soluble substances
Intermediary metabolism and respiration	Glucose production
	Lipolysis
	Blood coagulation
Reproduction	Ovum fertilization and sperm capacitation
	Ovum maturation and meiosis

TABLE 5-8 Intracellular Calcium-Dependent Changes Relating to Aging

Phenomena	Examples of regulation
Intermediary metabolism and respiration	Activation of oxygen radicals
	Obesity and diabetes
	Arthritis and other diseases
Tissue calcification	Loss of bone calcium (osteoporosis)
	Abnormal deposition on normal and injured tissues (e.g., atherosclerotic lesions)
Cell excitability	Changes in cell potentials
	Changes in response to drugs
Cell secretion	Alterations in neurotransmitter and hormone production
Phagocytosis	Alterations in immune responses

REFERENCES

1. Timiras, P. S., Neuroendocrinology of aging: retrospective, current, and prospective views, in *Neuroendocrinology of Aging,* Meites, J., Ed., Plenum Press, New York, 1983, 5.
2. Ooka, H. and Shinkai, T., Effects of chronic hyperthyroidism on the lifespan of the rat, *Mech. Ageing Dev.,* 33, 275, 1986.
3. Ooka, H., Fujita, S., and Yoshimoto, E., Pituitary-thyroid activity and longevity in neonatally thyroxine-treated rats, *Mech. Ageing Dev.,* 22, 113, 1983.
4. Crewe, F., Rejuvenation of the aged fowl through thyroid medication, *Proc. Roy. Soc.,* 45, 252, 1924-1925.
5. Hegedus, L., Perrild, H., Poulsen, L. R., Andersen, J. R., Holm, B., Schnohr, P., Jensen, G., and Hansen, J. M., The determination of thyroid volume by ultrasound and its relationship to body weight, age, and sex in normal subjects, *J. Clin. Endocrinol. Metab.,* 56, 260, 1983.
6. Hintze, G., Windeler, J., Baumert, J., Stein, H., and Kobberling, J., Thyroid volume and goitre prevalence in the elderly as determined by ultrasound and their relationships to laboratory indices, *Acta Endocrinol.,* 124, 12, 1991.
7. Berghout, A., Wiersinga, W. M., Smits, N. J., and Touber, J. L., Interrelationships between age, thyroid volume, thyroid nodularity, and thryoid function in patients with sporadic nontoxic goiter, *Am. J. Med.,* 89, 602, 1990.
8. Blumenthal, H. T. and Perlstein, I. B., The aging thyroid. I. A description of lesions and an analysis of their age and sex distribution, *J. Am. Geriatr. Soc.,* 35, 843, 1987.
9. Blumenthal, H. T. and Perlstein, I. B., The aging thyroid. II. An immunocytochemical analysis of the age-associated lesions, *J. Am. Geriatr. Soc.,* 35, 855, 1987.
10. Sampson, R. J., Woolner, L. B., Bahn, R. C., and Kurland, L. T., Occult thyroid carcinoma in Olmsted County, Minnesota: prevalence at autopsy compared with that in Hiroshima and Nagasaki, Japan, *Cancer,* 34, 2072, 1974.
11. Florini, J. R., Limitations of interpretation of age-related changes in hormone levels: illustration by effects of thyroid hormones on cardiac and skeletal muscle, *J. Gerontol.,* 44, B107, 1989.
12. Aizawa, T., Ishihara, M., Hashizume, K., Takasu, N., and Yamada, T., Age-related changes of thyroid function and immunologic abnormalities in patients with hyperthyroidism due to Graves' disease, *J. Am. Geriat. Soc.,* 37, 944, 1989.
13. Griffin, J. E., Hypothyroidism in the elderly, *Am. J. Med. Sci.,* 299, 334, 1990.
14. Runnels, B. L., Garry, P. J., Hunt, W. C., and Standefer, J. C., Thyroid function in a healthy elderly population: implications for clinical evaluation, *J. Gerontol.,* 46, B39, 1991.
15. Mintzer, M. J., Hypothyroidism and hyperthyroidism in the elderly, *J. Florida Med. Assoc.,* 79, 231, 1992.
16. Van Camp, G., Bourdoux, P. P., and Bonnyns, M. A., Age influence on clinical features in hospitalized thyroid patients: dissimilarity between clinical and laboratory findings in adulthood. A retrospective study, *Thyroidology,* 4, 75, 1992.
17. Cavalieri, T. A., Chopra, A., and Bryman, P. N., When outside the norm is normal: interpreting lab data in the aged, *Geriatrics,* 47, 66, 1992.
18. Melillo, K. D., Interpretation of laboratory values in older adults, *Nurse Practitioner,* 18, 59, 1993.
19. Gregerman, R. I. and Solomon, N., Acceleration of thyroxine and triiodothyronine turnover during bacterial pulmonary infections and fever: implications for the functional state of the thyroid during stress and in senescence, *J. Clin. Endocrinol. Metab.,* 27, 93, 1967.

20. Wenzel, K. W. and Horn, W. R., T3 and T4 kinetics in aged men, in *Thyroid Research: Proceedings of the Seventh International Thyroid Conference, Boston, MA, June 9-13, 1975*, Robbins, J. A., Braverman, L. E., Eds., Elsevier, New York, 1976, 270.
21. Schroffner, W. G., The aging thyroid in health and disease, *Geriatrics*, 42, 41, 1987.
22. Sawin, C. T., Castelli, W. P., Hershman, J. M., McNamara, P., and Bacharach, P., The aging thyroid. Thyroid deficiency in the Framingham Study, *Arch. Intern. Med.*, 145, 1386, 1985.
23. Sundbeck, G., Lundberg, P. A., Lindstedt, G., Svanborg, A., and Eden, S., Screening for thyroid disease in the elderly. Serum free thyroxine and thyrotropin concentrations in a representative population of 81-year-old women and men, *Aging*, 3, 31, 1991.
24. Choy, V. J., Klemme, W. R., and Timiras, P. S., Variant forms of immunoreactive thyrotropin in aged rats, *Mech. Ageing Dev.*, 19, 273, 1982.
25. Conn, P. M., Cooper, R., McNamara, C., Rogers, D. C., and Shoenhardt, L., Qualitative change in gonadotropin during normal aging in the male rat, *Endocrinology*, 106, 1549, 1980.
26. Snyder, P. J. and Utiger, R. D., Response to thyrotropin releasing hormone (TRH) in normal men, *J. Clin. Endocrinol. Metab.*, 34, 380, 1972.
27. Jacques, C., Schlienger, J. L., Kissel, C., Kuntzmann, F., and Sapin, R., TRH-induced TSH and prolactin responses in the elderly, *Age, Ageing*, 16, 181, 1987.
28. Naidoo, S. and Timiras, P. S., Effects of age on the metabolism of thyroid hormones by rat brain tissue in vitro, *Dev. Neurosci.*, 2, 213, 1979.
29. Eberhardt, N. L., Valcana, T., and Timiras, P. S., Triiodothyronine nuclear receptors: an in vitro comparison of the binding of triiodothyronine to nuclei of adult rat liver, cerebral hemisphere, and anterior pituitary, *Endocrinology*, 102, 556, 1978.
30. Leidig, F., Shepard, A. R., Zhang, W., Stelter, A., Cattini, P. A., Baxter, J. D., and Eberhardt, N. L., Thyroid hormone responsiveness in human growth hormone-related genes. Possible correlation with receptor-induced DNA conformational changes, *J. Biol. Chem.*, 267, 913, 1992.
31. Margarity, M., Valcana, T., and Timiras, P. S., Thyroxine deiodination, cytoplasmic distribution and nuclear binding of thyroxine and triiodothyronine in liver and brain of young and aged rats, *Mech. Ageing Dev.*, 29, 181, 1985.
32. Denckla, W. D., Role of pituitary and thyroid glands in decline of minimal O_2 consumption with age, *J. Clin. Invest.*, 53, 572, 1974.
33. Timiras, P. S., Thyroid hormones and the developing brain, in *Handbook of Human Growth and Developmental Biology*, Vol. I, part C., Meisami, E. and Timiras, P. S., Eds., CRC Press, Boca Raton, FL, 1988, 59.
34. Timiras, P. S. and Nzekwe, E. U., Thyroid hormones and nervous system development, *Biol. Neonate*, 55, 376, 1989.
35. Charrasse, S., Jehan, F., Confort, C., Brachet, P., and Clos, J., Thyroid hormone promotes transient nerve growth factor synthesis in rat cerebellar neuroblasts, *Dev. Neurosci.*, 14, 282, 1992.
36. Meisami, E., Complete recovery of growth deficits after reversal of PTU-induced postnatal hypothyroidism in the female rat: a model for catch-up growth, *Life Sci.*, 34, 1487, 1984.
37. Tamasy, V., Meisami, E., Vallerga, A., and Timiras, P. S., Rehabilitation from neonatal hypothyroidism: spontaneous motor activity, exploratory behavior, avoidance learning and responses of pituitary-thyroid axis to stress in male rats, *Psychoneuroendocrinology*, 11, 91, 1986.
38. Loosen, P. T., Effects of thyroid hormones on central nervous system in aging, *Psychoneuroendocrinology*, 17, 355, 1992.
39. Vaccari, A. and Timiras, P. S., Alterations in brain dopaminergic receptors in developing hypo- and hyperthyroid rats, *Neurochem. Intl.*, 3, 149, 1981.
40. Masoro, E. J., Metabolism, in *Handbook of the Biology of Aging*, 2nd ed., Finch, C. E. and Schneider, E. L., Eds., Van Nostrand Reinhold, New York, 1985, 540.
41. Chopra, I. J., Solomon, D. H., Chopra, U., Wu, S. Y., Fisher, D. A., and Nakamura, Y., Pathways of metabolism of thyroid hormones, *Recent Prog. Horm. Res.*, 34, 521, 1978.
42. Utiger, R. D., Decreased extrathyroidal triiodothyronine production in nonthyroidal illness: benefit or harm?, *Am J. Med.*, 69, 807, 1980.
43. Segall, P. E. and Timiras, P. S., Age-related changes in thermoregulatory capacity of tryptophan-deficient rats, *Fed. Proc.*, 34, 83, 1975.
44. Finch, C. E. and Landfield, P. W., Neuroendocrine and autonomic functions in aging mammals, in *Handbook of the Biology of Aging*, 2nd ed., Finch, C. E. and Schneider, E. L., Eds., Van Nostrand Reinhold, New York, 1985, 567.
45. Burrow, G. N., Thyroid hormone therapy in nonthyroid disorders, in *The Thyroid: A Fundamental and Clinical Text*, 4th ed., Werner, S. C. and Ingbar, S. H., Eds., Harper & Row, Hagerstown, MD, 1978, 947.
46. Sawin, C. T., Geller, A., Hershman, J. M., Castelli, W., and Bacharach, P., The aging thyroid. The use of thyroid hormone in older persons, *JAMA*, 261, 2653, 1989.

47. Melmed, S. and Hershman, J. M., The thyroid and aging, in *Endocrine Aspects of Aging*, Korenman, S. G., Ed., Elsevier, New York, 1982, 33.

48. Levy, E. G., Thyroid disease in the elderly, *Med. Clin. N. Am.*, 75, 151, 1991.

49. Francis, T. and Wartofsky, L., Common thyroid disorders in the elderly, *Postgrad. Med.*, 92, 225, 1992.

50. Mokshagundam, S. and Barzel, U. S., Thyroid disease in the elderly, *J. Am. Geriatr. Soc.*, 41, 1361, 1993.

51. Leovey, A., Sztojka, I., Paragh, G., and Mohacsi, A., Atypical clinical features of hypo- and hyperthyroidism in elderly age, *Terapia Hungarica*, 39, 167, 1991.

52. Felicetta, J. V., Thyroid changes with aging: significance and management, *Geriatrics*, 42, 86, 1987.

53. Robuschi, G., Safran, M., Braverman, L. E., Gnudi, A., and Roti, E., Hypothyroidism in the elderly, *Endocrine Rev.*, 8, 142, 1987.

54. Sap, J., Munoz, A., Damm, K., Goldberg, Y., Ghysdael, J., Leutz, A., Beug, H., and Vennstrom, B., The c-erb-A protein in a high-affinity receptor for thyroid hormone, *Nature*, 324, 635, 1986.

55. Gullo, D., Sinha, A. K., Bashir, A., Hubank, M., and Ekins, R. P., Differences in nuclear triiodothyronine binding in rat brain cells suggest phylogenetic specialization of neuronal functions, *Endocrinology*, 120, 2398, 1987.

56. Thompson, C. C., Weinberger, C., Lebo, R., and Evans, R. M., Identification of a novel thyroid hormone receptor expressed in the mammalian central nervous system, *Science*, 237, 1610, 1987.

57. Walker, R. F. and Timiras, P. S., Pacemaker insufficiency and the onset of aging, in *Cellular Pacemakers*, Vol. 2, Carpenter, D. O., Ed., John Wiley & Sons, New York, 1982, 345.

58. Everitt, A. V., Hormonal basis of aging: antiaging action of hypophysectomy, in *Regulation of Neuroendocrine Aging*, Everitt, A. V. and Walton, J. R., Eds., Karger, New York, 1988, 51.

59. Ooka, H., Segall, P. E., and Timiras, P. S., Neural and endocrine development after chronic tryptophan deficiency in rats. II. Pituitary-thyroid axis, *Mech. Ageing Dev.*, 7, 19, 1978.

60. Cooper, D. S., Thyroid hormone and the skeleton: a bone of contention, editorial, *JAMA*, 259, 3175, 1988.

61. McKenna, M. J. and Frame, B., Hormonal influences on osteoporosis, *Am. J. Med.*, 82, 61, 1987.

62. Benker, G., Breuer, N., Windeck, R., and Reinwein, D., Calcium metabolism in thyroid disease, *J. Endocrinol. Invest.*, 11, 61, 1988.

63. Goldring, S. R. and Krane, S. M., The skeletal system, in *Werner's The Thyroid: A Fundamental and Clinical Text*, 5th ed., Part IV, Section A, Ingbar, S. H. and Braverman, L. E., Eds., Lippincott, Philadelphia, 1986, 930.

64. Eriksen, E. F., Normal and pathological remodeling of human trabecular bone: three dimensional reconstruction of the remodeling sequence in normal and in metabolic bone disease, *Endocrinol. Rev.*, 7, 379, 1986.

65. Raue, F, Zink, A., and Scherubl, H., Regulation of calcitonin secretion and calcitonin gene expression, *Recent Results Cancer Research*, 125, 1, 1992.

66. Stevenson, J. C., Hillyard, C. J., MacIntyre, I., Cooper, H., and Whitehead, M. I., A physiological role for calcitonin: protection of the maternal skeleton, *Lancet*, 2, 769, 1979.

67. Bell, N. H., Vitamin D-endocrine system, *J. Clin. Invest.*, 76, 1, 1985.

68. Blumenthal, H. T. and Perlstein, I. B., The biopathology of aging of the endocrine system: the parathyroid glands, *J. Am. Geriatr. Soc.*, 41, 1116, 1993.

69. Endres, D. B., Morgan, C. H., Garry, P. J., and Omdahl, J. L., Age-related changes in serum immunoreactive parathyroid hormone and its biological action in healthy men and women, *J. Clin. Endocrinol. Metab.*, 65, 724, 1987.

70. Wiske, P. S., Epstein, S., Bell, N. H., Queener, S. F., Edmondson, J., and Johnston, C. C., Jr., Increases in immunoreactive parathyroid hormone with age, *N. Engl. J. Med.*, 300, 1419, 1979.

71. Liang, C. T., Hanai, H., Ishida, M., Cheng, L., and Sacktor, B., Regulation of renal sodium calcium exchange by PTH: alteration with age, *Environ. Health Perspectives*, 84, 137, 1990.

72. Fujita, T., Calcium, parathyroids and aging, *Contr. Nephrol.*, 90, 206, 1991.

73. Peacock, M., Interpretation of bone mass determinations as they relate to fracture: implications for asymptomatic primary hyperparathyroidism, *J. Bone Mineral Res.*, 6(Suppl. 2), S77, 1991.

74. Silver, J., Russell, J., and Sherwood, L. M., Regulation by vitamin D metabolites of messenger ribonucleic acid for preproparathyroid hormone in isolated bovine parathyroid cells, *Proc. Natl. Acad. Sci. U.S.A.*, 82, 4270, 1985.

75. Clemens, T. L., Zhou, X. Y., Myles, M., Endres, D., and Lindsay, R., Serum vitamin D_2 and vitamin D_3 metabolite concentrations and absorption of vitamin D_2 in elderly subjects, *J. Clin. Endocrinol. Metab.*, 63, 656, 1986.

76. Wongsurawat, N. and Armbrecht, H. J., Comparison of calcium effect on in vitro calcitonin and parathyroid hormone release by young and aged thyroparathyroid glands, *Exp. Gerontol.*, 22, 263, 1987.

77. Clissold, S. P., Fitton, A., and Chrisp, P., Intranasal salmon calcitonin. A review of its pharmacological properties and potential utility in metabolic bone disorders associated with aging, *Drugs and Aging*, 1, 405, 1991.

78. Fujita, T., Aging and calcium metabolism, *Advances in Second Messenger and Phosphoprotein Research*, 24, 542, 1990.

79. Felicetta, J. V., Age-related changes in calcium metabolism. Why they occur and what can be done, *Postgrad. Med.*, 85, 85, 1989.

80. Disterhoft, J. F., Moyer, J. R., Jr., Thompson, L. T., and Kowalska, M., Functional apsects of calcium-channel modulation, *Clin. Neuropharmacol.*, 16(Suppl. 1), S12, 1993.

6

Diffuse Endocrines and Chemical Mediators

Wilbur B. Quay

CONTENTS

I. INTRODUCTION

Advances in techniques and concepts of molecular and cell biology have expanded greatly the number of known chemical mediators in the body, and knowledge of how they are synthesized, processed, secreted, transported, and have specific actions at target cells. Many of these chemical mediators behave in part like hormones, but most of these same molecules have mediator actions of other kinds, too (autocrine, paracrine, neurotransmitter, etc.). What we consider here as "diffuse endocrines" are *chemical mediators that have hormonal characteristics* in some circumstances. However, these mediators:

0-8493-2446-7/95/$0.00+$.50
© 1995 by CRC Press Inc.

- Do not originate from classically known endocrine glands, or
- Are produced as hormones, or from hormone precursors, by organs or tissues having primary functions that are nonendocrine.

It is an artificial, ever-growing assemblage of compounds as we discover more hormone-like chemical mediators being produced by organs and tissues that had previously been considered to be nonendocrine.

II. GASTROINTESTINAL HORMONES IN AGING AND DISEASE

Gastrointestinal (GI) or gastroenteric hormones, as usually considered, are peptides. Many of these peptides function as chemical mediators not only in the GI tract but also elsewhere — such as the nervous system (neurotransmitters, neuromodulators, neuroendocrines). A few have endocrine and/or paracrine functions as component cell products within the endocrine pancreas (Chapters 3 and 10). This has led to the concept of a gastro-entero-pancreatic (GEP) endocrine system. Endocrine cells of this system are predominantly isolated cells within the epithelial lining and exocrine glands of specific parts of the GI tract and related duct systems. Within the pancreas, certain of these cells types occur as well within clusters known as pancreatic islets. The currently better known GEP endocrine cells are listed in Table 6-1, with their locations, hormones, and some of their distinguishing characteristics.

These cells also have sensory capabilities responsive to specific chemical stimuli within the gut lumen, and sometimes to the physical state of that region of the GI tract. These and other primary physiologic characteristics of these cells are summarized in Table 6-2. Physiologic actions of gut hormones include paracrine and endocrine modes of chemical mediator transport; they usually involve complex and multiple mediator-target cell interactions. Some GI endocrine cells are also known to secrete some of their peptide mediators into the gut lumen, but the physiologic meaning of this remains obscure.[1,2]

The complexity of the regulatory actions on the tissues of the gut wall is augmented by the presence of nerve fibers and their endings. Some of these endings are close to GI endocrine cells, but usually do not have typical synaptic relations with them (Figure 6-1).[3] Their chemical mediator contents, generally categorized as neurotransmitters, occur with similar functional localizations in the CNS. Somatostatin (Tables 6-1 and 6-2) in the gut occurs both as a GI hormone and as a putative transmitter in some of the nerve fibers and endings. Degenerative changes with age have been reported in intestinal peptidergic nerve fibers in laboratory rats and can be expected to affect physiologic gut mechanisms to which the GI hormones contribute (Table 6-3).[4]

A. Gastrin

A number of conditions affecting older people lead to abnormally elevated blood levels of gastrin. Very low gastrin levels are far less common. However, therapeutic oral doses of lithium can suppress release of gastrin. Abnormally high blood gastrin is often seen with duodenal ulcer, partial gastrectomy (gastrin-secreting G-cells in the remaining duodenal stump are no longer under the inhibitory control of gastric acid), pernicious anemia, obstruction of the stomach's outlet (chronic gastric distension can be one of the causes), renal insufficiency, rheumatoid arthritis, and hyperthyroidism. The etiology of some of these has a logical basis (see Table 6-2), but for the last three, interpretation of cause remains difficult. Other conditions can be noted:

- Hypercalcemia tends to enhance release of gastrin, but only when associated with hyperparathyroidism, and most notably in patients who have additionally a gastrinoma.[5]

TABLE 6-1 Gastro-Entero-Pancreatic (GEP) Endocrine Cells in Humans (and/or Other Mammalian Species)

Cell type	Anatomical distribution	Secretory granules (diameter in nm)	Peptide hormone(s)	Biogenic amine content[a]	Ref.
A	Pancreas, (stomach-dog), small intestine	Round, dark core, clear halo (200–400)	Glucagon	(DA, 5-HT)	3,78
B	Pancreas, fetal intestine	Round sac with angular core (200-400)	Insulin	(DA, 5-HT)	3,78
D	Stomach, small intestine, pancreas	Round, gray (300-450)	Somatostatin		3
D_1	Small intestine	Round, gray (150-200)	GIP + ?		3
EC[Δ]	Stomach, intestine	Distorted, very dark (200-400)	Substance P[b], Motilin	5-HT	3,5,79, 80
ECL	Stomach fundus	Vacuolated, eccentric core (400)	?	(Histamine)	3,7
G	Pyloric antrum, duodenum	Round sac with flocculent contents (300)	Gastrin	DA	3
K	Small intestine	Slightly distorted, dark (350)	[Δ]GIP, (Secretin, dog)		3,5,81
L	Intestine (pancreatic A cells)	Round, dark (300-400)	Glicentin		3,5
M (or I)	Small intestine	Round, dark (150-250)	Cholecystokinin (CCK)		3,5,82
N	Intestine, stomach	Round, dark (300)	Neurotensin		3,5,83-85
PP (or F)	Pancreas, stomach, upper small intestine	Round, gray (150-170)	Pancreatic poly-peptide (PP)	DA	3,5,78
S	Small intestine	Round (100-150)	Secretin (CCK, dog)		3,81, 82

[a] Content generally small in amount; amount and type vary with species; DA = dopamine; 5-HT = serotonin; [Δ]Enterochromaffin cell; includes relatives or subtypes.

[b] Possibly only in nerve fibers and paracrine rather than endocrine.

• Long-term hypoacidity (achlorhydria), as in pernicious anemia, causes G-cell hyperplasia in the antrum of the stomach. This is then responsible for increases in both basal and stimulated levels of gastrin.

High levels of gastrin are characteristic of Zollinger-Ellison syndrome (ZES). Hallmarks of ZES are recurrent and intractable peptic ulcers and diarrhea. The ulcers are caused by excessive secretion of gastric acid and are usually (>75%) in or near the duodenal bulb.[5] This disease has peak occurrence in the fifth decade of life. Chronically high gastrin levels are often coextant with hyperplasia of the gastric mucosa, as might be expected (Table 6-2). Gastrinomas are the usual basis of ZES; most often they are non-B-cell pancreatic islet tumors, less commonly (about 10%) duodenal or gastric tumors.[6] They often produce several other hormones in addition to gastrin. The diagnosis of ZES is to be considered in all patients with duodenal ulcer because symptoms of gastrinomas and of ordinary duodenal ulcers may be essentially the same and differentiation between the two is still difficult.[7,8]

B. Gastric Inhibitory Polypeptide (GIP)

Abnormal levels of the intestinal peptide hormone, GIP, occur in several disease conditions. However, a definite pathophysiologic role for it has not been demonstrated.[5] GIP blood levels are especially high in some obese subjects and in patients with chronic pancreatitis,[9] but causes are unknown. In response to a 50 g oral glucose tolerance test, elderly (66 to 98 years) females

TABLE 6-2 Physiologic Characteristics of Major Gastroenteric Peptide Hormones in Humans (and/or Other Mammalian Species)

Hormone	Secretion of Stimulated by meal contents	Inhibited by (and other agents)	Actions	Normal blood levels	Half-life (mins)	Major (lesser) sites of metabolism
[a]CCK	Peptides and some amino acids; fatty acids $>C_{10}$ positive feedback by effects of stimulated bile secretion)		Gall bladder contraction; ↑ secretion pancreatic digestive enzymes (depending usually on hormonal and/or neural potentiation); etc.	<0.2 to 1.0 pmol/1		
[a]Gastrin	Proteins, peptides, some amino acids and other amines (luminal distension); ↑, vagal discharge	(↓ Gastric pH; bloodborne secretin GIP, VIP, glucagon, calcitonin)	↑ Gastric acid and pepsin secretion; ↑ antral motility; trophic to GI mucosa	20 to 200 pg/ml	8 to 40	Kidneys (liver and intestine)
[a]GIP	Carbohydrate, fat, some amino acids		Potentiates insulin release mediated by glucose (or amino acid); ↓ gastric acid secretion and motility)		20	
[a]Glicentin			May modify development and functional activity of GI tract; (inhibit gastrin-stimulated gastric acid release — rats)			
Motilin	Fat; (distension with water)	Food intake inhibits its cyclic ↑ secretion	Accelerates gastric emptying; stimulates colonic motility may (?) initiate interdigestive myoelectric complexes	Cyclical with period of 90 to 120 min		
Neurotensin	Fat and mixed meals but not glucose nor amino acids		(Many pharmacologic actions; physiologic actions not yet known)			
PP	Fat, protein, or mixed meals	(Atropine, cholinergic transmission (?)	Physiologic role? Many pharmacologic actions, mostly opposite to those of CCK	54 to 207	6 pg/ml	Kidneys
Secretin	Acidified content; products of protein digestion	(Somatostatin)	In concert with CCK (and/or ?) stimulates pancreatic biliary ductal bicarbonate secretion; ↓ gastric acid	<10 pg/ml	3	Kidneys
Somatostatin	Mixed meals; glucose, amino acids, free fatty acids; (gastrin, secretin, CCK); (obesity); (by isoproterenol, and this blocked by propranolol — indicating adrenergic control)	(Metenkephalin; substance P; starvation)	Tonic inhibition of release of several hormones (incl. glucagon gastrin, insulin, secretin); regulation of rate of nutrient entry to circulation; inhibition of gastric acid and pepsin secretion; plus others (pharmacologic; ? physiologic)	10 to 80 pg/ml	<3	Liver and kidneys

[a] Includes several molecular forms, some differing in levels of activity/potency.

Sources: Data from Boden and Shelmet,[5] Reichlin,[20] Ganong,[86] and Solcia et al.[87]

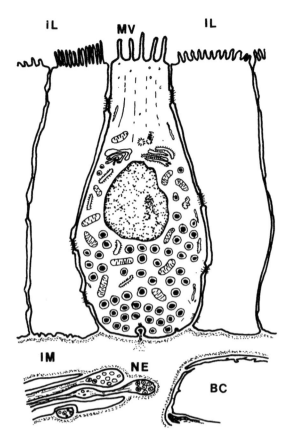

FIGURE 6-1 Diagram of a gut endocrine cell as seen in vertical section. The apical ends of most gut endocrine cells are in contact with the lumen (IL), and have specialized microvilli (MV) which have been suggested to be involved in chemical sensing of lumen contents. The basal cytoplasm often has an abundance of secretory granules, whose contents when released diffuse across the intercellular material (IM) with uptake by capillaries (BC), and possibly has interactions with adjacent cells and tissues, including nerve endings (NE).

have higher responses of increased blood GIP levels than do elderly males; but the physiologic significance of this is unclear.[10] High blood concentrations of GIP have been also noted in patients with duodenal ulcer; this may be related to accelerated emptying of the stomach.[11] Increased secretion of GIP may be the cause of postprandial hypoglycemia in some cases with idiopathic reactive hypoglycemia.[12] This remains a confusing and controversial topic in metabolic and endocrine pathophysiology (Chapters 10 and 11).

TABLE 6-3 Density of Immunoreactive Peptidergic Nerve Fibers in the Small Intestine of the Rat in Relation to Age (Number/100 μm² Tissue Area)

Peptide Mediator	Age (months)		
	Young (6)	Old (24)	Senile (36)
Substance P	10 ± 2.05	9 ± 2.57	1 ± 0.50
VIP	15 ± 3.05	14 ± 4.52	2 ± 12.5
Somatostatin	17 ± 2.86	18 ± 3.75	2 ± 1.08

From Feher, E. and Penzes, L., *Gerontology*, 33, 341, 1987, with permission.

C. Pancreatic Polypeptide (PP)

Plasma PP rises within minutes after oral but not after intravenous administration of nutrients. This indicates that PP release into the blood is mediated by direct action of nutrients or their digestive products on D-cells of the intestinal mucosa and not by absorbed nutrients delivered to pancreatic PP-containing cells by the blood (Table 6-1).[5] Human plasma PP (hPP) concentration increases with age. Basal hPP in normal subjects increased from 54 ± 28 pg/ml in the third decade of life to 207 ± 129 pg/ml in the seventh.[13] Elderly (66 to 98 years) subjects have higher hPP levels than younger adults (21 to 39 years), both during fasting and after glucose stimulation, and in both males and females.[10]

Other factors and conditions may lead to increased plasma hPP, and some of these are of interest in relation to the life habits of the elderly:

1. Hypoglycemia;
2. Exercise;
3. Prolonged fasting as well as ingestion of fat, protein, or mixed meals; and
4. Parasympathetic stimulation.[13-15]

Patients with renal deficiency generally have elevated hPP levels since the kidneys are the most important sites of its metabolism (Table 6-2).[16] High hPP levels are also observed frequently in patients with tumors involving one or more parts of the GEP system. Such tumors include: insulinomas, glucagonomas, VIP-secreting tumors, gastrinomas, and carcinoid tumors (see below). In addition, some pancreatic tumors with excessive hPP content and/or output have been noted.[17,18] Since the chronically high blood concentrations of hPP in patients with these tumors are not tied to a definable clinical "PPoma"-type syndrome, it is suspected that many of the so-called "nonfunctional endocrine tumors" of the pancreas, seen in older individuals, may be in fact PP-secreting tumors.[17]

D. Secretin

Elevated plasma concentrations of secretin occur in patients with chronic renal failure due to decreased metabolism of the hormone. Increased gastric acid secretion and intestinal acidification are causative agents in the high blood secretin levels seen in patients with ZES (see above).[19] Patients with ordinary duodenal ulcer usually have normal secretin levels, except in the presence of basal gastric acid outputs of more than 15 meq/h; in this instance secretin levels may be high.[5] Secretin is used in provocative tests for the diagnosis of ZES, and for the evaluation of the functional state of the exocrine pancreas.

E.   Somatostatin

Somatostatin (S) is widespread in the body and has a multitude of biologic (Table 6-2) and clinical actions.[20] The sources of plasma S are D-cells of pancreatic islets, GI tract, and from synapses of the peripheral nervous system, such as those in the gut wall (Table 6-3). Somatostatin is excreted in the urine. The normal half-life of SLI (somatostatin-like immunoreactive substances) (Table 6-2) is increased about 50% by chronic renal failure.[21]

Basal blood levels of S are greater ($p <0.01$) in the elderly (76 to 90 years) than in young adults (22 to 30 years) (20.0 ± 1.5 vs. 14.1 ± 0.6 pg/ml, respectively).[22] Likewise the mean 24-h S levels are greater ($p <0.01$) in the elderly (21.3 ± 0.8 pg/ml) than in young adults (16.7 ± 0.5 pg/ml) (same subject ages as above). Likewise, daytime variations in concentration and responses to meal tests are lower in amplitude in the elderly.[22]

Somatostatinomas, tumors containing and/or secreting excessive amounts of S, have been extensively studied.[23,24] Males and females are affected in similar numbers, and occurrences peak in the fifth decade. About 20% of these tumors occur in the duodenum or jejunum.[25] At

TABLE 6-4   Reduced Products of Carcinoid Tumors or Their Metastases

Relatively common	Less common	
Serotonin (5-HT)	ACTH	MSH
5-Hydroxytryptophan	Kallikrein	PTH
Histamine	Prostaglandins	ADH
Bradykinin	Calcitonin	Neurotensin
5-HIAA (normally the major	Growth hormone (GH)	Enteroglucagon
and biologically inactive	Motilin	Glucagon
metabolite of 5-HT)	Substance P	Insulin
	Dopamine (DA)	Gastrin
	Norepinephrine (NE)	HCG-α
	VIP	Pancreatic polypeptide

Modified from Boden, G. and Shelmet, J. J., *Endocrinology and Metabolism,* 2nd ed., Felig, P., Baxter, J. D., Broadus, A. E., and Frohman, L. A., Eds., McGraw-Hill, New York, 1987.

diagnosis, metastases from somatostatinomas have often spread to the liver or regional lymph nodes or both. Malignancy was attested to in one study by death of 8 out of 12 patients at from 1 week to 14 months after diagnosis.[5] Clinical findings in patients with somatostatinomas include: diabetes mellitus, gall bladder disease, diarrhea with steatorrhea, hypochlorhydria, weight loss, anemia, and elevated blood SLI concentrations (averaging 15,500 pg/ml and ranging to 107,000 pg/ml). About half of such patients with somatostatinoma have other, diverse, kinds of endocrinopathies. These include insulinoma, gastrinoma, Cushing's syndrome, pheochromocytoma, and goiter.

F.   Carcinoid Tumors and Their Hormonal Products

Carcinoids are neoplasms of the alimentary tract and related organs. They usually can release a number of peptide and amine chemical mediators (Table 6-4). These and other attributes suggest a relationship with, if not a derivation from, the diffuse endocrine cells of the gut and other viscera. Although they are located most often in the jejuno-ileal intestine (75% of 201 autopsied cases),[26] they have also been found in many nonenteric organs,[27] presumably not always as metastases.

The peak incidence of these hormone-releasing tumors occurs in the fifth and sixth decades of life, but the tumors have been reported in patients of less than one year to 98 years of age. Most are small (< 2 cm diameter) and asymptomatic, being discovered at autopsy or during surgery for other concerns. Carcinoid tumors often coexist with other neoplasms (37% in 390 autopsied carcinoid cases, and 18% in 374 surgically treated carcinoids).[28] There is a classical roster of clinical signs of the carcinoid syndrome, which is notable, however, in only about 5% of diagnosed patients (Table 6-5).[29] Major and typical carcinoid symptoms often have complex causes, not attributable simply to the hormonal mediators secreted at excessive levels. High concentrations of particular amine and/or peptide contents of carcinoid cells

TABLE 6-5   Major Clinical Manifestations of the Carcinoid Syndrome

Manifestation	Percent of patients showing
Episodic cutaneous flushing	84
GI hypermotility (diarrhea/cramps)	79
Signs of heart disease (right-sided valvular disease, etc.)	37
Bronchoconstriction	17
Abnormal pigmentation (pellegra-like)	5

Modified from Boden, G. and Shelmet, J. J., *Endocrinology and Metabolism,* 2nd ed., Felig, P., Baxter, J. D., Broadus, A. E., and Frohman, L. A., Eds., McGraw-Hill, New York, 1987.

provide the basis for pathological cellular and tissue characteristics useful for classification and for recognition of carcinoid cells, both at primary sites and in some metastases.[30]

III. OTHER DIFFUSE SENSORY/ENDOCRINE CELLS

Gastrointestinal endocrine cells are not the only diffuse sensory/endocrine cells in the body. There are others, generally lying within or near specific epithelia in other organs. Like the GI endocrine cells they show structural characteristics and, less often, physiologic evidence consistent with the ability to sense the nature of luminal contents or of changes within the surrounding epithelium. Endocrine activity of these cells is typically inferred from an abundance of "secretory" granules in the cell base not far from subjacent capillaries, and from the cytoplasmic content of amine and/or peptide chemical mediator(s).

A. Merkel Cells of the Skin

Merkel cells occur individually and in groups, usually between or below epidermal epithelial cells. Their microvillous processes extending between adjacent epidermal cells, and the sensory nerve ending (tactile meniscus) synapsing at their base, provide the basis for their mechano-receptor function. Metenkephalin-like and a number of other opioid peptides, as well as VIP-like peptides, are present in the abundant granules of the basal cytoplasm. Paracrine and endocrine fates have been suggested for their contents, in addition to the structurally more obvious sensory neurotransmission.[3,31] Physiologic evidence is slight.

B. Sensory/Secretory Cells of the Respiratory System

These, like the Merkel cells above, are basi-granular cells and occur as solitary and aggregated types. They occur in larynx, trachea, bronchi, bronchioles, and pulmonary alveoli. Some, but not all, have sensory innervations and also release neurotransmitter/secretory granule contents exocytotically during hypoxia.[32-35] The paracrine and endocrine functional relations suggested for certain of these substances remain largely inferential.[5,36-37] Little has been reported concerning possible changes during old age.

C. Urogenital Sensory/Secretory Cells

Basi-granular cells superficially resembling EC cells (Table 6-1) and some others above, are distributed in epithelia of many parts of the urogenital system of males and females.[5,38] Serotonin (5-HT) occurs most often in these cells, and peptides rarely. The report of somatostatin-immunoreactive cells in human prostatic epithelium is the best evidence for the latter.[39] It is likely that the 5-HT and somatostatin-like secretory material subserve paracrine rather than endocrine function. Again, little information is available about possible changes in old age.

IV. ATRIOPEPTINS (ATRIAL NATRIURETIC PEPTIDES OR FACTORS [ANP])

Myocytes of cardiac atria were reported in 1956 to contain secretory-like granules and to secrete chemical mediators.[40,41] Currently, a large family of peptides, atriopeptins (with many synonyms still in use), are produced predominantly by the cardiac atria and have physiological and pharmacological actions. This has led to the understanding, extensively supported by experimental evidence, "that the heart is a major endocrine organ".[42]

Human atriopeptin is produced under the influence of a single gene. Its mRNA is transcribed with the encoding of a 151-amino-acid protein (preproatriopeptin).[43-46] A signal peptide sequence is split from the precursor at the time of its translation and passage into the cisternae of the endoplasmic reticulum. The resulting prohormone, a 126-amino-acid peptide, is the major storage form within cardiac tissue.[41,47-49] Cleavage of this proatriopeptin gives rise to a 28-amino-acid peptide with a carboxyl terminal, which is the predominant biologically active form in humans.[41,49-51]

The importance of the cardiac atrial source of atriopeptins is supported by the finding that the requisite mRNA is the most abundant atrial mRNA, equalling about 2% in the rat.[43,47] It has been concluded that the protein synthetic activity of atrial tissue is directed more to this molecule than to any other protein.[42] Atriopeptin concentrations in coronary sinus venous plasma are two to eight times those in peripheral arterial or venous blood, further supporting the importance of the cardiac atrial source.[40]

Atriopeptins are produced in much smaller amounts in a number of other tissues, where they and their mRNAs are found. These sites include: ventricular subendothelial cells, particular cells within the lungs, the aorta, autonomic ganglia,[52] salivary glands,[53] pituitary,[54] adrenals[54] and corpus luteum,[55] spinal cord,[52] and parts of the brain,[56] including choroid plexus epithelium[52] and hypothalamus.[58-60]

This pattern of occurrence suggests that atriopeptin presence is often associated with tissues or regions that are sensitive and respond to pressure changes.[42] Atriopeptin, in these sites of relatively low concentrations, probably subserves mainly neurotransmitter and paracrine functions.

Although the major actions of atriopeptins are complex, they chiefly stimulate excretion of sodium and water and are vasorelaxants. In this capacity they oppose the effects of sodium- and water-retaining and pressor stimuli and agents and inhibit renin release.[42] In aged rats, the biologic potency of atriopeptin fractions declines significantly. This cannot be explained on the basis of lowered atrial stores, since the quantity per amount of tissue DNA actually increases steadily with age in this species. Rather, the potency decrease appears to be due to age-related changes in the biologic activity of some of the atriopeptin molecules, with probably important consequences in regulation of mean arterial pressure.[61] Such an age-related decrease in hormonal bioactivity is considered by some to be uncommon (however, see below). In a number of other endocrine tissues, too, aging is accompanied by increased hormonal molecular heterogeneity, with gradual augmentation of biologically less active and inactive hormonal peptide molecules (Chapters 5 and 7).[62-67]

Atriopeptins have been isolated also from human cardiac atria (hANP).[50,68] As in rats (above), high concentrations have been found in aged human males;[69] there is also an enhanced response in plasma hANP in aged subjects following loading with NaCl. However, a diminished cellular response to endogenous hANP has been reported in healthy elderly men.[69] The response of plasma cGMP (cyclic 3',5'-guanosine monophosphate), a putative second messenger of hANP, is the same in old and young after NACl loading; thus, the increased hANP concentration in the elderly has been associated with a lowered cellular uptake of hANP.[69] A reduced metabolic clearance rate for hANP in healthy old (71 to 77 years) as compared with young adult (25 to 28 years) men has been reported. It has been tentatively concluded on the basis of the latter finding that high concentrations of hANP in blood of elderly men can be due in part to reduced metabolic clearance rates for hANP in these subjects.[70]

V. GROWTH FACTORS — "MEDIATORY HORMONES"

The tenet that classical hormones *directly* regulate growth and maturation has been gradually and largely replaced by the concept that growth is normally controlled by a diversity of classical hormone-dependent "growth or mediatory factors" in specific tissues.[71]

The known growth factors are mostly, if not all, polypeptides. As with many of the above-noted diffuse endocrine systems, they act through different routes to targets (autocrine, paracrine, endocrine, etc.) along with diffuse or not yet well-defined physiologic origins. Attention has been directed, and the available information almost exclusively pertains to their occurrence, actions, and significance at early ages and in related developing cells and tissues of importance in human growth. Therefore they will not be considered individually here. Actions and interactions of growth factors and other mediators are important in the control or *inhibition* of growth in both normal and neoplastic kinds of growth (Chapter 18).[72,73] There are still few published data concerning these topics in the elderly.

VI.   HEMOCYTIC AND LYMPHOCYTIC HORMONES AND MEDIATORS

Most of these important chemical mediators, often transported like hormones by blood and other body fluids, are generally considered, as here, in the physiologic domain of the immune system (Chapter 20).

VII.   ECTOPIC HORMONES

Ectopic (out of place, displaced) hormones, most simply, are hormones produced by:

- Neoplasms of nonendocrine origin, and/or
- Endocrine neoplasms not closely related to the usual endocrine tissue or cell of origin of the hormone.[74,75]

The ectopic synthesis, usually accompanied by release, of polypeptides by neoplasms arising from nonendocrine tissues is considered to be "a universal concomitant of neoplasia."[76] These ectopic compounds usually have biologic activities but often their potencies may be different from those of the "normal" hormones. Their molecular structure may differ sufficiently from the "normal" hormone to account for a difference in rate of metabolism and excretion and, hence, for a difference in biologic life time and duration of activity. Therefore, the precise interpretation of endocrine changes and their mechanisms in a particular aged individual is usually extremely difficult.

Many neoplasms are at least superficially asymptomatic in older subjects and are not discovered without a comprehensive autopsy accompanied by detailed microscopic pathologic study. These neoplasms nevertheless may have been releasing biologically active and deviant polypeptide molecules. "Quantitatively, neoplasia is a disease of the aged, and ample evidence indicates aneuploidy increases with age."[77] The occurrence of somatic mutations in neoplasia is supported by the finding of chromosomal (karyotype) abnormalities in the resulting tumor cells. Yet, although "certain benign as well as malignant neoplasms possess morphologically normal karyotypes, aneuploidy is the rule rather than the exception."[77]

REFERENCES

1. Arnold, R., Koop, H., Simson, G., Bedell, R. A., and Creutzfeldt, W., Luminar secretion of gastrointestinal peptides. Release of gastrin and somatostatin into the gastric lumen in rats, in *Frontiers of Hormone Research. The Entero-Insular Axis*, Creutzfeldt, W., Ed., S. Karger, Basel, 1980, 72.
2. Goldschmiedt, M., Barnett, C. C., Schwarz, B. E., Karnes, W. E., Redfern, J. S., and Feldman, M., Effect of age on gastric acid secretion and serum gastrin concentrations in healthy men and women, *Gastroenterology*, 101, 977, 1991.
3. Fujita, T., Kanno, T., and Kobayashi, S., *The Paraneuron*, Springer-Verlag, Tokyo, 1988.
4. Feher, E. and Penzes, L., Density of substance P, vasoactive intestinal polypeptide and somatostatin-containing nerve fibers in the ageing small intestine of the rat, *Gerontology*, 33, 341, 1987.
5. Boden, G. and Shelmet, J. J., Gastrointestinal hormones and carcinoid tumors and syndrome, in *Endocrinology and Metabolism*, 2nd ed., Felig, P., Baxter, J. D., Broadus, A. E., and Frohman, L. A., Eds., McGraw-Hill, New York, 1987, 1629.
6. Jensen, R. T., Zollinger-Ellison syndrome: current concepts and management, *Ann. Intern. Med.*, 98, 59, 1983.

7. Krudy, A. G., Doppman, J. L., Jensen, R. T., Norton, J. A., Collen, M. J., Shawker, T. H., Gardner, J. D., McArthur, K., and Gorden, P., Localization of islet cell tumors by dynamic CT: comparison with plain CT, arteriography, sonography, and venous sampling, *Am. J. Roentgenol.*, 143, 585, 1984.

8. Malagelada, J. R., Davis, C. S., O'Fallon, W. M., and Go, V. L., Laboratory diagnosis of gastrinoma. I. A prospective evaluation of gastric analysis and fasting serum gastrin levels, *Mayo Clin. Proc.*, 57, 211, 1982.

9. Bardram, L., Hilsted, L., and Rehfeld, J. F., Progastrin expression in mammalian pancreas, *Proc. Natl. Acad. Sci., USA.*, 87, 298, 1990.

10. McConnell, J. G., Alam, M. J., O'Hare, M. M. T., Buchanan, K. D., and Stout, R. W., The effect of age and sex on the response of enteropancreatic polypeptides to oral glucose, *Age and Ageing*, 12, 54, 1983.

11. Khalil, T., Poston, G. J., and Thompson, J. C., Effects of aging on gastrointestinal hormones, *Prog. Clin. Biol. Res.*, 326, 39, 1990.

12. Hadji-Georgopoulos, A., Schmidt, M. I., Elahi, D., Hershcopf, R., and Kowarski, A. A., Increased gastric inhibitory polypeptide levels in patients with symptomatic postprandial hypoglycemia, *J. Clin. Endocrinol. Metab.*, 56, 648, 1983.

13. Floyd, J. C. and Vinik, A. I., Pancreatic polypeptide, in *Gut Hormones*, Bloom, S. R. and Polak, J. M., Eds., Churchill Livingstone, New York, 1981, 195.

14. Schwartz, T. W., Holst, J. J., Fahrenkrug, J., Jensen, S. L., Nielsen, O. V., Rehfeld, J. F., Schaffalitzky de Muckadell, O. B., and Stadil, F., Vagal, cholinergic regulation of pancreatic polypeptide secretion, *J. Clin. Invest.*, 61, 781, 1978.

15. Gettys, T. W., Tanaka, J., and Taylor, I. L., Modulation of pancreatic exocrine function in rodents by treatment with pancreatic polypeptide, *Pancreas*, 7, 705, 1992.

16. Boden, G., Master, R. W., Owen, O. E., and Rudnick, M. R., Human pancreatic polypeptide in chronic renal failure and cirrhosis of the liver: role of the kidneys and liver in pancreatic polypeptide metabolism, *J. Clin. Endocrinol. Metab.*, 51, 573, 1980.

17. O'Dorisio, T. M. and Vinik, A. I., Pancreatic peptide and mixed peptide producing tumors of the gastrointestinal tract, in *Contemporary Issues in Gastroenterology: Hormone Producing Tumors of the Gastrointestinal Tract*, Cohen, S. and Soloway, R. D., Eds., Churchill Livingstone, New York, 1985, 117.

18. Strodel, W. E., Vinik, A. I., Lloyd, R. V., Glaser, B., Eckhauser, F. E., Fiddian-Green, R. G., Turcotte, J. G., and Thompson N. W., Pancreatic polypeptide-producing tumors. Silent lesions of the pancreas? *Arch. Surg.*, 119, 508, 1984.

19. Straus, E., Radioimmunoassay of gastrointestinal hormones, *Gastroenterology*, 74, 141, 1978.

20. Reichlin, S., Somatostatin, *N. Engl. J. Med.*, 309, 1495, 1983.

21. Sheppard, M., Shapiro, B., Pimstone, B., Kronheim, S., Berelowitz, M., and Gregory, M., Metabolic clearance and plasma half-disappearance time of exogenous somatostatin in man, *J. Clin. Endocrinol. Metab.*, 48, 50, 1979.

22. Rolandi, E., Franceschini, R., Messina, V., Cataldi, A., Salvemini, M., and Barreca, T., Somatostatin in the elderly: diurnal plasma profile and secretory response to meal stimulation, *Gerontology*, 33, 296, 1987.

23. Ganda, O. P., Weir, G. C., Soeldner, J. S., Legg, M. A., Chick, W. L., Patel, Y. C., Ebeid, A. M., Gabbay, K. H., and Reichlin, S., 'Somatostatinoma': a somatostatin-containing tumor of the endocrine pancreas, *N. Engl. J. Med.*, 296, 963, 1977.

24. Larsson, L.I., Hirsch, M. A., Holst, J. J., Ingemansson, S., Kuhl, C., Jensen, S. L., Lundqvist, G., Rehfeld, J. F., and Schwartz, T. W., Pancreatic somatostatinoma. Clinical features and physiological implications, *Lancet*, 1, 666, 1977.

25. Boden, G. and Shimoyama, R., Somatostatinoma, in *Contemporary Issues in Gastroenterology: Hormone Producing Tumors of the Gastrointestinal Tract*, Cohen, S. and Soloway, R. D., Eds., Churchill Livingstone, New York, 1985, 85.

26. Berge, T. and Linell, F., Carcinoid tumors — frequency in a defined population during a 12-year period, *Acta Pathol. Microbiol. Scand.*, 84, 322, 1976.

27. DeLellis, R. A., Dayal, Y., and Wolfe, H. J., Carcinoid tumors. Changing concepts and new perspectives, *Am. J. Surg. Pathol.*, 8, 295, 1984.

28. Moertel, C. G., Sauer, W. G., Dockerty, M. B., and Baggenstoss, A. H., Life history of the carcinoid tumor of the small intestine, *Cancer*, 14, 901, 1961.

29. Beaton, H., Homan, W., and Dineen, P., Gastrointestinal carcinoids and the malignant carcinoid syndrome, *Surg. Gynecol. Obstet.*, 152, 268, 1981.

30. Soga, J., Carcinoids: their changing concepts and a new histological classification, in *Gastro-entero-pancreatic Endocrine System; A Cell Biological Approach*, Fujita, T., Ed., Williams & Wilkins, Baltimore, MD, 1974, 101.

31. Hartschuh, W., Weihe, E., and Reinecke, M., The Merkel cell, in *Biology of the Integument*, Vol. 2, Bereiter-Hahn, J., Matoltsy, A. G., and Richards, K. S., Eds., Springer-Verlag, Berlin, 1986, 605.

32. Hernandez-Vasquez, A., Will, J. A., and Quay, W. B., Quantitative characteristics of the Feyrter (APUD) cells of the neonatal rabbit lung in normoxia and chronic hypoxia, *Thorax*, 32, 449, 1977.

33. Hernandez-Vasquez, A., Will, J. A., and Quay, W. B., Quantitative characteristics of the Feyrter cells and neuroepithelial bodies of the fetal rabbit lung in normoxia and short term chronic hypoxia, *Cell Tissue Res.*, 189, 179, 1978.
34. Lauweryns, J. M. and Cokelaere, M., Intrapulmonary neuro-epithelial bodies: hypoxia-sensitive neuro(chemo-) receptors, *Experientia*, 29, 1384, 1973.
35. Lauweryns, J. M. and Cokelaere, M., Hypoxia-sensitive neuro-epithelial bodies: intrapulmonary secretory neuroreceptors, modulated by the CNS, *Z. Zellforsch. Mikrosk. Anat.*, 145, 521, 1973.
36. Heinemann, H. O., Ryan, J. W., and Ryan, U. S., Is the lung a para-endocrine organ?, *Am. J. Med.*, 63, 595, 1977.
37. Sorokin, S. P., The respiratory system, in *Cell and Tissue Biology. A Textbook of Histology*, 6th ed., Weiss, L., Ed., Urban & Schwarzenberg, Baltimore, MD, 1988, 751.
38. Lendon, R. G., Dixon, J. S., and Gosling, J. A., The distribution of endocrine-like cells in the human male and female urethral epithelium, *Experientia*, 32, 377, 1976.
39. di Sant'Agnese, P. A. and de Mesy Jensen, K. L., Endocrine-paracrine cells of the prostate and prostatic urethra: an ultrastructural study, *Human Pathol.*, 15, 1034, 1984.
40. Cantin, M. and Genest, J., The heart as an endocrine gland, *Sci. Am.*, 254, 76, 1986.
41. de Bold, A. J., Atrial natriuretic factor: a hormone produced by the heart, *Science*, 230, 767,1985.
42. Baxter, J. D., Perloff, D., Hsueh, W., and Biglieri, E. G., The endocrinology of hypertension, in *Endocrinology and Metabolism*, 2nd ed., Felig, P., Baxter, J. D., Broadus, A. E., and Frohman, L. A., Eds., McGraw-Hill, New York, 1987, 693.
43. Greenberg, B. D., Bencen, G. H., Seilhamer, J. J., Lewicki, J. A., and Fiddes, J. C., Nucleotide sequence of the gene encoding human atrial natriuretic factor precursor, *Nature*, 312, 656, 1984.
44. Oikawa, S., Imai, M., Ueno, A., Tanaka, S., Noguchi, T., Nakazato, H., Kangawa, K., Fukuda, A., and Matsuo, H., Cloning and sequence analysis of cDNA encoding a precursor for human atrial natriuretic polypeptide, *Nature*, 309, 724, 1984.
45. Schwartz, D., Geller, D. M., Manning, P. T., Siegel, N. R., Fok, K. F., Smith, C. E., and Needleman, P., Ser-Leu-Arg-Arg-atriopeptin III: the major circulating form of atrial peptide, *Science*, 229, 397, 1985.
46. Seidman, C. E., Bloch, K. D., Zisfein, J., Smith, J. A., Haber, E., Homcy, C., Duby, A. D., Choi, E., Graham, R. M., and Seidman, J. G., Molecular studies of the atrial natriuretic factor gene, *Hypertension*, 7, 131,1985.
47. Ballermann, B. J. and Brenner, B. M., Biologically active atrial peptides, *J. Clin. Invest.*, 76, 2041, 1985.
48. Needleman, P., Adams, S. P., Cole, B. R., Currie, M. G., Geller, D. M., Michener, M. L., Saper, C. B., Schwartz, D., and Standaert, D. G., Atriopeptins as cardiac hormones, *Hypertension*, 7, 469, 1985.
49. Needleman, P. and Greenwald, J. E., Atriopeptin: a cardiac hormone intimately involved in fluid, electrolyte, and blood-pressure homeostasis, *N. Engl. J. Med.*, 314, 828, 1986.
50. Kangawa K., Fukuda, A., and Matsuo, H., Structural identification of beta- and gamma-human atrial natriuretic polypeptides, *Nature*, 313, 397, 1985.
51. Yamaji, T., Ishibashi, M., and Takaku, F., Atrial natriuretic factor in human blood, *J. Clin. Invest.*, 76, 1705, 1985.
52. Morii, N., Nakao, K., Itoh, H., Shiono, S., Yamada, T., Sugawara, A., Saito, Y., Mukoyama, M., Arai, H., Sakamoto, M., and Imura, H., Atrial natriuretic polypeptide in spinal cord and autonomic ganglia, *Biochem. Biophys. Res. Commun.*, 145, 196, 1987.
53. Cantin, M., Gutkowska, J., Thibault, G., Milne, R. W., Ledoux, S., MinLi, S., Chapeau, C., Garcia, R., Hamet, P., and Genest, J., Immunocytochemical localization of atrial natriuretic factor in the heart and salivary glands, *Histochemistry*, 80, 113, 1984.
54. McKenzie, J. C., Tanaka, I., Misono, K. S., and Inagami, T., Immuno-cytochemical localization of atrial natriuretic factor in the kidney, adrenal medulla, pituitary, and atrium of rat, *J. Histochem. Cytochem.*, 338, 828, 1985.
55. Vollmar, A. M., Mytzka, C., Arendt, R. M., and Schulz, R., Atrial natriuretic peptide in bovine corpus luteum, *Endocrinology*, 123, 762, 1988.
56. Gardner, D. G., Deschepper, C. P., Ganong, W. F., Hane, S., Fiddes, J., Baxter, J. D., and Lewicki, J., Extra-atrial expression of the gene for atrial natriuretic factor, *Proc. Natl. Acad. Sci. USA*, 83, 6697, 1986.
57. Steardo, L. and Nathanson, J. A., Brain barrier tissues: end organs for atriopeptins, *Science*, 235, 470, 1987.
58. Jacobowitz, D. M., Skofitsch, G., Keiser, H. R., Eskay, R. L., and Zamir, N., Evidence for the existence of atrial natriuretic factor-containing neurons in the rat brain, *Neuroendocrinology*, 40, 92, 1985.
59. Morii, N., Nakao, K., Sugawara, A., Sakamoto, M., Suda, M., Shimokura, M., Kiso, Y., Kihara, M., Yamori, Y., and Imura, H., Occurrence of atrial natriuretic polypeptide in brain, *Biochem. Biophys. Res. Commun.*, 127, 413, 1985.
60. Skofitsch, G., Jacobowitz, D. M., Eskay, R. L., and Zamir, N., Distribution of atrial natriuretic factor-like immunoreactive neurons in the rat brain, *Neuroscience*, 16, 917, 1985.
61. Inscho, E. W., Wilfinger, W. W., and Banks, R. O., Age-related differences in the natriuretic and hypotensive properties of rat atrial extracts, *Endocrinology*, 121, 1662, 1987.

62. Choy, V. J., Klemme, W. R., and Timiras, P. S., Variant forms of immunoreactive thyrotropin in aged rats, *Mech. Ageing Dev.*, 19, 273, 1982.

63. Klug, T. L. and Adelman, R. C., Evidence for a large thyrotropin and its accumulation during aging in rats, *Biochem. Biophys. Res. Commun.*, 77, 1431, 1977.

64. Krieger, D. T., Glandular and organ deficiency associated with secretion of biologically inactive pituitary peptides, *J. Clin. Endocrinol. Metab.*, 38, 964, 1974.

65. Lewis, U. J., Variants of growth hormone and prolactin and their posttranslational modifications, *Annu. Rev. Physiol.*, 46, 33, 1986.

66. Morris, B. J., New possibilities for intracellular renin and inactive renin now that the structure of the human renin gene has been elucidated, *Clin. Sci.*, 71, 345, 1986.

67. Owens, R. E., Casanueva, F. F., and Friesen, H. G., Comparison between rat prolactin radioimmunoassay and bioassay values under different experimental and physiological conditions, *Mol. Cell. Endocrinol.*, 39, 131, 1985.

68. Kangawa, K. and Matsuo, H., Purification and complete amino acid sequence of α-human atrial natriuretic polypeptide (α-hANP), *Biochem. Biophys. Res. Commun.*, 118, 131, 1984.

69. Ohashi, M., Fujio, N., Nawata, H., Kato, K., Ibayashi, H., Kangawa, K., and Matsuo, H., High plasma concentrations of human atrial natriuretic polypeptide in aged men, *J. Clin. Endocrinol. Metab.*, 64, 81, 1987.

70. Ohashi, M., Fujio, N., Nawata, H., Kato, K., Matsuo, H., and Ibayashi, H., Pharmacokinetics of synthetic α-human atrial natriuretic polypeptide in normal men; effect of aging, *Regulatory Peptides*, 19, 265, 1987.

71. MacGillivray, M. H., Disorders of growth and development, in *Endocrinology and Metabolism*, 2nd ed., Felig, P., Baxter, J. D., Broadus, A. E., and Frohman, L. A., Eds., McGraw-Hill, New York, 1987, 1581.

72. Barnes, D. M., Cells without growth factors commit suicide, *Science*, 242, 1510, 1988.

73. Pelech, S., Cellular security, *The Sciences*, 29, 39, 1994.

74. Liddle, G. W., Island, D., and Meador, C. K., Normal and abnormal regulation of corticotropin secretion in man, *Recent Prog. Horm. Res.*, 18, 125, 1962.

75. Leake, A., and Ferrier, I. N., Alterations in neuropeptides in aging and disease. Pathophysiology and potential for clinical intervention, *Drugs and Aging*, 3, 408, 1993.

76. Odell, W., Wolfsen, A., Yoshimoto, Y., Weitzman, R., Fisher, D., and Hirose, F., Ectopic peptide synthesis: a universal concomitant of neoplasia, *Trans. Assoc. Am. Physicians*, 90, 204, 1977.

77. Pitot, H. C., *Fundamentals of Oncology*, 3rd ed., Marcel Dekker, New York, 1986, 120.

78. Sundler, F., Hakanson, R., Loren, I., and Lundquist, I., Amine storage and function in peptide hormone-producing cells, *Invest. Cell. Pathol.*, 3, 87, 1980.

79. Alumets, J., Hakanson, R., Sundler, F., and Chang, K. J., Leu-enkephalin-like material in nerves and enterochromaffin cells in the gut. An immunohistochemical study, *Histochemistry*, 56, 187, 1978.

80. Nihei, K., Iwanaga, T., Fujita, T., Mochizuki, T., and Yanaihara, N., Distribution of Met-enkephalin-Arg6-Gly7-Leu8-like immunoreactivity in the gut of rats and pigs, *Endorphin Enkephalin.*, 3, 434, 1984.

81. Usellini, L., Capella, C., Malesci, A., Rindi, G., and Solcia, E., Ultrastructural localization of cholecystokinin in endocrine cells of the dog duodenum by the immunogold technique, *Histochemistry*, 83, 331, 1985.

82. Bussolati, G., Capella, C., Solcia, E., Vassallo, G., and Vezzadini, P., Ultrastructural and immunofluorescent investigations of the secretin cell in the dog intestinal mucosa, *Histochemistry*, 26, 218, 1971.

83. Polak, J. M., Sullivan, S. N., Bloom, S. R., Buchan, A. M. J., Facer, P., Brown, M. R., and Pearse, A. G. E., Specific localization of neurotensin to the N-cell in human intestine by radioimmunoassay and immunocytochemistry, *Nature*, 270, 183, 1977.

84. Rosell, S., Substance P and neurotensin in the control of gastrointestinal function, in *Peptides: Integrators of Cell and Tissue Function*, Bloom, F. E., Ed., Raven Press, New York, 1980, 147.

85. Sundler, F., Hakanson, R., Leander, S., and Uddman, R., Light and electron microscopic localization of neurotensin in the gastrointestinal tract, *Ann. N.Y. Acad. Sci.*, 400, 94, 1982.

86. Ganong, W. F., *Review of Medical Physiology*, 16th ed., Appleton & Lange, Norwalk, CT, 1993.

87. Solcia, E., Creutzfeldt, W., Falkmer, S., Fujita, T., Greider, M. H., Grossman, M. I., Grube, D., Hakanson, R., Larsson, L. I., Lechago, J., Lewin, K., Polak, J. M., and Rubin, W., Human gastroenteropancreatic endocrine-paracrine cells. Santa Monica 1980 classification, in *Cellular Basis of Chemical Messengers in the Digestive System*, Grossman, M.I., Brazier, M.A.B., and Lechago, J., Eds., Academic Press, New York, 1981, 159.

7

Aging of the Female Reproductive System

Paola S. Timiras and Jacqueline Sentenac

CONTENTS

I. INTRODUCTION

The initiation and cessation of reproductive function in the female have been taken as signposts of physiologic maturity and senescence, respectively. At puberty, in the human female, the initiation of menstruation is associated with somatic, neurologic, and psychologic changes — harbingers of adulthood. At menopause, the cessation of menstruation indicates termination of ovarian function and profound alterations in pituitary-ovarian relationships.

Just a few years ago it also used to mark the beginning of senescence, but today, with an average lifespan of approximately 80 years for women in most economically developed countries (Chapter 1), it merely marks the passage from one endocrine state to the next. Indeed, termination of the reproductive function is often viewed as a welcomed event, beneficial to an overpopulated society and offering a greater choice of activities (life patterns) for women.

The relationship between cessation of reproduction and aging of the entire organism has been studied in a number of species, but correlations have not been found between the generalized effects of hormone deficiency and most of the involutional changes associated with old age. Although a decline in the production of sex hormones and loss of sexual vigor with aging are common to both female and male, none of the research thus far conducted has established that the loss of sexual function represents a primary cause of aging nor has any treatment been devised that is capable of permanently restoring the sexual vigor of youth. Since the very early claims that sex hormones possess "rejuvenating" effects, it has been tempting to pursue the idea that restoration of sexual potency may reduce many of the "ravages of time" on the organism as a whole. Such a panacea has not been found! However, the demonstrated similarity in several parameters (e.g., organ weights, hormonal secretion, fat deposition, metabolic activity) between the aged and the castrated male or female and the temporary restorative effects of replacement hormonal therapy have been taken as suggestive of a secondary causative relationship between aging and endocrine insufficiency (involving other endocrine glands, in addition to gonads).

Given the many important actions of pituitary and ovarian hormones, in addition to those related exclusively to reproduction, loss of endocrine function has significant somatic and neuropsychologic repercussions capable of influencing the physiologic state and, eventually, of contributing to aging-related pathology. With aging, the decline in gonadal secretions may be expected to affect not only reproductive but also nonreproductive functions.

This chapter is concerned with the menopause and aging of the ovary and secondary sex organs in women, comparison with other animal species, and the relationship to aging of the hypothalamo-pituitary-ovarian axis. Clinical (reproductive and nonreproductive) symptoms of menopause and treatment thereof are considered next in Chapter 8.

II. THE MENOPAUSE

A. Definitions

The menopause is the permanent cessation of menses in women. It designates the loss of ovarian function with advanced age, particularly, the depletion of a woman's complement of ovarian follicles. It also refers to cessation of menstruation due to surgical removal of the ovaries at younger ages. In the latter case, when both ovaries are removed with or without hysterectomy (i.e., removal of the uterus), the term used is surgical menopause.[1]

Ovarian function does not cease abruptly and completely at a specific age, but rather declines progressively to gradual termination. The terms "premenopause" and "postmenopause" have been adopted to indicate those periods of gradual changes before or after menopause (Table 7-1).

B. Comparative Aspects

The menopause appears restricted to the human female, although if they live long enough, some species of monkeys (e.g., macaca, papio) may exhibit hormonal and physiologic changes similar to those of women.[2,3] In the wild state, senescence coincides with the reduction or cessation of reproductive capability and the postreproductive period is irrelevant to natural selection (Chapter 1). As long as the evolutionary value of the individual depends on the ability to produce the maximum number of offspring, selective pressures will favor survival

TABLE 7-1 Some Definitions of Menopause[1]

Menopause
  The permanent cessation of menstruation resulting from a loss of ovarian follicular activity.
Climacteric
  A critical stage in human life generally relating to the menopausal years.
Perimenopause of Climacteric
  The period immediately prior to and at least 1 year after the menopause, characterized by
  physiologic and clinical features of ovarian involution.
Premenopause
  An ambiguous term used variously to describe the 1 or 2 years previous to the menopause or the
  whole reproductive period prior to the menopause.
Postmenopause
  The period of life remaining after the menopause.

of young, reproductively active individuals. In women, until less than a century ago, in educationally and economically advanced countries and still today in several developing countries, menopause was (is) seen as a negative event of little importance to the life of the community: "when a woman's usefulness (in reproductive terms) was seen to be ended, she ceased to be a woman" (Chapter 8).[4]

In women, the origin of menopause is controversial. It could have evolved because the survival of women to an age when natural selection no longer favors the maintenance of reproductive ability may be the consequence of a gene or gene cluster with selective value early in life.[5] Alternatively, it may impart the advantage of providing for the care and protection of children by "surrogate mothers", that is, women themselves no longer capable of reproducing;[6] in this case, the increased morbidity and mortality of older women may outweigh any benefits from this "grandmotherly" function. The menopause could, then, be viewed as an artifact of human civilization which has emerged along with our increasing mastery of the environment and prolonged survivorship.[7]

C. Factors Influencing the Menopause

It is difficult to determine an age for menopause because of individual and population variability as well as sampling bias (e.g., retrospective sampling, sampling of hospitalized or self-selected individuals, tendency to round-up age at one- or five-year intervals). Using combined cross-sectional and longitudinal studies, the median age of Caucasian women at menopause has been established at between 49 and 51 years.[7] Less is known about other races. In the U.S., the median age for black women is about 49 years and for black women in South Africa it is also around 49 years. However, some populations of women in India, New Guinea, and Mexico all have a lower (40 years) median age at menopause. This difference may be due to factors related to nutrition, health, and socioeconomic status.

The importance of the nutritional status is reflected in the earlier age of menopause in women of malnourished populations and of thinner as compared to heavier women in a well-nourished population.[8,9] Parity, that is, the bearing of children, and status, single/married, employed/unemployed, may also play a role.[10] Smoking has been correlated with an early menopausal age,[11] perhaps through adverse effects of nicotine and carbon dioxide on ovarian circulation and/or on hemoglobin (reduced) and oocyte destruction (increased). Conversely, the use of oral (steroid) contraceptives delays the age of menopause.[9]

III. AGING OF THE OVARIAN FUNCTION

The gradual decline, and eventual cessation of reproductive function of the human female, with its involutional, regressive, and atrophic changes of reproductive organs, constitutes a classic example of the aging of a physiologic system. Such changes occur earlier and far more markedly in the ovary than in most other organs and are responsible for the degenerative changes in the secondary sex organs as well as numerous endocrine imbalances characteristic of the menopausal and postmenopausal state. Given the regulatory role of ovarian hormones on several systemic functions, a decline in their secretion would also be reflected in the impairment of several extragonadal functions (e.g., metabolic, cardiovascular, nervous). To facilitate the discussion of changes with aging the reader is referred to Chapter 2 for a short summary of the reproductive function in the young adult human female and its neuroendocrine regulation.

A. Structural Changes

Changes in the ovary may be observed as early as 30 years of age when a decline in weight is progressively accompanied by generalized atrophy, proliferation of fibrous tissue, a tendency to form follicular cysts (i.e., cavities) and various degrees of vascular sclerosis (i.e., narrowing and hardening of blood vessels) (Figure 7-1).[12]

The most striking changes, however, are represented by:

- The continuing reduction in the total number of ova,
- The continuing reduction in the number of ova shed per cycle,
- The increase in the number of abnormal ova, and
- The disruption of the hormonal environment.

In the human female and in most other mammals, the number of primitive ova is established prenatally and this original stock is progressively depleted by ovulation and loss through continuing atresia (involution of follicles that failed to mature) (Table 7-2). Of the original complement of two million ovarian follicles at five months of intrauterine life, most are lost before or at birth. Only 300,000 to 400,000 follicles actually participate in the process of ovulation.

The rate of oocyte loss varies depending on the genetic make-up of the species or strain.[13,14] In humans, the oocyte number decreases rapidly from birth to 25 years, more slowly until 38 years, and again at a rapid rate from 38 to 45 years when only a few ova may persist.[12] Among mammals, the human female exhibits a certain uniqueness in that the loss of reproductive capacity coincides with exhaustion of ova. By contrast, in most rodents, reproduction is terminated long before the ovaries are depleted of oocytes.[15]

The causes underlying the loss of oocytes are not understood. Ovulation does not significantly affect the rate of loss since only a few ova are lost by ovulation with every cycle as compared to the several hundreds lost by atresia. Thus, the rate of atresia is the major factor controlling oocyte loss.

Hypophysectomy reduces the rate of loss of oocytes by slowing down the rate of atresia. Similarly, a restricted diet in rats and mice delays the onset of aging-related abnormalities of the estrous cycle: it abolishes the increase in cycle length and the rate of atresia.[16-18]

The progressive oocyte loss with advancing age is associated with an increasing rate of ovarian abnormalities. These are manifested by the paucity of active corpora lutea and, among the follicles that remain after age 40 (premenopausal), by cysts and cell atrophy. Follicle alterations during late reproductive life may lead to *preovulatory aging,* perhaps through prolongation of menstrual cycles. Such prolongation is preceded and associated with changes in levels of ovarian steroids which are known to impair chromosomal meiosis in vitro with a possible risk of abortion and consequences detrimental to development.[19]

Chromosomal aberrations may also result from *postovulatory aging* of the ova, that is, to delayed fertilization of "overripe" ova, a condition that may, in part, be a cause of Down's syndrome. This syndrome, characterized by abnormal somatic features (hence the alternate designation of mongolism), arrest of neurologic development and maturation with severely

TABLE 7-2   Changes With Age in the Total Number of Follicles in the
Human Ovaries

Prenatal	Childhood	Adolescence	Adulthood
2,000,000	**0–5**[a]	**11–15**	**21–25**
	318,000	383,500 + 11,200[b]	118,800 + 34,200
	6–10	**16–20**	**26–30**
	484,000 + 99,900	186,200 + 66,200	70,700 + 39,500
			31–35
			49,800 + 18,100
			36–40
			63,300 + 41,600
			41–45
			4,690 + 2,000

[a] Numbers in **bold** represent age range in years.

[b] Mean + standard error.

Adapted from Block, E., *Acta Anat.*, 14, 108, 1952.

impaired learning and intellectual capability, arises from a trisomy of chromosome 21 (hence the other designation of Trisomy 21). It is the most common age-related chromosomal disorder in humans, increasing from an incidence of 1:2500 in women under 30 years to 1:300 between the ages of 35 to 39 years and as high as 1:45 after 45 years. Other age-related chromosomal disorders involve chromosomes 18 (Edward's syndrome) and 13 (Patau's syndrome) as well as sex chromosome trisomies (e.g., Klinefelter's syndrome).[20]

The mechanism(s) involved in the production of genetically abnormal offspring with increased maternal age are little known: several have been suggested (e.g., increased exposure to radiation chemicals, autoantibodies, infectious agents, genetic predisposition) in addition to pre- and postovulatory aging, already mentioned. Extra-ovarian factors acting on transport and implantation of the fertilized ovum in the aged uterine wall as well as factors affecting the embryo and fetus may also be responsible for a possible increased risk of abnormal pregnancy and offspring past age 35.

B. Hormonal Changes

1. Estrogens

All hormones of the hypothalamo-pituitary-ovarian axis undergo changes with aging.[21-23] Estrogen levels (essentially those of estradiol, the more potent estrogen) in normal, regularly cycling women 45 years and older are significantly more variable but always lower (50 to 75%) than in younger women. Plasma or serum levels of estradiol decrease from premenopausal average values of 620 pmol/L to postmenopausal values of 40 pmol/L; those for estrone from 440 to 110. This decline is dependent on the age-related loss of follicles. It is in the cells of follicles that most estrogen is produced by aromatization of weak androgens synthesized *in situ*. Some estrogen (essentially estrone, the less potent estrogen) is also formed in various tissues (fat, muscle, hair, bone, brain) from aromatization of circulating androgens (from the ovary and adrenal cortex). In postmenopausal women, estrogen production is exclusively extragonadal in origin and depends on several factors, such as the amount of body fat.[24,25]

The major portion of circulating ovarian steroids is specifically bound to high affinity serum proteins such as sex-hormone-binding globulins (SHBG). While an association between age and SHBG has not been demonstrated, in obese postmenopausal women the percent decrease in free estrogen correlates with a decrease in serum SHBG capacity. Since postmenopausal women with breast or endometrial cancer tend to have a higher percent of free estrogen than women without these cancers, it is possible that the higher frequency of these neoplasms

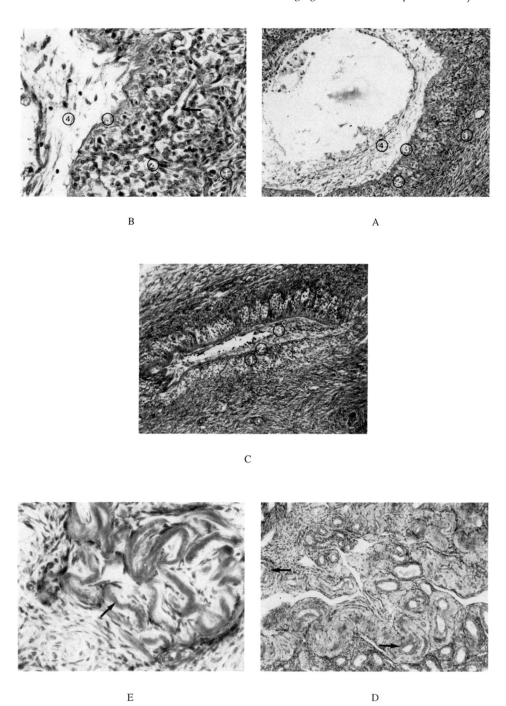

B

A

C

E

D

FIGURE 7-1 Atresia and vascular changes in the ovary of a menopausal 48-year-old woman.

in obese postmenopausal women is related to increased production of estrogen (a known mitogenic, carcinogenic hormone) and reduced SHBG capacity. The consequent prolonged stimulation of estrogen receptors in target cells (including the presence of estrogen receptors in about 70% of primary or metastatic breast cancers) would create a chronic proliferative state that may set the stage for neoplastic transformations.[26] Chronic estrogen stimulation is further enhanced by the fact that progesterone, which normally reduces estrogen receptor number, is no longer produced in the ovary of postmenopausal women.

2. Progesterone

Failure of progesterone production is one of the earliest demonstrable endocrine changes in the aging ovary. It is due to the increasing frequency of anovulatory (without ovulation) cycles prior to menopause. A nearly 50% decline in the urinary excretion of pregnanediol, a product of progesterone breakdown, is observed in the urine of women between the ages of 30 and 80 years. This decline in the production of progesterone seems to result from the decreased number of corpora lutea which, in turn, is due to the decreased number of follicles associated with the increased incidence of anovulation.

3. Androgens

The postmenopausal ovary, while not secreting any estrogen, continues to produce small but significant amounts of two male steroid hormones, testosterone (from premenopausal average values of 1000 pmol/L to postmenopausal of 800 pmol/L) and androstenedione (from 6300 pmol/L to 3100 pmol/L).[27] These, then, become the major ovarian hormones. They are secreted at the same (testosterone) or a lower rate (androstenedione) than before the menopause. Dehydroepiandrosterone, mainly of adrenocortical origin, is also significantly reduced (from 17,000 nmol/L to 5500 nmol/L) (Chapter 2). As estrogen levels fall, the unopposed male sex steroids may be responsible for the apparent masculinization (e.g., growth of hair on chin and upper lip; increased agressiveness?) of some elderly women.

4. Gonadotropins

The decline in estrogens and progesterone secretion is not due to hypofunction of the anterior pituitary. On the contrary, the anterior pituitary exhibits all the signs of hypersecretion (e.g., prominent cytoplasmic vacuoles and Golgi apparatus, increased RNA and mitochondria), presumably in response to the low levels of plasma estrogens. Some of these changes are also observed in premenopausal ovariectomized women. In laboratory animals, the pituitary does not exhibit any significant and sudden changes with aging but may undergo subtle and progressive alterations (Chapter 3) in conformity with the gradual nature of the loss of ovarian function and reproductive capacities.

FIGURE 7-1 Atresia and vascular changes in the ovary of a menopausal 48-year-old woman.

A. Illustrated in this figure are atresic changes involving primarily the internal layers of the ovarian follicle: (1) cells of the theca externa (surrounding externally the follicle) which are still unaltered; (2) cells of the theca interna (representing the innermost follicular cells) showing hyperplasia (i.e., proliferation) and hypertrophy (i.e., enlargement); (3) basal membrane undergoing proliferation and thickening of connective fibers to generate a thicker "membrane of atresia"; and (4) follicular cavity which is being invaded by macrophages and connective fibers.

B. A higher magnification of the same area as in A. Note proliferation of thecal cells (1 and 2) of connective fibers in basal membrane (3) and central cavity (4). Also note (arrow) an enlarged blood vessel.

C. Same ovary but another follicle which has undergone more severe atresia. Note greater hypertrophy and hyperplasia of internal thecal cells (1), thicker basal membrane (2), and almost complete disappearance of the follicular cavity (3).

D. Atresia is associated with (or preceded by ?) vascular changes. Blood vessels (arrows indicate two among many altered arteries) show thickening of arterial wall due to proliferation of smooth muscle and connective tissue cells and infiltration of vascular cavity by hyaline (proteoglycans) degeneration.

E. Higher magnification of same area as in D with extensive vascular degeneration.

(Courtesy of Professor R. Canivenc and Dr. J. Lobry, Laboratoire d'Histoplogie et Embryologie, University of Bordeaux Medical School, Bordeaux, France.)

With the onset of menopause, serum levels of FSH and LH rise so that one year after menopause FSH and LH levels are considerably higher than in young women, more so FSH (about 10 to 15 times) than LH (about 3 times).[28] This elevation persists for several years, but declines with advanced age — first LH (after age 60) and then FSH (after age 70 to 80). An explanation for this reduction in postmenopausal elevation of FSH and LH levels is not currently available. The cause may be a late age decline in overall anterior pituitary secretion associated, for example, with alterations in the antigenicity of these hormones as well as that of TSH and perhaps ACTH . Or it may be due to aging of the hypothalamus which no longer becomes sensitive to the loss of the negative feedback (due to the extremely low circulating levels of estrogen), or it may be due to both an hypothalamic and pituitary deficiency.[29]

Both FSH and LH levels retain a certain pulsatility (i.e., rhythmicity), pulsing every 1 to 2 h with a frequency similar to that of young women but with a much greater amplitude. This larger amplitude would be due to increased stimulation from hypothalamic GnRH, probably in response to the low circulating levels of estrogens and the ensuing decrease in negative feedback). With the increased circulating and stored levels, gonadotropins, particularly LH, exhibit some structural changes (e.g., increased molecular weight, polymorphism, immunoreactivity) associated with decreased biological activity, reminiscent of the aging changes in TSH (Chapter 5).

C. Functional Changes

Both gonadal and extragonadal tissues and organs undergo functional changes. With menopause, the cyclicity of the hypothalamo-pituitary-ovarian axis gradually ceases but amenorrhea (i.e., absence of menstruation) is preceded by a period of irregularities indicative of alterations in ovulation and hormonal cycles. They are characterized by a decline in length of the cycle and, particularly, of the follicular phase, an increase in the number of anovulatory cycles, and lowered estrogen levels together with an increase in FSH (but not LH) levels.

The fall in female ovarian hormones results, as expected, in profound atrophy of those organs and female sex characteristics that are stimulated most directly by their presence (see below). Changes in other functions are also induced by the declining ovarian hormonal levels. Among those most affected are the cardiovascular and nervous systems, the bone, and skin (Chapter 8).

1.   Changes in Cyclicity

As cyclicity is one of the essential characteristics of ovarian function, changes in this function represent one of the important signs of the imminence of menopause. As already discussed above, the onset of menstrual irregularities is taken as an indication of the failing ovarian function. The difficulty of decoding the nature and level of neuroendocrine changes contributing to or responsible for the menopause in humans has led to the frequent use of laboratory animals, usually rodents, as models. Although the end of the reproductive life of animals is not signaled by any phenomenon similar to the menopause, like humans, the aging animal begins to demonstrate irregularities in estrous cycles preceding and following cessation of reproduction. Such irregularities have been ascribed to aging changes of those CNS centers, like the hypothalamus and limbic system, that normally regulate reproductive function and cyclicity. These centers would undergo the same structural (e.g., loss of neurons, dendrites, and synapses), neurochemical (e.g., neurotransmitter imbalance) and functional changes (e.g., EEG alterations, loss of memory, sensory impairment) as other CNS areas. In addition, hypothalamic and limbic structures are particularly sensitive to steroid hormones.[30] With aging, they would lose the ability to orchestrate ovarian cyclicity.[29]

2.   Rodents as Models for the Study of Reproductive Aging

Rodents (rats, mice, guinea pigs, hamsters) possess estrous cycles associated with hormonal changes somewhat resembling the human menstrual cycle. In these animals, interventions —

hormonal, nutritional, psychologic, pharmacologic — can alter the rhythmicity and duration of reproductive function and interact with age in triggering both onset and termination of reproduction.[31-34] In the rat, estrous cycles lasting 3 to 5 days are repeated throughout the year except during pregnancy: eggs are released from the ovary during "heat" or estrus, corresponding to sexual interest and receptivity. The days of the cycle are numbered from that of estrus (day 1) followed by diestrus, proestrus, and again estrus. Each stage has its own functional and hormonal characteristics which are translated at the vagina by specific changes of the mucosa; such vaginal changes can be easily detected and permit the investigator to follow many cycles with little discomfort to the animal.

At 10 to 15 months (the lifespan of the laboratory rat is approximately 3 years) estrous cycles lenghten due to the prolongation of estrus. Despite the diminished number of total oocytes, the number of eggs ovulated and corpora lutea formed are normal during this period of "presenile" irregularity.[35] With continued irregularity, increased anovulation and lengthening of the cycles, the animal becomes acyclic and enters a period of constant estrus, probably due to the uninterrupted secretion of estrogens with little or no progesterone (corpora lutea are lacking in the ovary); as in postmenopausal women, levels of FSH are elevated, although less so than in older women, and levels of LH may be increased as well.[36]

At a later age, around 20 months and older, the rat undergoes a period of so-called "repetitive pseudopregnancy". In this period, the duration of diestrus is prolonged to 1 to 2 weeks: numerous corpora lutea but few or no follicles are present in the ovary with consequent high levels of progesterone in the absence of estrogen. At still older ages, 28 months and older, corpora lutea are no longer present and the animal is anestrous, that is, no longer undergoes any ovarian and vaginal cycles.

With the rat or mouse as models, the complexity of the signals that regulate the hypothalamo-pituitary-ovarian interactions has begun to unravel. Major findings include:

- The responsiveness of the hypothalamus to ovarian hormones is decreased in aging animals, probably as part of overall CNS changes;
- This decreased responsiveness with aging may be related to alterations of neurotransmission (e.g., neurotransmitter imbalance) as manifested by decreased catecholamine levels and altered timing of the serotonin peak (responsible for triggering LH secretion and ovulation);
- The cumulative effects of estrogens throughout life, particularly, high estrogen levels during constant estrus may induce neurotoxic damage in the hypothalamus;[33]
- The neurotoxicity of estrogens may affect, also, the structures of the limbic system,[33] a CNS area anatomically and functionally closely related to the hypothalamus and reproductive function; a similar selective neurotoxicity has been described for glucocorticoid hormones from the adrenal cortex (Chapter 14)
- The neurotoxicity is manifested by neuronal degeneration and loss with (compensatory?) gliosis, neurotransmitter, and hormonal alterations (e.g., decreased dopamine, the neurotransmitter involved in inhibition of the hormone prolactin, results in increased circulating levels of prolactin)[39] and changes in number and affinity of estrogen receptors;[37,38]
- These structural and neurochemical alterations may result in "deafferentation", that is, functional separation of the hypothalamic nuclei one from the other so that integration of signals among them and with limbic structures for normal function is no longer possible.

3. Experimental Interventions to Delay Aging-Related Changes in Reproductive Function

As the factors which regulate ovarian function in adulthood and determine its cessation at menopause are better understood, it becomes possible to envision ways in which physiologic competence may be enhanced or prolonged and reproductive pathology prevented or treated.

These interventions may be hormonal, nutritional, and pharmacologic. They may influence the hypothalamo-pituitary-ovarian axis by several, perhaps synergistic, mechanisms:

- The cumulative adverse impact of estrogen on the hypothalamus may be prevented by ovariectomy at a young age; or
- The length of estrus is shortened or prolonged by the administration of selected neurotransmitters to modify the timing of signals necessary for maintenance of cyclicity; or
- The neonatal administration of hormones such as testosterone prevents the cyclic differentiation of the hypothalamus; or
- Dietary restriction (involving total calories or specific constituents) delays the onset of ovarian maturation and aging.

Although these interventions cannot, so far, be adopted for humans, they demonstrate the importance of neuroendocrine controls on reproduction. In humans, replacement therapy with estrogens (or progestins) improves considerably the quality of life of a great number of postmenopausal women by ameliorating sexual and some nonsexual functions; it also may prolong the duration of life by reducing the severity of age-associated pathologic processes (e.g., osteoporosis, cardiovascular diseases) which are among the main causes of death (Chapter 8).

IV. AGING OF THE FEMALE SECONDARY SEX ORGANS

A. Oviducts

After menopause, these organs shorten and their diameter decreases. The lining epithelium atrophies and its cells gradually lose their cilia. With the atrophy of the epithelium, the underlying (stromal) tissue forms blunted villi and the smooth muscle layer is replaced by fibrous tissue.[40] After 60 years of age, tubal secretions cease and peristaltic movements are decreased or absent.[41]

B. Uterus and Cervix

With the fall of estrogen levels, the uterus gradually decreases in size, concomitant with a decrease in muscle content and an increase in fibrous tissue. From age 30 to 50 years changes are minimal, but in the following 15 years they are more drastic with a 30 to 50% reduction; in very old women, the uterus may atrophy to 1 cm. The uterine endometrium becomes atrophic with flattening of the lining epithelium and, sometimes, cystic dilation of the glands, leading to glandular hyperplasia.[42-44]

Such changes may be due to the progressive decline in estrogen. Intrinsic uterine changes may also be responsible for the reduced sensitivity to hormones. The senescent uterus exhibits receptor loss, decreased receptor activation, impaired stimulation of RNA polymerase II, and defects in nuclear translocation (or enhanced association) of receptor-estradiol complexes.[37,38,45]

With appropriate estrogen therapy, uterine structure and function may be restored, at least partially. Persistence of circulating estrogen (after increased extragonadal production) in obese women or after decreased metabolism due to severely impaired liver function, or administration of exogenous estrogen (as in replacement therapy) may result in a more juvenile appearance with proliferation and secretory activity of the glands.

The cervix, the lower portion of the uterus, undergoes atrophy similar to that of the remainder of the uterus, with frequent closure of the uterine orifice, thinning of the epithelium, increased connective tissue (collagen), and little secretory activity of the glands.[46] With the concomitant atrophy of the vagina, the cervix no longer protrudes in the vagina but often becomes flush with the apex of the vaginal vault, making it almost impossible to be located when attempting to perform a diagnostic (Papanicolau) smear (or an eventual neoplastic transformation). The accumulation of specific types of "parabasal" cells also makes difficult the interpretation of smears for diagnosis.

C. Vagina and Vulva

In the vagina, atrophy of the epithelium causes shortening with reduction of elasticity. Epithelial cells flatten and lose glycogen (necessary for lactobacilli activity). The consequent reduced lactobacilli population results in a rise of vaginal pH (or decreased acidity), thereby increasing the risk of bacterial infections.[47] Treatment of such bacterial infections by antibiotics may encourage the growth of yeasts responsible for menopausal (senile or atrophic) vaginitis. The thinner epithelium makes the vagina more vulnerable to mechanical injury and bleeding. Associated with vaginal dryness (due to failure of mucous secretion), this condition may lead to painful intercourse (but is responsive to topical estrogen treatment).[48] The efficacy of vaginal absorption of steroids is well demonstrated and seems to be enhanced in the atrophic vagina.[49]

Changes in the vulva include: loss and whitening of pubic hair, atrophy of labia minora and limpiness of majora, atrophy of vulvar skin, and reduction in glycogen content of epithelial cells.[50,51] These changes lead to frequent skin alterations such as lichen sclerosis (a distressingly itchy condition) and hyperplastic dystrophy prevalent in elderly women.

D. Mammary Gland

The mammary glands are modified skin (sweat) glands specialized for milk production. In humans, two glands (or breasts) develop only on the pectoral region, whereas in other mammals several glands develop along the so-called "milk lines" (extending from axilla to groin). Their growth and function are controlled by hormones from the pituitary, adrenal cortex, ovary, and placenta. Each gland in women consists of 15 to 20 lobes, further subdivided into lobules comprised of a duct surrounded by cords of secretory cells forming acini and alveoli. The small ducts open into a main duct leading to the nipple. Lobes and lobules are supported by a network of connective tissue and adipose tissue deposits.

At puberty, the rising levels of estrogens are responsible for the development of adipose and connective tissue and the proliferation of ducts, and progesterone for that of lobules and alveoli. Growth hormone and glucocorticoids are also necessary for mammary growth.

During pregnancy, all these hormones plus some prolactin from the pituitary and growth hormone-prolactin (i.e., somatomammotropic hormone) from the placenta induce full alveolar development and some milk production. After delivery, increased secretion of prolactin combined with declining estrogen and progesterone levels bring about copious secretion of milk. In the presence of oxytocin (also from the pituitary and secreted by the suckling reflex, Chapter 3) ejection of milk occurs and thereby completes the process of lactation.

After menopause, mammary glands usually decrease in size due to atrophy, although in some women they may enlarge together with increasing obesity. Rates of atrophy or enlargement greatly vary with each individual. Atrophy is due to resorption of adipose stores (which, on the contrary, greatly increase in obese women) and disappearance of secretory cells and ducts and their replacement by connective tissue (fibrosis) (the latter changes occur in obese women as well). The nipple loses pigmentation and erectibility.

1. Cancer of the Breast and Uterus

The breasts and uterus may be the site of cancer (usually carcinoma) in women, breast cancer being the most frequent. The incidence of the most frequent cancers in women increases with age from 40 to 70 years, almost doubling each 10 years for breast cancer and more than doubling for cancer of the lung, colon/rectum, and uterus. Annual incidence rates (per 100,000 white U.S. women) at all ages are highest for breast cancer, with cancer of the lung, colon/rectum, and uterus following in second, third, and fourth place, respectively (Table 7-3).[52-55]

TABLE 7-3 Annual Incidence and Age-Adjusted
Mortality Rates for Major Cancers in
White Women, U.S.

Annual (1985–1989) Incidence Rates per 100,000 for Major Cancers for U.S. White Women				
Organ	40–44[a]	50–54	60–64	70–74
Breast	129	230	356	450
Lung	13	67	162	228
Colon+Rectum	11	47	121	253
Corpus uterus	12	43	90	115

Age-Adjusted Mortality Rates per 100,000 for U.S. White Women, 1973 and 1989		
Organ	year: 1973	year: 1989
Breast	27	28
Lung	13	31
Colon + rectum	20	16
Corpus uterus	4	3

[a] Numbers in bold represent age ranges.

Data obtained courtesy of Dr. Warren Winkelstein, Jr., University of California, Berkeley.

When one considers age-adjusted mortality rates (rather than incidence of disease), the recent impact of lung cancer in women can be better appreciated by a rate that has doubled from 1973 to 1985 (Table 7-3). During this period, death rates from breast, colon/rectum, and uterine cancer have remained about the same or have decreased (colon/rectum). Currently (1995), lung cancer probably kills more women than breast cancer. This morbidity and mortality is not exclusive to the U.S. Europe is facing the same trend and the data will probably be worse since more European women still smoke, the causal relationship between cigarette-smoking and lung cancer not being widely accepted.

The high incidence and mortality from mammary and uterine cancer, the important role of estrogen in development and maintenance of these two secondary sex organs, the well-known mitotic-promoting actions of estrogen and, therefore, the possible relation of estrogen to cancer must be kept in mind when evaluating the pros and contras of estrogen replacement therapy for the prevention or treatment of the symptoms and disorders of women after menopause.[56-58] Such considerations will be discussed further in Chapter 8.

REFERENCES

1. World Health Organization, WHO Scientific Group on Research on the Menopause, W.H.O., *Technical Report Series No. 670*, Geneva, WHO Publication Centre USA, Albany, New York, 1981.
2. Short, R., England, N., Bridson, W. E., and Bowden, D. M., Ovarian cyclicity, hormones, and behavior as markers of aging in female pigtailed macaques (*Macaca nemestrina*), *J. Gerontol.*, 44, B131, 1989.
3. Graham, C. F., Menstrual cycle of the great apes, in *Reproductive Biology of the Great Apes, Comparative and Biomedical Perspectives*, Graham, C. E., Ed., Academic Press, New York, 1981, 1.
4. Vertinsky, P., "Of no use without health": late nineteenth century medical prescriptions for female exercise through the life span, *Women and Health*, 14, 89, 1988.
5. Charlesworth, B., *Evolution in Age-Structured Populations*, Cambridge University Press, Cambridge, 1980.
6. Mayer, P. J., Evolutionary advantage of the menopause, *Hum. Ecol.*, 10: 477, 1982.
7. Gosden, R. G., *Biology of Menopause: the Causes and Consequences of Ovarian Ageing*, Academic Press, London, 1985.
8. Sherman, B. M., Wallace, R. B., and Treloar, A. E., The menopausal transition: endocrinological and epidemiological considerations, *J. Biosoc. Sci.*, Suppl. 6, 19, 1979.

9. van Keep, P. A., Brand, P. C., and Lehert, P., Factors affecting the age at menopause, *J. Biosoc. Sci.,* Suppl. 6, 37, 1979.

10. Brand, P. C. and Lehert, P., A new way of looking at environmental variables that may affect the age at menopause, *Maturitas,* 1, 121, 1978.

11. Kaufman, D. W., Slone, D., Rosenberg, L., Miettinen, O. S., and Shapiro, S., Cigarette smoking and age at natural menopause, *Am. J. Pub. Health,* 70, 420, 1980.

12. Canivenc, R., Lobry, J., and Scholler, R., Histophysiologie de l'ovaire á la peri- et la postmenopause, *Proc. Journees d'Endocrinologie Clinique,* 16-17 November, 1979, Fondation de Recherche en Hormonologie, SEPE Publ., Fresnes (France), 1980, 43.

13. Block, E., Quantitative morphological investigations of the follicular system in women. Variations at different ages, *Acta Anat.,* 14, 108, 1952.

14. Richardson, S. J. and Nelson, J. F., Follicular depletion during the menopausal transition, *Ann. N.Y. Acad. Sci.,* 592, 13, 1990.

15. Mandl, A. M. and Shelton, M., A quantitative study of oocytes in young and old nulliparous laboratory rats, *J. Endocrinol.,* 18, 444, 1959.

16. Segall, P. E., Timiras, P. S., and Walton, J. R., Low tryptophan diets delay reproductive aging, *Mech. Ageing Dev.,* 23, 245, 1983.

17. Goodrick, G. J. and Nelson, J. F., The decidual cell response in aging C57BL/6J mice is potentiated by long-term ovariectomy and chronic food restriction, *J. Gerontol.,* 44, B67, 1989.

18. Merry, B. and Holehan, A., Aging of the female reproductive system, in *Physiological Basis of Aging and Geriatrics,* Timiras, P. S., Ed., CRC Press, Boca Raton, FL, 1994.

19. Wertheim, I., Jagiello, G. M., and Ducayen, M. B., Aging and aneuploidy in human oocytes and follicular cells, *J. Gerontol.,* 41, 567, 1986.

20. Hook, E. B., Rates of chromosome abnormalities at different maternal ages, *Obstet. Gynecol.,* 58, 282, 1981.

21. Vagenakis, A. G., Endocrine aspects of menopause, *Clin. Rheumatol.,* 8 (Suppl. 2), 48, 1989.

22. Bates, G. W. and Boone, W. R., The female reproductive cycle: new variations on an old theme, *Curr. Opin. Obstet. Gynecol.,* 3, 838, 1991.

23. al-Azzawi, F., Endocrinological aspects of the menopause, *Br. Med. Bull.,* 48, 262, 1992.

24. Siiteri, P. K. and MacDonald, P. C., Role of extraglandular estrogen in human endocrinology, in *Handbook of Physiology, Section 7: Endocrinology,* Vol. II, Part I, Greep, R. O. and Astwood, E. B., Am. Physiol. Soc., Washington, D.C., 1973, 615.

25. Marshall, D. H., Crilly, R., and Nordin, B. E. C., The relation between plasma androstenedione and oestrone levels in untreated and corticosteroid-treated post-menopausal women, *Clin. Endocrinol.,* 9, 407, 1978.

26. Fernig, D. G., Smith, J. A., and Rudland, P. S., Relationship of growth factors and differentiation in normal and neoplastic development of the mammary gland, *Cancer Treat. Res.,* 53, 47, 1991.

27. Judd, H. L. and Korenman, S. G., Effects of aging on reproductive function in women, in *Endocrine Aspects of Aging,* Korenman, S. G., Ed., Elsevier, New York, 1982, 163.

28. Chakravarti, S., Collins, W. P., Forecast, J. J., Newton, J. R., Oram, D. H., and Studd, J. W., Hormonal profiles after the menopause, *Br. Med. J.,* 2, 784, 1976.

29. Wise, P. M., Weiland, N. G., Scarbrough, K., Sortino, M. A., Cohen, I. R., and Larson, G. H., Changing hypothalamopituitary function: its role in aging of the female reproductive system, *Horm. Res.,* 31, 39, 1989.

30. Terasawa, E. and Timiras, P. S., Electrical activity during the estrous cycle of the rat: cyclic changes in limbic structures, *Endocrinology,* 83, 207, 1968.

31. Nelson, J. F. and Felicio, L. S., Hormonal influences on reproductive aging in mice, *Ann. N.Y. Acad. Sci.,* 592, 8, 1990.

32. Bestetti, G. E., Reymond, M. J., Blanc, F., Boujon, C. E., Furrer, B., and Rossi, G. L., Functional and morphological changes in the hypothalamo-pituitary-gonadal axis of aged female rats, *Biol. Reprod.,* 45, 221, 1991.

33. Finch, C. E., Kohama, S. G., and Pasinetti, G. M., Ovarian steroid and neurotoxin models of brain aging in rodents, *Ann. N.Y. Acad. Sci.,* 648, 119, 1992.

34. Kalra, S. P., Sahu, A., and Kalra, P. S., Ageing of the neuropeptidergic signals in rats, *J. Reprod. Fertil. Suppl.,* 46, 11, 1993.

35. Aschheim, P., Relation of neuroendocrine system to reproductive decline in female rats, in *Neuroendocrinology of Aging,* Meites, J., Ed., Plenum Press, New York, 1983, 73.

36. Walker, R. F., Cooper, R. L., and Timiras, P. S., Constant estrus: role of rostral hypothalamic monoamines in development of reproductive dysfunction in aging rats, *Endocrinology,* 107, 249, 1980.

37. Cooper, R. L., McNamara, M. C., and Linnoila, M., Catecholaminergic-serotonergic balance in the CNS and reproductive cycling in aging rats, *Neurobiol. Aging,* 7, 9, 1986.

38. Belisle, S., Bellabarba, D., Lehoux, J. G., Robel, P., and Baulieu, E. E., Effect of aging on the dissociation kinetics and estradiol receptor nuclear interactions in mouse uteri: correlation with biological effects, *Endocrinology,* 118, 750, 1987.

39. Belisle, S., Bellabarba, D., and Lehoux, J.-H., Enhanced inhibition of estrogen receptor nuclear binding in the uterus of aged mice, *J. Steroid Biochem.,* 26, 521, 1989.

40. Gaddum-Rosse, P., Rumery, R. E., Blandau, R. J., and Thiersch, J. B., Studies on the mucosa of postmeno- pausal oviducts: surface appearance, ciliary activity, and the effect of estrogen treatment, *Fertil. Steril.,* 26, 951, 1975.

41. Hafez, E. S. E., Scanning electron microscopy of female reproductive organs during menopause and related pathologies, in *The Menopause: Clinical, Endocrinological and Pathophysiological Aspects,* Fiorette, P., Martini, L., Melis, G. B., and Yen, S. S. C., Eds., Academic Press, New York, 1982, 201.

42. Ferenczy, A. and Bergeron, C., Histology of the human endometrium: from birth to senescence, *Ann. N.Y. Acad. Sci.,* 622, 6, 1991.

43. Meldrum, D. R., Female reproductive aging — ovarian and uterine factors, *Fertil. Steril.,* 59, 1, 1993.

44. Mulholland, J. and Jones, C. J., Characteristics of uterine aging, *Microsc. Res. Tech.,* 25, 148, 1993.

45. Roth, G. S., Altered estrogen action in the senescent rat uterus: a model for steroid resistance during aging, *Advan. Exp. Med. Biol.,* 196, 347, 1986.

46. Roberts, A. D., Cordiner, J. W., Hart, D. M., Barlow, D. H., MacRae, D., and Leggate, I., The variation in cervical hydroxyproline and cervical water with age, *Br. J. Obstet. Gynaecol.,* 95, 1159, 1988.

47. Milsom, I., Arvidsson, L., Ekelund, P., Molander, U., and Erticksson, O., Factors influencing vaginal cytology, pH and bacterial flora in elderly women, *Acta Obstet. Gynecol. Scand.,* 72, 286, 1993.

48. Key, E. and Smith, S., Management of vaginal dryness, *Nursing Standard,* 5, 24, 1991.

49. Pschera, H., Hjerpe, A., and Carlstrom, K., Influence of the maturity of the vaginal epithelium upon the absorption of vaginally administered estradiol-17 beta and progesterone in postmenopausal women, *Gynecol. Obstet. Invest.,* 27, 204, 1989.

50. Voet, R. L., End organ response to estrogen deprivation, in *The Menopause,* Buchsbaum, H. J., Ed., Springer-Verlag, New York, 1983, 9.

51. Semmelink, H. J., de Wilde, P. C., van Houwelingen, J. C., and Vooijs, G. P., Histomorphometric study of the lower urogenital tract in pre- and post-menopausal women, *Cytometry,* 11, 700, 1990.

52. Dix, D., The role of aging in cancer incidence: an epidemiological study, *J. Gerontol.,* 44, 10, 1989.

53. Newell, G. R., Spitz, M. R., and Sider, J. G., Cancer and age, *Semin. Oncol.,* 16, 3, 1989.

54. Stewart, J. A. and Foster, R. S., Jr., Breast cancer and aging, *Semin. Oncol.,* 16, 41, 1989.

55. Byrne, A. and Carney, D. N., Cancer in the elderly, *Curr. Prob. Cancer,* 17, 145, 1993.

56. Satariano, W. A., Comorbidity and functional status in older women with breast cancer: implications for screening, treatment and prognosis, *J. Gerontol.,* 47, 24, 1992.

57. Shay, J. W., Wright, W. E., and Werbin, H., Toward a molecular understanding of human breast cancer: a hypothesis, *Breast Cancer Res. Treat.,* 25, 83, 1993.

58. Satariano, W. A., Aging, comorbidity and breast cancer survival: an epidemiologic view, *Adv. Exper. Med. Biol.,* 330, 1, 1993.

8

The Menopause: Clinical Aspects and Current Trends in Therapy

Jacqueline Sentenac and Paola S. Timiras

CONTENTS

I. INTRODUCTION

The menopause, included within the general framework of the female "climacteric period", represents a major, critical, turning point in a woman's lifespan. The concept of "critical age" originally indicated those changes that occurred during embryogenesis and resulted in the differentiation and growth of a specific organ or tissue. This concept, later extended to include the postnatal period from infancy to adolescence, identifies periods of accelerated growth and maturation. Critical periods are particularly responsive and vulnerable to environmental influences, and any intervention at a critical age may have long-term beneficial or damaging effects on the adult individual.

Menopause, as a critical climacteric age, refers both to the vulnerability of this period and the impact of physiologic events at this time on subsequent senescence. The terms menopause and female climacteric are used interchangeably to cover gonadal and extragonadal events in women's transition from maturity to senescence.

Cessation of reproductive function is associated with:

- Progressive physiologic changes,
- Increasing pathologic risks that reflect:
  - The gradual disappearance of the ovarian hormones, and
  - The continuous aging of their targets.

Of these targets, the most affected are the secondary sex organs (Chapter 7). Changes occur as well in organs and tissues (cardiovascular, nervous, skeletal, tegumental, and excretory systems) unrelated to reproductive function but extremely important for adaptation and survival. Extrareproductive actions will be considered briefly in the first part of this chapter. In the second part, replacement therapy will be presented with a brief discussion of its major indications and contraindications.

II. SOCIOCULTURAL ASPECTS INFLUENCING MENOPAUSE

Early studies of menopause focused on irregularities and abnormal abundance of menstrual flow (menorrhagia) during the pre- and perimenopausal years.[1,2] From the 17th and 18th centuries on in Western Europe, menstrual irregularities were associated with a large number of diseases often included under the category of "female mergrims and miasms of difficult classification."[3] Signs and symptoms ascribed to menopause were numerous and varied, but usually trivial, although they could be in some cases quite severe. They were more frequent in "upper class women" and, later, "middle class" as well (with, occasionally, promiscuous and self-indulgent lifestyles) than in peasant women (of the same country): "the latter's complete freedom from climacteric complications, including menorrhagia, was regarded as proof of the health promoting qualities of an uncomplicated life close to nature, of moderation in food and drink, and of abstinence from the pleasures of (promiscuous) love."[2]

Towards the end of the 19th century, with more rigorous diagnostic methods, the "menopausal syndrome" was divested of most of its agglomerated primary, secondary, or incidental manifestations. However, despite vigorous clinical "pruning" the menopause remains, for many women, a period in the lifespan often marked by physiologic vulnerability and increasing pathology.[4-7] Even today, a number of women, their physicians, and certainly representatives of the pharmaceutical industry, consider menopause as a disabling and pathological period of life that requires vigorous medical intervention for restoration of normal function. This approach may be viewed as "medicalization" of menopause, from the sociologic term for defining and treating human experiences as medical problems.[8-10] It belies the experiences of the many women for whom the menopause represents merely a period of transition, virtually devoid of any specific subjectively disturbing sign.[11-13]

Socioeconomic and cultural factors strongly influence all biomedical aspects of human life. Variations in the characteristics of the menopause between women categorized as "Western" (from socioeconomically developed countries) and "non-Western" (from developing countries) aptly illustrate the importance of such influences. In the past, a woman born in a non-Western society often did not reach or survive beyond the age of menopause. Today, with the prolongation of the average lifespan even in the less developed countries, such a woman will enter the menopausal years but with a past reproductive and endocrine history quite different from that of her Western counterpart. Married soon after the menarche, most non-Western women will become pregnant and miss menses during gestation and lactation. After one or two menses, they may become pregnant again, a process that will then repeat itself until the menopause will supervene silently during lactation.[14] This contrasts with the Western lifestyle where the widespread use of contraception has created what has been termed "incessant ovulation".[15,16] Hormonal cyclicity in the absence of pregnancy in Western women can then be contrasted with the consistently high levels of sex hormones in pregnancy in non-Western women. The very question has been raised of whether menstruation represents a "natural, biologic function" or an abnormal physiologic condition;[15] menses have been poetically viewed as "the tears shed by the uterus for the sorrow of not being pregnant."

The consequences of such different hormonal profiles individually among women of the same cultural background, and collectively among women of widely different cultures remains to be evaluated by future studies. Given the important gonadal and extragonadal actions of sex hormones, a wide range of functions may be affected with long-term influence on both the quality and length of life.

III. SYMPTOMS OF MENOPAUSE ASSOCIATED WITH NONREPRODUCTIVE SYSTEMS AND FUNCTIONS

In addition to aging of the ovaries, oviducts, uterus, vagina, vulva, and mammary glands discussed in the preceding Chapter 7, the menopause affects a number of nonreproductive organs and functions, with the resulting most common symptoms grouped under three major categories:

- Those related to the autonomic nervous system, such as hot flashes, perspiration, and palpitations;
- Those related to the central nervous system (CNS), such as headaches, insomnia, depression, irritability, and mood changes, and
- Those related to circulatory and metabolic changes such as hypertension, atherosclerosis, obesity, diabetes, osteoporosis, osteoarthritis, autoimmune disease, and some skin and hair changes.

Not all women undergoing the menopause become chronic invalids and experience years of ill health. A few are genuinely miserable and lack vigor and initiative, but many report to be free of any subjective symptom, and many tolerate the event quite well.

A. Hot Flashes

Hot flashes (or flushes), that is, a rapid and intense increase in blood flow in the face, ears, arms, and in some cases, the entire upper portion of the body with reddening and increased skin temperature, represent the most common (occurring in 70 to 75% of women) and well-known symptom of menopause.[17-19] Flashes are often associated with tachycardia (i.e., accelerated cardiac beat), anxiety, chilling sensations, inappropriate sweating, and paresthesias (i.e., abnormal sensations such as formication, sensation of ants creeping on the skin). Symptoms vary in type and severity from woman to woman and even in the same woman from one occurrence to the other. They usually lessen and disappear with time. Some 15 to 25% of menopausal women seek medical advice and treatment.

Why some women flash frequently and why others never flash or do so for only a short time is not understood. Hot flashes may result from instability of the autonomic control of vasomotor tone, with the peripheral circulation (e.g., selective vasodilation of the forearm) differing in menopausal women experiencing the flashes.[20] Metabolic changes are implicated as well (e.g., increased plasma free fatty acids, increased norepinephrine and LH levels).[21]

The flashing may have a CNS, particularly hypothalamic, origin. After hypothalamic damage, flashes have been experienced by boys and girls at the onset of puberty.[22] Centers for thermoregulation are located in the hypothalamus in proximity of LHRH-containing neurons. Inappropriate activity of these thermoregulatory centers — either due to their intrinsic aging or altered levels of estrogens and gonadotropins — would be responsible for the vasomotor symptoms.[23] Other causes implicated in these vasomotor disturbances may involve alterations in neurotransmitters (i.e., dopamine, norepinephrine, endorphin) of hypothalamic and limbic structures, as well as in prostaglandins (i.e., unsaturated fatty acids with multiple actions on secretions, muscle contraction, neurotransmission, and others).[24,25]

Whether the flashing is a direct and specific effect of estrogen deficiency remains controversial. In most cases, treatment with estrogens (with or without progestins) appears to be specific and effective. However, other compounds (e.g., clonidine, nalazone) and sometimes placebos may also be effective.[26]

B. Psychologic Symptoms

A large proportion of women enter menopause with equanimity, as a new life period heralding its own advantages (e.g., freedom from child-bearing and rearing) and disadvantages (e.g., loneliness, declining physical attractiveness). Others find it a period of considerable stress viewing it as signaling the termination of physiologic and psychologic youth. They suffer, with varying degrees of severity, loss of self-image, unwarranted apprehension and anxiety, amnesia, and difficulty in concentrating and in making decisions. Alterations of mood and behavior (e.g., nervousness, irritability, depression) may result from fear of a future construed to be devoid of a well-defined purpose, with only the certainty of senescence, disease, and death. Often, loss of reproductive capability is interpreted as functional castration and is associated with disturbances of sexual behavior.[27-29]

While sexual activity declines in men continuously from puberty, the sexual abilities of (unmarried) women remain practically unchanged until 55 to 60 years of age,[30] and well into older ages upon regular stimulation.[31] In postmenopausal (married) women, decline in coital rates is due primarily to decreasing libido in the male.[32] In some women, however, vaginal dryness and fragility (Chapter 7) may cause painful intercourse and this, in turn, a secondary decline in sexual enjoyment and interest.[33]

In most cases, when postmenopausal symptoms are present, a variety of so-called "conditioning" or "predisposing" factors related to ethnic background, personality, socioeconomic conditions, employment and professional status, marriage and family network, and others will considerably influence onset, frequency, duration, and severity of all psychologic symptoms. Treatment and prevention, therefore, should include not only specific pharmacologic and hormonal therapy but must also address the need to improve the quality of the environment and life style.[34,35]

1.   Role of Estrogens in Normal and Abnormal CNS Development and Aging

That estrogens affect brain development at neonatal and adolescent ages is demonstrated experimentally in laboratory animals (e.g., rats) and clinically in humans. Particularly susceptible to the actions of estrogens are the limbic structures (e.g., amygdala and hippocampus) responsible for maturation and maintenance of sexual behavior and reproductive function as well as memory and adaptive responses. Estrogens bind to receptors, abundant in limbic structures, and stimulate neuronal plasticity (e.g., electrical activity, synaptogenesis, cyclicity, and behavior).[36] With aging, the number of dendrites decreases in several areas of the CNS, including limbic structures. This neuronal "denudation" is due not to an absolute loss of dendrites but, rather, to a slower (than at younger ages) replacement of continually renewing dendrites. With estrogen deprivation the anabolic stimulation of dendritic growth would be attenuated or lost. When these changes involve the hippocampus, memory and cognitive functions may be impaired.

Degenerative disorders of the brain associated with aging such as dementia of the Alzheimer's type (AD) are more frequent in women than in men, a difference originally attributed to the longer lifespan of women and the close relationship between advancing age and AD incidence. However, estrogens may influence hippocampal neurons directly by stimulating the number of receptors and expression of Nerve Growth Factor (NGF), a local promoter of neural cell growth.[37] Thus, administration of estrogens may improve cognitive performance of elderly women with probable AD.[38]

C. The Skin

Changes of the skin are due both to estrogen deficiency and the unopposed levels of androgens secreted by the ovary and the adrenal cortex (Chapter 2).

Estrogen receptors in the skin actively bind estrogen; the hormone is internalized and carried to the nucleus where it stimulates protein production (protoglycans, collagen, elastin), and influences water content and hyaluronic acid (major skin components). With aging, the skin becomes:

- Thinner (due to loss of collagen fibers),
- Dryer (due to water loss),
- Less elastic, and
- More wrinkled (due to loss of elastic fibers).

These changes are more evident in the face, the skin area richest in estrogen receptors and the one most exposed to the environment, particularly the sun. The loss of cutaneous collagen parallels the loss of bone collagen (matrix) characteristic of osteoporosis (Chapter 13).

The effects of unopposed androgens are especially upsetting to postmenopausal women as they are responsible for a certain degree of masculinization reflected in both appearance and behavior, the jestingly so-called "mother-in-law syndrome".[39] Hair grows on the lip and chin (rarely on the body), but it becomes sparse on the pubis and scalp (due to loss of sebaceous secretion) and changes color to gray and then to white (due to loss of pigment). The voice becomes deeper and the behavior acquires a certain degree of aggressiveness and "bossiness" generally attributed more to males than females.

As in other tissues, age pigments (lipofuscin) accumulate and give rise to dark brown "aging spots" alternating with pale areas (vitiligo) where pigment has been lost. Thinning of the skin makes it more susceptible to solar damage, temperature, humidity, and trauma.[40,41]

D. The Skeletal System

The causes, manifestations, and eventual treatment of osteoporosis, a progressive and severe bone loss frequent in postmenopausal women, are discussed in Chapter 13. Osteoporosis results from thinning and weakening of the bones due to loss of both hydroxyapatite (calcium phosphate complexes) and protein matrix (e.g., loss of collagen as in the skin). It results in fractures which occur in 1 of 5 postmenopausal women by the age of 90.[42,43] However, not all postmenopausal women will suffer a fracture since some have a higher initial bone mass, a better calcium intake and less severe estrogen deficiency because of endogenous hormone production in subcutaneous fat in the more obese. Prevention and treatment of osteoporosis by estrogens[44] and other interventions are discussed in Chapter 13.

In addition to osteoporosis, other skeletal and musculoskeletal disorders increase in frequency and severity with old age.[45] Among these, osteoarthritis (of unknown origin), gout (of metabolic origin), and rheumatoid arthritis (an autoimmune disease) are the most frequent.

The relation between ovarian hormones and the immune system remains to be further explored despite the well-known ability of estrogens to induce thymus atrophy. Cells of the immune system such as monocytes and macrophages are abundant in bone tissue and may play a role in bone metabolism and the inflammatory processes involving collagen and connective joint membranes. Monocytes secrete interleukin-1 which acts on bone and collagen. Estrogens do not affect *in vitro* interleukin-1 release by monocytes, but their deficiency in menopause or excess by replacement therapy may, in some women, alter interleukin-1 release[46] and increase autoimmune susceptibility to rheumatoid arthritis.[47]

E.　The Cardiovascular System

Myocardial infarction, that is, functional loss of an area of cardiac muscle (myocardium) due to occlusion of a coronary (cardiac) artery (also designated as Coronary Heart Disease, CHD), rarely occurs in women before the age of menopause. The high levels of estrogens in adult women protect them against atherosclerosis, the most frequent cause of CHD; when estrogen levels fall, this protection fails and CHD incidence increases. Atherosclerosis, in brief, is an age-associated alteration of the arteries characterized by hardening of the arterial wall, narrowing of arterial lumen, and the presence on the wall of lipid, fibrotic (often calcified) deposits, the most advanced called atheroma (hence the name "atherosclerosis").[48-50]

Sex difference in adulthood between males (at a higher risk for CHD) and females (at a lower risk for CHD) varies throughout life, peaking around the time of menopause and then gradually disappearing.[48,51] The decline in male-to-female ratio after menopause has also been interpreted as a slowing down of CHD in males rather than an acceleration in the rate of morbidity and mortality in women.[51] This interpretation agrees with the lowering of plasma cholesterol and triglycerides levels in men aged 60 years and older to reach values similar to those of women of the same age. The presence of such sex difference is noted primarily in affluent societies in which other risk factors such as hyperlipidemia, diabetes, cigarette smoking, and hypertension also prevail.

Before the menopause, females tend to have lower total blood cholesterol than males, but the most functionally significant difference is the higher levels of high density lipoprotein (HDL) cholesterol in females. Lipoproteins are lipid-protein complexes that transport insoluble lipids, principally cholesterol and triglycerides, in blood and interstitial fluids. The density of lipoproteins is inversely proportional to their lipid content so that HDLs have the lowest total lipid and the highest protein (the apoproteins) content; the reverse occurs in the low density lipoproteins (LDL),

Lipoproteins are important structural and metabolic components of cells and are necessary for the maintenance of overall body functions. However, certain lipoproteins may predispose to atherosclerosis, while others have a protective role. In women, the higher HDL cholesterol is in a specific subclass of HDL, the HLD2. The HDL2 are lighter than the HDL3, which represent the primary HDL subclass in men. Epidemiologic studies suggest that HDL2 plays a protective role in atherosclerosis and that estrogens are responsible for their high levels in women.[48,52-54] Cholesterol and LDL levels (in both males and females) rise with aging.[48] In females, a moderate age-associated rise in HDL after the menopause has been associated with the high levels of gonadotropins.[55]

Despite biochemical (lipoprotein levels) and epidemiological (CHD incidence and prevalence) evidence, the role of estrogens in reducing the incidence of cardiovascular disease and, thereby, morbidity and mortality, is not unanimously accepted. The majority of reports support a protective action for estrogen.[50,56-59] However, an increased risk of cardiovascular disease after estrogen treatment and a decreased effectiveness of estrogen therapy were reported, especially in smoking women.[60-62]

The biologic actions of estrogens are numerous but the most likely explanation for their beneficial effects in reducing the risk of cardiovascular disease is their ability to favorably alter lipid and liproprotein levels. Adults show sex differences in plasma lipid levels as discussed above, with higher levels of the "good" lipoproteins (HDL, HDL2) in women before the menopause, as compared to men who have higher levels of the "bad" lipoproteins (LDL). Overproduction of LDL or underproduction of HDL due to genetic or metabolic factors (e.g., deficiencies in metabolic enzymes, alterations in receptors) would increase the risk of cardiovascular disease. With estrogens, diet, exercise, life style, and a variety of drugs (e.g., nicotinic acid, clofibrate, Mevinolin) influence liproprotein levels and metabolism.[48]

Mortality due to CHD has been considerably reduced in the 1980s, especially due to the awareness of contributing factors (e.g., estrogen deficiency) and their prevention or amelioration (e.g., estrogen administration to postmenopausal women). New developments in the area of CHD management demonstrate that it is possible to induce regression/reversal or at least to arrest the progression of atherosclerotic lesions by appropriate dietary, hormonal, and pharmacologic interventions.[63]

Long-term estrogen administration may also affect blood pressure by lowering diastolic blood pressure in normotensive and, possibly, hypertensive women, thereby protecting them from hypertension.[64] However, the frequency of some electrocardiogram abnormalities (e.g., alterations of the ST segment) may increase at rest and in response to exercise, postural shifts, and hyperventilation in postmenopausal women receiving estrogen therapy. The mechanisms of this higher frequency of ST-segment abnormalities are not known, although the presence of estrogen receptors on the myocardium and arterial smooth muscle cells and the effects of estrogens on the autonomic nervous system may be implicated.[65]

F. The Urinary System

The structures of the lower urinary tract, the two ureters (carrying the urine from the kidney to the bladder), the bladder (a smooth muscle chamber storing the urine), and the urethra (the canal for the external excretion of urine) are progressively altered in elderly women. As a consequence, the function of micturition (i.e., the voiding of urine) is impaired with resulting urinary incontinence (i.e., inability to retain urine). This is one of the most frequent as well as embarrassing and distressing problems of old age.[66-68] Incontinence would occur in 10 to 15% of community-dwelling elderly and 50 to 60% of those living in institutions. However, such statistics are not accurate as people often fail to disclose the condition.

Many consider urinary incontinence inevitable but many refuse to admit to it. Normal control of bladder and urethral function is often taken for granted by the majority of individuals and, in fact, remains efficient in many individuals well into old age. However, when it occurs, failure of this control represents a main threat to the welfare of those affected. Therefore, hormonal supplementation with estrogens, which in many cases may prevent or diminish incontinence, must be viewed as critical to the clinical relief of this functional impairment.[69-74]

There are different types of incontinence (e.g., acute vs. chronic) and different causes (e.g., infections, muscle weakness, neurologic and psychiatric disorders). In females, the most frequent types are stress and urge incontinence.

Stress incontinence may occur in 1 out of 10 women of 60 years and older. It is due to increased intra-abdominal pressure (such as in coughing or laughing) on a weakened pelvic musculature, slackened bladder ligaments, and the presence of less contractile scar tissue (following muscle tearing at parturition).[75]

Urge incontinence is due to the inability to delay voiding after perception of bladder fullness and may be associated with increased urine production (polyuria) during the day and, sometimes, also at night (nocturia). It may be caused by mild but recurrent infections of the urinary tract, although these are relatively rare in older women. Usually, it is associated with histologic alterations of bladder muscle cells and ligaments and, functionally, with altered nervous control of micturition.

The smooth muscles of the bladder walls and sphincters (circular rings to open or close bladder orifices) are regulated by the autonomic nervous system and this regulation may be impaired by low estrogen levels; the resulting progressive hyperexcitability of bladder muscle cells, probably due to shifts in sympathetic control, responds well to drugs acting on the autonomic nervous system (as discussed earlier in Section III.A).

Management of incontinence varies with the type and the cause of the incontinence and ranges from the use of special undergarments and exercise of pelvic muscles, to administration of estrogen and parasympatholytic and sympathomimetic drugs, bladder catheterization, and surgery. Topical (intravaginally) or systemic (orally) administration of estrogens ameliorates greatly both urge and stress incontinence, perhaps through increased collagen strength.[70-74] Drugs, agonists, or antagonists of autonomic nervous control of bladder contractility and sphincter function are also effective, alone or in combination with estrogens.

G. The Gastrointestinal System and Metabolism

Changes in gastrointestinal function with aging are varied, appear to affect both sexes similarly, and generally reflect the overall health of the elderly.[76] Gender differences, when present, do not seem to be related to ovarian hormones and, therefore, are not significantly affected by cessation of their secretion at menopause. For example, gastric emptying and motility may be slower in women than men at all ages before and after the menopause; administration of estrogen and progesterone in postmenopausal women further slows down gastric emptying as these hormones inhibit gastric motility.[77]

Gallbladder emptying appears slower in postmenopausal women as compared to young adults. This hypomotility may contribute to the pathogenesis of gallstones, more frequent after menopause.[78] Fecal incontinence, that is, the inability of retaining the feces, is a problem similar to that of urinary incontinence and occurs in older women for the same reasons (e.g., weakness of pelvic muscles). Whether estrogen strengthens rectal muscles as it does those of the bladder and whether its administration prevents or improves incontinence remains unclear.

The major metabolic effects of estrogen were discussed earlier under blood lipid (lipoprotein) profile and their beneficial consequences for cardiovascular disease. Other metabolic actions involve glucose metabolism. While only a few elderly individuals have a higher fasting blood glucose level, about 50% of those aged 65 and older have significantly altered glucose tolerance as compared to younger individuals. The mechanisms of this glucose intolerance are controversial, although the most currently accepted is an increased insulin resistance of target tissues (Chapters 10 and 11).

IV. HORMONAL REPLACEMENT THERAPY IN MENOPAUSE

Given the cessation of ovarian function at menopause, the rearrangement of hormonal balance that it entrains, the simultaneous senescent alterations in target cells and organs, and the availability of natural and synthetic ovarian steroids, hormonal replacement therapy seems the logical intervention to prevent, delay, or reverse at least some of the symptoms of menopause. Yet, despite the justifiable rationale for the administration of estrogens (eventually associated with progestins) and the evidence for their beneficial effects, several objections both theoretical and practical continue to be raised with respect to the extension of this treatment to a large segment of the menopausal and postmenopausal population.

The efficacy and specificity of the treatment is undisputed. What is still debated is whether "all" or "nearly all" postmenopausal women, with or without overt signs of discomfort and dysfunction, should be given estrogen therapy.[79-85] To definitely answer this question more precise knowledge is needed on:

- The exact mechanism of action of the hormones,
- The best possible means of administration,
- The most appropriate doses and hormonal preparations,
- The methods (continuous vs. discontinuous) and routes (oral vs. percutaneous) of administration,
- The age at onset, and duration of treatment,
- The administration of estrogen alone or in combination with progestins,
- The benefits to be derived from the treatment, and
- The occurrence of undesirable side effects.

Currently, the debate remains open and is further complicated by the association of menopause with other factors besides hormones, such as genetic makeup, life style, diet, exercise, smoking, alcohol, social habits, and the limited availability of alternative approaches to treatment.

A. Support for the Routine Use of Estrogen Therapy

Estrogen therapy is recognized as needed and effective in preventing the involution of secondary sex organs (Chapter 7). Atrophy of the vagina and vulva (with accompanying bleeding, itching, and painful intercourse) is prevented by estrogen therapy. Likewise, estrogen treatment maintains the tone of the supporting structures (muscles and ligaments) of the vagina and uterus. Overall, estrogens are more effective in preventing than in reversing atrophic changes of secondary sex organs. Hence, their administration must start early during the perimenopausal period.

Treatment with estrogens is also effective in relieving the hot flushes and other vasomotor symptoms. Beneficial effects have also been reported with respect to certain psychologic symptoms of the menopause (e.g., related to sexual behavior), but their consistency and efficacy remain controversial.[29] Little evidence exists for the rejuvenating effects of topical estrogens on the skin, so loudly (and profitably for business!) advertised by many beauty products from the cosmetic industry.

The major beneficial effect of estrogen therapy is the slowing of the bone loss and of bone fragility associated with aging that leads to osteoporosis and, consequently, to bone fractures — leading causes of morbidity and death among elderly women (Chapter 13).[42-44]

Current estrogen use is associated with lower body weight, diastolic blood pressure, and plasma glucose. It also lowers LDL cholesterol levels and raises HDL cholesterol levels, the specific lipoprotein profile most effective in reducing the risk of atherosclerotic damage and its consequences.[52-59,86-88] It is well demonstrated today that such beneficial effects can be obtained with low doses of estrogens. Addition of progestins, despite some potential adverse effects on body fluids and blood pressure (see below), adds a measure of safety in reducing the risk of uterine carcinoma.

Overall, estrogen therapy (with or without progestins) would exert a protective action toward all causes of death in nonsmoking women but not in the smokers.[61,62,89,90] This is particularly true for those women who started to smoke at an early age. The increased mortality is related to an increased number of deaths from cancer.

B. Opposition to the Routine Use of Estrogen

Theoretical and practical arguments have been put forward against the administration of estrogens (with or without progestins) as a routine replacement therapy for women during and after the menopause:

- The majority of women do not experience adverse reactions from the menopause or these are minimal and transitory, therefore therapy is not necessary;

- After menopause, estrogens (i.e., estrone) are still present in blood and tissues although at a low level and potency — therefore, administration of estrogens (and progesterone) may be better described as "additive" rather than as "replacement" therapy and is often based on pharmacologic rather than physiologic doses;
- The progressive changes in cellular and organismic functions with aging (e.g., reduced number and affinity of steroid receptors, changed cell enzymatic activity, decline in hormone secretion and metabolism, storage and excretion) make it difficult, if not currently impossible, to identify the "physiologic" dose appropriate to the senescing individual;
- Those conditions of menopause such as osteoporosis and cardiovascular disease, for which estrogen therapy is most indicated, are multifactorial and heavily influenced by other factors besides estrogens (e.g., genetic makeup, life style) which are also amenable to prevention and treatment.

Women who enter the menopause with adequate bone mass and continue a good regimen of physical exercise do not inevitably develop osteoporosis severe enough to represent a real risk for bone fracture. Postmenopausal women who are normotensive, have appropriate lipid and lipoprotein profiles, are physically active, are not obese, and do not smoke are unlikely to experience an increased incidence of cardiovascular accidents. Why then should one treat all postmenopausal women with hormonal replacement therapy?

1. Adverse Effects of Estrogen Replacement Therapy With or Without Progestins

The question raised above is particularly pertinent as estrogen therapy has a number of well-recognized untoward side effects. According to several epidemiological studies, long-term administration of estrogen alone significantly increases the incidence of hyperplasia and cancer of the uterus.[80,81,91-93] The increased risk is proportional to both dosage and duration of treatment. The danger is reduced by the associated treatment with progestins.[94] Progestins would oppose the binding of estrogen on the endometrial receptors and thus diminish the hormonal induction of hyperplasia and cancer. However, while progestins may protect the endometrium from the mitogenic actions of estrogen, they have an adverse effect of their own by stimulating cholesterol and LDL levels, thereby reversing or diminishing the beneficial effects of estrogens in raising HDL. Administration of estrogens would also increase the incidence of breast cancer although the majority of studies on estrogen treatment with or without progestins remain controversial.[95-99]

2. Dose, Duration, Route of Administration, and Combination With Progestins

The types, doses, and routes of administration of the major estrogens currently in use in the U.S. and other Western countries (e.g., France) are listed in Table 8-1. The efficacy of treatment varies with:

- The individual and population treated,
- The dose (physiologic vs. pharmacologic),
- The type of hormone administered (natural or synthetic, free or conjugated),
- The route of administration (orally, passing through the liver; or topically, for slow, extrahepatic systemic absorption).

Progestins are associated with estrogen because they reduce the risk of uterine and, eventually, breast cancer as discussed above. The major progestins utilized as anti-estrogens, their doses, and untoward effects are listed in Table 8-2. The usefulness of progestins is still under study. If the prediction of a reduction in the benefit of cardiovascular disease with estrogen-progestin therapy is correct, there would be no justification for the use of progestins.

Insufficient hormonal doses will lead to the reappearance of the symptoms and risks of menopause. An excessive dosage will result in adverse effects some of which may relate to

TABLE 8-1 Estrogens[a] Administered for Replacement Therapy at and After Menopause

Hormones	Source	Route of administration	Dose
17-β estradiol (micronized)	Ovary	Oral	2 mg
		Percutaneous (arms, thighs, abdomen)	1.5 mg
		Patch	25, 50 (preferred), or 100 μg[b]
17-β estradiol valerionate (micronized)	Semisynthetic, metabolized to 17-β estradiol	Oral	Same dose as 17-β estradiol
Conjugated estradiol estrone and estriol (Premarin[c])	Urine of pregnant mare	Oral	0.33, 0.625, or 1.25 mg
Ethinylestradiol[d]	Synthetic	Oral	50 μg

[a] In the blood, estrogen is found free or bound to proteins or conjugated (as sulfate or glucuronate); in tissues, estradiol the most biologically active estrogen, is metabolized to estrone, less biologically active (Chapters 2 and 7). Estrogens taken orally will be absorbed in the gut and carried to the liver where they are conjugated and, from there, enter the systemic circulation where they reach an early peak. Hormonal levels in blood will decay more or less slowly depending on tissue uptake and excretion rate. Estrogens given parenterally (in the vagina, skin, or muscle) are absorbed locally first and then slowly in the circulation; they lack a characteristic peak but their systemic levels may vary markedly not only among individuals but also within the same individual.[73,74,91,100]

[b] Patch is replaced every 4 days.

[c] Trade name of representative drug.

[d] The relatively slow rate of metabolism and excretion may explain some of the untoward effects (nausea, diarrhea).

the actions of hormones on the uterus (e.g., bleeding or amenorrhea), on metabolism (e.g., increased body weight), or on the CNS (e.g., headache, nausea).

3. To Whom Should Hormonal Therapy After Menopause Be Recommended?

Hormonal treatment should be proposed to women with low plasma estradiol (<50 pg/l) and high gonadotropins (FSH: >15–20 IU/l) whether due to menopause or to cessation of ovarian function (e.g., by surgical removal of ovaries) at an age preceding the menopause. Hormonal treatment is advisable unless there are special contraindications involving reproductive and extrareproductive organs and functions, as summarized in Table 8-3. The decision to initiate hormonal treatment at all ages and with all hormones must always be based on the complete assessment of the physical conditions of the individual requiring the treatment. This certainly applies to the choice of ovarian hormonal therapy, which can be decided only after assessment has revealed the need for the therapy and the absence of contraindications (Table 8-4). Once treatment has been initiated, it is necessary to adhere to a consistent follow-up schedule which should be continued as long as the treatment (Table 8-5).

4. For How Long Should Hormonal Therapy Continue?

Despite continuing advances in hormonal treatment of menopause, satisfactory answers to a number of important questions are still lacking in the literature. These questions are:

- Does long-term hormonal therapy lose its protective value to elderly women and, if so, at what age should estrogen therapy be terminated?
- If estrogen therapy does not lose its protective value with advancing age should not all elderly women (the 80-year-and-older segment of the population that is currently growing the fastest in the U.S.) at risk for osteoporosis (and without contraindications) receive estrogen therapy to reduce the risk of fractures? and

TABLE 8-2 **Progestins Utilized With Estrogens for Replacement Therapy at and After Menopause[a]**

Hormone	Source	Daily oral dose	Untoward side effects
Progesterone (micronized)	Ovary Adrenal cortex	100 mg	None, (very short half-life)
Didrogesterone	Synthetic	20 mg	None
Pregnane derivatives:	Synthetic		Hypertension
Medrogestone		10 mg	Masculinizing, anabolic and
Medroxyprogestone acetate		10–20 mg	diabetogenic actions
Nonpregnane derivatives:	Synthetic		None(?) Short-acting (24 h)
Demegestone		0.500 mg	
Promegestone		0.500 mg	
Nomegestrol acetate		10 mg	
19-Nortestosterone derivatives	Synthetic	Not to be used	Hypertension LDL elevation, anabolic and masculinizing actions

[a] Oral estrogens and progestins can be taken following different actions schedules and therapeutic strategies. The most usual strategy involves the *sequential administration* of estrogen for 22–24 days with an interval of a few days without hormone to mimic the menstrual 28-day cycle: estrogen may be 17-β estradiol given orally or percutaneously. Progestins can be added starting on days 10–14 of estrogen treatment, corresponding to the second half of a preexisting monthly cycle. Examples of such combined treatment may include: conjugated estrogens given orally in a dose which can range from 0.3 to 0. 625 mg/day for 25 days to which are added, starting from day 10–14 and continuing until day 25, 10 mg/day of medroxyprogesterone acetate. The *continuous schedule* is less popular and is used in certain cases when monthly bleeding is to be avoided. Estrogen is administered daily without interruption. Whether the treatment is continuous or sequential, there is some bleeding (e.g., from hormone withdrawal) in 30% of cases. A pause of 10 days (after 20 days of estrogens) appears no longer advisable as some of the symptoms for which the treatment was prescribed may reappear and the risk of fractures due to osteoporosis may not be effectively reduced.

- Should estrogen therapy (eventually combined with progestins) be initiated to arrest osteoporosis and improve cardiovascular function in women who are 65 years old and have never taken estrogens before?

There is no rationale to determine a limited duration for hormonal treatment nor to establish a termination date. Often the treatment is interrupted by the recipient herself because of negligence or lack of interest.[101-103] Although some women are generally willing to accept the view that they may have to take hormonal treatment for life, the rate of noncompliance in the overall population is high.[101] For osteoporosis, prevention needs long-term treatment starting

TABLE 8-3 **Indications and Contraindications of Hormonal Replacement Therapy**

Indications
  Early menopause (secondary to surgery)
  Menopausal symptoms
  High risk of osteoporosis
Contraindications
  Related to reproductive system:
  History of breast and uterine cancer
  Uterine fibroma
  Endometriosis
  Proliferating tumor of the breast with malignant tendency
Unrelated to reproductive system:
  Obesity
  Liver insufficiency

TABLE 8-4 Recommended Assessment for
Women Considered for Hormonal
Therapy

History:	Hypertension
	Vascular diseases
	Cancer (breast, colon)
	Fractures
	Osteoporosis risk factors:
	Alcohol
	Smoking
	Low calcium intake
	Date of last menstrual period
Physical exam:	Blood pressure
	Breast exam
	Mammography
	Gynecologic exam
Chemistry profile:	Lipid profile
	Hormonal profile:
	FSH, LH
	Estrogens
	Test for bone mass:
	Dual photon
	Absorptiometry

early, possibly even before menopause, and continuing for many years, perhaps throughout life.[104] The early onset of treatment is made possible by the sensitivity of current tests for assessing bone mass and structure and the availability of early screening. As bone loss is a continuing process, it is conceivable that treatment may be useful even when started in later years, although prevention is less efficient when bone destruction is more advanced.[104]

Likewise, for protection of the cardiovascular system (e.g., maintenance of high HDL and low LDL cholesterol), continuing treatment appears advisable. However, how long, for example for life, is impossible to affirm today due to the lack of appropriate long-term epidemiological studies.

C. Nonhormonal Treatment of Menopause

When hormonal treatment is not advisable, interventions are directed primarily to alleviate some of the symptoms of menopause. They consist in:

- Psychotherapy for support (always useful at menopause but often ineffective when utilized alone);

TABLE 8-5 Recommendations for Follow-Up
of Women on Hormonal
Replacement Therapy

Period (months)	Purpose
3	To assess symptoms
6	To measure:
	Body weight
	Blood pressure
	Breast exam
12 (repeat)	Gynecologic check-up
	Blood chemistry profile
18–24 (repeat)	Mammogram
	Bone mass (for osteoporosis)

- Tranquillizers and sedatives to relieve insomnia and anxiety;
- A diet low in calories (in case of obesity) and sugars and fats (in case of hyperglycemia and hypercholesteremia);
- Dietary supplementation with high calcium (to minimize bone loss and risk of fractures); and
- Increased physical activity to prevent obesity and bone loss.

All of these treatments can be taken separately or in combination, depending on the number of symptoms displayed by the menopausal woman. None is as effective as hormonal therapy. Several can be used advantageously in combination with the hormonal therapy presented above.

Still largely ignored are "alternative" solutions to the medical/physical aspects of menopause (rather than estrogen administration). Thus, "women who exercise daily, eat healthy food and work on achieving emotional balance, usually manage to avoid the ills of midlife."[11] As indicated earlier, the menopause provides some potential positive feelings such as freedom from menstruation and fear of pregnancy. Yet the potential effectiveness of social and psychological interventions has so far been overlooked in favor of the more medically oriented view of menopause as an "estrogen deficiency syndrome". A safer and certainly physiologically and clinically sounder path would be to consider each case individually and from both a comprehensive psychosocial and medical approach.

V. OVERALL CONCLUSIONS

Whether to undertake hormonal therapy with estrogens (in combination with progestins) or not should remain the decision of the woman entering menopause and should be taken in agreement with her physician. Except in the presence of overt medical contraindications, the choice of undertaking treatment should always be considered, especially when a number of symptoms are present and, in general, for the prevention of osteoporosis. The effectiveness of the treatment and the absence of undesirable side effects will depend on the type of the hormone (and hormone combination) selected and the dose administered. In all cases, hormone therapy should be associated with good health practices (e.g., no smoking, diet low in calories) and support therapy for the concomitant pathology associated with aging processes.

Appropriate hormonal (replacement) therapy (eventually associated with other nonmedical interventions) will provide those menopausal and postmenopausal women affected by a complex symptomatology with a number of benefits:

- An overall more youthful (for their age) appearance with better skin and hair,
- More satisfactory sexual life in the absence of vaginal and vulvar atrophy,
- Freedom from hot flashes and maintenance of a more balanced behavior without anxiety and insomnia,
- A decreased risk of atherosclerosis, CHD, and high blood cholesterol, and
- Prevention or slowing down of osteoporosis and reduction of the resulting risk of fractures.

Given the 30 and more years that women in the developed countries are likely to live after menopause, such benefits of hormonal therapy are critically important not only for the quality of life of each elderly woman but also for the impact on socioeconomic conditions and health services for the entire community.

REFERENCES

1. Wilbush, J., Menorrhagia and menopause: a historical review, *Maturitas,* 10, 5, 1988.
2. Wilbush, J., Menopause and menorrhagia: a historical exploration, *Maturitas,* 10, 83, 1988.

3. Rutherford, R. N. and Rutherford, J. J., The climacteric years in the woman, man and family, in *Counseling in Marital and Sexual Problems. A Physician's Handbook*, Klemer, R. H., Ed., Williams & Wilkins, Baltimore, MD, 1965, 220.

4. Pavelka, M. and Fedigan, L., Menopause. A comparative life history perspective, *Yearb. Phys. Anthropol.,* 34, 13, 1991.

5. Flint, M. and Samil, R. S., Cultural and subcultural meanings of the menopause, *Ann. N. Y. Acad. Sci.*, 592, 134, 1990.

6. Delaney, J., Lupton, M., and Toth, E., November of the body: The menopause and literature, in *The Curse: A Cultural History of Menstruation*, Lupton, M. J., Delaney, J., and Toth, E., Eds., University of Illinois Press, Chicago, 1988, 213.

7. Matthews, K. A., Myths and realities of menopause, *Psychosom. Med.,* 54, 1, 1992.

8. McCrea, F., The politics of menopause: The "discovery" of a deficiency disease, *Soc. Probl.,* 31, 111, 1983.

9. Bell, S. E., Changing ideas: the medicalization of menopause, *Social Science and Medicine*, 24, 535, 1987.

10. Bell, S. E., Sociological perspectives on the medicalization of menopause, *Ann. N. Y. Acad. Sci.*, 592, 173, 1990.

11. Greenwood, S., *Menopause, Naturally*, Volcano Press, San Francisco, CA, 1984.

12. Greer, G., *The Change: Women, Aging and the Menopause,* A. A. Knopf, New York, 1992.

13. Sheehy, G., *The Silent Passage,* Simon and Schuster, New York, 1993.

14. Wilbush, J., Historical perspectives. Climacteric expression and social context, *Maturitas*, 4, 195, 1982.

15. Mishell, D. R., Jr., Noncontraceptive health benefits of oral steroidal contraceptives, *Am. J. Obstet. Gynecol.,* 142, 809, 1982.

16. Asso, D., *The Real Menstrual Cycle*, John Wiley & Sons, New York, 1983.

17. Bider, D., Mashiach, S., Serr, D. M., and Ben-Rafael, Z., Endocrinological basis of hot flushes, *Obstet. Gynecol. Surv.*, 44, 495, 1989.

18. Ravnikar, V., Physiology and treatment of hot flushes, *Obstet. Gynecol.,* 75 (Suppl. 4), 3S, 1990.

19. Lomax, P. and Schonbaum, E., Postmenopausal hot flushes and their management, *Pharmacol. Therap.,* 57, 347, 1993.

20. Ginsburg, J., Hardiman, P., and O'Reilly, B., Peripheral blood flow in menopausal women who have hot flushes and in those who do not, *Br. Med. J.,* 298, 1488, 1989.

21. Cignarelli, M., Cicinelli, E., Corso, M., Cospite, M. R., Garruti, G., Tafaro, E., Giorgino, R., and Schonauer, S., Biophysical and endocrine-metabolic changes during menopausal hot flashes: increase in plasma free fatty acid and norepinephrine levels, *Gynecol. Obstet. Invest.,* 27, 34, 1989.

22. Witt, M. F. and Blethen, S. L., The endocrine evaluation of three children with vasomotor flushes following hypothalamic surgery, *Clin. Endocrinol.,* 18, 551, 1983.

23. Tataryn, I. V., Lomax, P., Bajorek, J. G., Chesarek, W., Meldrum, D. R., and Judd, H. L., Postmenopausal hot flushes: a disorder of thermoregulation, *Maturitas,* 2, 101, 1980.

24. Cagnacci, A., Melis, G. B., Paoletti, A. M., Soldani, R., and Fioretti, P., Interaction between veralipride and the endogenous opioid system in the regulation of body temperature in postmenopausal women, *Life Sci.,* 42, 547, 1988.

25. Lightman, S. L., McGarrick, G., Maguire, A. K., Jeffcoate, S., and Jacobs, H. S., Reproduction of the frequency of climacteric flushing and LH pulses by blockade of opiate receptors, in *The Menopause: Clinical, Endocrinological and Pathophysiological Aspects,* Fioretti, P., Martini, L., Melis, G. B., and Yen, S. S. C., Eds., Serono Symposia Vol. 39., Academic Press, New York, 1982, 575.

26. Judd, H. L., Pathophysiology of menopausal hot flushes, in *Neuroendocrinology of Aging,* Meites, J., Ed., Plenum Press, New York, 1983, 173.

27. Hunter, M. S., Predictors of menopausal symptoms: psychosocial aspects, *Baillierés Clin. Endocrinol. Metabol.,* 7, 33, 1993.

28. Ballinger, C. B., Psychiatric aspects of the menopause, *Br. J. Psychiatry,* 156, 773, 1990.

29. Montgomery, J. C. and Studd, J. W., Psychological and sexual aspects of menopause, *Br. J. Hosp. Med.*, 45, 300, 1991.

30. Kinsey, A. C., Pomeroy, W. B., Martin, C. E., and Gebhard, P. H., *Sexual Behavior in the Human Female,* W.B. Saunders, Philadelphia, 1953.

31. Masters, W. H. and Johnson, V. E., *Human Sexual Response,* Churchill, London, 1966.

32. James, W. H., Marital coital rates, spouses' ages, family size and social class, *J. Sex Res.,* 10, 205, 1974.

33. Goldstein, M. K. and Teng, N. N., Gynecologic factors in sexual dysfunction of the older woman, *Clin. Geriat. Med.,* 7, 41, 1991.

34. Hunter, M. S., Emotional well-being, sexual behavior and hormone replacement therapy, *Maturitas,* 12, 299, 1990.

35. Sarrel, P. M., Sexuality and menopause, *Obstet. Gynecol.*, 75 (Suppl. 4), 26S, 1990.

36. Terasawa, E. and Timiras, P. S., Electrical activity during the estrous cycle of the rat: cyclic changes in limbic structures, *Endocrinology,* 83, 207, 1968.

37. Toran-Allerand, C. D., Ellis, L., and Pfenninger, K. H., Estrogen and insulin synergism in neurite growth enhancement in vitro: mediation of steroid effects by interactions with growth factors?, *Brain Res.*, 469, 87, 1988.

38. Buckwalter, J. G., Sobel, E., Dunn, M. E., Diz, M. M., and Henderson, V. W., Gender differences on a brief measure of cognitive functioning in Alzheimer's disease, *Arch. Neurol.*, 50, 757, 1993.

39. Bolognia, J. L., Dermatologic and cosmetic concerns of the older woman, *Clin. Geriat. Med.*, 9, 209, 1993.

40. Bolognia, J. L., Aging skin, epidermal and dermal changes, *Prog. Clin. Biol. Res.*, 320, 121, 1989.

41. Timiras, M. L., The skin and connective tissue, in *Physiological Basis of Aging and Geriatrics*, 2nd ed., Timiras, P. S., Ed., CRC, Boca Raton, FL, 1994, 273.

42. Dequeker, J., Detection of the patient at risk for osteoporosis at the time of the menopause, *Maturitas*, 11, 85, 1989.

43. Notelovitz, M., Osteoporosis: screening, prevention, and management, *Fertil. Steril.*, 59, 707, 1993.

44. Lindsay, R., Criteria for successful estrogen therapy in osteoporosis, *Osteoporosis Int.*, 3 (Suppl. 2), S9, 1993.

45. Timiras, P. S., Aging of the skeleton, joints and muscles, in, *Physiological Basis of Aging and Geriatrics*, 2nd ed., Timiras, P. S., Ed., CRC Press, Boca Raton, FL, 1994, 259.

46. Stock, J. L., Coderre, J. A., McDonald, B., and Rosenwasser, L. J., Effects of estrogen in vivo and in vitro on spontaneous Interleukin-1 release by monocytes from postmenopausal women, *J. Clin. Endocrinol. Metab.*, 68, 364, 1989.

47. Hernandez-Avila, M., Liang, M. H., Willett, W. C., Stampfer, M. J., Colditz, G. A., Rosner, B., Chang, R. W., Hennekens, C. H., and Speizer, F. E., Oral contraceptives, replacement oestrogens and the risk of rheumatoid arthritis, *Br. J. Rheumatol.*, 28 (Suppl. 1), 42, 1989.

48. Forte, T., Plasma lipoproteins: their metabolism and role in atherosclerosis, in *Physiological Basis of Aging and Geriatrics*, 2nd ed., Timiras, P. S., Ed., CRC Press, Boca Raton, FL, 1994, 215.

49. Timiras, P. S., Cardiovascular alterations with aging, in *Physiological Basis of Ageing and Geriatrics*, 2nd ed., Timiras, P. S., Ed., CRC Press, Boca Raton, FL, 1994, 199.

50. Stampfer, M. J., Colditz, G. A., and Willett, W. C., Menopause and heart disease. A review, *Ann. N. Y. Acad. Sci.*, 592, 193, 1990.

51. Heller, R. F. and Jacobs, H. S., Coronary heart disease in relation to age, sex, and menopause, *Br. Med. J.*, 1, 472, 1978.

52. Wren, B. G., The effect of oestrogen on the female cardiovascular system, *Med. J. Aust.*, 157, 204, 1992.

53. Sarrel, P. M., Ovarian hormones and the circulation, *Maturitas*, 12, 287, 1990.

54. Lobo, R. A., Cardiovascular implications of estrogen replacement therapy, *Obstet. Gynecol.*, 75 (Suppl. 4), 18S, 1990.

55. Krauss, R. M., Regulation of high density lipoprotein levels, *Med. Clin. North Am.*, 66, 403, 1982.

56. LaRosa, J. C., Lipids and cardiovascular disease: do the findings and therapy apply equally to men and women?, *Women's Health Issues*, 2, 102, 1992.

57. Stampfer, M. J., Willett, W. C., Colditz, G. A., Rosner, B., Speizer, F. E., and Hennekens, C. H., A prospective study of postmenopausal estrogen therapy and coronary heart disease, *N. Engl. J. Med.*, 313, 1044, 1985.

58. Barrett-Connor, E. and Miller, V., Estrogens, lipids, and heart disease, *Clin. Geriat. Med.*, 9, 57, 1993.

59. Ross, R. K., Paganini-Hill, A., Mack, T. M., and Henderson, B. E., Cardiovascular benefits of estrogen replacement therapy, *Am. J. Obstet. Gynecol.*, 160, 1301, 1989.

60. McCrea, F. and Markle G., The estrogen replacement controversy in the USA and UK. Different answers to the same question?, *Soc. Stud. Sci.*, 14, 1, 1984.

61. Wilson, P. W., Garrison, R. J., and Castelli, W. P., Postmenopausal estrogen use, cigarette smoking and cardiovascular morbidity in women over 50, The Framingham Study, *N. Engl. J. Med.*, 313, 1038, 1985.

62. Jensen, J. and Christiansen, C., Effects of smoking on serum lipoproteins and bone mineral content during postmenopausal hormone replacement therapy, *Am. J. Obst. Gynecol.*, 159, 820, 1989.

63. Kane, J. P., Malloy, M. J., Ports, T. A., Phillips, N. R., Diehl, J. C., and Havel, R. J., Regression of coronary atherosclerosis during treatment of familial hypercholesterolemia with combined drug regimens, *JAMA*, 264, 3007, 1990.

64. Henderson, B. E., Paganini-Hill, A., and Ross, R. K., Estrogen replacement therapy and protection from acute myocardial infarction, *Am. J. Obstet. Gynecol.*, 159, 312, 1988.

65. Vaitkevicius, P., Wright, J. G., and Fleg, J. L., Effect of estrogen replacement therapy on the ST-segment response to postural and hyperventilation stimuli, *Am. J. Cardiol.*, 64, 1076, 1989.

66. Semmelink, H. J., de Wilde, P. C., van Houwelingen, J. C., and Vooijs, G. P., Histomorphometric study of the lower urogenital tract in pre- and post-menopausal women, *Cytometry*, 11, 700, 1990.

67. Molander, U., Urinary incontinence and related urogenital symptoms in elderly women, *Acta Obstet. Gynecol. Scand.*, 158, 1, 1993.

68. Timiras, M. L., The kidney, the lower urinary tract, the prostate and body fluids, in *Physiological Basis of Aging and Geriatrics,* 2nd ed., Timiras, P. S., Ed., CRC Press, Boca Raton, FL, 1994, 239.

69. Bent, A. E., Etiology and management of detrusor instability and mixed incontinence, *Obstet. Gynecol. Clin. North Am.*, 16, 853, 1989.

70. Cardozo, L., Role of estrogens in the treatment of female urinary incontinence, *J. Am. Geriatr. Soc.*, 38, 326, 1990.

71. Sand, P. K. and Brubaker, L., Nonsurgical treatment of detrusor overactivity in postmenopausal women, *J. Reprod. Med.*, 35, 758, 1990.

72. Elia, G. and Bergman, A., Estrogen effects on the urethra: beneficial effects in women with genuine stress incontinence, *Obstet. Gynecol. Sur.*, 48, 509, 1993.

73. Smith, P., Estrogens and the urogenital tract. Studies on steroid hormone receptors and a clinical study on a new estradiol-releasing vaginal ring, *Acta Obstet. Gynecol. Scand.*, 157, 1, 1993.

74. Smith, P., Heimer, G., Lindskog, M., and Ulmsten, U., Oestradiol-releasing vaginal ring for treatment of postmenopausal urogenital atrophy, *Maturitas,* 16, 145, 1993.

75. Stanton, S. L., Stress urinary incontinence, *Ciba Foundation Symposium,* 151, 182, 1990.

76. Timiras, P. S., Aging of the gastronintestinal tract and liver, in *Physiological Basis of Aging and Geriatrics,* 2nd ed., Timiras, P. S., Ed., CRC Press, Boca Raton, FL, 1994, 247.

77. Hutson, W. R., Roehrkasse, R. L., and Wald, A., Influence of gender and menopause on gastric emptying and motility, *Gastroenterology,* 96, 11, 1989.

78. Petroianu, A., Gallbladder emptying in perimenopausal women, *Med. Hypotheses,* 30, 129, 1989.

79. Birkenfeld, A. and Kase, N. G., Menopause medicine: current treatment options and trends, *Comprehensive Therapy,* 17, 36, 1991.

80. Jones, K. P., Estrogens and progestins: what to use and how to use it, *Clin. Obstet. Gynecol.*, 35, 871, 1992.

81. Greendale, G. A. and Judd, H. L., The menopause: health implications and clinical management, *J. Am. Geriatr. Soc.*, 41, 426, 1993.

82. Kelly, J., Effects and treatment of the menopause, BJN, 2, 123, 1993.

83. Rosenberg, L., Hormone replacement therapy: the need for reconsideration, *Am. J. Publ. Health*, 83, 1670, 1993.

84. Session, D. R., Kelly, A. C., and Jewelewicz, R., Current concepts in estrogen replacement therapy in the menopause, *Fertil. Steril.*, 59, 277, 1993.

85. Speroff, L., Menopause and hormone replacement therapy, *Clin. Geriatr. Med.*, 9, 33, 1993.

86. Krauss, R. M. and Burkman, R. T., Jr., The metabolic impact of oral contraceptives, *Am. J. Obstet. Gynecol.*, 167, 1177, 1992.

87. Vaziri, S. M., Evans, J. C., Larson, M. G., and Wilson, P. W., The impact of female hormone usage on the lipid profile, The Framingham Offspring Study, *Arch. Intern. Med.*, 153, 2200, 1993.

88. Farish, E., Rolton, H. A., Barnes, J. F., Fletcher, C. D., Walsh, D. J., Spowart, K. J., and Hart, D. M., Lipoprotein(a) and postmenopausal oestrogen, *Acta Endocrinol.*, 129, 225, 1993.

89. Zubialde, J. P., Lawler, F., and Clemenson, N., Estimated gains in life expectancy with use of postmeno-pausal estrogen therapy: a decision analysis, *J. Fam. Pract.*, 36, 271, 1993.

90. Brinton, L. A., Barrett, R. J., Berman, M. L., Mortel, R., Twiggs, L. B., and Wilbanks, G. D., Cigarette smoking and the risk of endometrial cancer, *Am. J. Epidemiol.*, 137, 281, 1993.

91. Utian, W. H., The menopause in perspective. From potions to patches, *Ann. N.Y. Acad. Sci.*, 592, 1, 1990.

92. Crosignani, P. G., Effects of hormone replacement therapy, *Int. J. Fertil.*, 37 (Suppl. 2), 98, 1992.

93. Adami, H. O., Long-term consequences of estrogen and estrogen-progestin replacement, *Cancer Causes and Control,* 3, 83, 1992.

94. Samsioe, G., Introduction to steroids in the menopause, *Am. J. Obstet. Gynecol.*, 166, 1980, 1992.

95. Harris, R. E., Namboodiri, K. K., and Wynder, E. L., Breast cancer risk: effects of estrogen replacement therapy and body mass, *J. Natl. Cancer Inst.*, 84, 1575, 1992.

96. Sitruk-Ware, R., Estrogens, progestins and breast cancer risk in post-menopausal women: state of the ongoing controversy in 1992, *Maturitas,* 15, 129, 1992.

97. Hulka, B. S., Hormone-replacement therapy and the risk of breast cancer, CA, 40, 289, 1990.

98. Brinton, L. A., Menopause and the risk of breast cancer, *Ann. N.Y., Acad. Sci.,* 592, 357, 1990.

99. Lundgren, S., Progestins in breast cancer treatment. A review, *Acta Oncol.,* 31, 709, 1992.

100. Tzingounis, V. A., Perdikaris, A. G., Lioutas, G., and Dimopoulos, D., Subcutaneous hormone replacement therapy, *Eur. J. Obstet., Gynecol. Reprod. Biol.,* 49, 64, 1993.

101. Hahn, R. G., Compliance considerations with estrogen replacement: withdrawal bleeding and other factors, *Am. J. Obstet. Gynecol.,* 161, 1854, 1989.

102. Draper, J. and Roland, M., Perimenopausal women's views on taking hormone replacement therapy to prevent osteoporosis, *Br. Med. J.,* 300, 786, 1990.
103. Ferguson K. J., Hoegh, C., and Johnson, S., Estrogen replacement therapy. A survey of women's knowledge and attitudes, *Arch. Intern. Med.,* 149, 133, 1989.
104. Quigley, M. E., Martin, P. L., Burnier, A. M., and Brooks, P., Estrogen therapy arrests bone loss in elderly women, *Am. J. Obstet. Gynecol.,* 156, 1516, 1987.

9

Reproductive Hormonal Changes in the Aging Male

Fran E. Kaiser and John E. Morley

CONTENTS

I. INTRODUCTION

In 1889, C.E. Brown-Sequard noted that a day would come when the "degenerations" of age could be mitigated by the use of testosterone, bringing forth a "rejuvenation" that would approximate that of a younger individual.[1] Over a hundred years have passed, and we are slightly closer in our understanding of hormonal repletion in elderly men than Brown-Sequard was. However, for the reproductive hormonal changes of age per se, our knowledge has certainly increased. Data have accumulated showing that older males develop hypogonadism, with concomitant changes in the hypothalamic-pituitary axis contributing to these changes. This decrease in male hormones has been termed male "menopause" by some, "andropause", or "andrngenopause" by others.[2,3] While there is no cessation of a particular phenomenon, such as with female menopause, the decline of hormones that can be seen in men may be likened to the years of altered (and decreasing) hormone levels of the perimenopause. There is no clearly defined clinical marker to note these hormonal changes in males.

    This chapter will review the changes in reproductive hormones in the aging male and explore some of the evidence that implicates hypogonadism as part of the pathophysiology of the aging process.

II. MALE REPRODUCTIVE HORMONES

At every level, from testicular histology and function to pituitary and hypothalamic function, age-related changes have been noted. With aging, testicular weight and Leydig cell numbers decrease; and histologic aberrancy of Leydig cells can be found with degenerative changes, vacuolization, and pigment accumulation.[4-6] Leydig cells, which predominantly produce testosterone, decrease from about 700 million cells at age 20 to 200 million by age 80.[4] Atherosclerosis of testicular blood vessels, and perhaps impaired tissue oxygenation, may contribute to Leydig cell death.[7] Total testicular steroid concentration diminishes in conjunction with the fall in Leydig cell number,[6] but occurs in the absence of any specific enzymatic defects in the testis.

Testosterone exists in the circulation bound to sex hormone binding globulin (SHBG), bound to albumin, or as "free" testosterone. Several studies have reported an increase in SHBG with age, presumably due to increased synthesis by the liver.[8-10] However, Tenover et al.,[11] have noted no age-related changes of SHBG in healthy elderly males. Circulating testosterone falls with advancing age in the majority of studies, with differences becoming apparent by the fifth decade[12-16] and further noted in a meta-analysis;[17] but testosterone levels may remain normal in elderly individuals selected for optimal health.[4,18,-21] However, some studies of "no change" in testosterone with age are due to afternoon sampling for hormone levels, or relate to the frequency of sampling. In the Massachusetts Male Aging study, testosterone decreased between the ages of 39 and 70 in the 1709 subjects studied.[22] With aging, there is attenuation of normal daily variability in testosterone concentrations in the elderly[11,13,23-25] and 24-h sampling has documented a decreased total testosterone concentration.[26]

Free testosterone (FT) concentration falls with age,[13] and while FT was previously thought to be the tissue "bioavailable" moiety, it has become apparent that what is bioavailable testosterone (BT) is both free testosterone and testosterone that is weakly bound to albumin (non-SHGB-bound testosterone).[27] BT has been reported to decrease with age[11,28] and in impotent individuals the fall in BT is present by age 50.[29] The decline in BT is even more marked with aging than that of total testosterone. Additionally, there is a loss of circadian variation in BT in older subjects.[25,30] Compared to males aged 20 to 40, >50% of men between ages 50 to 70 will have bioavailable testosterone concentrations below the lowest level of their younger counterparts.[14]

Dihydrotestosterone (DHT) which is formed from the conversion of testosterone by 5-alpha reductase (see Figure 9-1) has been reported to fall with age,[31-33] though some studies reported either no change or an increase in this potent metabolite.[34,35] This latter finding may have been due to the increased conversion of testosterone to DHT seen in a group of subjects with prostatic hyperplasia. No age-related hormonal changes have been found in normal prostatic tissue in subjects up to 75 years of age.[36]

Tissue levels of testosterone and some of its metabolites (DHT and 5-alpha androsterone 3-alpha, 17-beta-diol) show age-related changes in pubic skin but no change in some tissue areas studied such as skeletal muscle or scrotal or thigh skin.[37]

Another peripheral metabolite of testosterone, estradiol, has been reported to increase or remain unchanged with age.[9,15,26,29,38] However, these data are not consistent with other reports of a decrement in estradiol with age.[39] Fatty tissue is an important site of aromatization, and obesity is associated with increased estrogen (estrone) concentrations.[40,41] It is not surprising to find some data suggesting an increase in estrogenic concentration with age, as the percent of body fat in normal individuals increases as an age-related phenomenon. Additionally, the metabolic clearance of estradiol decreases with age.[42] As testosterone decreases, the testosterone/ estradiol ratio declines. Testosterone and androstenedione undergo an increase in peripheral aromatization to estrogens in aging men.[43,44] Androstenedione, as well as dehydroepiandrosterone

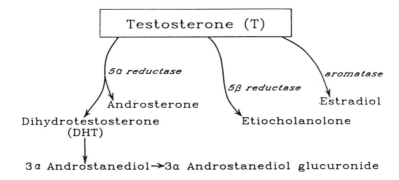

FIGURE 9-1 Steroidogenesis.

and its sulfate (DHEAS), decrease with age.[22,31,37,44,45] Total production rates for testosterone diminish from a mean of 6.6 mg/24 h down to a mean of 4mg/24 h for those over age 70, but this is partially offset by the decreases in the plasma clearance rate seen with aging.[46,47] These hormonal changes are listed in Table 9-1.

The age-related alterations of testosterone, bioavailable testosterone, and their relationship to relatively unchanged or increased levels of estradiol, may add to the impact of hormonal change. Sex hormone binding globulin binds testosterone more avidly than estradiol, and estradiol further enhances secretion of SHGB. As a result, the ratio of T or E_2 certainly changes with age[29] — falling rapidly after age 40 — and the ratio of BT to free estradiol also diminishes. This may further affect testosterone as well as gonadotropin secretion.

The clinical effect(s) of the age-related decrease in bioavailable testosterone and testosterone appear to be multiple. Effects of testosterone on erythropoiesis, sebaceous gland secretion, hair growth, maintenance of bone mass in men, and maintenance of libido have been extensively reviewed in Reference 48. The loss of these hormones (or at least their diminished concentration) and their putative role in aging is further discussed below.

A. Gonadotropins/Gonadotropin Releasing Hormone

Until recent studies, with what appeared to be an appropriate response to the lowered androgen levels seen with aging (described in the previous section), basal circulating levels of pituitary and urinary gonadotropins were thought to increase with age in most, but not all data.[13,15,18,20,21,38,42,49-51] Figure 9-2, taken from Baker et al.,[42] shows the age-related changes in gonadotropins that led many to believe that primary testicular failure was common with aging.

TABLE 9-1 Age-Related Reproductive Hormonal Changes

↓ Mean Serum Testosterone
↓ Bioavailable Testosterone
↓ Clearance/Production of Testosterone
↑ Aromatization
↓ Androstenedione/ ↓ Dehydroepiandrosterone (DHEA)/↓ DHEAS
Normal or Slight ↑ in Sex Hormone Binding Globulin
Normal Slightly ↑ Mean (LH) Concentration
↓ Bioactive LH
↓ Mean LH Response to Gonadotropin Releasing Hormone (GnRH)
↓ LH Response to GnRH
↓ LH Amplitude and/or Frequency (Altered Pulse Generation)
↑ Follicle Stimulating Hormone Concentration
↓ Inhibin Concentration

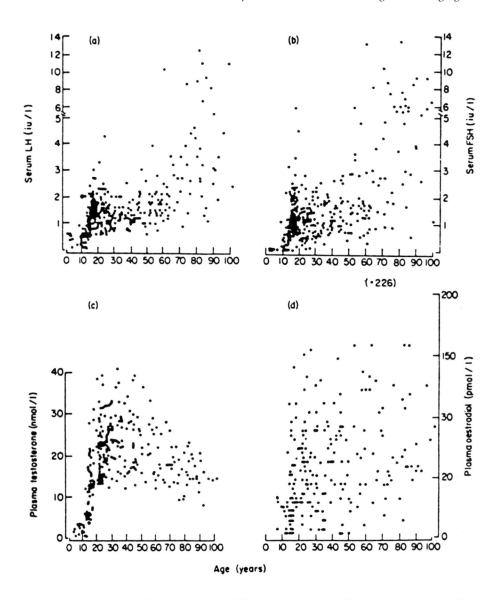

FIGURE 9-2 (a) Serum LH (IU/l), (b) serum FSH (IU/l), (c) testosterone (nmol/l), and (d) estradiol (pmol/l) as a function of age in normal males. (From Baker, H.W.G. et al., *Clin. Endocrinol.,* 5:349–372, 1976, with permission.)

Furthermore, diminished response to HCG (human chorionic gonadotropin) added support to the notion of diminished testicular reserve. This led to the concept that the hypogonadism of aging was due to primary testicular failure.

Yet it has become clear that the majority of hypogonadal older males, whether they have a problem such as impotence[29] or are chosen for health,[14] have secondary hypogonadism.[52] These men have low testosterone and bioavailable testosterone levels accompanied by low luteinizing hormone (LH) and follicle stimulating hormone (FSH) concentrations. In the study by our group,[14] 48% of healthy men over the age of 50 were found to have levels of bioavailable testosterone far below those of young healthy subjects, but none had elevated levels of luteinizing hormone (LH). Reviewing older studies that noted primary testicular failure, it seems a few subjects with primary hypogonadism appeared to increase the mean LH out of proportion, while the majority of subjects with low testosterone had LH levels below

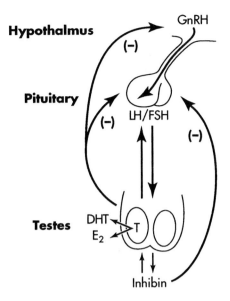

Hypothalmus

GnRH

(-)

Pituitary

(-) LH/FSH

(-)

Testes DHT T

E₂

Inhibin

FIGURE 9-3 Schematic of hormonal feedback/regulation.

the mean of that for younger subjects. Figure 9-3 shows a schematic version of feedback on the hypothalamic-pituitary axis.

Additionally, altered sensitivity of the hypothalamic-pituitary axis to exogenous androgens occurs with aging, further supporting an altered hypothalamic-pituitary state.[53,54] This suggests that in the continuum of hormonal changes with aging, along with a decrease in endogenous testosterone and bioavailable testosterone one sees primarily a low LH and FSH. The hypothalamic pituitary unit exhibits a differential response — in some cases showing no response to low levels of target organ hormones, and in others exhibiting an appropriate rise in gonadotropins to these low concentrations of T and BT. Slight or no alteration in the ratio of biologic to immunologic LH activity has been reported by some, while other data suggest a decrease in bioactive/immunologically active LH as a function of age.[55-57] The decrement in bioactive to immunoreactive ratio would be in concordance with the fact that androgens increase and estrogens decrease the ratio.[58-61] LH, a glycoprotein, is composed of an alpha subunit (similar to FSH), and a beta subunit, which makes LH specific. A rise in alpha subunits can be seen with aging, and may be in part responsible for an age-related decrease in bioactive LH.[62,63]

The response to gonadotropin releasing hormone (GnRH) shows a diminution with age[14,19,52,64] and a decrease in bioactive LH in response to GnRH stimulation may occur.[63,65] Prolonged stimulation of the pituitary may improve response.[11,65] However, short-term "priming" with more physiologic levels of GnRH results in a less robust response in elderly men with secondary hypogonadism, when compared to eugonadal healthy elderly or to young individuals.[66] These diminished responses seen in the face of the increased pituitary content of LH that occurs with aging,[67] suggest that despite apparently adequate pituitary reserves some alteration has occurred at the pituitary level, perhaps an alteration in receptor number or characteristics. The response to GnRH appears to be dependent on the degree of the underlying GnRH defect, and it is possible that appropriate exposure to LH may be a prerequisite for normal responsivity for GnRH, though a linear relationship between GnRH dose and LH secretory rate and LH mass released per secretory event, regardless of steroid level, has been found.[68-70] In feedback regulation, androgens appear to slow the gonadotropin releasing hormone generator, resulting in a decrease in pulse frequency;[70-72] while estrogen appear to affect amplitude.[73-76]

With aging, there is certainly no agreement regarding LH pulse characteristics. Desylpere et al. have suggested that LH pulse frequency is reduced, but amplitude maintained, when elderly men are compared with young controls.[72] Other data, including our own, have suggested that LH pulse frequency does not change with age, but amplitude is altered, and diminishes with aging.[11,25,66,77] Vermuelen and co-workers[78,79] have suggested that a decreased frequency of large amplitude pulses occurs with aging, while Veldhuis and colleagues have suggested that increased pulse frequency and decreased pulse amplitude may occur.[61] Certainly, however, pulse frequency does not *markedly* increase with age, despite low testosterone and bioavailable testosterone concentrations. The variability in data relating to pulse characteristics may reflect LH assay sensitivity, sampling frequency, and the model used to detect pulsatility.

The use of an antiestrogen (tamoxifen) in elderly males, while increasing bioactive LH pulse frequency in both young and old men, resulted in less of a response of a 12-h mean concentration of bioactive LH in the elderly group.[72] This suggests that relative changes in the concentration of estrogen to testosterone may impact on hypothalamic-pituitary function.[76] Additionally, it also suggests that alterations in pulse generation occur with aging, or it is possible that GnRH diminishes in the amount being released with each burst of activity. Other modulators of pulse generation, such as neuropeptide Y and dopamine which inhibit LH secretion, substance P and endogenous opioids, which decrease LH, may play a role in age-related change.[79-83] Prolactin, which increases with age, has inhibitory gonadotropin effects at both the hypothalamic and pituitary level.[84-86] Disease states such as diabetes and renal failure are associated with elevated prolactin levels as well.[77,85] Recently, another novel neurotransmitter, nitric oxide, has been found in gonadotrophs, with *in vitro* studies suggesting an inhibitory effect of nitric oxide on GnRH stimulated LH release.[86] Alternatively, the response at the pituitary level may be altered. These studies, despite lack of consensus on the types of changes seen with aging, imply that a transformation in pulse hypothalamic-pituitary generation occurs with aging.

Therefore, with aging (Table 9-1) there is evidence for the occurrence of testicular failure, with an inability to secrete testosterone, as well as mounting evidence for failure of the hypothalamic-pituitary axis, with an inability to respond appropriately to the lowered T and BT concentrations that occurs with aging (Figure 9-3).

III. SPERMATOGENESIS

Men retain sufficient seminiferous function to allow paternity to continue in most elderly males. Along with biblical reports, there is apparently one documented case of paternity at age 94.[51] Despite histological changes that include basement membrane thickening, peritubular fibrosis, and impairment in sperm maturation, this occurs in various degrees and in a patchy distribution such that overall function is maintained.[87]

Reports of sperm counts as a function of age have presented varying results — decreased, normal, or increased (perhaps related to length of abstinence).[20,88-90] In one study, a 30% decrease in sperm number in the ejaculate was noted in 52 to 68 year olds compared to younger men.[88] Neaves et al.[4] found a marked change in sperm number with age, with most men over age 40 producing less than 200 million sperm per day and those under 40 producing more than 200 million sperm per day (Figure 9-4). An inverse correlation between FSH and daily sperm production appears to exist. Alterations, not only in sperm number but sperm morphology and motility, have been reported to occur with aging.[89,90]

Inhibin, a glycoprotein produced by Sertoli cells of the testes in response to FSH, feeds back to inhibit FSH secretion at the pituitary level. The role of LH on regulating inhibin levels remains to be clarified, but at pharmacologic concentrations LH can raise inhibin levels. With aging, the number of Sertoli cells diminishes.[91] Tenover et al.[56] have shown a decrease in inhibin concentrations in men aged 65 to 85, compared to men aged 22 to 35, despite a higher level of both immunoreactive FSH and LH in the elderly, but comparable levels of bioactive

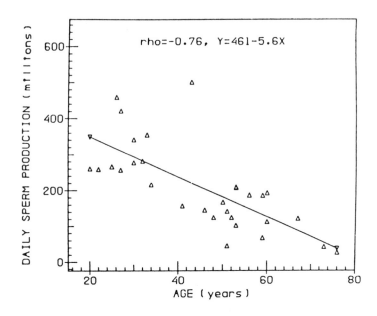

FIGURE 9-4 Daily sperm production by both testes of 30 men in relation to age. The correlation coefficient and equation of the regression line are shown. (From Neaves, W.B. et al., *J. Clin. Endocrinol. Metab.*, 55:756–763, 1984; with permission.)

FSH (Figure 9-5). The low levels of inhibin would suggest that there is either a defect in inhibin production or, alternatively, that there is accelerated clearance of this substance with advancing age. Ativan, produced by Leydig cells and involved in Sertoli cell function sperm proliferation, and acts to increase FSH, has not been studied in older individuals.[92]

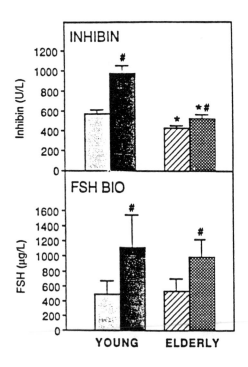

FIGURE 9-5 Mean ($\pm$ SEM) serum inhibin and bioactive FSH levels in 11 young and 13 elderly men before ($\square$ and $\boxtimes$) and after ($\blacksquare$ and $\blacksquare$) 1 week of clomiphene citrate administration; * $p < 0.01$ compared to young, # $p < 0.01$ compared to baseline. (From Tenover, J.S. et al., *J. Clin. Endocrinol. Metab.*, 67:455–459, 1988; with permission.)

TABLE 9-2 Potential Effects of Hypogonadism

$\downarrow$ Muscle Mass
$\downarrow$ Strength
$\uparrow$ Body fat
Osteoporosis
Cognitive (Memory) Impairment
$\downarrow$ Appetite
$\downarrow$ Libido
$\downarrow$ Body Hair
$\uparrow$ Waist/Hip Ratio
Anemia
$\downarrow$ Libido and Sexual Function

IV. TESTOSTERONE EFFECTS

Many of the effects of testosterone deficiency appear almost to be a paradigm for age-related problems in older men (Table 9-2). Testosterone effects have been extensively reviewed.[48] The implications of low hormone levels for any given individual may vary. Testosterone has clear implications in terms of bone mass maintenance in younger hypogonadal individuals, while in older males testosterone levels correlate with bone mass, but age per se is a confounder.[93-97] Hypogonadism confers a 6.5 times greater risk of hip fracture following minimal trauma in elderly males.[98] In our study,[99] a marker of bone formation, osteocalcin, increased in older individuals receiving testosterone therapy for a 3-month period. Tenover[100] reported a decrease in urinary hydroxyproline excretion with testosterone therapy in 13 hypogonadal men, suggesting a decrease in bone turnover. Certainly, these data suggest a role for testosterone deficiency in the pathogenesis of osteoporosis/hip fracture in older men, but the long-term effect of therapy has not been evaluated.

While lean body mass decreased with age, androgenic treatment has been shown to increase new myofibril formation and increase muscle fiber area.[101-103] Loss of muscle mass may contribute to weakness, immobility, and gait and balance instability, resulting in a syndrome of "frailty". Testosterone produces primarily changes in upper limb musculature.[103] Our data also noted increased grip strength.[99]

With age, hemoglobin and hematocrit decrease in older men. Testosterone is well known to increase hematocrit through both direct and indirect effects on erythropoietin.[104-105]

Visual spatial ability has been linked to testosterone levels in younger men, and in animals, testosterone has been shown to enhance visual-spatial task retention in mice.[27,50] In senescent accelerated mice with marked memory impairment, the levels of testosterone are lower than those of aged matched controls (Flood, J.F., Kaiser, F.E., and Morley, J.E., unpublished observations). A strong correlation of bioavailable testosterone and testosterone for a number of memory tests has also been found in males (Kaiser, F.E., Morley, J.E., and Jensen, J., unpublished observations). Further long-term studies will need to be undertaken to examine the role of testosterone repletion on cognitive performance.

V. IMPOTENCE

Impotence is defined as the inability to achieve an erection sufficient for successful intercourse in 75% or more attempts, or cessation of attempts at intercourse.[29] The prevalence of sexual dysfunction among the elderly is unknown, but up to 55% of men at the age of 75 were reported to be impotent or sexually inactive by Kinsey.[108] Depending on the population studied, over the age of 70, >95% of those may report impotence.[109] It has become increasingly clear that the etiology of impotence is multifactorial[29,109-114] and that organic factors, rather than psychogenic ones, underlie the pathogenesis of impotence, especially in the elderly.

Illness, aside from the psychic stress, may result in gonadal dysfunction. "Stress" may result in release of endogenous opioids, which inhibits the release of hypothalamic GnRH, which then results in inhibition of LH release. Depression, in addition to psychic change, may result in hormonally mediated impotence in that the decreased LH and testosterone seen[115] may relate to the increased levels of corticotropin releasing factor that occur in depression. The effects of medication on sexual function are numerous, but the specific alterations by various medications are far from clear.[112,116-120]

Some studies have shown a correlation between serum testosterone and sexual activity in older men.[29,49,121] However, the major correlation appears to be with libido, with lesser effects on erectile function. Sexual thoughts, frequency of sexual desire, ease of arousability and the degree of erections have been linked to bioavailable testosterone concentrations in older men.[122] Both libido and activity may improve with testosterone administration[123,124] though extensive studies have not been performed in older men. However, other therapeutic alternatives exist for relief of potency problems and should also be considered for older individuals.[1,99,125-127]

In other men, 17-β testosterone actually lowers cholesterol,[99,100] whereas 17-α alkylated androgens decrease HDL. In our study,[99] LDL decreased while HDL concentrations were maintained in those receiving 17-β therapy.

Testosterone trials in older men are few (reviewed in Reference 1). Positive effects seen in the study of Tenover[100] and our group[99] have both shown an increase in hematocrit, positive effects on bone metabolism, and decreases in cholesterol; concerns remain, however, over the use of testosterone in the large numbers of hypogonadal men that exist. Adverse effects (Table 9-2) may include a marked increase in hematocrit, which can lead to stroke. Prostatic growth has been thought to occur at a more rapid rate in testosterone-treated subjects. At least in young hypogonadal men, testosterone treatment results in prostate volume and prostate specific antigen comparable to that of age-matched controls.[128] No data exist to suggest that prostate carcinoma will occur as a direct effect of testosterone therapy. It is important that prostatic examinations and measures of prostate specific antigen should be obtained periodically (we generally suggest at least every 6 months). Sleep apnea may be aggravated in younger hypogonadal men treated with testosterone, but again, this remains unstudied in older men.[129] Other phenomena such as gynecomastia and salt and fluid retention reverse when testosterone is stopped.

The effects of short-term testosterone therapy in preliminary studies are an invitation to long-term placebo-controlled trials of therapy in older hypogonadal men. While it is unclear at present if these hormonal changes of aging are "adaptive" or part of the pathogenesis of aging, hope for hormonal intervention to forestall or even prevent problems that may contribute to frailty, or at least improve the quality of life for an older individual, makes this an area worth further investigation.

VI. CONCLUSION

With aging, it appears that testosterone and bioavailable testosterone decrease, and evidence exists not only for primary testicular failure in elderly males, but hypothalamic-pituitary perturbations. These changes may represent a continuum of the pattern seen in a given individual.

The role of reproductive hormonal alterations in the aging male may have significant implications for the aging process per se. Many questions remain. Do the benefits of hormonal intervention outweigh long-term risks? Which group of older men are optimal targets for intervention, and for how long? Long-term randomized trials are needed to address these issues.

REFERENCES

1. Morley, J.E. and Kaiser, F.E., Hypogonadism in the elderly man, *Adv. Endocrinol. Metab.*, 4, 241, 1993.
2. Mastrogiacomo, I., Feghali, G., Foresta, C. and Ruzza, G., Andropause: incidence and pathogenesis, *Arch. Androl.*, 9, 293, 1982.
3. Werner, A.A., The male climacteric, *J. Am. Med. Assoc.*, 112, 1441, 1939.
4. Neaves, W.B., Johnson, L., Porter, J.C., Parker, C.R. and Petty, C.S., Leydig cell numbers, daily sperm production and serum gonadotropin levels in aging men, *J. Clin. Endocrinol. Metab.*, 59, 756, 1984.
5. Sarjent, J.W. and McDonald, J.R., A method for the quantitative estimate of Leydig cells in the human testes, *Mayo Clin. Proc.* 23, 249, 1948.
6. Tillenger, K.G., Testicular morphology, *Acta. Endocrinol.* (Copenh) Suppl. 24, 1, 1957.
7. Sasano, N. and Ichijo, S., Vascular patterns of the human testis with special reference to its senile changes, *Tohuku J. Exp. Med.*, 99, 269, 1969.
8. Horst, H.J., Becker, H. and Voigt, K.D., The determination in human males of specific testosterone and 5alpha-dihydrotestosterone binding to sex hormone binding globulin by a differential dissocation technique, *Steroids* 23, 833, 1974.
9. Kley, H.K., Nieschlag, E., Bidlingmaier, F. and Kruskemper, H.L., Possible age-dependent influence of estrogens on the binding of testosterone in plasma of adult men, *Horm. Metab. Res.*, 6, 213, 1974.
10. Vermeulen, A. and Verdonck, L., Some studies on the biological significance of free testosterone, *J. Steroid Biochem.*, 3, 421, 1972.
11. Tenover, J.S., Matsumoto, A.M., Plymate, S.R. and Bremner, W.J., The effects of aging in normal men on bioavailable testosterone and luteinizing hormone secretion: response to clomiphene citrate, *J. Clin. Endocrinol. Metab.* 65, 1118, 1987.
12. Davidson, J.M., Chen, J.J., Crapo, L., Gary, G.D., Greenleaf, W.J. and Catania, J.A., Hormonal changes and sexual function in aging men, *J. Clin. Endocrinol. Metab.*, 57, 71, 1983.
13. Deslypere, J.P. and A. Vermeulen, Leydig cell function in normal men: effect of age, life-style, residence, diet, and activity, *J. Clin. Endocrinol. Metab.*, 59, 955, 1984.
14. Korenman S.G., Morley, J.E., Mooradian, A.D., Davis, S.S., Kaiser, F.E., Silver, A.J., Viosca, S.P. and Garza, D., Secondary hypogonadism in older men: its relation to impotence, *J. Clin. Endocrinol Metab.*, 71, 963, 1990.
15. Stearns, E.L., MacDonnell, J.A., Kaufman, B.J., Padua, R., Lucman, T.S., Winter, J.S.D. and Faiman, C., Declining testicular function with age: hormonal and clinical correlates, *Am. J. Med.*, 57, 761, 1974.
16. Vermeulen, A., Androgens in the aging male, *J. Clin. Endocrinol. Metab.*, 73, 221, 1991.
17. Gray, A., Berlin, J.A., McKinley, J.B. and Longcope, C., An examination of research design effects on the association of testosterone and male aging: results of a meta-analysis, *J. Clin. Epidemiol.* 44, 671, 1991.
18. Harman, S.M. and Tsitouras, P.D., Reproductive hormones in aging men: I. Measurement of sex steroids, basal luteinizing hormone, and Leydig cell response to human chorionic gonadotropin, *J. Clin. Endocrinol. Metab.*, 51, 35, 1980.
19. Harman, S.M., Tsitouras, P.D., Costa, P.T. and Blackman, M.R., Reproductive hormones in aging men. II. Basal pituitary gonadotropins and gonadotropin responses to luteinizing hormone-releasing hormone, *J. Clin. Endocrinol. Metab.*, 54, 547, 1982.
20. Nieschlag, E., Lammers, U., Freischem, C.W., Langer, K. and Wickings. E.J., Reproductive functions in young fathers and grandfathers, *J. Clin. Endocrinol. Metab.*, 55, 676, 1982.
21. Sparrow, D., Bosse, R. and Rowe, J.W., The influence of age, alcohol consumption and body build on gonadal function in men, *J. Clin. Endocrinol. Metab.*, 51, 508, 1980.
22. Gray, A., Feldman, H.A., McKinlay, J.B., and Longcope, C., Age, disease, and changing sex hormone levels in middle-aged men: results of the Massachusetts Male Aging Study, *J. Clin. Endocrinol. Metab.*, 73, 1016, 1991.
23. Bremner, W.J., Vitiello, M.V. and Prinz, P.N., Loss of circadian rhythmicity in blood testosterone levels with aging in normal men, *J. Clin. Endocrinol. Metab.*, 56, 1278, 1983.
24. Tenover, J.S., Matsumoto, A.M., Clifton, D.K., and Bremner, W.J., Age related alterations in the circadian rhythms of pulsatile luteinizing hormone and testosterone secretion in healthy men, *J. Gerontol.*, 43, M163, 1988.
25. Kaiser, F.E., Viosca, S.P., Mooradian, A.D., Morley, J.E. and Korenman, S.G., Impotence and aging: alterations in hormonal secretory patterns with age, *Endo. Soc.*, 778A, 215, 1988.
26. Zumoff, B., Strain, G.W., Kream, J., O'Connor, J., Rosenfeld, R.S., Levin, J. and Fukushima, D.K., Age variation of the 24-hour mean plasma concentration of androgens, estrogens and gonadotropins in normal adult men, *J. Clin. Endocrinol. Metab.*, 54, 534, 1982.
27. Manni, A., Pardridge, W.M., Cefalu, W., Nisula, B.C., Bardin, C.W., Santner, S.J. and Santen, R.J., Bioavailability of albumin-bound testosterone, *J. Clin. Endocrinol. Metab.*, 61, 705, 1985.

28. Nankin, H.R. and Calkins, J.H., Decreased bioavailable testosterone in aging normal and impotent men, *J. Clin. Endocrinol. Metab.*, 63, 1418, 1986.

29. Kaiser, F.E., Viosca, S.P., Morley, J.E., Mooradian, A.D., Davis, S.S. and Korenman, S.G., Impotence and aging, clinical and hormonal factors, *J. Am. Geriatr. Soc.*, 36, 511, 1988.

30. Plymate, S.R., Tenover, J.S. and Bremner. W.J., Circadian variation in testosterone sex hormone-binding globulin and calculated non-sex hormone-binding globulin bound testosterone in healthy young and elderly men, *J. Androl.*, 10, 366, 1989.

31. Giusti, G., Gonnelli, P., Borrelli, D., Fiorelli, G., Forti, G., Pazzagli, M. and Serio, M., Age-related secretion of androstenedione, testosterone and dihydrotestosterone by the human testis, *Exp. Geront.*, 10, 241, 1975.

32. Lewis, J.G., Ghanadian, R. and Chisholm, G.D., Serum 5-alpha-dihydrotestosterone and testosterone changes with age in man, *Acta. Endocrinol.* (Copenh), 82, 444, 1976.

33. Pirke, K.M. and Doerr, P., Age related changes in free plasma testosterone dihydrotestosterone and oestradiol, *Acta. Endocrinol.* (Copenh), 80, 171, 1975.

34. Horton, R., Hsieh, P., Barberia, J., Pages, L. and Cosgrove, M., Altered blood androgens in elderly men with prostate hyperplasia, *J. Clin. Endocrinol. Metab.*, 41, 793, 1975.

35. Pirke, K.M., Doerr, P., Sintermann, R. and Vogt, H.J., Age dependence of testosterone precursors in plasma of normal adult males, *Acta. Endocrinol.* (Copenh), 86, 415, 1977.

36. Lamberigts, G., Dierickx, P., DeMoor, P. and Verhoeven, G., Comparison of the metabolism and receptor binding of testosterone and 17-beta-hydroxy-5-alpha-androstan-3-one in normal skin fibroblast cultures: influence of origin and passage number, *J. Clin. Endocrinol. Metab.*, 48, 924, 1979.

37. Deslypere, J.P. and Vermeulen, A., Aging and tissue androgens, *J. Clin. Endocrinol. Metab.*, 53, 430, 1981.

38. Rubens, R., Dhont, M. and Vermeulen, A., Further studies on Leydig cell function in old age. *J. Clin. Endocrinol. Metab,* 39, 40, 1974.

39. Simon, D., Preziosi, P., Barrett-Conner, E., Roger, M., Saint-Paul, M., Nahoul, K. and Papaz, L., The influence of aging on plasma sex hormones in men: The Telecom Study, *Am. J. Epidemiol.*, 135, 783, 1992.

40. Kley, H.K., Solbach, H.G., McKinnan, J.C. and Kruskemper, H.L., Testosterone decrease and oestrogen increase in male patients with obesity. *Acta Endocrinol.*, 91, 553, 1979.

41. Stanik, S., Dornfeld, L.P., Maxwell, M.H., Viosca, S.P. and Korenman, S.G., The effect of weight loss on reproductive hormones in obese men, *J. Clin. Endocrinol. Metab.*, 53, 828, 1981.

42. Baker, H.W., Burger, H.G., de Kretser, D.M., Hudson, B., O'Connor, S., Wang, C., Mirovics, A., Court, J., Dunlop, M. and Rennie, G.C., Changes in the pituitary-testicular system with age, *Clin. Endocrinol.*, 5, 349, 1976.

43. Hemsell, D.L., Grodin, J.M., Brenner, P.F., Siiteri, P.K. and MacDonald, P.C., Plasma precursors of estrogen. II. Correlation of extent of conversion of plasma androstenedione to estrone with age, *J. Clin. Endocrinol. Metab.*, 38, 476, 1974.

44. Montanini, V., Simoni, M., Chiossi, G., Baraghini, G.F., Velardo, A., Baraldi, E. and Marrama, P., Age-related changes in plasma dehydroepiandrosterone sulphate, cortisol, testosterone and free testosterone circadian rhythms in adult men, *Horm. Res.*, 29, 1, 1988.

45. Orentreich, N., Brind, J.L., Rizer, R.L. and Vogelman, J.H., Age changes and sex differences in serum dehydroepiandrosterone sulfate concentrations throughout adulthood, *J. Clin. Endocrinol. Metab.*, 59, 551, 1984.

46. Kent, J.Z. and Acone, A.B., Plasma androgens and aging, in *Androgens in Normal and Pathological Conditions*, Exley, D. and Vermeulen, A., Eds., Excerpta Medica Foundation, Amsterdam, 1966, 31.

47. Vermeulen, A., Rubens, R. and Verdonck, L., Testosterone secretion and metabolism in male senescence, *J. Clin. Endocrinol. Metab.*, 34, 730, 1972.

48. Mooradian, A.D., Morley, J.E. and Korenman, S.G., Biological actions of androgens, *Endocr. Rev.*, 8, 1, 1987.

49. Davidson, J.M., Camargo, C.A. and Smith, E.R., Effects of androgen on sexual behavior in hypogonadal men, *J. Clin. Endocrinol. Metab.*, 48, 955, 1979.

50. Slag, M.F., Morley, J.E., Elson, M.K., Trence, D.L., Nelson, C.J., Nelson, A.E., Kinlaw, W.B., Beyer, H.S., Nuttal, F.Q. and Shafer, R.B., Impotence in medical clinic outpatients, *JAMA*, 249, 1736, 1983.

51. Tsitouras, P.D., Effects of age on testicular function, *Endocrinol. Metab. Clin. N. Am.*, 16, 1045, 1987.

52. Winters, S.J. and Troen, P., Episodic luteinizing hormone (LH) secretion and the response of LH and follicle-stimulating hormone to LH-releasing hormone in aged men: evidence for coexistent primary testicular insufficiency and an impairment in gonadotropin secretion, *J. Clin. Endocrinol. Metab.*, 55, 560, 1982.

53. Muta, K., Kato, K., Akamine, Y. and Ibayashi, H., Age-related changes in the feedback regulation of gonadotrophin secretion by sex steroids in men, *Acta Endocrinol.* 96, 154, 1981.

54. Winters, S.J., Sherins, R.J. and Troen, P., The gonadotropin-suppressive activity of androgen is increased in elderly men, *Metab. Clin. Exp.*, 33, 1052, 1984.

55. Marrama, P., Montanini, V., Celani, M.F., Carani, C., Cioni, K., Bazzani, M., Cavani, D. and Baraghini, G.F., Decrease in luteinizing hormone biological activity/immunoreactivity ratio in elderly men, *Maturitas* 5, 223, 1984.

56. Tenover, J.S., McLachlan, R.I., Dahl, K.D., Burger, H.G., de Kretser, D.M. and Bremner, W.J., Decreased serum inhibin levels in normal elderly men: evidence for a decline in Sertoli cell function with aging, *J. Clin. Endocrinol. Metab.*, 67, 455, 1988.

57. Warner, B.A., Dufau, M.L. and Santen, R.J., Effects of aging and illness on the pituitary testicular axis in men: qualitative as well as quantitative changes in luteinizing hormone, *J. Clin. Endocrinol. Metab.*, 60, 263, 1985.

58. Solano, A.R., Garcia-Vela, A., Catt, K.J. and Dufau, M.L., Modulation of serum and pituitary luteinizing hormone bioactivity by androgen in the rat, *Endocrinology*, 106, 1941, 1980.

59. Carani, C., Celani, M.F., Zini, D., Baldini, A., Della Casa, L. and Marrama, P., Changes in the bioactivity to immunoreactivity ratio of circulating luteinizing hormone in impotent men treated with testosterone undecanoate, *Acta Endocrinol.* 120, 284, 1989.

60. Lucky, A.W., Rebar, R.W., Rosenfield, R.L., Roche-Bender, N. and Helke, J., Reduction of the potency of luteinizing hormone by estrogen, *N. Engl. J. Med.* 300, 1034, 1979.

61. Veldhuis, J.D., Urban, R.J., Lizarralde, G., Johnson, M.L. and Iranmanesh, A., Attenuation of luteinizing hormone secretory burst amplitude as a proximate basis for the hypoandrogenism of healthy aging in men, *J. Clin. Endocrinol. Metab.*, 75, 52, 1992.

62. Ceda, G.P., Denti, L., Ceresini, G., Torsiglieri, W., Hoffman, A.R. and Valenti, G., The effects of aging on the secretion of the common alpha-subunit of the glycoprotein hormones in men, *J. Am. Geriatr. Soc.*, 39, 353, 1991.

63. Blackman, M.R., Tsitouras, P.D. and Harman, S.M., Reproductive hormones in aging men. III: Basal and LHRH-stimulated serum concentrations of the common alpha-subunit of the glycoprotein hormones, *J. Gerontol.*, 42, 476, 1987.

64. Jarjour, L.T., Handelsman, D.J. and Swerdloff, R.S., Effects of aging on the in vitro release of gonadotropin-releasing hormone, *Endocrinology*, 119, 1113, 1986.

65. Urban, R.J., Veldhuis, J.D., Blizzard, R.M. and Dufau, M.L., Attenuated release of biologically active luteinizing hormone in healthy aging men, *J. Clin. Invest.*, 81, 1020, 1988.

66. Kaiser, F.E., Morley, J.E., Viosca, S.P., Garza, D. and Korenman. S.G., Effects of low dose GnRH in healthy potent elderly and impotent elderly subjects with secondary hypogonadism, *Endo. Soc.*, 1295A, 1989.

67. Ryan, R.J., The luteinizing hormone content of human pituitaries. I. Variations with sex and age, *J. Clin. Endocrinol. Metab.*, 22, 300, 1962.

68. Barkan, A.L., Reame, N.E., Kelch, R.P. and Marshall, J.C., Idiopathic hypogonadotropic hypogonadism in men: dependence of the hormone responses to gonadotropin-releasing hormone (GnRH) on the magnitude of the endogenous GnRH secretory defect, *J. Clin. Endocrinol. Metab.*, 61, 1118, 1985.

69. Spratt, D.I., Crowley, W.R. Jr., Butler, J.P., Hoffman, A.R., Conn, P.M. and Badger, T.M., Pituitary luteinizing hormone responses to intravenous and subcutaneous administration of gonadotropin-releasing hormone in men, *J. Clin. Endocrinol. Metab.*, 61, 890, 1985.

70. Veldhuis, J.D., Rogol, A.D., Samojlik, E. and Ertel, N.H., Role of endogenous opiates in the expression of negative feedback actions of androgen and estrogen on pulsatile properties of luteinizing hormone secretion in man, *J. Clin. Invest.*, 74, 47, 1984.

71. Winters, S.J., Janick, J.J., Loriaux, D.L. and Sherins. R.J., Studies on the role of sex steroids in the feedback control of gonadotropin concentrations in men. II. Use of the estrogen antagonist, clomiphene citrate, *J. Clin. Endocrinol. Metab.*, 48, 222, 1979.

72. Deslypere, J.P., Kaufman, J.M., Vermeulen, T., Vogelaers, D., Vandalem, J.L. and Vermeulen, A., Influence of age on pulsatile luteinizing hormone release and responsiveness of the gonadotrophs to sex hormone feedback in men, *J. Clin. Endocrinol. Metab.*, 64, 68, 1987.

73. Spijkstra, J.J., Spinder, T., Gooren, L. and Van Kessel, H., Divergent effects of the antiestrogen tamoxifen and of estrogens on luteinizing hormone (LH) pulse frequency, but not on basal LH levels and LH pulse amplitude in men, *J. Clin. Endocrinol. Metab.*, 66, 355, 1988.

74. Winters, S.J. and Troen, P., Evidence for a role of endogenous estrogen in the hypothalamic control of gonadotropin secretion in men, *J. Clin. Endocrinol. Metab.*, 61, 842, 1985.

75. Veldhuis, J.D., Rogol, A.D., Perez-Palacios, G., Stumpf, P., Kitchin, J.D. and Dufau, M.L., Endogenous opiates participate in the regulation of pulsatile luteinizing hormone release in an unopposed estrogen milieu: studies in estrogen-replaced, gonadectomized patients with testicular feminization, *J. Clin. Endocrinol. Metab.*, 61, 709, 1985.

76. Veldhuis, J.D. and Dufau, M.L., Estradiol modulates the pulsatile secretion of biologically active luteinizing hormone in man, *J. Clin. Invest.*, 80, 631, 1987.

77. Kaiser, F.E. and Morley, J.E., Gonadotropins, testosterone, and the aging male, *Neurobiol. of Aging*, 15, 559, 1994.

78. Vermeulen, A. and Kaufman, J.M., Role of the hypothalamo-pituitary function in the hypoandrogenism of healthy aging, *J. Clin. Endocrinol. Metab.*, 74, 1226A, 1992.

79. Vermeulen, A., Deslypere, J.P. and Kaufman, J.M., Influence of antiopioids on luteinizing hormone pulsatility in aging men, *J. Clin. Endocrinol. Metab.*, 68, 68, 1989.

80. Allen, L.G., Crowley, W.R. and Kalra, S.P., Interactions between neuropeptide Y and adrenergic systems in the stimulation of luteinizing hormone release in steroid-primed ovariectomized rats, *Endocrinology*, 121, 1953, 1987.

81. Huseman, C.A., Kugler, J.A. and Schneider, I.G., Mechanism of dopaminergic suppression of gonadotropin secretion in men, *J. Clin. Endocrinol. Metab.*, 51, 209, 1980.

82. Morley, J.E., Neuroendocrine effects of endogenous opioid peptides in human subjects: a review, *Psychoneuroendocrinol.* 8, 361, 1983.

83. Morley J.E., Baranetsky, N.G., Wingert, T.D., Carlson, H.E., Hershman, J.M., Melmed, S., Levin, S.R., Jamison, K.R., Weitzman, R., Chang, R.J. and Varner, A.A., Endocrine effects of naloxone-induced opiate receptor blockade, *J. Clin. Endocrinol. Metab.*, 50, 251, 1980.

84. Billington, C.J., Shafer, R.B. and Morley, J.E., Effects of opioid blockade with nalmefene in older impotent men, *Life Sci.*, 47, 799, 1990.

85. Morley, J.E. and Melmed, S., Gonadal dysfunction in systemic disorders, *Metab. Clin. Exp.*, 28, 1051, 1979.

86. Ceccatelli, S., Hulting, A.L., Zhang, X., Gustafsson, L., Villar, M. and Hokfelt, T., Nitric oxide synthase in the rat anterior pituitary gland and the role of nitric oxide in regulation of luteinizing hormone secretion, *Proc. Natl. Acad. Sci. USA*, 90, 11292, 1993.

87. Engle, E.T., The male reproductive system stem, in *Problems of ageing: biological and medical aspects* (3rd Ed.), Lansing, A.I., Eds., Williams and Wilkins, Baltimore, 1952, 708.

88. Homonnai, Z.T., Fainman, N., David, M.P. and Paz, G.F., Semen quality and sex hormone pattern of 29 middle aged men, *Andrologia*, 14, 164, 1982.

89. McLeod, J. and Gold, R.Z., The male factor in fertility and infertility. II. Semen quality in relation to age and sexual activity, *Fertil. Steril.*, 4, 194, 1953.

90. Natoli, A., Riondino, G. and Brancati, A., Studio della funzione gonadale ormonica e spermatogenica nel corso delta senescenza muschille, *G. Gerontol.*, 20, 1103, 1972.

91. Johnson, L., Zane, R.S., Petty, C.S. and Neaves, W.B., Quantification of the human Sertoli cell population: its distribution relation to germ cell numbers, and age-related decline, *Biol. Reprod.*, 31, 785, 1984.

92. Mather, J.P., Woodruff, T.K. and Krummen, L.A., Paracrine regulation of reproductive function by inhibin and activan, *Proc. Soc. Exp. Biol. Med.*, 201, 1, 1992.

93. Spencer, H., Lewin, I. and Friedland, J.A., Action of androgens and related substances on mineral metabolism and bone, *Pharmaceut. Ther. C.* 1, 207, 1976.

94. Baran, D.T., Bergfeld, M.A., Teitelbaum, S.L. and Avioli, L.V., Effect of testosterone therapy on bone formation in an osteoporotic hypogonadal male, *Calcif. Tissue Res.*, 26, 103, 1978.

95. Foresta, C., Ruzza, G., Mioni, R., Guarneri, G., Gribaldo, R., Meneghello, A. and Mastrogiacomo, I., Osteoporosis and decline of gonadal function in the elderly male, *Horm. Res.*, 19, 18, 1984.

96. McElduff, A., Wilkinson, M., Ward, P. and Posen, S., Forearm mineral content in normal men: relationship to weight, height and plasma testosterone concentrations, *Bone* 9, 281, 1988.

97. Meier, D.E., Orwoll, E.S., Keenan, E.J. and Fagerstrom, R.M., Marked decline in trabecular bone mineral content in healthy men with age: lack of association with sex steroid levels, *J. Am. Geriatr. Soc.*, 35, 189, 1987.

98. Stanley, H.L., Schmitt, B.P., Poses, R.M. and Deiss, W.P., Does hypogonadism contribute to the occurrence of a minimal trauma hip fracture in elderly men?, *J. Am. Geriatr. Soc.* 39, 766, 1991.

99. Morley, J.E., Perry, H.M. III, Kaiser, F.E., Kraenzle, D., Jensen, J., Houston, K., Mattammal, M. and Perry, H.M. Jr., Effects of testosterone replacement in old hypogonadal males: a preliminary study, *J. Am. Geriatr. Soc.* 41, 149, 1993.

100. Tenover, J.S., Effects of testosterone supplementation in the aging male, *J. Clin. Endocrinol. Metab.*, 75, 1092, 1992.

101. Chumlea, W.C., Roche, A.F. and Webb, P., Body size, subcutaneous fatness and total body fat in older adults, *Int. J. Obes.*, 8, 311, 1984.

102. Carlson, K.E., Alston, W. and Feldman. D.J., Electromyographic study of aging in skeletal muscle, *Am. J. Physiol.*, 43, 141, 1964.

103. Hamilton, J.B., The role of testicular secretions as indicated by the effects of castration in man and studies of pathologic conditions and the short lifespan associated with maleness, *Rec. Prog. Horm. Res.*, 3, 257, 1948.

104. Ammus S.S., The role of androgens in the treatment of hematologic disorders, *Adv. Intern. Med.*, 34, 191, 1989.

105. Alexanian R., Erythropoietin and erythropoiesis in anemic man following androgens, *Blood* 33, 564, 1969.

106. Flood, J.F., Morley, J.E. and Roberts, E., Memory-enhancing effects in male mice of pregnenolone and steroids metabolically derived from it, *Proc. Natl. Acad. Sci. USA*, 89, 1567, 1992.
107. Kimura, D., Sex differences in the brain, *Sci. Am.*, 267, 118, 1992.
108. Kinsey, A.C., Pomeroy, W.B. and C.E. Martin, *Sexual behavior in the human male*, W.B. Saunders, Philadelphia, 1948.
109. Kaiser, F.E. and Korenman, S.G., Impotence in diabetic men, *Am. J. Med.* 85, 147, 1988.
110. Morley, J.E, Impotence, *Am. J. Med.*, 80, 897, 1986.
111. Morley, J.E., Impotence in older men, *Hosp. Pract.*, 23, 139, 1988.
112. Papadopoulos, C., Cardiovascular drugs and sexuality, *Arch. Intern. Med.*, 140:1341, 1980.
113. Persson, G. Sexuality in a 70-year-old urban population, *J. Psychosom. Res.*, 24, 335, 1980.
114. Van Unnik, J.G. and Marsman. J.W., Impotence due to external iliac steal syndrome treated by percutaneous transluminal angioplasty, *J. Urol.*, 131, 544, 1984.
115. Yesavage, J.A., Davidson, J., Widrow, L. and Berger, P.A., Plasma testosterone levels, depression, sexuality, and age, *Biol. Psychiatry*, 20, 222, 1985.
116. Anonymous, Drugs that cause sexual dysfunction, *Med. Lett. Drugs Ther.*, 29, 65, 1987.
117. Buffum, J., Pharmacosexology update: prescription drugs and sexual function, *J. Psychoact. Drugs*, 18, 97, 1986.
118. Croog, S.H., Levine, S., Sudilovsky, A., Baume, R.M. and Clive, J., Sexual symptoms in hypertensive patients. A clinical trial of antihypertensive medications, *Arch. Intern. Med.*, 148, 788, 1988.
119. Hogan, M.J., Wallin, J.D. and Baer, R.M., Antihypertensive therapy and male sexual dysfunction, *Psychosomatics*, 21, 234, 1980.
120. Billington, C.J., Levine, A.S. and Morley, J.E., Zinc status in impotent patients., *Clin. Res.* 31, 714A, 1983.
121. Tsitouras P.D., Martin, C.E. and Harman, S.M., Relationship of serum testosterone to sexual activity in healthy elderly men, *J. Gerontol.* 37, 288, 1982.
122. Schiavi, R.C., Schreiner-Engel, P., White, D. and Mandeli, J., The relationship between pituitary-gonadal function and sexual behavior in healthy aging men, *Psychosom. Med.*, 53, 363, 1991.
123. Carani, C., Zini, D., Baldini, A., Della Casa, L., Ghizzani, A. and Marrama, P., Effects of androgen treatment in impotent men with normal and low levels of free testosterone, *Arch. Sex. Behav.* 19, 223, 1990.
124. O'Carroll, R. and Bancroft, J., Testosterone therapy for low sexual interest and erectile dysfunction in men: a controlled study, *Br. J. Psychiatry* 145, 146, 1984.
125. Kaiser, F.E., Sexuality and impotence in the aging man, *Clin. Geriatr. Med.*, 7, 63, 1991.
126. Korenman, S.G., Viosca, S.P., Kaiser, F.E., Mooradian, A.D. and Morley, J.E., Use of a vacuum tumescence device in the management of impotence, *J. Am. Geriatr. Soc.* 38, 217, 1990.
127. Michal, V., Kramar, R, Pospichal, J. and Hejhal, L., Direct arterial anastomosis on corpora cavernosa penis in the therapy of erectile impotence, *Rozhl. Chir.*, 52, 587, 1973.
128. Behre, H.M., Bohmeyer, J. and Nieschlag, E., Prostate volume in testosterone-treated and untreated hypogonadal men in comparison to age-matched normal controls, *Clin. Endocrinol.*, 40, 341, 1994.
129. Matsumoto, A.M., Sandblom, R.E., Schoene, R.B., Lee, K.A., Giblin, E.C., Pierson, D.J. and Bremner, W.J., Testosterone replacement in hypogonadal men: effects on obstructive sleep apnoea, respiratory drives and sleep, *Clin. Endocrinol.*, 22, 713, 1985.

PART III

PATHOLOGY
AND HORMONAL ACTION
IN THE AGED

10

Pancreatic Regulation of Nutrient Metabolism

Wilbur B. Quay

CONTENTS

I. INTRODUCTION

Human nutritional needs change with aging and have a major impact on health (Chapter 12). The factors responsible for these changes are complex and involve the intervention of various physiologic processes in the pathways of metabolism of nutrients. Hormones have a major role

TABLE 10-1 **Prevalence of Diabetes Mellitus in the U.S. (Per 1000 Individuals in the Population)**

Age group (years)	<17	17-44	45-64	>65	All ages
Males	1.2	8.1	47.9	77.9	20.1
Females	0.9	10.7	52.4	86.6	25.4
Both sexes	1.1	9.4	50.3	83.0	22.9

Note: Self-reported diabetes during U. S. Health Interview Survey.

From Bennett, P. H., *Diabetes Mellitus,* Vol. V, Robert J. Brady Co./Am. Diabetes Assoc., Bowie, MD, 1981, with permission.

in the regulation of these metabolic pathways, and hormonal aberrations that occur with aging underlie many of the age-related changes in the elderly.

Hormones of the endocrine pancreas (the islets of Langerhans) are of importance in this regard, particularly insulin; insufficient insulin secretion, or insensitivity of target tissue to the hormone, leads to clinical manifestations of diabetes mellitus (sugar diabetes) which reflect altered metabolism of carbohydrate, fat, and protein. Currently, there are no cures for diabetes, only palliative measures, and the high incidence and cost of this disease (to the victims and society, in terms of suffering and money) are of great concern (Tables 10-1 and 10-2).

Various other chemical mediators (Chapter 6) intervene in the regulation of nutrient metabolism including neurotransmitters and pancreatic islet hormones other than insulin; some of these modulate the secretion of insulin and some participate more directly in the complex network of neuroendocrine metabolic mechanisms. Because of difficulties in conducting long-term controlled studies and interpreting the resulting data, there is uncertainty about whether the detrimental metabolic changes are due to specific disease states or are inherent in the aging process.

II. PANCREATIC ISLETS AND THEIR HORMONES

Hormones of the pancreatic islets have a central role in the regulation of nutrient metabolism. The human pancreas contains approximately one million islets of Langerhans, each about 0.2 mm in diameter, scattered through the exocrine portion of the gland. Each islet consists of anastomosing cords of endocrine cells separated from surrounding exocrine tissue by connective tissue. Each islet is supplied with a network of afferent blood capillaries and drained by efferent capillaries which then comprise some of the blood supply to the exocrine pancreas.

TABLE 10-2 **Diabetes Mellitus in the U.S. in 1987: Impacts and Estimated Costs**

Total patients with diabetes:		6,510,000
Newly diagnosed diabetics:		564,868
Deaths caused by diabetes:		40,078
Monetary costs:		
Direct:	Hospitals and nursing homes:	$7,871,400,000
	Outpatient:	$1,727,800,000
Indirect:	Short-term morbidity:	$ 141,900,000
	Long-term disability:	$3,143,200,000
	Mortality:	$7,488,800,000
Total:		$20,373,100,000

Note: From a study by the Center for Economic Studies in Medicine (a division of Pracon, Inc.), published by the American Diabetes Association (also in *Diabetes Spectrum,* 2(1), 54, 1989. With permission.

TABLE 10-3 The Major Pancreatic Hormones

| Hormone | Chemical nature | Pancreatic cell of origin | | |
		Name(s) of cell	%	Total weight per adult pancreas (mg)
Insulin	Two polypeptide chains (A&B) connected by disulfide bridges; 51 amino acids; MW = 5733	B (β, beta, insulin)	10–80	761–1097
Glucagon	Single polypeptide chain; 29 amino acids, MW = 3485	A (α, alpha, A_2, glucagon)	15–40	185–355
Somatostatin	Two related peptides; 14, 28 amino acids, respectively; 14, MW = 1368; 28, MW = 3149	D (δ, delta, A_1, somatostatin)	6–20	83–187

Note: Based chiefly on data reviewed in References 179 and 206.

This angioarchitecture provides a pathway for islet cell hormones to participate in the regulation of pancreatic acinar (exocrine) tissue. Islets contain four major types of secretory cells as follows:

- A-cells secrete glucagon;
- B-cells secrete insulin;
- D-cells secrete somatostatin; and
- PP-cells secrete pancreatic polypeptide.

In each islet, the B-cells usually have a central location, and the other cell types a more peripheral distribution. The cellular disposition is heterogeneous as a function of position in the pancreas.

Characteristics and frequency of occurrence of the various cells of the islets and their hormones (insulin, glucagon, somatostatin) are listed in Table 10-3. The physiology of the 36-amino-acid pancreatic polypeptide is not well understood but includes inhibitory effects on the secretory activity of the exocrine and endocrine pancreas and on gastrointestinal motility.

Each cell type secretes its own hormone to the blood capillaries, but also to islet extracellular space where each probably has direct access to the various other islet cell types and can mediate and influence secretory activity of the others (paracrine effects) (Figure 10-1). Somatostatin is the chief inhibitory paracrine mediator of the islets and locally inhibits both insulin and glucagon release.[1] Some islet mediators, for example 5-HT (5-hydroxytryptamine, serotonin) in B-cells, contribute to intracellular regulatory mechanisms for hormone synthesis and release; they therefore participate in autocrine type mediation.

A. Aging Changes in Islet Cells

Changes with age in mammalian islet cells have been most studied in laboratory rats. Islets in old rats are larger than in younger rats, and contain more B-cells and more insulin per B-cell, an observation that may be interpreted as compensatory growth.[2] However, in a study comparing 11-week- and 12-month-old rats, although total islet cell mass increased with age, maximum glucose-stimulated insulin secretion decreased with age in both males and females when expressed in terms of unit weight of islet tissue. At either end of the age range, although female as compared with male rats had less islet tissue, the former secreted more insulin per unit amount of islet tissue.[3]

Aging rats show decrements in both exocrine[4] and endocrine pancreatic function. B-cells in older age often have a relative insensitivity to glucose[5] including reduced glucose-induced (either maximal or submaximal glucose) margination of secretion vesicles at B-cell plasma membranes and a smaller insulin secretory response.[6]

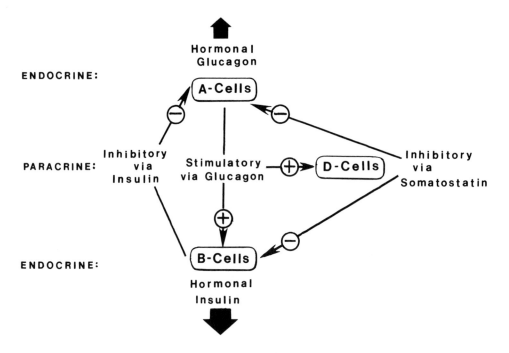

FIGURE 10-1 Paracrine interactions of major islet cells and their humoral (endocrine + paracrine) secretory products.

Humans show a similar age-related decrement in pancreatic endocrine function. The inability of aging B-cells to respond normally to a glucose stimulus represents an intrinsic loss of an adaptive mechanism.[7] Also, the enteric hormonal enhancement of glucose-stimulated insulin release, which remains unchanged in either obesity or non-treated diabetes mellitus (Chapter 6), decreases with age despite the increased blood levels of immunoreactive gastric inhibitory polypeptide (GIP).[8]

B. Regulation of Hormone Output

The well-recognized physiologic regulators of insulin secretion are listed in Table 10-4. These include ingested foodstuffs or their metabolic products, other hormones of the endocrine

TABLE 10-4 Major Endogenous Chemical Signals Regulating Insulin Release by B-Cells

Source	Stimulating	Inhibiting
Nutrition	Glucose	
	Amino acids (leucine, arginine, etc.)	
	Fatty acids	
GI tract	GI peptide hormones (GIP, gastrin, secretin, CCK, VIP [Chap. 6])	
Pancreas	Glucagon	Somatostatin
Autonomic and adreno-medullary systems	Catecholamine, β-adrenergic mediation	Catecholamine, α-Adrenergic mediation
	Acetylcholine, cholinergic mediation	
Local tissue (autocrine and paracine mediation)		5-Hydroxytryptamine (5-HT, serotonin)
		Prostaglandin E

Note: Based in part on References 48,179, and 207.

TABLE 10-5 Major Endogenous Signals Regulating Glucagon Release By A-Cells

Source	Stimulating	Inhibiting
Nutrition	Proteins and amino acids (especially: alanine, serine, glycine, cysteine, and threonine)	Glucose (as in hyperglycemia)
		Free fatty acids
		Ketones
GI tract	CCK and gastrin [Chap. 6]	Secretin [Chap. 6]
Pancreas		Somatostatin and insulin
Autonomic and adreno-medullary systems	Acetylcholine, cholinergic mediation	
(as with hypoglycemia and/or strenuous and/or prolonged physical exercise)	Catecholamines, mostly β-adrenergic mechanisms	Catecholamines (mostly α-Adrenergic mechanisms)

pancreas, hormones of the gastrointestinal mucosa, neurotransmitters, and prostaglandins. Hormones and related factors that inhibit insulin release or augment blood glucose are often designated as "counterregulatory".

In some older persons, insulin secretion stimulated by glucose may be aberrant, defective, or distorted, and often associated with other metabolic and/or hormonal disturbances characteristic of human noninsulin-dependent diabetes (or Type II diabetes mellitus).[9-15] There is extensive evidence that chronic sustained hyperglycemia in the rat has deleterious effects on B-cell function.[16-19] Reversal of the hyperglycemia is followed promptly by recovery of normal insulin-secretory activity.[20,21] The underlying intra-islet molecular mechanism remains obscure, but impaired phosphoinositide hydrolysis may be involved.[22]

Regulation of A-cell secretion of glucagon is summarized in Table 10-5. The response of A- and B-cells to some signals, for example to blood glucose, are essentially opposite, while to others they are similar. It is important, also, to be aware of the actions of various therapeutic agents and of stress-related hormones and factors that can alter the secretory activity of the B-cell and/or insulin-sensitivity of the target cells or in some other way alter blood sugar levels. This is particularly important in the interpretation of regulatory mechanisms in older people, who often follow multiple drug regimens for diverse purposes. Periodic review of the **total** therapeutic program, prescribed and nonprescribed, with or without diabetes, should be required in an evaluation of the metabolic states of such subjects.

C. Aging of Pancreatic Hormone Output

Insulin secretion in the rat generally decreases with age. Although dietary manipulation can change the mass of islet tissue, it does not alter the age-related decline in insulin secretion per B-cell in the perfused pancreas.[23] This defect may involve both biosynthetic and secretory mechanisms. Comparison of the response of insulin biosynthesis and of secretion to a glucose signal in 2-, 4-, 8-, and 12-month-old rats did not indicate an age-related uncoupling of biosynthesis, and secretion.[24] However, there is evidence for differential effects of aging on levels of pre-pro-insulin messenger RNA, proinsulin biosynthesis, and secretion of newly made and preformed insulin in the rat.[25]

Age-associated decreases both in secretion of insulin and in sensitivity of peripheral tissues to the hormone may be partly responsible for the age-associated decrease in cholesterol turnover in the rat.[26] Decreased cholesterol turnover in several animal species including humans has been related to the increasing severity of atherosclerotic lesions and incidence of cardiovascular diseases with aging. However, the decreased insulin secretion in response to glucose and consequent decreased cholesterol turnover may be attributable to indirect effects of other hormonal and mediator systems on the B-cell.

Changes in human insulin dynamics with age are more variable and controversial than those described in laboratory rats.[27-30] The frequent association of human aging with hyperinsulinemia[29] has been noted for some time and has been noted in postprandial, postabsorptive, and fasting subjects.[31,32] Also, the ratio of serum immunoreactive (IR) proinsulin to IR-insulin rises with older age.[33,34] Although the hyperinsulinemia observed in old people (66 ± 4 vs. 30 ± 5 years of age) may result more from increased insulin secretion than from decreased insulin clearance,[35] there was a lower metabolic clearance rate (MCR) of insulin in the elderly (70 ± 2 vs. 35 ± 2 years of age)[36] when low levels of the hormone were infused. MCR was estimated from insulin infusion rate, steady-state insulin levels, and the degree of suppression of plasma C-peptide. In the B-cell, insulin is synthesized in a "pro" form which contains, in addition to the amino acid sequence of insulin, a connecting peptide (C-peptide); conversion of proinsulin to insulin by cleavage of C-peptide from the molecule occurs within the B-cell and both insulin and C-peptide are secreted to the blood. Blood levels of C-peptide can be used as an index of insulin secretion rate in diabetic subjects who receive exogenous insulin.

Age changes in somatostatin (S) levels and in responses of the islet D-cells to stimuli may contribute to modifications in metabolism and utilization of nutrients in older people. The source of circulating S is not only D-cells but also endocrine cells of the GI mucosa (Chapter 6) and synapses in the peripheral neurons.[37] Plasma S levels, and changes in these levels in response to secretory stimuli in the elderly (70 to 90 years) vs. the young (22 to 30 years), indicate an increased basal production of S in the former and less variability in levels throughout the 24-h day and in relation to the timing of meals (Chapter 6).[38]

D. Physiologic Action of Insulin

Insulin is the chief mediator of storage and metabolism of nutrient fuels. Soon after the start of a meal, secreted insulin expedites cellular uptake, utilization, and storage of glucose, fat, and amino acids arriving in the blood from the GI tract. In contrast, lower blood levels of insulin lead to depressed uptake of ingested nutrient fuels, and increased mobilization of previously stored fuels. Within each of the major target tissues, liver, adipose tissue, and muscle, the actions of insulin on the major cellular fuels (carbohydrate, protein, and fat) are both anabolic and anticatabolic (Table 10-6).

In mammalian target cells, insulin stimulates hexose transport and alters the state of seryl phosphorylation and the activities of many enzymes involved in regulating metabolism; insulin also functions as a growth factor and alters gene transcription.[39]

TABLE 10-6 Major Insulin Actions in Metabolically Important Target Tissues

Tissues	Muscle	Adipose tissue	Liver
Increase of:	Uptake of:	Uptake of:	
	Glucose	Glucose	
	K+	K+	
	Amino acids		
	Ketones		
	Synthesis of:	Synthesis of:	Synthesis of:
	Protein on	Fatty acids	Glycogen
	ribosomes	Glycerol phosphate	Lipid
			Protein
		Activity of:	
		Lipoprotein lipase	
Decrease of:	Release of:	Activity of:	
	Gluconeogenic	Hormone-sensitive	Gluconeogenesis
	amino acids	lipase	and glucose output
	Protein breakdown		Cyclic AMP
			Ketogenesis

TABLE 10-7 Target Cell Binding of Insulin and Changes of Insulin
Sensitivity in Some Physiologic and Pathophysiologic States

	Athletic training Growth hormone deficiency Glucocorticoid deficiency Anorexia nervosa	Obesity Growth hormone excess Glucocorticoid excess Type II diabetes
Insulin binding:	↑	↓
Insulin sensitivity:	↑	↓

Although much remains to be discovered about the mechanisms of action of insulin,[40] the initiation of its actions depends, as is the case of other polypeptide hormones, on its binding to specific plasma membrane receptors of the target tissue cells:[41]

- Insulin binding to an extracellular region of the receptor tetrameric glycoprotein (the subunits are linked by disulfide bonds) initiates a signal that is transduced into the target cell, resulting in activation or enhancement of particular enzymatically catalyzed metabolic pathways.
- Endocytotic internalization of the insulin-receptor molecular complex then occurs, followed by lysosomal breakdown (proteolysis) of the hormone.[42]
- The internalized receptor may be recycled to the plasma membrane,[43] completing several such cycles from plasma membrane into cell before it is degraded.[44] This degradation is enhanced by insulin; the receptor half-life is 2 to 3 h in the presence of the hormone and 7 to 10 h in its absence.[45]

The dynamics of insulin receptors have an important role in regulation of insulin action. For example, with hyperinsulinemia (common in obesity), the number of insulin receptors is decreased ("down-regulated"); "up-regulation" occurs following hypoinsulinemia, for example, in starvation. Decreased and increased target cell sensitivity, respectively, would be expected in these circumstances. Some changes in insulin binding and tissue sensitivity to the hormone in various physiologic and pathophysiologic conditions are listed in Table 10-7. In conditions where there is relative insulin resistance, or the converse, relative hypersensitivity, the underlying mechanisms are complex and are not explainable only on the basis of changing numbers of receptors.

Intracellular actions of insulin depend on at least four kinds of postreceptor events which are not fully understood:

- Stimulation of intracellular transport of glucose by glucose transporters which cycle between a cytoplasmic pool and the plasma membrane;[46,47]
- Modification of the activities of a variety of intracellular enzymes, through a cAMP-independent phosphorylation cascade following autophosphorylation of the receptor before or during internalization;
- Synthesis and propagation of cytoplasmic mediators including low molecular weight peptides[48] and/or phospholipids[49,50] which may interact with intracellular enzyme systems, causing them to be phosphorylated or stimulating their dephosphorylation;[51,52]
- Internalization of the receptor-insulin complex allowing access of the hormone to microsomal and nuclear protein synthetic systems.

Actions of insulin involve changes in nutrient uptake, especially of glucose, in some, but not all tissues (Table 10-8), and many of the diverse effects on metabolite synthesis and breakdown or utilization stem from the cellular entry and utilization of glucose in insulin-sensitive tissues (Figure 10-2). Insulin actions can be described as both **anticatabolic** (inhibiting the breakdown, metabolism, or loss of particular nutrient molecules and/or their macromolecular sources), and **anabolic** (stimulating the synthesis of storage forms of nutrients [e.g., glycogen etc.], and of macromolecular forms required by cells for structural and other special purposes).

TABLE 10-8 Glucose Uptake Is Insulin-
             Dependent in Some Tissues But
             Not in Others

Glucose uptake	
Insulin dependent:	Not insulin dependent:
Muscle:	Brain (most of)
Skeletal	
Cardiac	Kidney: tubules
Smooth	
Connective tissue:	Intestine: mucosa
Fibroblasts	
Adipose cells	
Vascular system (parts):	Vascular system (part):
Aorta	erythrocytes
Leukocytes	
Glands (some):	
Mammary gland	
Pituitary	
Pancreatic A-cells	

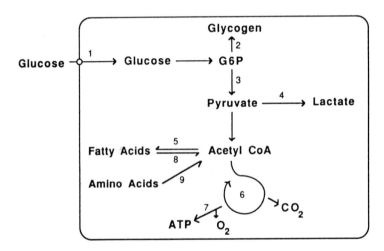

FIGURE 10-2 Metabolic fate of glucose in insulin-sensitive tissues. Glucose, transported into cell (pathway 1), may be metabolized by nonoxidative or oxidative pathways. Nonoxidative metabolism includes glycogen formation (pathway 2), glycolysis and conversion to lactate (pathways 3 and 4), and glycolysis followed by lipogenesis (pathways 3 and 5). Oxidative metabolism occurs when pyruvate formed by glycolysis is converted to acetyl coenzyme A and oxidized via the tricarboxylic acid cycle (pathway 6) and oxidative phosphorylation (pathway 7). Fatty acids (pathway 8) and amino acids (pathway 9) are oxidized in a similar manner. (From Thorburn, A. W., Gunbiner, B., Brechtel, G., and Henry, R. R., *Diabetes,* 39, 22, 1990, with permission.)

E.   Physiologic Action of Glucagon

In contrast to insulin, the secretion of glucagon in normal human beings does not vary greatly during the course of a day or with the ingestion of meals of mixed or normal composition. Physiologic increases in levels of blood glucagon, due to stimuli noted in Table 10-5, augment hepatic glycogenolysis and gluconeogenesis and cause an increase in blood glucose; glucagon is also lipolytic. Thus, glucagon is a hormone of energy mobilization and release. Because insulin and glucagon have largely opposite metabolic effects, the molar ratio of their blood levels closely correlates with relative nutrient storage vs. mobilization (Table 10-9).

TABLE 10-9 Relation of Blood Insulin/Glucagon Molar Ratio (I/G) to Relative Storage
(Glucose Available) and Production-Release (Glucose Needed) of Liver Glucose

Glucose available			Glucose needed		
Through:	I/G Ratio	Relative glucose[a] storage resulting	Through:	I/G Ratio	Relative glucose[a] production — release resulting
Large ingestion of carbohydrate	70	4	Starvation	0.4	4
Glucose i.v. administration	25	2	Low carbohydrate diet or meal	1.8	2
Small meal, mixed composition	7	1	Fasting overnight	2.3	1

Note: Modified from Reference 169.

[a] On an increasing scale of 1 to 4.

III. GLUCOSE TOLERANCE AND TARGET CELL MECHANISMS

A. Glucose Tolerance Decrease With Aging

Glucose intolerance, the inability of a subject to lower blood glucose after ingestion of a standard acute dosage of glucose, has served to diagnose diabetes mellitus. Glucose tolerance is assessed by determination of glucose levels at given times after a usually oral glucose challenge (Table 10-10 and Figure 10-3, top panel). The results of such "oral glucose tolerance tests" (OGTT) are interpreted arbitrarily in relation to glucose levels at stated times after the glucose challenge and lead to arbitrary diagnosis of impaired glucose tolerance (IGT) and diabetes, as illustrated by the differences (shown in Table 10-11) between data of WHO (World Health Organization) and of NDDG (National Diabetes Data Group). Those with IGT (undiagnosed diabetics in this example), and in older age groups, are fewer by NDDG than by WHO criteria. Of the 191 subjects who were judged diabetic by WHO criteria, 11 did not

TABLE 10-10 Age-Related Changes in Plasma Glucose
Concentrations of Subjects Without Medical
History of Diabetes

Age range (years)	20–44	45–64	65–74
mg/dl (mean ± SE)			
Both sexes:			
Fasting:[a]	89.5 ± 0.3	96.8 ± 0.8	97.9 ± 0.7
Oral glucose:[b]			
1 hour	130.3 ± 1.1	160.9 ± 1.9	170.0 ± 1.9
2 hours	100.2 ± 0.8	119.1 ± 1.9	133.3 ± 1.9
Men:			
Fasting:	92.3 ± 0.3	97.9 ± 0.7	99.5 ± 1.0
Oral glucose:			
1 hour	136.1 ± 1.7	168.6 ± 2.3	177.4 ± 3.0
2 hours	97.8 ± 1.2	116.4 ± 2.3	133.6 ± 3.2
Women:			
Fasting:	87.3 ± 0.5	95.9 ± 1.2	96.7 ± 0.8
Oral glucose:			
1 hour	125.4 ± 1.5	154.1 ± 2.8	164.1 ± 2.4
2 hours	102.3 ± 1.1	121.5 ± 2.6	133.1 ± 2.4

[a] Overnight fast of 10 to 16 hours.

[b] Hours after a 75 mg oral glucose challenge.

Note: Extracted from data of Reference 54.

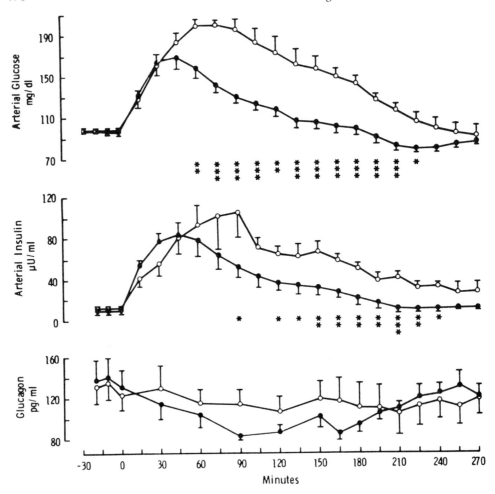

FIGURE 10-3 Responses to oral glucose loading in young (•) and elderly (o) subjects. Asterisks (*) indicate
significance of difference between matched points in the two curves: *$p < 0.05$, **$p < 0.01$, ***p
< 0.001. From Jackson, R. A., Roshania, R. D., Hawa, M. J., Sim, B. M., DiSilvio, L., and Jaspan,
J. B., *Diabetes*, 37, 119, 1988, with permission.)

satisfy the NDDG specification that the midtest blood glucose level be equal to or greater
than 200 mg/dl. Only about one-fourth of the undiagnosed would be judged diabetic
according to the criterion of elevated fasting blood glucose (i.e., = or >140 mg/dl), while
the diabetes diagnosis of the remainder had to be based upon posttest glucose levels of 200
mg/dl or more.[53]

Diagnosis of diabetes mellitus is also made on other criteria including such classic signs
as polyuria, polydipsia, and polyphagia. Several studies in diverse U.S. communities indicate
that the ratio of undiagnosed diabetes to physician-diagnosed diabetes is approximately 1:1.
Thus, not only is there a large reservoir of undiagnosed diabetics in the U.S.,[54] but the
transition for many, especially Type II or NIDDM (noninsulin-dependent) diabetics, from
marginally positive OGTTs to frank or overt diabetes is often wavering and drawn out over
time. This situation, then, is represented by many individuals at any one time.

The hyperglycemia associated with a decreased ability to lower heightened blood glucose
levels can lead to insidious long-term pathophysiologic changes in many tissues. Deterioration
in glucose homeostasis is not an inevitable consequence of aging in all mammalian species,
for example, laboratory mice (*Mus musculus*).[55] Nevertheless, plasma glucose levels and the
incidence of impaired glucose tolerance generally increase with human aging (Tables 10-10

TABLE 10-11   Age-Related Increase of Impaired Glucose Tolerance (IGT) in U.S. Citizens

Age range (years)	20–44	45–54	55–64	65–74
Percent of population (mean ± SE)				
By WHO criteria:				
All races:				
Both sexes:	6.4 ± 0.59	14.8 ± 1.48	15.1 ± 1.23	22.8 ± 1.70
White:				
Men:	4.6 ± 0.72	12.6 ± 2.25	17.2 ± 1.79	22.8 ± 2.04
Women:	6.5 ± 1.05	14.5 ± 2.38	13.7 ± 2.04	23.0 ± 2.55
Black:				
Men:	4.7 ± 1.80	18.8 ± 3.90	18.6 ± 6.02	22.6 ± 8.62
Women:	14.2 ± 2.98	15.8 ± 8.05	12.2 ± 1.94	8.2 ± 4.94
By NDDG criteria:				
All races:				
Both sexes:	2.1 ± 0.39	7.0 ± 0.93	7.4 ± 0.91	9.2 ± 0.85
White:				
Men:	1.0 ± 0.34	6.3 ± 1.79	10.1 ± 1.48	9.0 ± 1.55
Women:	2.8 ± 0.73	6.2 ± 1.15	5.5 ± 1.43	9.9 ± 1.20
Black:				
Men:	1.4 ± 1.30	18.3 ± 3.90	7.0 ± 4.78	5.4 ± 3.80
Women:	1.1 ± 1.11	5.1 ± 4.86	3.1 ± 2.07	1.9 ± 2.22

Note: Extracted from data of Reference 54.

and 10-11). This is especially true in many affluent Western societies and includes subjects with and without medical histories of diabetes mellitus.[29,56-59]

Impairment of glucose tolerance with human aging was first recognized 70 years ago by Spence[60] and confirmed repeatedly since. This decline in glucose tolerance measured after a glucose challenge usually begins during the third decade of life and continues throughout adulthood (Figure 10-3, top panel).[27,29,61] Although most investigators have failed to demonstrate a significant change in fasting blood glucose with aging (for references see Jackson[59]), a rise of about 1 to 2 mg/dl per decade of life has been found by several others.[54,62-64] In contrast, venous blood glucose, measured 1 or 2 h after glucose loading, increases about 6 to 13 mg/dl per decade of life[59] in women at all ages; the reported values are about 10 mg/dl higher than in men.[27,59,61,65] In another study, the blood glucose levels 1 h after a glucose load were significantly higher in men than in women (Table 10-10).

B.   Diverse Aging Changes: Causative of Glucose Intolerance?

A wealth of experimental data support the idea that old age defects in glucose metabolism are both intrinsic and specific to the aging process, and are not merely reflections or metabolic concomitants of obesity and/or noninsulin-dependent diabetes (NIDDM).[59] This is illustrated by a comparison of the metabolic characteristics of these three conditions (aging, obesity, and NIDDM) (Table 10-12).

Age-associated glucose intolerance has a multifactorial pathogenesis in humans. Although such factors as impaired glucose-induced insulin secretion and impaired insulin-mediated suppression of hepatic glucose output (HGO) are sometimes evident, the major defect appears to be a lowered insulin-mediated glucose uptake by target cells. This is especially true of skeletal muscle, and the most important cause appears to be faulty postreceptor mechanisms.[56,57,66-71]

Before discussing the changes of specific insulin-target cell mechanisms that occur with aging, it is necessary to consider the factors that are concerned in the complex glucose regulatory system, their changes in older age, and the possible extent to which they might contribute to the observed impairment of glucose tolerance during aging:

TABLE 10-12   Comparative Differences in Metabolic Characteristics
of Three Conditions Often or Generally Associated
With Defects in Glucose Metabolism

Metabolic parameter	Aging	Obesity	NIDDM
Glucose:			
Basal level	NCC	NCC	NCC or ↑
Tolerance	↓	NCC	↓↓↓
Insulin:			
Basal level	NCC	↑	NCC
With glucose loading:			
Initial response	Delayed	↑	Delayed
Later response	↑	↑↑↑	Variable
Feedback inhibition of secretion	↓	↓	↓
B-cell sensitivity to GIP	↓	NCC	NCC
Probable site of defect:			
Number of insulin receptors	NCC	↓	↓
In postreceptor component(s)	Yes	? to yes	Yes
Lipids:			
Triglyceride	NCC	↑	↑
Free fatty acids (FFA):			
Basal levels	↑	↑	↑
Basal lipid oxidation	↓	↑	↑
Basal glucose oxidation	↓	↓	↓
Respiratory quotient (RQ)	NCC	↓	↓

Note: ↑ = increase; ↓ = decrease; multiple arrows = much greater such response; NCC=
no consistent change

Modified from Reference 59.

- *Delayed and/or impaired glucose absorption from the aged gut* is reported in most[72-75] but not all[75-77] studies and is consistent with the observed delay in posthepatic glucose output following oral glucose[78] and the slowed systemic appearance of ingested glucose in the elderly.[69] Although these changes in handling of glucose by the gut should improve glucose tolerance,[59] tolerance to intravenously administered glucose is decreased in the elderly.[29]

- In the older human, although the circulating *levels of insulin after glucose ingestion equal or exceed those in younger individuals,*[61,69] glucose tolerance is not improved. In addition, impaired insulin secretion in the absence of increased target tissue resistance to insulin does not account for the age-associated glucose intolerance.[59]

- *Age reduction of the body's muscle mass,* a major compartment for uptake, storage, and metabolism of a carbohydrate load, does not account for the impaired glucose tolerance of aging. Lean body mass decreases with age about 11 to 13% expressed in relation to body weight. In terms of skeletal muscle mass, this reflects a decrement of about 30% from the third to seventh decades, and of 40 to 45% by the end of the eighth decade.[79] However, sex and age differences in muscle mass do not follow the age-based pattern of lowered glucose tolerance. That is, healthy 70- to 79-year-old men have a greater average muscle mass than healthy women in their third decade.[79] Furthermore, only slight changes occur in the glucose tolerance of nonobese patients with problems (e.g., neuromuscular) leading to a 29 to 36% reduction in muscle when compared with that of the elderly with similar disease.[25,80] Finally, elderly subjects may have marked impairment of glucose tolerance despite no significant decrease in lean body mass.[68]

- *Increased adiposity with aging* is a common feature in many of our Western cultures or populations. Although impaired glucose tolerance is usually associated with such adiposity, it is unlikely that the impaired glucose tolerance in the elderly results from obesity[59] because fasting hyperinsulinemia, characteristic of obesity, is generally absent in **healthy** elderly humans (Table 10-12).[61,69] Even after glucose ingestion, blood insulin levels are not as high as those found in the obese, and most current studies on age-associated changes in glucose metabolism now are with nonobese subjects.[29,57,61,67-69,71]

- *Immobilization or greatly diminished physical activity* may decrease glucose tolerance and insulin resistance/sensitivity in both animals and humans.[29,81-84] Physical training induces a rise in insulin-mediated glucose uptake in both young and old men.[85,86] In physically trained subjects, basal and glucose-stimulated insulin levels are much reduced yet glucose tolerance is unaltered, suggesting increased sensitivity of tissues.[59] *Physical inactivity* can not fully account for the glucose intolerance of aging.[59] Closely coordinated reciprocal changes in B-cell sensitivity to glucose (for insulin output) and target cell sensitivity to insulin (for uptake of glucose) should operate in tandem to maintain normal glucose tolerance even during great changes in physical activity. Metabolic changes associated with physical inactivity and with aging appear unrelated.[59] This follows in part from the fact that aging-related decrements in sensitivity of target tissue to insulin are accompanied by decreases in sensitivity of the B-cell to glucose. Moreover, mechanisms of exercise-induced and of insulin-mediated augmentation of glucose uptake by muscle are different, though they may interact synergistically. Insulin action, not *adaptation to exercise*, becomes defective during aging. In fact, exercise adaptation is relatively preserved in the old, and to some extent can counteract the age-related decline in insulin action.[87] In recent studies, major differences in levels of physical activity of the test subjects have been avoided; young subjects were selected who had sedentary occupations, the old were fully ambulatory, and athletes were not included.[59,61,67,69,71,88]

- *Increase in fasting plasma free fatty acid (FFA) concentrations with older age* has usually, but not always, been noted.[61,89-91] As proposed more than 25 years ago, increased plasma FFA levels in some diabetics are causally related to lowered insulin sensitivity of target cells.[92,93] This idea was based in part upon the demonstration that when FFA levels were high there was inhibition of glucose phosphorylation, glycolysis, and glucose oxidation.[93] Evidence indicates that, after acutely increased FFA concentrations, glucose tolerance declines due to inhibition of the oxidation and storage of glucose.[94] Aged-related increases in fasting FFA levels would lead to glucose intolerance in the elderly and lowered FFA levels may improve glucose tolerance.[95]

- *Diets high in carbohydrate may prevent or reverse insulin resistance and the islet defect related to aging.*[62,96,97] Nevertheless, it is likely that high FFA levels merely denote a new metabolic steady state in the older person's regulation of FFA metabolism[59] and do not have a significant role in the etiology of aging-associated glucose intolerance.

- *Insulin action on skeletal muscle in vivo* has been correlated with both the density of *capillary blood supply* and the relative proportions of *muscle fibers* of different types;[98] the capillary to muscle fiber diffusion distance could modify, and be inversely related to, the level of insulin action. However, there are uncertainties and contradictions about several aspects of these studies, and about the probability of a relationship between such changes in skeletal muscle and insulin sensitivity.[59,99]

C. Insulin Sensitivity: Decrease With Aging

Recent research, in the main, supports the concept of lowered sensitivity or responsiveness to insulin in older people. With advancing older age, humans given insulin intravenously show a less rapid but more prolonged fall in blood sugar.[100] However, in relatively early studies, older subjects were apparently not always controlled for chronic drug intakes that could have had metabolic side effects. Moreover, the older available subjects were usually chronically bedridden and had metabolic abnormalities due to inactivity.[101]

Some earlier studies, however, did not report a decrease in the sensitivity to the hormone in the elderly. Part of this variance may arise from differences in times after glucose loading when the measurements were made (Table 10-12).[102-104] There are instances in which glucose intolerance is apparently accompanied by normal peripheral tissue insulin sensitivity (PTIS)

TABLE 10-13   Interrelation of Insulin Sensitivity (S_I) and Glucose Effectiveness (S_G) in Different Subjects, Ages, and Metabolic Conditions

Subject sample and condition	S_I	S_G
White men (young non-Hispanics)	7.56 ± 1.13	0.026 ± 0.008
Healthy women	5.61 ± 0.51	0.023 ± 0.002
Postpartum/pregnant	4.63 ± 0.44	0.023 ± 0.002
Aged with high carbohydrate diet	4.40 ± 1.30	0.027 ± 0.004
Mexican Americans	4.06 ± 0.72	0.022 ± 0.002
Aged with *ad libitum* diet	2.40 ± 0.70	0.026 ± 0.003
Obese and nondiabetic	2.30 ± 0.16	0.024 ± 0.003
Women on oral contraceptives	2.40 ± 0.36	0.018 ± 0.004
Noninsulin-dependent diabetics	0.61 ± 0.16	0.014 ± 0.002

Note: $S_I = \times\ 10^{-4} \cdot min^{-1} \cdot \mu U^{-1} \cdot ml$; $S_G = \times\ min^{-1}$
Adapted from Reference 89.

in healthy older (65- to 85- vs. 20- to 30-year-old) subjects; this perhaps reflects a greater importance than previously recognized of such factors as hepatic uptake of glucose and hepatic-peripheral tissue interaction.[105]

Quantitative analysis of relative glucose tolerance has led to models in which insulin sensitivity (SI) of target tissues and glucose effectiveness (or sensitivity) (SG) in stimulating insulin secretion are major components. Their interrelations in different human populations and at different ages are illustrated in Table 10-13. The range in insulin sensitivity differs by a factor greater than 10, while that of SG by a factor of about 2. These two parameters have been studied recently in relation to a "minimal model" of the system — essentially a mathematical representation of insulin action *in vivo*.[89] The basic procedure is to administer glucose and then analyze resultant plasma glucose and insulin concentrations. Instead of the popular OGTT (oral glucose tolerance test), a FSIGT (frequently sampled intravenous glucose tolerance test) is employed, avoiding the uncertainty in the assay due to the highly variable rates of glucose absorption from the gastrointestinal tract.[106,107] The "minimum model" depends upon three generally accepted assumptions:[89]

1. Glucose inhibits its own production and increases its utilization in proportion to its concentration in plasma;[108-110]
2. Insulin synergizes these glucose effects; and
3. Insulin's lowering of plasma glucose levels depends upon insulin concentration in a compartment separate from that of plasma.[111,112]

Insulin-sensitive tissue appears to be responding to a signal equivalent to insulin concentration of lymph; this is generally taken to be essentially the same as the concentration of insulin in the interstitial (extracellular) fluid within the target tissues.[89] Insulin sensitivity usually has been estimated from results with a so-called "euglycemic clamp" procedure.[88,113] However, important advantages accrue from the "minimum model" procedure based upon FSIGT.[89] A computer program based on the latter can be utilized to estimate both insulin sensitivity and SG from the dynamic interrelations of plasma insulin and the time course of plasma glucose levels. SG in these studies represents the fractional glucose turnover at basal insulin levels. Thus, in man, 2.1% of the body's extracellular glucose pool will disappear per minute, and this percentage will remain constant with increased plasma glucose so long as no increase in plasma insulin concentration occurs.[89] Despite the above relationships profound genetically and/or environmentally derived changes in SI may occur in the absence of concurrent defects or changes in SG (Table 10-13).[89]

D. Glucagon-Target Cell Mechanisms: Age Changes

The postabsorptive serum level of glucagon is not significantly influenced by older age (Figure 10-3, bottom panel), nor is the secretion of glucagon in response to intravenously administered arginine.[31] However, age differences have been observed in the target cell response to glucagon. Subcutaneous adipose tissue from 20- to 30-year-old humans responds to glucagon *in vitro* by an increased release of glycerol and a decreased release of FFAs; in comparison, there is no increased release of glycerol from adipose tissue from 50- to 70-year-old subjects when glucagon is added *in vitro*, but there is increased release of FFAs.[114] Additional observations support the occasional occurrence of age changes in the glucagon axis. Overall, the progressive impairment in the disposal of a glucose load in older people appears more likely to be due to aberrations in the B-cell insulin target cell axis than in the glucagon system.

E. Insulin-Target Cell Mechanisms: Age Changes

Glucose intolerance associated with human aging has been attributed by some investigators primarily to impaired peripheral tissue utilization of glucose, which can be viewed as due to impaired insulin-mediated glucose uptake.[59,69,78] Investigators in one study (elderly 73- to 80- vs. young adult men 20- to 23-years-old) concluded that age-related glucose intolerance:

1. Develops despite slowed GI absorption of glucose;
2. Is characterized by delays in:
   a. The initial rise in arterial insulin levels after an oral glucose load (Figure 10-3, middle panel),
   b. The suppression of hepatic glucose output (HG0), and
   c. The rise in peripheral glucose uptake, but
3. Results chiefly from impaired peripheral tissue utilization of glucose.

Whereas the last of these hypotheses indicates a net increased insulin resistance by target tissues, the delayed fall in HG0 may result mainly from delayed insulin secretion.[69]

In other studies, normal aging in (65- to 83- vs. 24- to 39-year-old) human males is associated with delayed but overall equivalent posthepatic delivery of oral glucose (Figure 10-4). This is consistent with the greater effect of age on the 2-h glucose levels rather than the early postprandial, or postglucose-challenge levels of the sugar (Figure 10-3, top panel). Such data also support the primary role of impaired peripheral utilization of glucose in the intolerance of aging.[78]

The cellular actions of insulin are mediated by a variety of reactions that include the intervention of second messengers after insulin binding to its receptors.[39,48,59,115,116] In this sense, one speaks of receptor (plasma membrane) and postreceptor (intracellular) mechanisms.

Although both decreased[117,118] and increased insulin binding[119] with aging have been reported, most investigators have not found an age-related change in insulin binding.[57,61,71,120-122] In an *in vitro* study, the amount of insulin bound by human fibroblasts increased during either normal or precocious aging.[119] In a study of human adipose cells, there was a decrease in insulin sensitivity and responsiveness and in the number of insulin receptors (Table 10-14).[117]

It is unknown to what extent the age changes are attributable to age-related changes in the insulin receptor. Insulin receptors are heterogeneous and their subunits can be glycosylated either through internal (biosynthetic) or external (exogenous) labeling.[44] Other hormones can participate in age modification of insulin receptors and their mechanisms. For example, glucocorticoids can participate in the regulation of insulin receptor messenger RNA (mRNA) levels.[123]

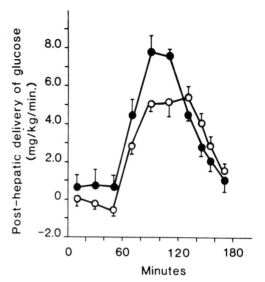

FIGURE 10-4 Time course of posthepatic delivery or oral glucose (PHDG) in younger (•) and older (o) men. The delay in PHDG of older men during the 60- to 180-minute period was significant (*p* <0.0001 by analysis of variance). (From Tonino, R. P., Miniker, K. L., and Rowe, J. W., *Diabetes Care,* 12, 394, 1989, with permission.)

TABLE 10-14   Differences in Insulin Actions (*In Vitro*) on Human Subcutaneous Adipose Cells as a Function of Age

Age - mean years: (range)	23 (23–24)	38 (30–46)	57 (51–59)
Receptor number $\times$ 10^{-3}	647 ± 62	396 ± 76	232 ± 42
Insulin concentration (μU/ml) required for half max. (ED_{50}):			
Stimulation of glucose oxidation:	5	165	1500
Inhibition of lipolysis	0.3	6.5	45
Insulin responsiveness:	1.20 ± 0.34	0.77 ± 0.22	0.17 ± 0.06

Note: Receptor number = sites [mean ± SEM] / cell × 10^3 (see Figure 10-2). Glucose oxidation, using ($U^{14}C$)-glucose and measuring ^{14}C-glucose output (see Figure 10-3). Lipolysis based on glycerol release. Insulin responsiveness = $mM^{14}CO_2$ [mean ± SEM] produced/ 10^7 cells/2 h.

Modified from References 117 and 208.

Alterations in the postreceptor steps in the intracellular action of insulin are currently being examined as possible sources of age-related defects in glucose metabolism and tolerance.[59] Rat adipose cells show modification in receptor kinase activity with aging.[124] In rat liver, the age defect may be distal to the insulin receptor tyrosine kinase.[125] The intrinsic tyrosine-specific kinase activity of the insulin receptor has been implicated in the induction of diverse biological responses to insulin, including stimulation of glucose uptake, glycogen synthesis, ribosomal protein S6 phosphorylation, thymidine synthesis, and receptor internalization.[39,126] The kinase activity (with respect to some substrates) of purified preparations of insulin receptors can be increased as much as 250-fold by other proteins.[127] This suggests that the possibility of aging-related protein modulation of receptor kinase activities merits study.

1.   Three Intracellular Dynamic Molecular Systems

Three intracellular responses to insulin, distal to the binding of the hormone to its plasma membrane receptor, are now being considered causes of aging deficits. They include:

1. *The internalization, processing, and recycling of the insulin receptor complex.*[128,129] The presence of this complex in the target cell would increase glucose transport into the cell. Thus,

glucose transport is decreased by drugs that inhibit intracellular processing of the insulin-receptor complex.[129] Insulin-mediated recruitment of glucose transporters within the target cells appears to depend on internalization of the insulin-receptor complex. Insulin-receptor recycling has been reported defective in adipose cells of older rats. In this regard, an age-associated abnormality in intracellular processing of insulin and its receptor may inhibit the initiation of intracellular actions of insulin (such as translocation of glucose transporters from the cytoplasm to the plasma membrane), and the recycling of the insulin receptors back to the cell surface for the renewed binding of extracellular hormone.[104]

2. *The glucose-transport system in human adipose cells undergoes age changes;*[68] the maximum glucose uptake capacity of the target cells declines 34% with aging, but affinity of the uptake system for glucose remains unaltered. This may be interpreted to mean that the number of glucose transport units per target cell declines in the aged, but that each remaining unit functions normally. These observations are consistent with the concept that the insulin-stimulated increase in the maximum velocity (Vmax) of glucose transport is mediated by the translocation of glucose transporters from the intracellular low-density microsomal (LDM) compartment to the vicinity of the plasma membrane.[47,59,130] Thus, either depletion of the number of glucose transporters in their LDM pool, or defective insulin-stimulated recruitment and translocation from this pool to the plasma membrane, could lead to a compromised Vmax. The cause of insulin resistance in old obese rats might conceivably stem from changes of one or both of these phenomena.[131] It seems likely that a major defect early in the glucose intracellular pathway, such as in the transport system, is the problem in aging rather than multiple defects along distal glucose metabolic pathways. Adipocytes from elderly humans and rats show decreased glucose metabolism with respect to diverse pathways (e.g., oxidation, lactate production, triglyceride synthesis) without change in the proportion represented by each of them.[117,132] Insulin increases glucose-transporter mRNA and stimulates synthesis of glucose transporters in cultured human fibroblasts.[133] These effects should be examined with respect to aging changes.

3. *Activities along some intracellular enzymatic pathways distal to the glucose transporter systems are decreased with aging* (e.g., hexokinase type II and phosphofructokinase in human adipocytes;[134] hexokinase in rat adipocytes;[135] hexokinase[136] and glycogen synthetase[137] in rat muscle).

If we take a broader perspective with regard to reductions and defective metabolic adaptations in each of insulin's chief target tissues in the aged, we find reductions along carbohydrate, lipid, and protein pathways.[138-145] Since increased insulin administration can apparently overcome these defects, insulin resistance in target cells can be suggested as a major component in, and the basis for, the adaptational metabolic problems in the aged.[59]

IV. SECONDARY MEDIATORS AND COUNTER-REGULATION

A. Secondary Mediators and Factors

A diverse group of mediators, less important than insulin and glucagon, contribute to regulation of nutrient metabolism. Some of these change in level and/or in significance in older age. Two subgroups of these can be noted;

- Hormones that have counterregulatory roles with respect to insulin's glucoregulation and which will be considered as a group (see Section C) and,
- A disparate and miscellaneous group, that will be characterized briefly in the present subsection.

Hormones from the diffuse endocrine system of the gastrointestinal tract (Chapter 6), generally peptide in nature, constitute a major part in this subsection. With the probable exception of gut-derived glucagon, the actions of these hormones on nutrient metabolism are not counterregulatory and their physiologic significance are poorly understood. The concentrations of some of them change with aging, in fasting, and during oral glucose tolerance tests (Chapter 11).[146]

This subsection also includes tissue humors or nonendocrine local intercellular mediators whose roles in regulation of nutrient metabolism remain to be elucidated. Endogenous prostaglandins comprise one chemical family of such mediators. Some of these have a role in eliciting a selective decrease in the counterregulatory glucagon response to hypoglycemia in Type I (IDDM) diabetes.[147]

B. Calcium Ion Relations and Actions

Calcium ion (Ca^{2+}) is an important mediator of insulin's cellular actions.[148-150] Physiologic insulin concentrations augment intracellular Ca^{2+} concentrations,[151,152] and experimental lowering of intracellular calcium with chelating or sequestering agents compromises some of insulin's metabolic actions.[153]

A plasma membrane (Ca^{2+}/Mg^{2+})ATPase, an important regulator of intracellular calcium ion, is regulated, in turn, by insulin.[154-158] The activity of this enzyme in several tissues is altered in streptozytocin-induced diabetic rats, in obese nondiabetic rats,[157,159-162] and in human diabetic subjects.[163] Insulin resistance in noninsulin-dependent diabetics (NIDD) and in obese rats may be due in part to loss of this ATPase activity.[157,160] Lowered insulin resistance in NIDD rats is associated with a restoration of insulin's ability to stimulate the activity of this ATPase.[164]

Insulin-like growth factor II (IGF-II) stimulates fibroblast DNA replication when added to cells pretreated sequentially with platelet-derived and epidermal growth factors; this effect involves the opening of voltage-independent calcium-permeable channels and a consequent increase of IGF-II-mediated calcium entry into target cells.[165]

The above observations, considered with other data, suggest that lowered insulin sensitivity is related to a decrease in intracellular calcium ion. This follows from:

1. Ca^{2+} is a second messenger for insulin;
2. Ca^{2+} serves as an activator of the intracellular glucose transport system; and
3. The concentration of calmodulin, an intracellular protein mediator of the action of Ca^{2+} in a wide array of cellular processes,[166] decreases in some cells with older age, and in others in age-matched diabetics.[167]

A large number of other factors that influence the levels and actions of calcium ion have not yet been evaluated in aging changes and possible relations in insulin-target cell systems.

C. Counterregulation, Adaptive and Stress-Related

A number of so-called counterregulatory hormones, in addition to glucagon, oppose the hypoglycemic actions of insulin.[168,169] Under normal (nonpathologic) conditions, counterregulatory hormones are elicited for relatively short-term and adaptive purposes (Table 10-15). Circumstances such as stress that require increased mobilization of metabolic fuels provoke increased secretion and blood levels of the counterregulatory hormones (Table 10-15), a dominance of their action over that of insulin, a tendency to hyperglycemia, and in some cases to overt diabetes especially in older persons (see above). In the diabetic subject already hyperglycemic they augment the hyperglycemia, often with life-threatening consequences. Results of chemically poor control of hyperglycemia are insidious, especially as seen most frequently in long undiagnosed, usually Type II, diabetes.

Hypoglycemia, due to high levels of insulin, presents an acute clinical problem because the brain requires adequate uptake of glucose from the blood for its normal function, for consciousness,

TABLE 10-15 Relative Changes in Plasma Concentrations of Insulin and Counterregulatory Hormones in Selected Adaptive and Stress-Associated Conditions

Condition	Counterregulatory hormones			
	Glucagon	Growth hormone	Epinephrine	Cortisol
With Fuel Intake: Insulin ↑ in all: Ingestion of:				
Glucose	↓	↓	NCC	NCC
Protein	↑	↑	NCC	NCC
Mixed meal	NCC	NCC	NCC	NCC
With Marked Fuel Need and/or Stress: Insulin ↓ in all				
Starvation	↑	NCC	↑ / NCC	↓
Acute hypoglycemia	↑	↑	↑	↑
Exercise	↑	↑	↑	↑
Most other stress states, including:	↑	↑ / NCC	↑ (rapid and brief)	↑ (slow and chronic)
Fever (bacterial pyrogen-induced)	↑	↑	↑	↑
Surgical (and/or trauma stress)	↑ / NCC	↑	↑	↑
Myocardial infarction	↑	↑	↑	↑

Note: ↑ = increase; ↓ = decrease; NCC = no consistent change.

Based upon References 179,209, 214.

and for survival. The critical time for recovery after the induced hypoglycemia is an hour or a little longer, depending upon the depth of the fall in blood sugar and the rapidity of effective administration of exogenous glucose.

Marked hypoglycemia is a stress-provoking state which normally stimulates the output of hormones and mobilization of hepatic fuels, especially glucose. However, in many older diabetics, and in some not overtly diabetic seniors, this counterregulatory response to hypoglycemia is impaired. Not only is the ability to raise blood sugar by the counterregulatory hormone system impaired, but also the sensory and other neural response (especially sympathoadrenal) systems can be compromised in varying degrees and ways that diminish the subject's ability to become aware of the life-threatening hypoglycemia unless an appropriately knowledgeable observer or companion is present.

Actions and age-associated changes in individual counterregulatory hormones are included in some of the other chapters: cortisol/glucocorticoids in Chapters 2 and 14, growth hormone (GH) in Chapter 3, and epinephrine in Chapter 4. For example, in man, GH secretion[170] and the response of GH secretion to GHRH[171] may decline progressively with age from the third decade onward.[170] In old rats there is reduction in the pulsatile release of GH,[172] and in CNS-mediated pituitary secretion of GH.[158,173-175] This emphasizes the difficulty of interpreting age changes in the regulatory hormonal systems, for changes with aging can occur both in the insulin and the counterregulatory systems.

V. DIABETES MELLITUS

Studies of the nutrient metabolism of the elderly, especially in Western industrialized societies, are concerned mostly with aberrations in the transport, uptake, and utilization of glucose.

TABLE 10-16   Classification and Characteristics of the Major Types of Diabetes Mellitus (DM)

Type	Characteristics
A.	Primary DM

A. Primary DM
   I.   Type I Insulin dependent DM (IDDM)
        (also = juvenile-onset DM; ketosis-prone DM; unstable or brittle DM)
        Common in youth but can occur at any age.
        Loss of most, if not all, islet B-cells, with corresponding loss of insulin output, and need for insulin replacement therapy.
        Often associated with specific HLA types, predisposing to viral insulitis or autoimmune (islet cell antibody) attack
   II. Type II Non-insulin-dependent DM (NIDDM)
        (also = maturity-onset DM; ketosis-resistant DM)
        More frequent in adults and increasing in older age, but can occur at any age; majority are overweight; may occur in familial aggregates as an autosomal dominant genetic trait.
        Progressive insulin resistance in target tissues common; slow and insidious progression; in older age and/or extreme conditions and/or stress may require insulin therapy in addition to usual dietary and exercise program.
B. Secondary DM (= DM associated with, or following effects of, certain other diseases, syndromes, or problems)
   I.   Pancreatic disease or damage (as due to pancreatectomy [surgical removal, etc.], pancreatic functional insufficiency, hemochromatosis, etc.)
   II. Insulin receptor (peripheral target cells) abnormalities
   III. Hormonal problems. Commonly with excess secretion of counterregulatory hormones (e.g., as in acromegaly, Cushing's syndrome, pheochromocytoma, etc.)
   IV. Drug- or chemical-induced (e.g., following: toxins [alloxan, streptozocin, etc.]; potassium-losing diuretics, some psychoactive drugs, phenytoin, etc.)
   V.   Certain complex genetic syndromes, including ataxia, telangiectasia, Laurence-Moon-Biedl syndrome, myotonic dystrophy, Friedrich's ataxia
C. Gestational Diabetes (GDM) (a usually transient glucose intolerance with onset during pregnancy)

Based in part on References 99, 177–179.

However, this should not obscure the importance of changes that occur in metabolism of lipids and proteins in the aged and in diabetic subjects.

Diabetes mellitus (DM) is a multifaceted, heterogeneous set of diseases. Its human and monetary costs were noted in the introduction and in Tables 10-1 and 10-2. The most prevalent kind of DM in the elderly, noninsulin-dependent diabetes mellitus (NIDDM, or Type II DM) is examined in detail in Chapter 11. Here, we provide only a brief overview of the disease to facilitate understanding of this problem, its terminology, and its current prospects.

A. Multiple Types

Classifications of types of DM differ in their purposes and points of emphasis and are endless if they include related and transitional states. The eclectic classification presented in Table 10-16 is based largely upon several recently published ones, but omits some of the less frequent and less well-defined syndromes.[176-179]

The collective diversity and frequency of the types and subtypes of DM and the increased frequency (to about 90%) of the most common type, Type II, with age, reinforces one central impression — the importance of glucoregulation in normal physiology, in aging and in disease.

B. Diverse Factors and Etiologies

Glucose intolerance, and to some degree its pathologic sequelae in various tissues, are common to DM of different types or subtypes. However, there are varieties of etiologies and

TABLE 10-17   Genetic Syndromes in Which There is Glucose Intolerance or Clinical Diabetes Mellitus

Category of syndrome Syndrome name/description	Suggested inheritance
A. Syndromes associated with pancreatic degeneration	
Hereditary relapsing pancreatitis	AD
Cystic fibrosis	AR
Polyendocrine deficiency disease	AR
Hemochromatosis	AR
B. Hereditary endocrine disorders with glucose intolerance	
Isolated growth hormone deficiency	AR, AD
Hereditary panhypopituitary dwarfism	sporadic, AR, X-linked
Pheochromocytoma	AD
Multiple endocrine adenomatosis	AD
C. Inborn errors of metabolism with glucose intolerance	
Glycogen storage disease type 1	AR
Acute intermittent porphyria	AD
Hyperlipidemias	AR, AD
D. Syndromes with nonketotic, insulin-resistant, early onset DM	
Ataxia telangiectasia	AR
Myotonic dystrophy	AD
Lipoatrophic diabetes syndromes	AR
E. Hereditary neuromuscular disorders with glucose intolerance	
Muscular dystrophy	AD, X-linked
Late onset proximal myopathy	AR
Huntington chorea	AD
Machado disease	AD
Herrmann syndrome	AD
Optic atrophy-diabetes mellitus syndrome	AR
Friedreich's ataxia	AR
Alstrom syndrome	AR
Laurence-Moon-Biedl syndrome	AR
Pseudo-Refsum syndrome	AD
F. Progeroid syndromes with glucose intolerance	
Cockayne syndrome	AR
Werner syndrome	AR
G. Syndromes with glucose intolerance secondary to obesity	
Prader-Willi syndrome	AR, sporadic
Achondroplasia	AD
H. Miscellaneous syndromes with glucose intolerance	
Steroid-induced ocular hypertension	Multifactorial
Mendenhall syndrome	AR
Epiphyseal dysplasia and infantile-onset DM	AR

Notes: Indications of inheritance are often tentative and do not signify that every case is inherited in the designated way. AD = autosomal dominant; AR = autosomal recessive.

Based mainly on Reference 215.

distinctive differences in clinical manifestations depending on the type of DM. Two kinds of factors participate in the etiology:

- The endogenous or genetic, and
- The exogenous or environmental.

Neither is sufficient in itself to account for initiation of the disease.

The genetic component in DM is heterogeneous. Resulting syndromes (Table 10-17) are often rare. Many have early rather than late onsets in life. They represent effects of mutations occurring at different genetic loci,[180] but all have the symptomatic commonalty of glucose intolerance.

When one considers the two primary types of DM, Types I and II, it is clear that their etiologies are distinct.[181] Greater genetic involvement seems to underlie Type II than Type I, judged most compellingly on the basis of studies of monozygotic twins. For example, in one study there was concordance of 50% of the 64 monozygotic twins in which DM was diagnosed before the age of 40 vs. 93% for the 31 such twins who became diabetic after 40.[182] High concordance rates for NIDDM in monozygotic twins are found even when there is wide geographic separation, suggesting that intrinsic rather than extrinsic or environmental factors have the greater etiological significance in this older age-associated type of DM.[181] Identification of genetic markers and overriding proof of a primary defect remain to be established. There is also evidence that factors concerning nutrition, physical activity, and stress are causally involved.

Diverse evidence currently supports the idea that a virus-triggered autoimmune disease may be the central causal problem in many cases of Type I or IDDM. In IDDM, as compared with NIDDM, there is a prevalence, or unbalanced occurrence, of certain of the histocompatability antigens (HLA) which are encoded by chromosome 6. The immunologic reactions, particularly during early phases of the disease include:

- Lymphocytic infiltration of the islets,
- Signs of cell-mediated immune reactions, and
- Circulating antibodies against islet or islet B-cell plasma membranes and/or cytoplasmic components, with consequent
- Destruction of islet cells and arrest of their insulin production.

Onset of IDDM shows some seasonal variation and clustering consistent with the timing of certain viral epidemics. References regarding these other alternative interpretations are available.[179,181,183-189]

C. Cascading Pathologies — Common Mechanisms?

Pathological changes are widespread and progressive in diabetic subjects but their severity seems to be inversely related to the success achieved in correcting the chronic hyperglycemia and in controlling its duration. Lesions in the diabetic include micro- and macroangiopathies and neuropathies, and the organs usually affected are the retina, kidney, and peripheral nerves. Pathogenesis of the long-term microvascular and neuropathic complications of DM is still contested. Two schools of thought are notable:

1. "Metabolic hypotheses" — hyperglycemia and other abnormalities due to insulin deficiency are responsible for the microangiopathy and neuropathy.
2. "Genetic hypotheses" — peripheral and diverse lesions characteristic of DM are considered to be genetically determined abnormalities, occurring independently of either hyperglycemia or insulin deficiency.

A resolution of this disagreement is important. Advocates of the "genetic hypothesis" take a comparatively relaxed attitude about degree of control to be exerted over hyperglycemia. Those favoring the "metabolic hypothesis" hold that minimizing the magnitude of hyperglycemia will prevent or lessen the complications that occur progressively with DM.

The implications of this dispute are apparent in the therapeutic tactics proposed by some physicians for insulin-dependent diabetics, especially for those relatively newly diagnosed who have not yet been encumbered by major pathological complications[190] and by other researchers and therapists for patients with NIDDM.[191] Although in general this controversy persists, the author's present conclusion is that, at least for IDDM, the "metabolic hypothesis" and its aim of relatively close control of blood sugar has gained major acceptance.[192]

Metabolic mechanisms that may be involved both in general pathological changes in aging and in more specific changes in diabetics have been investigated intensively. An early and major focus in this research is basement membrane thickening, the key structural abnormality of diabetic microangiopathy.[193] This pathology is one manifestation of "AGEs" (advanced glycosylation end products),[194,195] which is thought to result from progressive nonenzymatic protein glycation (term preferred by the Joint Committee of the IUB and IUPAC over the more commonly used "glycosylation" and "glucosylation").[196] The high levels of glucose in poorly controlled diabetics and in some nondiabetic elderly subjects favor this protein glycation. For example, the degree of glycation of hemoglobin (HbA1c) is now used as a clinical indicator of the level of control of hyperglycemia integrated over the several weeks that precede the sampling and analysis of the hemoglobin.[197]

Although glycation occurs similarly in some basement membranes of diabetics (2+ years of disease) and of some non-diabetics (20 to 91 years of age), the degree of glycation has been reported to correlate neither with age nor with the known duration of diabetes.[196,198] However, the controversies about these interpretations[196,199] may stem from still imperfect understanding of mechanisms affecting glycation *in vivo*.[200] In spite of this, some major conclusion seem clear:

1. In diabetics, capillary basement membrane thickening (involving glycation and AGEs) appears to follow rather than precede the diabetic state.[66,201]
2. In both the elderly and the diabetic, the AGEs in some tissues, and in association with some other important pathological processes, can have markedly detrimental effects.[202-204]

ACKNOWLEDGMENT

The editors wish to thank Dr. Lawson L. Rosenberg, University of California, Berkeley, CA for his valuable editorial and updating contributions to this chapter.

REFERENCES

1. Kanutsuka, A., Makino, H., Osegawa, M., Kasanuki, J., Suzuki, T., Yoshida, S. and Horie, H., Is somatostatin a true local inhibitory regulator of insulin secretion?, *Diabetes*, 33, 510, 1984.
2. Bonner-Weir, S., Deery, D., Leahy, J. L. and Weir, G. C., Compensatory growth of pancreatic β-cells in adult rats after short-term glucose infusion, *Diabetes*, 38, 49, 1989.
3. Reaven, E. P., Curry, D. L. and Reaven, G. M., Effect of age and sex on rat endocrine pancreas, *Diabetes*, 36, 1397, 1987.
4. Hollander, D. and Dadufalza, V. D., Aging-associated pancreatic exocrine insufficiency in the unanaesthetized rat, *Gerontology*, 30, 218, 1984.
5. Kitahara, A. and Adelman, R. C., Altered regulation of insulin secretion in isolated islets of different sizes in aging rats, *Biochem. Biophys. Res. Commun.*, 87, 1207, 1979.
6. Draznin, B., Steinberg, J. P., Leitner, J. W. and Sussman, K. E., The nature of insulin secretory defect in aging rats, *Diabetes*, 34, 1168, 1985.
7. American Diabetes Association, Loss of adaptive mechanisms during aging, *Fed. Proc.*, 38, 1968, 1979.
8. Elahi, D. andersen, D. K., Muller, D. C., Tobin, J. D., Brown, J. C. and Andres, R., The enteric enhancement of glucose-stimulated insulin release: the role of GIP in aging, obesity, and non-insulin-dependent diabetes mellitus, *Diabetes*, 33, 950, 1984.
9. Brunzell, J. D., Robertson, R. P., Lerner, R. L., Hazzard, W. R., Ensinck, J. W., Bierman, E. L. and Porte, D., Jr., Relationships between fasting plasma glucose levels and insulin secretion during intravenous glucose tolerance tests, *J. Clin. Endocrinol. Metab.*, 46, 222, 1976.
10. Cerassi, E., Luft, R. and Efendic, S., Decreased sensitivity of the pancreatic beta cells to glucose in prediabetic and diabetic subjects. A glucose dose-response study, *Diabetes*, 21, 224, 1972.
11. DeFronzo, R. A., Bonadonna, R. C. and Ferrannini, E., Pathogenesis of NIDDM. A balanced overview, *Diabetes Care*, 15, 318, 1992.

12. Dimitriadis, G., Cryer, P. and Gerich, J., Prolonged hyperglycemia during infusion of glucose and soma-tostatin impairs pancreatic A- and B-cell reponses to decrements in plasma glucose in normal man: evidence for induction of altered sensitivity to glucose, *Diabetologia*, 28, 63, 1985.

13. Halter, J. B., Gray, R. J. and Porte, D., Jr., Potentiation of insulin secretory responses by plasma glucose levels in man: evidence that hyperglycemia in diabetes compensates for impaired glucose potentiation, *J. Clin. Endocrinol. Metab.*, 48, 946, 1979.

14. Robertson, R. P. and Porte, D., Jr., The glucose receptor. A defective mechanism in diabetes mellitus distinct from the beta adrenergic receptor, *J. Clin. Invest.*, 52, 870, 1973.

15. Ward, W. K., Bolgiano, D. C., McKnight, B., Halter, J. B. and Porte, D., Jr., Diminished B-cell secretory capacity in patients with noninsulin-dependent diabetes mellitus, *J. Clin. Invest.*, 74, 1318, 1984.

16. Grill, V. and Rundfeldt, M., Abnormalities of insulin responses after ambient and previous exposure to glucose in streptozocin-diabetic and dexamethasone-treated rats. Role of hyperglycemia and increased B-cell demands, *Diabetes*, 35, 44, 1986.

17. Leahy, J. L., Bonner-Weir, S. and Weir, G. C., Beta cell dysfunction induced by chronic hyperglycemia. Current ideas on mechanism of impaired glucose-induced insulin secretion, *Diabetes Care,* 15, 442, 1992.

18. Leahy, J. L. and Weir, G. C., Evolution of abnormal insulin secretory responses during 48-h of in vivo hyperglycemia, *Diabetes*, 37, 217, 1988.

19. Rossetti, L., Shulman, G. I., Zawalich, W. and DeFronzo, R. A., Effect of chronic hyperglycemia on in vitro insulin secretion in partially pancreatectomized rats, *J. Clin. Invest.*, 80, 1037, 1987.

20. Kosaka, K., Kuzuya, T., Akanuma, Y. and Hagura, R., Increase in insulin response after treatment of overt maturity-onset diabetes is independent of the mode of treatment, *Diabetologia*, 18, 23, 1980.

21. Stanik, S. and Marcus, R., Insulin secretion improves following dietary control of plasma glucose in severely hyperglycemic obese patients, *Metabolism*, 29, 346, 1980.

22. Zawzlich, W. S., Zawalich, K. C., Shulman, G. I. and Rossetti, L., Chronic in vivo hyperglycemia impairs phosphoinositide hydrolysis and insulin release in isolated perfused rat islets, *Endocrinology,* 126, 253, 1990.

23. Reaven, E. P., Curry, D. L., Moore, J. and Reaven, G. M., Effect of age and environmental factors on insulin release from the perfused pancreas of the rat, *J. Clin. Invest.*, 71, 345, 1983.

24. Curry, D. L. and MacLachlan, S. A., Synthesis-secretion coupling of insulin: effect of aging, *Endocrinology*, 121, 241, 1987.

25. Wang, S. Y., Halban, P. A. and Rowe, J. W., Effects of aging on insulin synthesis and secretion: differential effects on preproinsulin messenger RNA levels, proinsulin biosynthesis, and secretion of newly made and preformed insulin in the rat, *J. Clin. Invest.*, 81, 176, 1988.

26. Hruza, Z., Decrease of cholesterol turnover in the blood and tissues during aging, *Federation Proc.*, 29, 452, 1970.

27. Andres, R., Aging and diabetes, *Med. Clin. North Am.*, 55, 835, 1971.

28. Chlouveraki, C., Jarrett, R. J. and Keen, H., Glucose tolerance, age and circulating insulin, *Lancet,* 7494(1), 806, 1967.

29. Davidson, M. B., The effect of aging on carbohydrate metabolism: a review of the English literature and a practical approach to the diagnosis of diabetes mellitus in the elderly, *Metabolism,* 28, 688, 1979.

30. Reed, M. J., Reaven, G. M., Mondon, C. E. and Azhar, S., Why does insulin resistance develop during maturation?, *J. Gerontol.*, 48, B139, 1993.

31. Dudl, R. J. and Ensinck, J. W., Insulin and glucagon relationships during aging in man, *Metabolism*, 26, 33, 1977.

32. Metz, R., Surmaczynska, B., Berger, S. and Sobel, G., Glucose tolerance, plasma insulin, and free fatty acids in elderly subjects, *Ann. Intern. Med.*, 64, 1042, 1966.

33. Duckworth, W. C. and Kitabchi, A. E., Direct measurement of plasma proinsulin in normal and diabetic subjects, *Am. J. Med.*, 53, 418, 1972.

34. Duckworth, W. C., The effect of age on plasma pro-insulin-like material after oral glucose, *J. Lab. Clin. Med.*, 88, 359, 1976.

35. Gumbiner, B., Polonsky, K. S., Beltz, W. F., Wallace, P., Brechtel, G. and Fink, R. I., Effects of aging on insulin secretion, *Diabetes*, 38, 1549, 1989.

36. Fink, R. I., Wallace, P., Brechtel, G. and Olefsky, J. M., Evidence that glucose transport is rate-limiting for in vivo glucose uptake, *Metab. Clin. Exp.*, 41, 897, 1992.

37. Reichlin, R. P., Somatostatin, *N. Engl. J. Med.*, 309, 1495, 1983.

38. Rolandi, E., Franceschini, R., Messina, V., Cataldi, A., Salvemini, M. and Barreca, T., Somatostatin in the elderly: diurinal plasma profile and secretory response to meal stimulation, *Gerontology*, 33, 296, 1987.

39. Rosen, O. M., After insulin binds, *Science*, 237, 1452, 1987.

40. Bliss, M., *The Discovery of Insulin*, University of Chicago Press, Chicago, 1982.

41. Rosen, O. M., Structure and function of insulin receptors, *Diabetes*, 38, 1508, 1989.

42. Carpentier, J.-L., Gordon, P. and Freychet, P., Lysosomal association of internalized ^{125}I-insulin in isolated rat hepatocytes. Direct administration by quantitative electron microscopic autoradiography, *J. Clin. Invest.*, 63, 1249, 1979.

43. Marshall, S., Kinetics of insulin receptor biosynthesis and membrane insertion: relationship to cellular function, *Diabetes*, 32, 319, 1983.

44. Marshall, S. and Olefsky, J. M., Separate intracellular pathways for insulin receptor recycling and insulin degradation in isolated rat adipocytes, *Cell Physiol.*, 117, 195, 1983.

45. Hedo, J. A., Kasuga, M., Van Obberghen, E., Roth, J. and Kahn, C. R., Direct demonstration of glycosylation of insulin receptor subunits by biosynthetic and external labeling: evidence for heterogeneity, *Proc. Natl. Acad. Sci. U.S.A.*, 78, 4791, 1981.

46. Cushman, S. W. and Wardzala, L. J., Potential mechanism of insulin action on glucose transport in the isolated rat adipose cell: apparent translocation of intracellular transport systems to the plasma membrane, *J. Biol. Chem.*, 255, 4758, 1980.

47. Suzuki, K. and Kono, T., Evidence that insulin causes translocation of glucose transport activity to the plasma membrane from an intracellular storage site, *Proc. Natl. Acad. Sci. U.S.A.*, 77, 2542, 1980.

48. Larner, J., Insulin signaling mechanisms. Lessons from the Old Testament of glycogen metabolism and the New Testament of molecular biology, *Diabetes*, 37, 262, 1988.

49. Gottschalk, W. K. and Jarrett, L., Intracellular mediators of insulin action, in *Diabetes/Metabolism Reviews*, DeFronzo, R. A., Ed., John Wiley & Sons, New York, 1985, 229.

50. Mato, J. M., Kelly, K. L., Abler, A. and Jarett, L., Identification of a novel insulin-sensitive glycophospholipid from H35 hepatoma cells, *J. Biol. Chem.*, 262, 2131, 1987.

51. Alexander, M. C., Kowaloff, E. M. and Witters, L. A., Purification of a hepatic 123,000-Dalton hormone-stimulated ^{32}P-peptide and its identification as ATP-citrate lyase, *J. Biol. Chem.*, 254, 8052, 1979.

52. Seals, J. R. and Czech, M. P., Characterization of a pyruvate dehydrogenase activator released by adipocyte plasma membranes in response to insulin, *J. Biol. Chem.*, 256, 2894, 1981.

53. Harris, M. I., Hadden, W. C., Knowler, W. C. and Bennett, P. H., International criteria for the diagnosis of diabetes and impaired glucose tolerance, *Diabetes Care*, 8, 562, 1985.

54. Harris, M. I., Hadden, W. C., Knowler, W. C. and Bennett, P. H., Prevalence of diabetes and impaired glucose tolerance and plasma glucose levels in U.S. population aged 20 – 74 yr., *Diabetes*, 36, 523, 1987, (reprinted in *Diabetes Spectrum*, 2, 156, 1989).

55. Leiter, E. H., Premdas, F., Harrison, D. E. and Lipson, L. G., Aging and glucose homeostasis in C57BL/6J male mice, *FASEB J.*, 2, 2087, 1988.

56. Chen, M., Bergman, R. N., Pacini, G. and Porte, D., Jr., Pathogenesis of age-related glucose intolerance in man: insulin resistance and decreased β-cell function, *J. Clin. Endocrinol. Metab.*, 60, 13, 1985.

57. DeFronzo, R. A., Glucose intolerance and aging: evidence for tissue insensitivity to insulin, *Diabetes*, 28, 1095, 1979.

58. Fink, R. I., Kolterman, O. G. and Olefsky, J. M., The physiological significance of glucose intolerance of aging, *J. Gerontol.*, 39, 273, 1984.

59. Jackson, R. A., Mechanisms of age-related glucose intolerance, *Diabetes Care*, 13 (Suppl. 2), 9, 1990.

60. Spence, J. W., Some observations on sugar tolerance with special reference to variations found at different ages, *Quart. J. Med.*, 14, 314, 1920-1921.

61. Jackson, R. A., Blix, P. M., Matthews, J. A., Hamling, J. B., Din, B. M., Brown, D. C., Beilin, J., Rubenstein, A. G. and Nabarro, J. D. N., Influence of ageing on glucose homeostasis, *J. Clin. Endocrinol. Metab.*, 55, 840, 1982.

62. Chen, M., Halter, J. B. and Porte, D., Jr., The role of dietary carbohydrate in the decreased glucose tolerance of the elderly, *J. Am. Geriatr. Soc.*, 35, 417, 1987.

63. O'Sullivan, J. B., Age gradient in blood glucose levels: magnitude and clinical implications, *Diabetes*, 23, 713, 1974.

64. Rosenthal, M., Doberne, L., Greenfield, M., Widztrom, A. and Reaven, G. M., Effect of age on glucose tolerance, insulin secretion, and in vivo insulin action, *J. Am. Geriatr. Soc.*, 30, 562, 1982.

65. Butterfield, W. J. H., The Bedford diabetes survey, *Proc. Roy. Soc. Med.*, 57, 196, 1964.

66. Bennett, P. H., The basement membrane controversy, *Diabetologia*, 16, 280, 1979.

67. Reaven, G. M., Role of insulin resistance in the pathophysiology of noninsulin dependent diabetes mellitus, *Diabetes/Metabolism Rev.*, 9 (Suppl. 1), 5S, 1993.

68. Fink, R. I., Wallace, P. and Olefsky, J. M., Effects of aging on glucose-mediated glucose disposal and glucose transport, *J. Clin. Invest.*, 77, 2034, 1986.

69. Jackson, R. A., Hawa, M. I., Roshania, R. D., Sim, B. M., DiSilvio, L. and Jaspan, J. B., Influence of aging on hepatic and peripheral glucose metabolism in humans, *Diabetes*, 37, 119, 1988.

70. Jackson, R. A., Roshania, R. D., Hawa, M. I., Sim., B. M. and DiSilvio, L., Impact of glucose ingestion on hepatic and peripheral glucose metabolism in man: an analysis based on simultaneous use of the foream and double isotope techniques, *J. Clin. Endocrinol. Metab.*, 63, 541, 1986.

71. Rowe, J. W., Minaker, K. L., Pallotta, J. A. and Flier, J. S., Characterization of the insulin resistance of aging, *J. Clin. Invest.*, 67, 1361, 1981.

72. Feibusch, J. M. and Holt, P. R., Impaired absorptive capacity for carbohydrate in the ageing human, *Digestive Dis. Sci.*, 27, 1095, 1982.

73. Hogan, D. B., Lambi, L. and Cape, R. D. T., Gastric emptying and aging, *J. Clin. Exp. Gerontol.*, 6, 145, 1984.

74. Montgomery, R. D., Haeney, M. R., Ross, I. N., Sammons, H. G., Barford, A. V., Balakrishnan, S., Mayer, P. P., Culank, L. S., Field, J. and Gosling, P., The aging gut: a study of intestinal absorption in relation to nutrition in the elderly, *Quart. J. Med.*, 47, 197, 1978.

75. Webster, S. G. P. and Leeming, J. T., Assessment of small bowel function in the elderly using a modified xylose tolerance test, *Gut*, 16, 109, 1975.

76. Guth, P. H., Physiological alterations in small bowel function with age: the absorption of D-xylose, *Am. J. Digestive Dis.*, 13, 565, 1968.

77. Kendall, M. J., The influence of age on the xylose absorption test, *Gut*, 11, 498, 1979.

78. Tonino, R. P., Minaker, K. L. and Rowe, J. W., Effect of age on systemic delivery of glucose in men, *Diabetes Care*, 12, 394, 1989.

79. Cohn, S. H., Vartsky, D., Yasumura, S., Savitsky, A., Zanzi, I., Vaswani, A. and Ellis, K. G., Compartmental body composition based on total-body nitrogen, potassium, and calcium, *Am. J. Physiol.*, 239, E524, 1980.

80. Moxley, R. T., Griggs, R. C., Forbes, G. B., Goldblatt, D. and Donohoe, K., Influence of muscle wasting on oral glucose tolerance testing, *Clin. Sci.*, 64, 601, 1983.

81. Blotner, H., Effect of prolonged physical inactivity on tolerance of sugar, *Arch. Internal Med.*, 75, 39, 1945.

82. Wasserman, D. H., Geer, R. J., Rice, D. E., Bracy, D., Flakoll, P. J., Brown, L. L., Hill, J. O. and Abumrad, N. N., Interaction of exercise and insulin action in humans, *Am. J. Physiol.*, 260, E37, 1991.

83. Lipman, R. L., Schnure, J. J., Bradley, E. M. and Lecocq, F. R., Impairment of peripheral glucose utilization in normal subjects by prolonged bed rest, *J. Lab. Clin. Med.*, 76, 221, 1970.

84. Seider, M. J., Nicholson, W. F. and Booth, F. W., Insulin resistance for glucose metabolism in disused soleus muscle of mice, *Am. J. Physiol.*, 242, E12, 1982.

85. Hollenbeck, C. B., Haskell, W., Rosenthal, M. and Reaven, G. M., Effect of habitual physical activity on regulation of insulin-stimulated glucose disposal in older males, *J. Am. Geriatr. Soc.*, 33, 273, 1984.

86. Rodnick, K. J., Haskell, W. L., Swislocki, A. L. M., Foley, J. E. and Reaven, G. M., Improved insulin action in muscle, liver and adipose tissue in physically trained human subjects, *Am. J. Physiol.*, 253, E489, 1987.

87. Seals, D. R., Hagberg, J. M., Allen, W. K., Hurley, B. F., Dalsky, G. P., Ehsani, A. A. and Holloszy, J. O., Glucose tolerance in young and older athletes and sedentary men, *J. Appl. Physiol.*, 56, 1521, 1984.

88. DeFronzo, R. A., Tobin, J. D. and Andres, R., Glucose clamp technique: a method for quantifying insulin secretion and resistance, *Am. J. Physiol.*, 237, E214, 1979.

89. Bergman, R. N., Toward physiological understanding of glucose tolerance, *Diabetes*, 38, 1512, 1989.

90. Chen, Y.-D. I., Swami, S., Skowronski, R., Coulston, A. and Reaven, G. M., Differences in postprandial lipemia between patients with normal gluocose tolerance and non-insulin dependent diabetes mellitus, *J. Clin. Endocrinol. Metab.*, 76, 347, 1993.

91. Golay, A., Schutz, Y., Broquet, C., Moeri, R., Felber, J. P. and Jequier, E., Decreased thermogenic response to an oral glucose load in older subjects, *J. Am. Geriatr. Soc.*, 31, 144, 1983.

92. Meneilly, G. S., Minaker, K., Elahi, D. and Rowe, J. W., Insulin action in aging man: evidence for tissue-specific differences at low physiologic insulin levels, *J. Gerontol.*, 42, 196, 1987.

93. Randle, P. J., Garland, P. B., Hales, C. N. and Newsholme, E. A., The glucose-fatty acid cycle: its role in insulin sensitivity and the metabolic disturbances of diabetes mellitus, *Lancet*, 1, 785, 1963.

94. Thiebaud, D., DeFronzo, R. A., Jacot, E., Golay, A., Acheson, K., Maeder, E., Jequier, E. and Felber, J.-P., Effect of long chain triglyceride infusion on glucose metabolism in man, *Metabolism*, 31, 1128, 1982.

95. Meylan, M., Henny, C., Temler, E., Jequier, E. and Felber, J. P., Metabolic factors in the insulin resistance in human obesity, *Metabolism*, 36, 256, 1987.

96. Chen, M., Bergman, R. N. and Porte, D., Jr., Insulin resistance and B-cell dysfunction in aging: the importance of dietary carbohydrate, *J. Clin. Endocrinol. Metab.*, 67, 951, 1988.

97. Pacini, G., Beccaro, F., Valerio, A., Nosadini, R., Cobelli, C. and Crebaldi, G., Age per se does not influence glucose intolerance in a population following typical Mediterranean diet, *Diabetes*, 34 (Suppl. 1), 192A, 1985.

98. Lillioja, S., Young, A. A., Culter, C. L., Ivy, J. L., Abbott, W. G. H., Zawadski, J. K., Yki-Jarvinen, H., Christin, L., Secomb, T. W. and Bogardus, C., Skeletal muscle capillary density and fiber type are possible determinants of *in vivo* insulin resistance in man, *J. Clin. Invest.*, 80, 415, 1987.

99. Brown, M., Change in fibre size, not number, in ageing skeletal muscle, *Age Ageing*, 16, 244, 1987.

100. Silverstone, F. A., Brandforbrener, M., Shock, N. W. and Yiengst, M. J., Age differences in the intravenous glucose tolerance tests and the response to insulin, *J. Clin. Invest.*, 36, 504, 1957.

101. Andres, R. and Tobin, J. D., Aging and the disposition of glucose, *Adv. Exp. Med. Biol.*, 61, 239, 1975.

102. Kimmerling, G., Javorski, W. C. and Reaven, G. M., Aging and insulin resistance in a group of non-obese male volunteers, *J. Am. Geriatr. Soc.*, 25, 349, 1977.

103. Schreuder, H. B., Influence of age on insulin secretion and lipid mobilization after glucose stimulation, *Israel J. Med. Sci.*, 8, 832, 1972.

104. Broughton, D. L., Alberti, K. G. M. M., James, O. F. W. and Taylor, R., Peripheral tissue insulin sensitivity in healthy elderly subjects, *Gerontology*, 33, 357, 1987.

105. Petrides, A. S., Strohmeyer, G. and DeFronzo, R. A., Insulin resistance in liver disease and portal hypertension, *Progr. Liver Dis.*, 10, 311, 1992.

106. Abumrad, N M., Cherrington, A. D., Williams, P. E., Lacy, W. W. and Rabi, D., Absorption and disposition of a glucose load in the conscious dog, *Am. J. Physiol.*, 242, E398, 1982.

107. Wahren, J. and Felig, P., Influence of somatostatin on carbohydrate disposal and absorption in diabetes mellitus, *Lancet*, 2, 1213, 1976.

108. Bergman, R. N. and Bucolo, R. J., Interaction of insulin and glucose in the control of hepatic glucose balance, *Am. J. Physiol.*, 227, 1314, 1974.

109. Best, J. D., Taborsky, G. J., Halter, J. B. and Porte, D., Jr., Glucose disposal is not proportional to plasma glucose level in man, *Diabetes,* 30, 847, 1981.

110. Bucolo, R. J., Bergman, R. N., Marsh, D. J. and Yates, F. E., Dynamics of glucose autoregulation in the isolated, blood-perfused canine liver, *Am. J. Physiol.*, 227, 209, 1974.

111. Insel, P. A., Liljenquist, J. E., Tobin, J. D., Sherwin, R. S., Watkins, P. andres, R. and Berman, M., Insulin control of glucose metabolism in man, *J. Clin. Invest.*, 55, 1057, 1975.

112. Sherwin, R. S., Kramer, K. J., Robin, J. D., Insel, P. A., Liljenquist, J. E., Berman, M. and Andres, R., A model of the kinetics of insulin in man, *J. Clin. Invest.*, 53, 1481, 1974.

113. Andres, R., Swerdloff, R., Posefsky, T. and Coleman, D., Manual feedback technique for the control of blood glucose concentration, in *Automation in Analytical Chemistry,* Skeggs, L.T., Jr., Ed., Mediad, New York, 1966, 286.

114. Gries, F. A., Berger, M., Priess, H., Liebermeister, H. and Johnke, K., Glucagon effect on human adipose tissue in vitro: dependence on body weight and age, *Verh. Dtsch. Ges. Inn. Med.*, 75, 796, 1969.

115. Goldfine, I. D., The insulin receptor: molecular biology and transmembrane signaling, *Endocr. Rev.*, 8, 235, 1987.

116. Standaert, M. L., Mojsilovic, L., Farese, R. V. and Pollet, R. J., Phorbol ester inhibition of insulin-stimulated deoxyribonucleic acid synthesis in BC_3H-1 myocytes, *Endocrinology*, 121, 941, 1987.

117. Bolinder, J., Ostman, J. and Arner, P., Influence of aging or insulin receptor binding and metabolic effects of insulin on human adipose tissue, *Diabetes*, 32, 959, 1983.

118. Pagano, G., Cassader, M., Cavallo-Perin, P., Bruno, A., Masciola, P., Ozzello, A., Dall'Omo, A. M. and Foco, A., Insulin resistance in the aged: a quantitative evaluation of *in vivo* insulin sensitivity and *in vitro* glucose transport, *Metabolism*, 33, 976, 1984.

119. Rosenbloom, A. L., Goldstein, S. and Yip, C. C., Insulin binding to cultured human fibroblasts increases with normal and precocious aging, *Science*, 193, 412, 1976.

120. Fink, R. I., Huecksteadt, T. and Karaghlanian, Z., The effects of ageing on glucose metabolism in adipocytes from Fischer rats, *Endocrinology,* 118, 1139, 1986.

121. Hollenberg, N. D. and Schneider, E. L., Receptor for insulin and epidermal growth factor-urogastrone in adult human fibroblasts do not change with donor age, *Mech. Ageing Dev.*, 11, 37, 1979.

122. McConnell, J. G., Buchanan, K. D., Avdill, J. and Stout, R. W., Glucose tolerance in the elderly: the role of insulin and its receptor, *Eur. J. Clin. Invest.,* 12, 55, 1982.

123. McDonald, A. R., Maddux, B. A., Okabayashi, Y., Wong, K. Y., Hawley, D. M., Logsdon, C. D. and Goldfine, I. D., Regulation of insulin-receptor mRNA levels by glucocorticoids, *Diabetes*, 36, 779, 1987.

124. Andres, A., Pulido, J. A., Satrustegui, J. and Carrascosa, J. M., The kinase activity of the insulin receptor is modified during aging, *Diabetologia*, 30, 494A, 1987.

125. Bryer-Ash, M. and Freidenberg, G., The insulin resistance of aging resides at a site distal to the insulin receptor kinase in the Fischer rat, *Diabetes*, 36 (Suppl. 1), 56A, 1987.

126. Yarden, Y. and Ullrich, A., Growth factor receptor tyrosine kinases, *Annual Rev. Biochem.*, 57, 443, 1988.

127. Yonezawa, K. and Roth, R. A., Various proteins modulate the kinase activity of the insulin receptor, *FASEB J.*, 4, 194, 1990.

128. McClain, D. A. and Olefsky, J. M., Evidence for two independent pathways of insulin-receptor internalization in hepatocytes and hepatoma cells, *Diabetes,* 37, 806, 1988.

129. Trischitta, V. and Reaven, G. M., Evidence of a defect on insulin-receptor recycling in adipocytes from older rats, *Am. J. Physiol.*, 254, E39, 1988.

130. Karnieli, E., Zarnowski, M. J., Hissin, P. J., Simpson, I. A., Salans, L. B. and Cushman, S. W., Insulin-stimulated translocation of glucose transport systems in the isolated rat adipose cell: time course, reversal, insulin concentration dependency and relationship to glucose transport activity, *J. Biol. Chem.*, 256, 4772, 1981.

131. Hissin, P. J., Foley, J. E., Wadzala, L. J., Karnieli, E., Simpson, I. A., Salans, L. B. and Cushman, S. W., Mechanism of insulin-resistant glucose transport activity in the enlarged adipose cell of the aged obese rat: relative depletion of intracellular glucose transport systems, *J. Clin. Invest.*, 70, 780, 1982.

132. Fink, R. I., Kolterman, O. G., Kao, M. and Olefsky, J. M., The role of the glucose transport system in the postreceptor defect in insulin action associated with human aging, *J. Clin. Endocrinol. Metab.*, 58, 721, 1984.

133. Kosaki, A., Kazuya, H., Okamoto, M., Yamada, K., Nishimura, H., Ida, T., Kakehi, T., Takeda, J., Seino, Y. and Imura, H., Regulation of glucose transporter gene expression by insulin in cultured human fibroblasts, *Diabetes*, 37 (Suppl. 1), 28A, 1988.

134. Belfiore, F., Vagroni, G., Napoli, E. and Rabuazzo, M., Effects of ageing on key enzymes of glucose metabolism in human adipose tissue, *J. Molec. Med.*, 2, 89, 1977.

135. Bernstein, R. S. and Kipnis, D. M., Regulation of rat hexokinase isoenzymes. I. Assay and effect of age, fasting and refeeding, *Diabetes*, 22, 913, 1973.

136. Goodman, M. N., Dluz, S. M., McElancy, M., Belur, E. and Ruderman, N. B., Glucose uptake and insulin sensitivity in rat muscle: changes during 3-96 weeks of age, *Am. J. Physiol.*, 244, E93, 1983.

137. Mondon, C. and Azhar, S., Differential responsiveness to insulin by slow and fast twitch rat skeletal muscle with increase in age, *Diabetes*, 35 (Suppl. 1), 163A, 1986.

138. Adelman, R. C., An age-dependent modification of enzyme regulation, *J. Biol. Chem.*, 245, 1032, 1970.

139. Adelman, R. C. and Freeman, C., Age-dependent regulation of glucokinase and tyrosine aminotransferase activities of rat liver in vivo by adrenal, pancreatic and pituitary hormones, *Endocrinology*, 90, 1151, 1972.

140. Azhar, S., Ho, H., Reaven, E. P. and Reaven, G. M., Evidence of an age-related decline in mitochondrial glycerophosphate dehydrogenase activity in isolated rat islets, *Metabolism*, 32, 1019, 1983.

141. Forciea, M. A., Schwartz, H. L., Towle, H. C., Mariash, C. N., Kaiser, F. E. and Oppenheimer, J. H., Thyroid hormone-carbohydrate interaction in the rat: correlation between age-related reductions in the inducibility of hepatic malic enzyme by triiodo-L-thyronine and a high carbohydrate, fat-free diet, *J. Clin. Invest.*, 67, 1739, 1981.

142. Gafni, A., Age-related effects on subunit interactions in rat muscle glyceraldehyde-3-phosphate dehydrogenase, *Curr. Top. Cell Regul.*, 24, 273, 1984.

143. Gold, G., Karoly, K., Freeman, C. and Adelman, R. C., A possible role for insulin in the altered capability for hepatic enzyme adaptation during ageing, *Biochem. Biophys. Res. Commun.*, 73, 1003, 1976.

144. Kaiser, F. E., Schwartz, H. L., Mariash, G. N. and Oppenheimer, J. H., Comparison of age-related decrease in the basal and carbohydrate inducible levels of lipogenic enzymes in adipose tissue and liver, *Metabolism*, 32, 838, 1983.

145. Schwartz, H. L., Forciea, M. A., Mariash, C. N. and Oppenheimer, J. H., Age-related reduction in response of hepatic enzymes to 3,5,3'-triiodothyronine administration, *Endocrinology*, 105, 41, 1979.

146. McConnell, J. G., Alam, M. J., O'Hare, M. M. T., Buchanan, K. D. and Stout, R. W., The effect of age and sex on the response of enteropancreatic polypeptides to oral glucose, *Age Ageing*, 12, 54, 1983.

147. Giugliano, D., Giannett, G., DiPinto, P., Cerciello, T., Ceriello, A. and D'Onofrio, F., Normalization by sodium salicylate of the impaired counterregulatory glucagon response to hypoglycemia in insulin-dependent diabetes. A possible role for endogenous prostaglandins, *Diabetes*, 34, 521, 1985.

148. Delfert, D. M., Graves, C. B. and McDonald, J. M., Interaction of insulin receptor with calcium and calmodulin, in *Insulin Receptors, Part A: Methods for the Study of Structure and Function,* (Series on Receptor Biochemistry and Methodology, Vol. 12A), Kahn, C. R. and Harrison, L. C., Eds., Alan R. Liss, New York, 1988, 189.

149. Draznin, B., Cytosolic calcium and insulin resistance, *Am. J. Kidney Dis.*, 21 (Suppl. 3), 32, 1993.

150. Pershadsingh, H. A. and McDonald, J. M., Hormone-receptor coupling and the molecular mechanisms of insulin action in the adipocyte: a paradigm for Ca^{2+} homeostasis in the initiation of the insulin-induced metabolic cascade, *Cell Calcium*, 5, 111, 1984.

151. Draznin, B., Kao, M. and Sussman, K. E., Insulin and glyburide increase cytosolic free-Ca^{2+} concentration in isolated rat adipocyte, *Diabetes*, 36, 174, 1987.

152. Draznin, B., Sussman, K. E., Eckel, R. H., Kao, M., Yost, T. and Sherman, N. A., Possible role of cystosolic free calcium concentrations in mediating insulin resistance of obesity and hyperinsulinemia, *J. Clin. Invest.*, 82, 1848, 1988.

153. Pershadsingh, H. A., Shade, D. L., Delfert, J. M. and McDonald, J. M., Chelation of intracellular calcium blocks insulin action in the adipocytes, *Proc. Natl. Acad. Sc. U.S.A.*, 84, 1025, 1987.

154. Gupta, M. P., Makino, M., Khatter, K. and Dhalla, N. S., Stimulation of Na^+-Ca^{2+} exchange in heart sarcolemma by insulin, *Life Sci.*, 39, 1077, 1986.

155. Hope-Gill, H. F. and Nanda, V., Stimulation of calcium ATPase by insulin, glucagon, cyclic AMP and clyclic GMP in Triton X-100 extracts of purified liver plasma membranes, *Horm. Metab. Res.*, 11, 698, 1979.

156. Levy, J., Grunberger, G., Karl, I. and Gavin, J. R., III, Effects of food restriction and insulin treatment on ($Ca2^+$ + $Mg2^+$)-ATPase response to insulin in kidney basolateral membranes of non-insulin-dependent diabetic rats, *Metabolism Clin. Exp.*, 39, 25, 1990.

157. Levy, J., Gavin, J. R., III, Hammerman, M. R. and Avioli, L. V., (Ca^{2+} - Mg^{2+})-ATPase activity in kidney basolateral membrane in non-insulin-dependent diabetic rats: effect of insulin, *Diabetes*, 35, 899, 1986.

158. Parenti, M., Dall'ara, A., Rusconi, L., Cocchi, D. and Muller, E. E., Different regulation of growth hormone-releasing factor-sensitive adenylate cyclase in the anterior pituitary of young and aged rats, *Endocrinology*, 121, 1649, 1987.

159. Ganguly, P. K., Mathur, S., Gupta, M. P., Beamish, R. E. and Dhalla, N. S., Calcium pump activity of sarcoplasmic reticulum in diabetic rat skeletal muscle, *Am. J. Physiol.*, 251, E515, 1986.

160. Levy, J. and Rempinski, D., A hormone specific defect in insulin regulation of the membrane (Ca^{2+} + Mg^{2+})-ATPase in obesity, *Clin. Res.*, 37, 455A, 1989.

161. Makino, N., Dhalla, K. S., Elimban, V. and Dhalla, N. S., Sarcolemmal Ca^{2+} transport in streptozotocin-induced diabetic cardiomyopathy in rats, *Am. J. Physiol.*, 253, E202, 1987.

162. Zemel, M. B., Levy, J., Shehin, S., Walsh, M. and Sowers, J. R., Role of impaired calcium transport in obesity-associated hypertension, *FASEB*, 253, 1990.

163. Schaefer, W., Priessen, J., Mannhold, R. and Gries, A. F., $(Ca^{2+} + Mg^{2+})$-ATPase activity of human red blood cells in healthy and diabetic volunteers, *Klin. Wochenschr.*, 65, 17, 1987.

164. Nagy, K., Grunberger, G. and Levy, J., Insulin antagonistic effects of insulin receptor antibodies on plasma membrane $(Ca^{2+} + Mg^{2+})$-ATPase activity: a possible etiology of Type II insulin resistance, *Endocrinology*, 126, 45, 1990.

165. Nishimoto, I. and Kojima, I., Calcium signalling system triggered by insulin-like growth factor II, *News in Physiol. Sci.*, 4, 94, 1989.

166. Dedman, J. R., The role of calmodulin in the mediation of intracellular calcium, in *Mechanisms of Intestinal Electrolyte Transport and Regulation by Calcium*, Alan R. Liss, New York, 1984, 135.

167. Morley, J. E., Levine, A. S., Beyer, H. S., Mooradian, A. D., Kaiser, F. E. and Brown, D. M., The effects of aging and diabetes mellitus on human red and white cell calmodulin levels (chemotaxis/phagocytosis/calcium), *Diabetes*, 33, 77, 1984.

168. Flier, J. and Roth, J., Diabetes in acromegaly and other endocrine disorders, in *Endocrinology*, Vol. 2, DeGroot, L. T. and Cahill, G. F., Jr., Eds., Grune & Stratton, New York, 1979, 1089.

169. Unger, R. H., Glucagon and the insulin:glucagon ratio in diabetes and other catabolic illnesses, *Diabetes*, 20, 834, 1971.

170. Rudman, D., Feller, A. G., Nagraj, H. S., Gergans, G. A., Lalitha, Y., Goldberg, A. F., Schlenker, R. A., Cohn, L., Rudman, I. W. and Mattson, D. E., Effects of human growth hormone in men over 60 years old, *N. Engl. J. Med.*, 323, 1, 1990.

171. Shibasaki, T., Shizume, K., Nakahara, M., Masuda, A., Jibiki, K., Demura, H., Wakabayashi, I. and Ling, N., Age-related changes in plasma growth hormone response to growth hormone-releasing factor in man, *J. Clin. Endocrinol. Metab.*, 58, 212, 1984.

172. O'Costa, A. P., Ingram, R. L., Lenham, J. E. and Sonntag, W. E., The regulation and mechanisms of action of growth hormone and insulin-like growth factor 1 during normal aging, *J. Reprod. Fertil.*, Suppl. 46, 87, 1993.

173. Ceda, G. P., Valenti, G., Butturini, V. and Hoffman, A. R., Diminished pituitary responsiveness to growth hormone-releasing factor in aging male rats, *Endocrinology*, 118, 2109, 1986.

174. Sonntag, W. E., Forman, L. J., Miki, N., Steger, R. W., Ramos, T., Arimura, A. and Meites, J., Effects of CNS acting drugs and somatostatin antiserum on growth hormone release in young and old male rats, *Neuroendocrinology*, 33, 73, 1981.

175. Sonntag, W. E., Hylka, V. W. and Meites, J., Impaired ability of old male rats to secrete growth hormone in vivo but not in vitro in response to hpGRF (1-44), *Endocrinology*, 113, 2305, 1983.

176. American Diabetes Association, Position statement: Office guide to diagnosis and classification of diabetes mellitus and other categories of glucose intolerance, *Diabetes Care*, 13 (Suppl. 1), 3, 1990.

177. Bennett, P. H., Classification of diabetes, in *Diabetes Mellitus,, Theory and Practice*, 3rd ed., Ellenberg, M. and Rifkin, H., Eds., Medical Examination Publ., New Hyde Park, NY, 1983, 409.

178. Fajans, S. S., Classification of diabetes mellitus, in *Diabetes Mellitus*, Vol. 5, Rifkin, H. and Raskin, P., Eds., Robert J. Brady Co./Amer. Diabetes, Assoc., Bowie, MD, 1981, 95.

179. Shafrir, E., Bergman, M. and Felig, P., The endocrine pancreas: diabetes mellitus, in *Endocrinology and Metabolism*, 2nd ed., Felig, P., Baxter, J. D., Broadus, A. E. and Frohman, L. A., Eds., McGraw-Hill, New York, 1987, 1043.

180. Rotter, J. I. and Rimoin, D. L., Genetic heterogeneity in diabetes mellitus and peptic ulcer, in *Genetic Epidemiology*, Morton, N. E. and Chung, C. S., Academic Press, New York, 1978, 381.

181. Freinkel, N., On the etiology of diabetes mellitus, in *Diabetes Mellitus*, Vol. V., Rifkin, H. and Raskin, P., Eds., Robert J. Brady Co./Am. Diabetes Assoc., Bowie, MD, 1981, 1.

182. Tattersall, R. B. and Pyke, D. A., Diabetes in identical twins, *Lancet*, 2, 1120, 1972.

183. Bleich, D., Jackson, R. A., Soeldner, J. S. and Eisenbarth, G. S., Analysis of metabolic progression to type I diabetes in ICA^+ relatives of patients with type I diabetes, *Diabetes Care*, 13, 111, 1990.

184. Cudworth, A. G. and Gorsuch, A. N., Autoimmunity and viruses in Type I (insulin-dependent) diabetes, in *Diabetes Mellitus, Theory and Practice*, 3rd ed., Ellenberg, M. and Rifkin, H., Eds., Medical Examination Publ., New Hyde Park, NY, 1983, 505.

185. Harrison, L. C., Campbell, I. L., Allison, J. and Miller, J. F. A. P., MHC molecules and β-cell destruction: immune and nonimmune mechanisms, *Diabetes*, 38, 815, 1989.

186. Nerup, J., Mandrup-Poulsen, T., Molvig, J., Helqvist, S., Wogensen, L. and Egeberg, J., Mechanisms of pancreatic β-cell destruction in Type I diabetes, *Diabetes Care*, 11 (Suppl. 1), 16, 1988.

187. Rabinovitch, A., Baquerizo, H. and Sumoski, W., Cytotoxic effects of cytokines on islet β-cells: evidence for involvement of eicosanoids, *Endocrinology*, 126, 67, 1990.

188. Todd, J., A most intimate foe. How the immune system can betray the body it defends, *The Sciences (New York Acad. Sci.)*, 30, 20, 1990.

189. Todd, J. A., Acha-Orbea, H., Bell, J. I., Chao, N., Fronek, Z., Jacob, C. O., McDermott, M., Sinha, A. A., Timmerman, L., Steinman, L. and McDevitt, H. O., A molecular basis for MHC Class-II-associated autoimmunity, *Science*, 240, 1003, 1988.

190. Ross, M. D., Bernstein, G. and Rifkin, H., Relationship of metabolic control of diabetes mellitus to long-term complications, in *Diabetes Mellitus, Theory and Practice*, 3rd ed., Ellenberg, M. and Rifkin, H., Eds., Medical Examination Publ., New Hyde Park, NY, 1983, 907.

191. Robertson, R. P., Type II diabetes, glucose "non-sense," and islet desensitization, *Diabetes*, 38, 1501, 1989.

192. American Diabetes Association, Position statement: Blood glucose control in diabetes, *Diabetes Care,* 13, 16, 1990.

193. Osterby, R., Basement membrane morphology in diabetes mellitus, in *Diabetes Mellitus, Theory and Paractice*, 3rd ed., Ellenberg, M. and Rifkin, H., Eds., Medical Examiniation Publ., New Hyde Park, NY, 1983, 323.

194. Sell, D. R. and Monnier, V. M., End-stage renal disease and diabetes catalyze the formation of a pentose-derived crosslink from aging human collagen, *J. Clin. Investig.,* 85, 380, l990.

195. Monnier, V. M., Vishwanath, V., Frank, K. E., Elmets, C. A., Danchot, P. and Kohn, R. R., Relation between complications of Type I diabetes mellitus and collagen-linked fluorescence, *N. Engl. J. Med.*, 314, 403, 1986.

196. Garlick, R. L., Bunn, H. F. and Spiro, R. G., Nonenzymatic glycation of basement membranes from human glomeruli and bovine sources: effect of diabetes and age, *Diabetes*, 37, 1144, 1988.

197. Gabbay, K. H. and Fluckiger, R., Clinical significance of glycosylated hemoglobin, in *Diabetes Mellitus*, Vol. V., Rifkin, H. and Raskin, P., Eds., Robert J. Brady Co./Am. Diabetes Assoc., Bowie, MD, 1981, 241.

198. Kabadi, U. M., Glycosylation of proteins: lack of influence of ageing, *Diabetes Care*, 11, 429, 1988.

199. Kilo, C., Vogler, N. and Williamson, J. R., Muscle capillary basement membrane changes related to aging and to diabetes mellitus, *Diabetes*, 21, 881, 1972.

200. Vlassara, H., Browlee, M. and Cerami, A., Activity of the specific macrophage receptor for advanced glycosylation end-products correlates inversely with the insulin levels in vivo, *Diabetes*, 37, 456, 1988.

201. Barnett, A. H., Spiliopoulos, A. J. and Pyke, D. A., Muscle capillary basement membrane in identical twins discordant for insulin-dependent diabetes, *Diabetes*, 32, 557, 1983.

202. Cerami, A., Vlassara, H. and Brownlee, M., Glucose and aging, *Sci. Amer.*, 256, 91, 1987.

203. Cerami, A., Vlassara, H. and Brownlee, M., Role of advanced glycosylation products in complications of diabetes, *Diabetes Care*, 11 (Suppl. 1), 73, 1988.

204. Schnider, S. L. and Kohn, R. R., Effects of age and diabetes mellitus on the solubility and nonenzymatic glucosylation of human skin collagen, *J. Clin. Invest.*, 67, 1630, 1981.

205. Bennett, P. H., The epidemiology of diabetes mellitus, in *Diabetes Mellitus*, Vol. V, Rifkin, H. and Raskin, P., Eds., Robert J. Brady Co./Am. Diabetes Assoc., Bowie, MD, 1981, 87.

206. Quay, W. B., Endocrine pancreas: development and growth, in *Handbook of Human Growth and Development Biology, Vol. 11, Part A*, Meisami, E. and Timiras, P. S., Eds., CRC Press, Boca Raton, Florida, 1989, 95.

207. Kahn, C. R. and Shechter, Y., Insulin, oral hypoglycemic agents, and the pharmacology of the endocrine pancreas, in *Goodman and Gilman's The Pharmacological Basis of Therapeutics*, 8th ed., Gilman, A. G., Rall, T. W., Nies, A. S. and Taylor, P., Eds., Macmillan, New York, 1990, 1463.

208. Bolinder, J., Lithell, H., Skarfors, E. and Arner, P., Effects of obesity, hyperinsulinemia, and glucose intolerance on insulin action in adipose tissue of sixty-year-old men, *Diabetes*, 35, 282, 1986.

209. Boden, G., Hormonal and metabolic disturbances during acute and subacute myocardial infarction in man, *Diabetologia*, 7, 240, 1971.

210. Christensen, N. J. and Videback, J., Plasma catecholamines and carbohydrate metabolism in patients with acute myocardial infarction, *J. Clin. Invest.*, 54, 278, 1974.

211. George, J. M., Reier, C. E., Lanese, R. R. and Rower, J. M., Morphine anethesia blocks cortisol and growth hormone response to surgical stress in humans, *J. Clin. Endocrinol. Metab.*, 38, 736, 1974.

212. Halter, J. B., Pflug, A. E. and Porte, D., Jr., Mechanisms of plasma catecholamine increases during surgical stress in man, *J. Clin. Endocrinol. Metab.*, 45, 936, 1977.

213. Laniado, S., Segal, P. and Esrig, P., The role of glucagon hypersecretion in the pathogenesis of hyperglycemia following acute myocardial infarction, *Circulation*, 48, 797, 1973.

214. Schade, D. S. and Eaton, R. P., The temporal relationship between endogenously secreted stress hormones and metabolic decompensation in diabetic man, *J. Clin. Endocrinol. Metab.*, 50, 131, 1980.

215. Anderson, C. E., Rotter, J. I. and Rimoin, D. L., Genetics of diabetes mellitus, in *Diabetes Mellitus, Vol. V.*, Rifkin, H. and Raskin, P., Eds., Robert J. Brady Co./Am. Diabetes Assoc., Bowie, MD, 1981, 79.
216. Thorburn, A. W., Gunbiner, B., Brechtel, G. and Henry, R. R., Effect of hyperinsulinemia and hyperglycemia on intracellular glucose and fat metabolism in healthy subjects, *Diabetes*, 39, 22, 1990.
217. Ferrannini, E., Bjorkman, O., Reichard, G. A., Pilo, A., Olsson, M., Wahren, J. and DeFronzo, R. A., The disposal of an oral glucose load in healthy subjects: a quantitative study, *Diabetes*, 34, 580, 1985.

11

An Overview of the Pathogenesis and Management of Noninsulin-Dependent Diabetes Mellitus

William C. Duckworth

CONTENTS

I. INTRODUCTION

The pathogenesis of Noninsulin Dependent Diabetes Mellitus, NIDDM, is beginning to be better understood.[1] In patients with established disease, two abnormalities are consistently present:

1. Decreased tissue and cellular response to insulin, or, insulin resistance,
2. Abnormalities in pancreatic content and secretion of insulin.

Although itself a controversial question for many years, the presence of insulin resistance in patients with NIDDM is universal. The concept of insulin resistance was established by Hinsworth and Kerr in their pioneering studies[2] and supported by the demonstration of elevated insulin levels by Yalow and Berson,[3] but appreciation of the degree and the contribution of insulin resistance to the development of NIDDM is a more recent development. Work by Reaven and collaborators and others, initially using multiple hormone infusions and, more recently, glucose clamps, has clearly established the presence of whole-body insulin resistance in NIDDM.[4] Much additional investigation has been directed at determining the tissue sites and cellular mechanisms of the decreased insulin action. The initial lesion appears to be in muscle (decreased glucose uptake), with subsequent abnormalities in the liver (increased basal glucose output). Multiple genetic abnormalities resulting in insulin resistance have been suggested, supporting the heterogeneous nature of NIDDM. A subtype of NIDDM (Maturity Onset Diabetes of Youth [MODY]) appears to be due to alterations in the glucokinase gene in certain families.

II. PATHOGENESIS OF NONINSULIN-DEPENDENT DIABETES MELLITUS

NIDDM is a heterogeneous disease with different initial abnormalities resulting ultimately in a similar clinical presentation, i.e., hyperglycemia and its sequellae. The mechanism of action of insulin is a complex process involving multiple steps, not all of which are well understood (for review see Reference 5 and Chapter 10). The initial step in insulin action is binding to a specific cell membrane receptor. The insulin receptor is composed of two subunits — an α subunit which is entirely extracellular and contains the insulin binding site, and a β subunit which is a transmembrane protein with both extracellular and cytoplasmic domains. The cytoplasmic domain contains a tyrosine kinase sequence. Typically, two α and two β subunits are connected by disulfide bonds in a heterotetrameric structure. The α and β subunits are encoded by a single gene and translated as a single proreceptor protein which is then processed into the two subunits. The insulin receptor gene has been isolated, the amino acid sequence of the receptor deduced, and altered receptors have been produced by site-directed mutagenesis. This has provided valuable information on insulin-receptor interactions.

After binding of insulin to its receptor, the next event is activation of the tyrosine kinase portion of the receptor, with resultant autophosphorylation of the receptor and tyrosine phosphorylation of other cellular substrates.[6,7] This process appears to be important in generating the cellular response but its exact role is unknown, although recent studies support the potential role of a cytoplasmic substrate. The actual signaling mechanism, however, is not fully understood and multiple signaling processes are probable. A full discussion of possible signaling mechanisms is outside the scope of this review, but candidates include a phosphorylation cascade, generation of a peptide mediator, generation of a glycolipid mediator, activation of a protease, alterations in ion transport, intracellular insulin, and others.

After binding and activation of the kinase, the insulin receptor complex is internalized into endosomes where insulin degradation is initiated (see Reference 8 for review). The internalized insulin and receptor can associate with intracellular organelles, be degraded, or recycle to the cell surface. Most of the hormone is degraded intracellularly, and most of the receptors are reinserted in the membrane, but some insulin is released intact and some receptors are degraded. A biological role for internalization and degradation has been recently supported.

The effect of insulin on cellular glucose uptake in peripheral tissues is due to an increase in number and activity of membrane glucose transporters. The primary mechanism is translocation of glucose transporters (Glut 4) from an intracellular pool to the plasma membrane, but activation of preexisting translocated transporters may occur (see Chapter 10).

In patients with NIDDM, defects in all of the above processes have been described.[9-17] Decreases in insulin binding, receptor tyrosine kinase activity, insulin-receptor internalization, generation of mediators, and glucose transporter translocation and activity have been observed. Most of the insulin resistance is due to a postbinding abnormality presumably secondary to genetic alterations. Decreased insulin receptor tyrosine kinase activity has been shown in the liver, muscle, and fat from patients with NIDDM, and two populations of insulin receptors have been described. At the time of this writing, however, no evidence showing that this is a primary event has been given. In addition, there is some evidence that not all insulin's effects in NIDDM are equally defective. For example, adipocytes from NIDDM patients may respond better in terms of antilipolysis than in glucose transport.[18] If tyrosine kinase activation is the essential primary event, then all actions of insulin should be equally affected. However, evidence exists showing that insulin action can occur without tyrosine kinase activation.

The simple explanation for the divergent observations is that NIDDM is a heterogeneous disease and multiple defects in insulin action (and insulin secretion) may result ultimately in a similar clinical presentation of hyperglycemia, insulin resistance, and defects in insulin secretion.

A. Role of the Liver

The role of the liver in the development and expression of NIDDM has been extensively studied.[19-23] The level of fasting hyperglycemia in NIDDM correlates highly with hepatic glucose output. The increased hepatic glucose output appears primarily due to increased gluconeogenesis. Although controversial for many years, accumulated evidence suggests a role for fatty acids in the increased gluconeogenesis. The Randle glucose-fatty acid cycle predicts that increased fatty acid oxidation results in decreased glucose utilization and hyperglycemia. More recent evidence shows that the hyperglycemia is predominantly due to a requirement for increased gluconeogenesis to accompany the fatty acid oxidation. Studies in patients with NIDDM show a strong correlation among fatty acid levels, gluconeogenesis, and fasting hyperglycemia. Animal studies show that inhibition of fatty acid oxidation or reduction in fatty acid levels decreases gluconeogenesis and hyperglycemia. Thus, elevated fatty acid levels and fatty acid oxidation may play an important role in the development and progression of fasting hyperglycemia in NIDDM.

B. Abnormality in Peripheral (Muscle) Glucose Utilization

In most NIDDM patients, however, the earliest detectable abnormality is in peripheral glucose utilization, primarily muscle. This abnormality may be present for years prior to the development of overt hyperglycemia. In fact, this abnormality may occur in individuals who never develop overt diabetes (which requires a decrease in insulin secretion). There is speculation that genetic abnormalities in insulin action resulting in insulin resistance and hyperinsulinemia may contribute to the development of cardiovascular disease even in the absence of diabetes.

C. Reduced and Delayed Response to Elevated Glucose Levels

As mentioned above, abnormalities in insulin secretion are a universal finding and an apparent prerequisite for developing NIDDM. The most common and best characterized abnormality in established NIDDM is a reduced and delayed response to elevated glucose levels.[24] An acute increase in glucose levels delivered to the normal β cell results in an immediate, sharp increase in insulin release (first phase) followed by a slower, progressive increase (second phase). In NIDDM, the first phase response to an i.v. glucose challenge is lost while the second phase is present and frequently increased as a result of the greater hyperglycemia in these patients as compared with controls. Of interest is that first phase insulin release is also lost in the early stages of IDDM prior to the development of hyperglycemia. The response of the NIDDM pancreas to other insulin secretagogues is preserved better than the response to glucose and frequently appears normal. This preservation, however, is in the presence of hyperglycemia in the NIDDM patient, which potentiates the β cell response to other secretagogues. If an arginine stimulus is given to an NIDDM patient whose glucose has been normalized, then typically the response is reduced as compared with controls. Thus, from many studies, the insulin secretion response is reduced in NIDDM. Recent proposals have suggested that glucose itself could be toxic to β cells, as hyperglycemia is harmful to other tissues. Sustained hyperglycemia may desensitize the β cell and this may be one mechanism for reduced responsiveness. Maintenance of euglycemia for a period of time (by exogenous insulin, diet, oral agents) will improve β cell responses to changes in glucose. Of interest is that β cell desensitization may also occur with prolonged exposure to other secretagogues. With chronic sulfonylurea therapy the β cell may cease responding to the agent, but recover after the medication is stopped for a few days.

D. Abnormalities in Insulin and Proinsulin Secretion

Other abnormalities in insulin secretion are also present in NIDDM. Normal insulin secretion occurs in a pulsatile fashion as does secretion of many other hormones. This secretory pattern may enhance the sensitivity of control systems. In patients with NIDDM, in addition to reduction in amplitude of insulin pulses there is a decrease in regularity and less coordination with the glucose changes.[25] Furthermore, in relatives of patients with NIDDM at increased risk for development of the disease, the regular oscillatory pattern of insulin secretion (a pulse every 12 to 15 min) was lost, suggesting that this may be an early abnormality in NIDDM.[25]

An additional abnormality in NIDDM is an increased release of proinsulin.[26-28] Insulin is synthesized in the form of a single-chain precursor, proinsulin, which is proteolytically cleaved in the β cell to form insulin and C peptide. While some uncleaved proinsulin is released normally from the pancreas, and in the fasting state proinsulin comprises a significant percentage of circulating insulin-like material, after a stimulus the great majority of secreted material is insulin. In patients with NIDDM the percentage of proinsulin is increased after a glucose challenge. Since proinsulin has much less biological activity than insulin, this results in a lessened glucose-lowering effect. The reason for the increased release of proinsulin is not known but may simply be due to decreased pancreatic reserves and thus the release of incompletely processed material.

From the above discussion, it is obvious that a number of abnormalities in both insulin secretion and insulin action are present in the patient with established NIDDM. Studies in established disease, however, do not necessarily reflect the initiating abnormality. What, therefore, is the initial defect in NIDDM? The simple and probably correct answer is that there may be multiple initial defects which can result ultimately in the appearance of the clinical entity, NIDDM. Support for the primacy of pancreatic abnormalities can be found both in animal and human studies.[29,30] An animal model which closely, but not completely, mimics the human disease can be produced by partial destruction of β cells by either streptozotocin or partial pancreatectomy. In a study of humans, subjects with previous gestational diabetes who returned to normal or near normal, defects in insulin secretion were more common than defects in insulin action, although both could be found, not necessarily in the same individuals. These studies would suggest that in some individuals a pancreatic defect can be the primary defect in NIDDM.

E. Genetic Alterations

Genetic studies offer supportive evidence for an abnormality in the insulin response system rather than in the insulin secretory process in most individuals.[30,31] NIDDM is a highly hereditary disease, approaching 100% concordance in identical twins. Although initial studies of the insulin gene appeared to show differences between NIDDM and controls, subsequent extensive analyses have failed to find genetic differences. Recent studies, which need confirmation, have suggested that approximately 25% of NIDDM subjects (as compared with 4% of controls) have a specific genetic restriction fragment length polymorphism in the insulin receptor gene. This suggests, although by no means proves, that the control of insulin receptor structure and function may be different in a subpopulation of patients with NIDDM.

As discussed earlier, however, most evidence supports the importance of genetic alterations in insulin action systems (such as glycogen synthase) in the development of NIDDM. Prospective studies in a number of populations at risk for the development of NIDDM show insulin resistance and hyperinsulinemia to be the earliest detectable abnormalities.

In summary, therefore, the primary event in the development of most cases of NIDDM is unknown. Given the heterogeneous nature of NIDDM, multiple initial defects could be present and over time affect other processes. Multiple defects in both insulin secretion and insulin action may be necessary for the clinical expression and the development of NIDDM.[1]

III. MANAGEMENT OF NONINSULIN-DEPENDENT DIABETES MELLITUS

At the present time the management of NIDDM involves the use of four modalities: i.e., diet, exercise, sulfonylureas, and insulin. Dietary therapy remains the cornerstone for the management of NIDDM. A hypocaloric weight reduction diet will, in many cases, restore blood glucose values to normal in the obese patient with NIDDM, at least for a period of time. The efficacy of hypocaloric diets and weight reduction is such that, in many patients, minimal lowering of total body weight will result in significant improvements in blood glucose values. In the mildly hyperglycemic obese individual, a weight loss of as little as 10% may restore glucose tolerance completely to normal. In fact, some studies have shown that institution of an appropriate dietary plan improves blood glucose levels without significant weight loss.[32]

A. Weight Loss Diet

In the thin or normal weight patient with NIDDM a weight loss diet is not indicated, but again, the initial approach to these patients requires institution of an appropriate dietary plan. Other than the importance of hypocaloric intake and weight reduction in the obese patient, specific aspects of dietary management of NIDDM remain controversial and are the subject of a great deal of ongoing investigation. The current recommendations are for a diet relatively high in carbohydrates (50 to 60%) and low in cholesterol and saturated fats.[33]

Some investigators have questioned the high carbohydrate intake as possibly detrimental to patients with a susceptibility to carbohydrate-induced hyperlipidemia and a recent study suggested that a lower carbohydrate diet with an increase in unsaturated fat improved both glucose and lipid levels. The use of simple sugars in the diabetic diet has also been a matter of controversy, and although the current recommendation is that a limited amount of simple sugar may be allowed as part of a meal in patients with NIDDM, others have questioned this as well. The role of dietary fiber in the management of patients with NIDDM also has not been established. While a large intake of fiber may decrease glucose and improve lipids in some patients with NIDDM, particularly those with normal or increased levels of serum insulin, the acceptability and practicality of such a large increase in fiber intake has been questioned. The possible long-term effects of increased fiber intake on other aspects of health, such as bone density, trace minerals, etc., have not been established.[34] As additional information is obtained, adjustments of our approach to patients in terms of their dietary intake will be necessary. In general, however, at the present time the published recommendations of the American Diabetes Association for dietary therapy in patients with NIDDM should be followed.[33] As with any treatment modality, dietary therapy in patients with NIDDM must be individualized and diet adjustments made as necessary for each patient. The assistance of a knowledgeable and experienced dietitian is essential for the appropriate initiation and long-term maintenance of dietary therapy in patients with NIDDM.

B.   Exercise

Exercise is also an essential component for the management of patients with NIDDM.[35] In addition to its beneficial effects on the cardiovascular system, regular exercise is an important adjunct to caloric restriction for weight reduction and is a means to improve insulin sensitivity in the insulin-resistant individual. Current evidence suggests that exercise has an additive effect on weight reduction in the treatment of patients with NIDDM. Although exercise in patients with mild NIDDM may not result in major improvements in glucose levels, studies have shown that glycosylated hemoglobin levels are significantly lower in patients on regular exercise as compared with those who are not. The apparent mechanism for the improvement in insulin sensitivity and glucose levels is an increase in glucose utilization by peripheral tissues, particularly muscle, although there is also an effect on hepatic glucose output. A regular exercise program is an important adjunct to dietary therapy and may result in significant improvement in glucose levels in patients with NIDDM. Recent evidence also suggests that a regular exercise program may delay the development of NIDDM in subjects with genetic predisposition to this disease.

C.   Sulfonylureas

Although biguanides are available in other countries and other oral agents are under investigation, in this country, sulfonylureas remain the only approved pharmacological agents, other than insulin, for the management of blood glucose in patients with NIDDM. The use of sulfonylureas has had a long and checkered history and these agents remain the topic of intense investigation. Although much more remains to be learned about the effects and properties of these agents, particularly in long-term use, our current information allows us to make a rational approach to the use of these materials. In spite of a great deal of investigation, the full mechanism of action of sulfonylureas is not yet known. In general, these agents increase insulin secretion, alter hepatic metabolism, and have peripheral effects on insulin sensitivity and glucose utilization. Which of these is the predominant effect in chronic therapy remains uncertain. Some of this uncertainty may be due to the fact that different sulfonylureas have different effects, or at least have different degrees of effectiveness on the primary mechanisms. Recent studies have clarified some of the differences between the two second-generation oral agents, glyburide and glipizide.[36] While both of these drugs have effects on insulin secretion and on glucose utilization, glyburide appears to have a somewhat greater effect on insulin resistance and on basal insulin levels, while glipizide has less of an effect on insulin action and more of an effect on acute insulin release from the pancreas. The effect of the sulfonylureas on hepatic metabolism may also explain, to some extent, the controversy about the chronic effects of sulfonylurea therapy on insulin secretion.[37] Some studies have suggested that chronic therapy with sulfonylureas does not result in an increase in peripheral insulin levels,[38] whereas others have found a continued increase in insulin levels after several years of sulfonylurea therapy.

The pharmacological properties of sulfonylureas make them an attractive approach to the management of the patient with NIDDM. The increased secretion of insulin and thus the delivery of more insulin to the liver for suppression of hepatic glucose output with less peripheral hyperinsulinemia than with exogenous insulin therapy has many theoretical advantages, including a reduced risk of atherosclerosis. In addition, with their effect on increasing peripheral tissue sensitivity to insulin action, oral agents also improve insulin resistance. Thus, the dual effect of the sulfonylureas result in improvement in both of the known primary abnormalities in NIDDM. In practical clinical use, however, the sulfonylureas may not achieve the theoretical advantages suggested by their pharmacological properties. While a significant number of patients with NIDDM may respond to sulfonylurea therapy and achieve adequate control of their blood glucose levels, many patients do not respond and many more do not achieve totally normal glucose levels with sulfonylureas. In particular, patients who fail to follow dietary and exercise prescriptions may have an inadequate response. Nevertheless, in most patients with NIDDM who do not respond adequately to diet and exercise, a trial of sulfonylureas is indicated.

As with any therapeutic modality, the response to the drugs should be monitored and patients who fail to respond or who respond and subsequently lose that response must have their therapy reevaluated and changes made to bring glucose levels to desired levels. Patient characteristics which indicate a greater likelihood of response to sulfonylureas include normal weight or obese patients over the age of 40 with mild to moderate hyperglycemia and with a relatively recent onset of their disease.

The general approach for using sulfonylureas in the management of patients with NIDDM is to start with the lowest effective dose of either glyburide (2.5 mg) or glipizide (5 mg) and increase the dose every one to two weeks until the desired therapeutic approach is achieved or until the maximum dose is reached. Diet and exercise should continue to be emphasized during the period.

Another approach, especially in elderly patients who are unwilling or unable to take insulin, which has been used by this author is to combine the two second-generation oral agents. This approach is based on the observations that glyburide has greater effects on basal glucose levels and glipizide has greater effects on postprandial levels. Thus, glyburide is given at bedtime and glipizide in the morning. While this needs to be examined in a controlled study, several elderly patients who had failed maximal doses of each separate agent have responded to this combination.

D. Insulin Administration

Insulin, if given in sufficient amounts, will control the blood glucose in essentially all patients with NIDDM. The presence of insulin resistance, however, means that many patients will require relatively large amounts or even very large amounts of insulin for glucose control. Recently, considerable attention has been given to the possible deleterious effects of large amounts of circulating insulin on hypertension and atherosclerotic heart disease.[36,39,40] Insulin may have a direct effect to elevate blood pressure and increase the development of atherosclerosis.[41] The therapeutic role of diet and exercise thus should be stressed even more.

Another consideration for the use of large amounts of insulin is the potential effect of hyperinsulinemia on obesity. One of the most sensitive effects of insulin is to decrease lipolysis in fat cells and thus maintain fat stores.[34] In the obese patient, obviously, an increased weight or increased difficulty in losing weight is not to be desired. Patients on intensive insulin therapy gain significantly more weight than those on conventional insulin therapy.[42] Insulin-treated patients also have more difficulty in losing weight.[34]

Nevertheless, the dangers of chronic hyperglycemia appear to outweigh the theoretical danger of hyperinsulinemia and thus insulin therapy for glucose control in the patient who fails to respond to other therapeutic modalities is indicated. Some patients with NIDDM require insulin therapy from the onset of their disease. In the thin, severely hyperglycemic patient, insulin levels are low and true insulin deficiency exists. These patients all require insulin for control of their hyperglycemia. In the patient with absolute insulin deficiency, multiple injections of insulin with therapeutic programs similar to those used in patients with insulin-dependent diabetes may well be necessary. In patients with significant endogenous insulin secretion and significant hyperinsulinemia, a single daily injection or at least a more simplified therapeutic program may be efficacious. A major abnormality in patients with NIDDM is failure of suppression of hepatic glucose output resulting in rises in glucose overnight, thus morning fasting hyperglycemia. This pattern suggests that insulin therapy in the evening to suppress hepatic glucose output is a rational approach and studies have shown that a single dose of intermediate-acting insulin, either NPH or Lente, given at bedtime, may greatly improve fasting hyperglycemia and result in improved glucose control throughout the day.

While institution of this program should be accompanied by checking early morning (2 to 4 a.m.) glucose levels, this simplified approach may be the best initial therapy for patients whose primary problem is early morning fasting hyperglycemia. This approach, however, should be used with special care in the elderly patient with diabetes and many of these patients may respond better to insulin regimens directed at control of postprandial hyperglycemia. In the elderly patient, particularly those without severe fasting hyperglycemia, an a.m. injection of intermediate insulin may be a better approach. Ultralente insulin to provide a basal insulin supplement may also be used in elderly patients as the sole therapy. All insulin-requiring, and in the opinion of this author, all patients with diabetes, should be on self blood-glucose monitoring, although the frequency of monitoring should be highly individualized.

The combination of insulin and sulfonylureas has received a great deal of attention during the past few years.[43,44] Although this remains an area of controversy, this approach is becoming more popular. Theoretically, the properties of the sulfonylureas by decreasing insulin resistance and increasing endogenous secretion of insulin, thus delivering more insulin directly to the liver, offer a number of advantages over simply continuing to increase peripheral insulin delivery to very large amounts. If adequate control of blood glucose levels could be achieved with lower peripheral insulin levels, one might expect some protection against the deleterious effects of hyperinsulinemia on atherosclerosis, blood pressure, and obesity. Several recent studies support the approach of bedtime intermediate-acting insulin plus daytime suflonylurea therapy. In one study, this approach resulted in lower peripheral insulin levels and less weight gain than insulin alone or daytime insulin and evening oral agents. Our general approach is to initiate bedtime insulin therapy in a patient who has failed diet, exercise, and sulfonylurea alone. If glucose control can be achieved with insulin doses of less than 20 to 30 units per day, insulin alone is used. For those patients whose control is inadequate then a morning oral agent is begun. This is increased slowly to maximum. If control is still not achieved, then the sulfonylurea is stopped and a.m. insulin begun. If control is achieved with less than 70 to 80 units (approximately twice the normal pancreatic output) then insulin alone is used. If not, a sulfonylurea is added, usually at bedtime, and control examined. If the addition of the sulfonylurea has no discernible effect on blood glucose values, then the sulfonylurea should be stopped and insulin dosages increased to achieve glucose control.[20] Several recent studies have supported the approach of bedtime intermediate-acting insulin plus daytime sulfonylurea therapy. In one study, this approach resulted in lower peripheral insulin levels and less weight gain than insulin alone or daytime insulin and evening oral agents.

IV. OVERALL VIEW OF THERAPY

In the therapy of patients with NIDDM, a logical sequence of approaches can thus be formulated. First of all, as in any patient with a chronic disease, therapeutic goals must be established. In the case of diabetes, the therapeutic goal is based on a number of considerations including the patient's motivation and ability, as well as medical considerations. In a patient who has inadequate motivation or insufficient ability to cooperate in the necessary day-to-day management of the disease, the primary approach must be in education and in encouragement of the patient to achieve proper glucose control. These patients may respond better to a simpler approach, even though that achieves less than ideal control, but attempts should be continued to improve the patient's attitude and control over time. In a highly motivated patient, again, education is an essential component, but therapeutic attempts can be pursued more vigorously and usually more successfully.

In the therapy of a patient with NIDDM, it is also frequently helpful to attempt to classify the patient so as to have a better idea of what will be a successful approach. While subclassification of NIDDM is still in its infancy, the staging described by Granner[45] is useful for correlating pathophysiological processes and clinical status. Glucose intolerance or mild

NIDDM (fasting 150 or less) is characterized by insulin resistance, impaired glucose uptake, and hyperinsulinemia. This group, especially if obese, will usually respond to diet and exercise alone. The next stage has further increases in hepatic glucose output, along with peripheral insulin resistance, and some lessening of the endogenous hyperinsulinemia. Sulfonylureas, along with diet and exercise, are appropriate in this group, because of their effect on lessening insulin resistance and increasing endogenous insulin secretion (hepatic delivery of insulin). As NIDDM progresses to the next stage, endogenous insulin secretion decreases further and exogenous insulin is usually required. By considering the stage of the disease and the corresponding pathophysiological abnormalities, a treatment plan can be developed more easily.

Although a full discussion is outside the scope of this presentation, the management of patients with diabetes must include consideration of associated abnormalities. Hypertension is far more common in patients with NIDDM, perhaps secondary to hyperinsulinemia, and a combination of increased blood pressure and diabetes greatly increases the risk for the development and progression of retinal disease, renal disease, atherosclerosis, and other complications. Thus, careful attention to blood pressure control in the patient with diabetes is essential. The specific management of hypertension in diabetes will not be discussed here, other than to emphasize the importance of selecting therapeutic modalities which will not have deleterious effects on either glucose or lipids. Evidence is accumulating that therapy with angiotensin-converting enzyme inhibitors may have particular protective effects on renal function in diabetes.

Attention must also be paid to other risk factors for the development of atherosclerosis. Lipid abnormalities are very common in patients with diabetes and restoration to normal of serum lipid levels is an important goal in the management of patients with diabetes. Other risk factors for the development of atherosclerosis, such as cigarette smoking, must be addressed.

Attention must be paid to the chronic complications of diabetes, and careful assessment of renal function and retinopathy with appropriate therapy is extremely important. Careful attention to foot care in the patient with diabetes may have a greater impact on morbidity and mortality than any single other factor. Thus, extensive patient education and professional monitoring of foot status is an essential component in the management of the patient with diabetes.

It must be recognized and emphasized by the health care professional than NIDDM is a chronic disease and requires a long-term commitment by the care deliverers, the patient, and the patient's family. The importance of education and lifestyle modifications for the successful long-term management of this disease cannot be overemphasized. While the deleterious effects of long-term hyperglycemia and the beneficial effects of glucose control, especially in NIDDM, remain an important area for continued research, sufficient evidence now exists to support the goal of achieving as near normal levels of glucose as possible in all diabetic patients. The Diabetes Control and Complications Trial has clearly shown the importance of glucose control in preventing complications in IDDM. All available information supports this concept in NIDDM as well, with the possible exception of cardiovascular disease. Glucose control should be the goal of all diabetic patients and all individuals involved in the care of these patients.

REFERENCES

1. DeFronzo, R. A., Lilly Lecture, 1987, The triumvirate: β-cell, muscle, liver. A collusion responsible for NIDDM, *Diabetes*, 37, 667, 1988.
2. Hinsworth, H. P. and Kerr, R. B., Insulin-sensitive and insulin-insensitive types of diabetes mellitus, *Clin. Sci.*, 4, 119, 1939.
3. Yalow, R. S. and Berson, S. A., Immunoassay of endogenous plasma insulin in man, *J. Clin. Invest.*, 39, 1157, 1960.

4. Reaven, G. M., Insulin resistance in noninsulin-dependent diabetes mellitus. Does it exist and can it be measured?, *Am. J. Med.*, 74, 3, 1983.

5. Goldfine, I. D., The insulin receptor: molecular biology and transmembrane signalling, *Endocr. Rev.*, 8, 235, 1987.

6. Kasuga, M., Karlsson, F. A., and Kahn, C. R., Insulin stimulates the phosphorylation of the 95,000-dalton subunit of its own receptor, *Science*, 215, 185, 1982.

7. Morgan, D. O., Ho, L., Korn, L. J., and Roth, R. A., Insulin action is blocked by a monoclonal antibody that inhibits the insulin receptor kinase, *Proc. Natl. Acad. Sci. U.S.A.*, 83, 328, 1986.

8. Duckworth, W. C., Insulin degradation: mechanisms, products, and significance, *Endocr. Rev.*, 9, 319, 1988.

9. Arner, P., Einarsson, K., Ewerth, S., and Livingston, J., Studies of the human liver insulin receptor in non-insulin-dependent diabetes mellitus, *J. Clin. Invest.*, 77, 1716, 1986.

10. Arner, P., Pollare, T., Lithell, H., and Livingston, J. N., Defective insulin receptor tyrosine kinase in human skeletal muscle in obesity and type 2 (non-insulin-dependent) diabetes mellitus, *Diabetologia*, 30, 437, 1987.

11. Arsenis, G. and Livingston, J. N., Alterations in the tyrosine kinase activity of the insulin receptor produced by in vitro hyperinsulinemia, *J. Biol. Chem.*, 261, 147, 1986.

12. Caro, J., Ittoop, O., Pories, W. J., Meelheim, D., Flickinger, E. G., Thomas, F., Jenquin, M., Silverman, J. F., Khanzanie, P. G., and Sinha, M. K., Studies on the mechanism of insulin dependent diabetes. Insulin action and binding in isolated hepatocytes, insulin receptor structure, and kinase activity, *J. Clin. Invest.*, 78, 249, 1986.

13. Comi, R. J., Grunberger, G., and Gorden, P., Relationship of insulin binding and insulin-stimulated tyrosine kinase activity is altered in type II diabetes, *J. Clin. Invest.*, 79, 453, 1987.

14. Freidenberg, G. R., Henry, R. R., Klein, H. H., Reichart, D. R., and Olefsky, J. M., Decreased kinase activity of insulin receptors from adipocytes of non-insulin-dependent diabetes subjects, *J. Clin. Invest.*, 79, 240, 1987.

15. Garvey, W. T., Huecksteadt, T. P., Matthaei, S., and Olefsky, J. M., Role of glucose transporters in the cellular insulin resistance of type II non-insulin-dependent diabetes mellitus, *J. Clin. Invest.*, 81, 1528, 1988.

16. Grunberger, G., Zick, Y., and Gorden, P., Defect in phosphorylation in insulin receptors in cells from an insulin-resistant patient with normal insulin binding, *Science*, 223, 932, 1984.

17. Sinha, M. K., Pories, W. J., Flickinger, E. G., Meelheim, D., and Caro, J. F., Insulin receptor kinase activity of adipose tissue from morbidly obese humans with and without NIDDM, *Diabetes*, 36, 620, 1987.

18. Yki-Jarvinen, H., Kubo, K., Zawadzki, J., Lillioja, S., Young, A., Abbott, W., and Foley, J. E., Dissociation of in vitro sensitivities of glucose transport and antilipolysis to insulin in NIDDM, *Am. J. Physiol.*, 253, E300, 1987.

19. Taylor, R. and Agius, L., The biochemistry of diabetes, *Biochem. J.*, 250, 625, 1988.

20. Firth, R. G., Bell, P. M., Marsh, H. M., Hansen, I., and Rizza, R. A., Postprandial hyperglycemia in patients with noninsulin dependent diabetes mellitus. Role of hepatic and extrahepatic tissues, *J. Clin. Invest.*, 77, 1525, 1986.

21. Golay, A., Swislocki, A. L., Chen, Y. D., and Reaven, G. M., Relationship between plasma fatty acid concentration, endogenous glucose production, and fasting hyperglycemia in normal and non-insulin-dependent diabetic individuals, *Metab. Clin. Exp.*, 36, 692, 1987.

22. Reaven, G. M., Chang, H., and Hoffman, B. B., Additive hypoglycemic effects of drugs that modify free fatty acid metabolism by different mechanisms in rats with streptozotocin-indiced diabetes, *Diabetes*, 37, 28, 1988.

23. Chen, Y.-D., Golay, A., Swislocki, A. L., and Reaven, G. M., Resistance to insulin suppression of plasma free fatty acid concentrations and insulin stimulation of glucose uptake in noninsulin-dependent diabetes mellitus, *J. Clin. Endocrinol. Metab.*, 64, 17, 1987.

24. Ward, W. K., Beard, J. C., and Porte, D., Jr., Clinical aspects of islet B-cell function in non-insulin-dependent diabetes mellitus, *Diabetes/Metabolism Reviews*, 2, 297, 1986.

25. Polonsky, K. S., Given, B. D., Hirsch, L. J., Tillil, H., Shapiro, E. T., Beebe, C., Frank, B. H., Galloway, J. A., and Van Cauter, E., Abnormal pattern of insulin secretion in non-insulin dependent diabetes mellitus, *N. Engl. J. Med.*, 318, 1231, 1988.

26. Duckworth, W. C. and Kitabchi, A. E., Direct measurement of plasma proinsulin in normal and diabetic subjects, *Am. J. Med.*, 53, 418, 1972.

27. Ward, W. K., LaCava, E. C., Paquette, T. L., Beard, J. C., Wallum, B. J., and Porte, D., Jr., Disproportionate elevation of immunoreactive proinsulin in type 2 (non-insulin-dependent) diabetes mellitus and in experimental insulin resistance, *Diabetologia*, 30, 698, 1987.

28. Duckworth, W. C. and Kitabchi, A. E., The effect of age on plasma proinsulin in response to oral glucose, *J. Lab. Clin. Med.*, 88, 359, 1976.

29. Weir, G. C., Clore, E. T., Zmachinksi, C. J., and Bonner-Weir, S., Islet secretion in a new experimental model for non-insulin-dependent diabetes, *Diabetes*, 30, 590, 1981.

30. Efentic, S., Hanson, U., Persson, B., Wajnot, A., and Luft, R., Glucose tolerance, insulin release, anti-insulin sensitivity in normal-weight women with previous gestational diabetes mellitus, *Diabetes*, 36, 413, 1987.

31. McClain, D. A., Henry, R. R., Ullrich, A., and Olefsky, J. M., Restriction-fragment-length polymorphism in insulin-receptor gene and insulin resistance in NIDDM, *Diabetes*, 37, 1071, 1988.

32. Streja, D., Boyko, E., and Rabkin, S. W., Nutrition therapy in non-insulin-dependent diabetes mellitus, *Diabetes Care*, 4, 81, 1981.

33. American Diabetes Association, 1986 Position Statement: Nutritional recommendations and principles for individuals with diabetes mellitus, *Diabetes Care*, 10, 126, 1987.

34. Torbay, N., Bracco, E. F., Geliebter, A., Stewart, I. M., and Hashim, S. A., Insulin increases body fat despite control of food intake and physical activity, *Am. J. Physiol.*, 248, R120, 1985.

35. Horton, E. S., Role and management of exercise in diabetes mellitus, *Diabetes Care*, 11, 201, 1988.

36. Groop, L., Wahlin-Boll, E., Groop, P. H., Totterman, K. J., Melander, A., Tolppanen, E. M., and Fyhrqvist, F., Pharmacokinetics and metabolic effects of Glibenclamide and Glipizide in type 2 diabetes, *Eur. J. Clin. Pharmacol.*, 28, 697, 1985.

37. Chen, H., Hamel, F. G., Siford, G., and Duckworth, W. C., Alteration of rat hepatic insulin metabolism by glyburide and glipizide, *J. Pharmacol. Exp. Ther.*, 264, 1293, 1993.

38. Duckworth, W. C., Solomon, S. S., and Kitabchi, A. E., Effect of chronic sulfonylurea therapy on plasma proinsulin levels, *J. Clin. Endocrinol. Metab.*, 35, 585, 1972.

39. Stolar, M. W., Atherosclerosis in diabetes: the role of hyperinsulinemia, *Metab. Clin. Exp.*, 37, 1, 1988.

40. Fournier, A. M., Gadia, M. T., Kubrusly, D. B., Skyler, J. S., and Sosenko, J. M., Blood pressure, insulin, and glycemia in nondiabetic subjects, *Am. J. Med.*, 80, 861, 1986.

41. Falholt, K., Cutfield, R., Alejandro, R., Heiding, L., and Mintz, D., The effects of hyperinsulinemia on arterial wall and peripheral muscle metabolism in dogs, *Metab. Clin. Exp.*, 34, 1146, 1985.

42. DCCT Research Group, Weight gain associated with intensive therapy in the diabetes control and complications trial, *Diabetes Care*, 11, 567, 1988.

43. Lardinois, C. K., Liu, G. C., and Reaven, G. M., Glyburide in non-insulin-dependent diabetes. Its therapeutic effect in patients with disease poorly controlled by insulin alone, *Arch. Int. Med.*, 145, 1028, 1985.

44. Longnekcer, M. P., Elsenhaus, V. D., Leiman, S. M., Owen, O. E., and Boden, G., Insulin and a sulfonylurea agent in non-insulin-dependent diabetes mellitus, *Arch. Int. Med.*, 146, 673, 1986.

45. Granner, D. K. and O'Brien, R. M., Molecular physiology and Genetics of NIDDM, *Diabetes Care*, 15, 369, 1992.

12

Clinical and Metabolic Aspects of Nutrition and Aging

Regina C. Casper and Carol Hutner Winograd

CONTENTS

I. INTRODUCTION

Most studies of nutrition and aging have been carried out in Western countries, where perhaps for the first time in the history of humankind, healthy, nourishing foods are not in short supply. Although substantial differences exist in food preferences and availability and in activity levels among various ethnic and economic groups, most older adults in Western countries are now well nourished.

Considerable evidence exists that cultural trends influence eating patterns. Young people often restrict fat intake to reduce body weight, and middle-age women are increasingly aware of the link between high fat diets and cancer.[1] Hallfrisch et al.[2] reported striking changes in the type and amount of fat consumed from the Baltimore Longitudinal Study of Aging. Fat intake declined from 42 to 34% and cholesterol intake declined 30% in an older population, and both older and younger women reduced their fat intake from 35% to 10 to 15% of total calories.

Since good nutrition is one of the crucial elements for maintaining health and optimal functioning, in this chapter we examine factors which promote or interfere with optimal nutrition for older adults. We consider the psychological and physical contribution to food intake and we review how the aging process affects nutrition under normal and pathological conditions.

II. REGULATION OF APPETITE AND APPETITIVE BEHAVIOR

Increasing age is associated with a decline in sleep, sexuality, and eating. However, large individual differences exist regarding the timing and degree of these functional changes. The regulation of sleep, sexuality, and eating is complex, involving multiple neurotransmitter and neuroendocrine systems as well as the opioid system, and so far not one particular neurotransmitter system has been related with certainty to age-related changes in appetite or eating.[3-5] Based on neuropeptide studies in aging rodents,[6] data have suggested that the decreased appetite associated with aging may be related to a decreased opioid feeding combined with an excess satiety action produced by elevated cholecystokinin secretion (see Chapter 6).[7,8]

Physically healthy and psychologically well-adjusted elderly people show little change in appetite with aging.[9] Low rates of reduced food intake of between 16 to 18% were found in the Health and Nutrition Examination (Ten State) Survey (HANES)[10] for Americans in the Seventies. Similarly, over 90% of an elderly population who participated as control subjects in a depression study (ages 70 to 81 years) asserted they had a good appetite.[11]

Reductions in thirst and water intake were described in 67- to 75-year-old men compared to 20- to 31-year-old men, although osmoreceptor responsiveness and vasopressin plasma levels were higher in old as opposed to the young men.[12] Other changes with aging in fluid regulation are discussed in Chapter 3.

III. SOCIAL FACTORS

The appetite for and appreciation of food depends on taste, aroma, texture, and on sensations of warmth or cold. Beautiful surroundings and cheerful company can substantially enhance the pleasure of eating, therefore it is essential to consider the impact of the social and cultural background on the nutrition of older adults (Table 12-1). Elders from ethnic

TABLE 12-1   Conditions Contributing to Nutritional Problems and Weight Loss in Older People

Social	Psychological	Physical
Immobility	Depression	Chronic disease
Poverty	Loneliness	Drug side effects
Safety considerations	Bereavement	Poor dentition
Lack of transportation	Anxiety	Taste/smell changes
Social isolation	Suspiciousness	Dysphagia
Poor cooking skills	Fat phobia	Loss of appetite
Food fads	Forgetfulness	Loss of vision
Restrictive diets	Dementia	Hyperthyroidism
Inconvenience	Confusion	Cancer
Neglect	Memory loss	Cardiovascular disease
	Alcoholism	

minority populations are growing even more rapidly than the total population of older adults and are projected to be over 20% of those 65-and-over in the U.S. and 40% in California by 2030. Unfortunately, very little research has been published on this topic, but several important clinical issues have been raised in anecdotal and pilot data. Knowledge of the role of acculturation in food preferences is important to understand the nutritional habits of elders who have immigrated to the U.S. Do older immigrants from populations prone to lactose intolerance increase their milk consumption successfully in congregate senior meal programs? Are there effective strategies to prevent the increase of sugar and fat in the diets of elders as they adopt Western lifestyles?

Chronic inadequacy of food choice stemming from adverse social and environmental factors can lead to malnutrition in older persons. These include lack of basic knowledge of the principles of nutrition (especially in widowed men unused to purchasing and preparing food), and social isolation leading to loss of interest in food preparation.[13] Older adults with limited financial resources may be unable to purchase an adequate diet. Urban populations raised on frozen processed meals heated in the microwave oven will be at higher risks for nutritional deficiencies because they will have lost the knowledge on how to prepare and cook a meal from staple food. Their reliance on processed, attractively packaged meals rather than on natural fiber, low-fat, low-calorie bread and vegetables and the preference of fitness fanatics for so-called health foods are just two examples of how earlier eating habits likely will affect nutritional habits in old age. Excess alcohol consumption may be a more common cause of nutritional deficiency than is commonly considered. Elderly alcohol users who drink, rather than eat nourishing foods, may also impair absorption of folic acid and utilization of thiamine.[14] Physical illness and disability may make shopping and food preparation difficult.

The myth that thinness is beautiful and youthful can be perpetuated into old age and lead to severe caloric restrictions without or with excessive exercise in both women and men. Cholesterol phobia, which at its worst results in elimination not only of animal fat but of all fat from the diet, can impair absorption of fat-soluble vitamins and commonly leads to weight loss and occasionally to excessive weight loss.

IV. EMOTIONAL AND MENTAL DISTURBANCES

Emotional distress and mental disturbances, notably confusion and depression, may render elderly persons incapable of providing themselves with adequate nutrition and may be associated with lack of motivation or interest in food. An increasing number of elderly persons are now living alone; even in Japan, with a tradition of reverence for the older generation, the number of aged people living alone has tripled.[15]

A. Depression

The most common cause of anorexia, which accounts for weight loss in the elderly aside from those attributable to organic illness, are depressive feelings or a depressive disorder characterized by feelings of sadness, a loss of a sense of pleasure, loss of interest and efficacy, motor retardation, and/or anxiety.[16] Between 5 to 20% of the elderly in the U.S. have been estimated to be depressed.[17] Among the diagnoses for unexplained weight loss, depression was more common than cancer.[18] Depression may underlie somatic complaints and among older adults is more often associated with memory loss and cognitive impairment. Less commonly, a sense of suspicion or paranoid tendencies may lead to avoidance of food in the false belief that food may be unsafe or poisoned. Sheikh and Yesavage[19] have developed a 15-item Mood Scale for assessing depression which excludes physical symptoms, and hence is useful for assessing depressive symptoms in the physically well and the physically sick elderly population.

B. Cognitive Function

Healthy, active older people show only small decrements on tests of cognitive function. Nevertheless, nutritional factors may subtly affect cognition. A significant association was observed between the bottom fifth and tenth percentile plasma levels of Vitamin C, B_{12}, and riboflavin and performance on cognitive tests controlling for age, gender, and level of education, but no relationship to overall nutritional intake.[20] Significant relationships were also reported between plasma thiamin, riboflavin, and iron levels and EEG parameters in healthy individuals over 60 years of age.[21] Dementia and confusion are not uncommon in the physically sick hospitalized elderly. If dementia is suspected, a simplified cognitive mental status examination, the Mini-Mental State, which requires 5 to 10 min to administer, provides a reliable screen for cognitive deficits.[22]

A number of studies have documented cholinergic deficits in Alzheimer Disease.[23] Since the severity of cholinergic cell loss has been correlated with memory and cognitive impairment, attempts have been made through nutrients to stimulate the cholinergic system. One approach has been to increase precursor molecules for acetylcholine synthesis through supplementation with choline, lecithin, and phosphatidyl choline. Some studies have shown temporary improvement.[24] Winograd et al.[25] documented that the nutritional intake and nutritional status of moderately impaired Alzheimer patients who lived in the community were comparable to healthy age-matched controls. Others reported increased energy intake in female patients hospitalized with Alzheimer's disease despite a low body weight and no change in energy expenditure compared to elderly women living at home, suggesting a hypermetabolic state.[26]

V. ENERGY INTAKE AND BODY COMPOSITION

Because nutrient needs of older persons have not been adequately studied, specific standards for the older population have not been developed.[27] Existing standards fail to account fully for changes in nutrient need associated with aging. In the U.S., recommended daily dietary allowances (RDAs) for adults are estimated for two age ranges: 23 to 50 and over 50.[28] Nutritional requirements may change dramatically between the ages of 50 and 95. For instance, the diet of 65- to 97-year-old Dutch lacto-ovo-vegetarians was found to be adequate in micronutrients and nutrient density, but deficient in zinc, iron, vitamin B_{12} and, remarkably, in water intake.[29] Recommendations for daily nutrient and vitamin intake based on RDAs adapted for older adults[30] are presented in Table 12-2.

The most important factor regulating energy intake is energy expenditure. Energy expenditure consists of two principal components: basal metabolic rate and activity level. The World Health Organization recommends for older adults an RDA of 1.5 times the resting energy expenditure, thus expecting little decline in activity. This estimate may be too high in view of

TABLE 12-2   Recommendations for Nutrient Intake[27,28,33,115]

Nutrient	RDA	Additional recommendations	Comments
Energy (kcal)	1200–2000 (Women) 1650–2450 (Men)	25 kcal/kg ideal body weight ± 20% to 30% for activity + addition for disease	Nutrient-dense food is preferred; limit refined carbohydrates and fat
Protein	46 gm (Women) 58 gm (Men) 0.8 gm/kg/Body weight	1.0–1.25 gm/kg body weight	With substandard weight increase to 1.5 gm/kg/body weight
Carbohydrate	None	50–60% of total caloric requirement. Minimum 50–100 g to prevent ketosis	Complex carbohydrates preferable to refined carbohydrates for improved glucose tolerance and lipoprotein synthesis
Fat	None	No more than 35% of total calories. Polyunsaturated fatty acids <10% of total energy; monounsaturated fats 10% of total energy	Fat intake may inversely correlate with lifespan
Vitamin A	2,500 IU Retinol, 2,500 IU – 5,000 IU carotene or 800 retinol equivalents		Deficiencies occur with low-fat diets, mineral oil as laxative, or steatorrhea
Vitamin A μg RE	1000 RE = 1 μg retinol or 6 μg betacarotene retinol equivalents		
B Vitamins:			Changes in mucous membranes and tongues of elderly patients seen in deficiency state
Thiamine	0.5 mg/1,000 kcal or at least 1 mg/d 1.0 mg Women 1.2 mg Men	Higher requirements may be necessary due to alcohol consumption	Deficiency associated with poverty, disease, and alcoholism causes ascending symmetric polyneuritis. Gastric secretions may inactivate thiamine: (1) absent hydrochloric acid; (2) altered intestinal flora bind thiamine
Riboflavin	0.6 mg/1,000 kcal or at least 1.2 mg/d women, 1.4 mg/d men	Base riboflavin on protein allowance rather than on calory allowances as in RDA	Close relationship between riboflavin and protein metabolism
Niacin	6.6 Niacin equivalents/ 1,000 kcal or at least 13 niacin equivalents/day, 13 mg women, 16 mg men		Deficiency causes intestinal hypermotility
Pyridoxine	2.2 mg (Men) 2.0 mg (Women)	2 mg 0.02 mg/gm protein	More than half of older adults consume <70% RDA
Folate	400 μg	100 mg	Megaloblastic anemia in deficiency; B_{12} and iron deficiencies interfere with folic acid utilization. Deficiency attributed to inadequate intake, destruction by cooking, or increased tissue demands

TABLE 12-2 (continued)   Recommendations for Nutrient Intake[27,28,33,15]

Nutrient	RDA	Additional recommendations	Comments
Vitamin B$_{12}$	3.0 μg	2–4 mg	Dietary intake varies considerably, no impairment of absorption
Vitamin C	60 mg	36 mg	Dietary intake varies considerably. Sublingual redness and increased vascularization in chronic deficiency may relate to GI bleeding, impaired wound healing, atherosclerosis, arthritis, and diverticula of colon. Levels to prevent scurvy much lower than those needed for tissue saturation
Vitamin D	200 IU 5 μg	600–800 IU. Sunlight and intact hepatic and renal function needed for *in vivo* conversion	Dietary intake often low, marginal status common Osteomalacia in deficient state, adequate intake needed to maintain bone health and decrease risk of osteomalacia
Vitamin E (mg a -TE)	α - tocopherol 10 equivalents 1 α -TE = 1ng D - α- tocopherol		Antioxidant, may play a role in prevention of cardiovascular and neoplastic disease
Calcium	800 mg	1,500 mg after menopause in women	Chronic deficiency leads to osteoporosis. Calcium absorption impaired with fat intake >150 or<50 gm/day; optimum with fat intake between 100–150 gm
Iron	10 mg	10–12 mg	Decreased iron absorption with achlorhydria. Vitamin C necessary for optimal iron and mobilization from transferrin to ferritin
Sodium	1,100–3,300 mg	Decrease to minimize fluid retention and blood pressure elevation	Dehydration may lead to hypernatremia. Sodium deficiency uncommon because kidneys preserve sodium unless vomiting, diarrhea, or excessive sweating occur
Potassium	1,875–5,625 mg	65–150 mEq/day, maybe higher if on potassium-losing diuretics	Deficiency occurs with loss of intestinal fluid, purgatives, posttrauma or surgery. Intake <60 mEq/d show normal serum K but depletion of whole body K as evidenced by decreased grip strength and minor psychiatric symptoms
Trace minerals	Estimated safe and adequate daily dietary intakes		Toxicity may occur when consumed in excess

TABLE 12-2 (continued) Recommendations for Nutrient Intake[27,28,33,15]

Nutrient	RDA	Additional recommendations	Comments
Manganese	2.5–5.0 mg		
Molybdenum	0.15-0.5		Unlikely to cause nutritional disease
Copper	2.0–3.0		Deficiency may be tied to age-related disease
Zinc	15 mg	30 mg/day	Higher levels can be toxic and cause renal failure
Fluoride	1.5–4.0		
Selenium	0.05–0.2	Deficiencies may cause clinical diseases	Associated with antioxidant systems
Chromium	0.05–0.2		Associated with glucose tolerance
Silicon			Associated with bone health
Fluids	None	1 ml/kcal or 5 to 8 glasses of fluid or enough to provide 1 to 1.5 quarts urine volume/24 hours.	Decreased thirst mechanism, and total body water decreases with aging. Chronic illness, familial, and cultural habits may discourage water drinking.

the fact that the energy intake of older men between 65 to 74 years old is nearly a third less (2100 to 2300 cal/day) than that of men between 24 to 34 years old (2700 cal/day).[31-33]

Cross-sectional studies have shown that total caloric requirements diminish with increasing age. Men who participated in the Baltimore Longitudinal Study had age-related decrements in caloric intake beginning in their forties due to decreases in basal metabolism and reduced energy needs because of greatly reduced physical activity.[34] A 3-cm reduction in height was observed between men aged 35 to 44 years and men aged 65 to 74 years, but weight showed no change. In contrast, weight declined by nearly 7 kg in those 75 to 99 years old. Strikingly, energy expenditure, expressed per unit of body weight, declined from 30 to 60 years of age, but changed little thereafter.

A. Reduction in Lean Body Mass

Several factors account for diminished caloric requirements with age. First, as lean body mass decreases the basal metabolic rate drops, decreasing caloric need (especially in sedentary individuals) (Chapter 5). Reductions in food intake with old age have been shown to be closely associated to a decline in lean body mass and energy expenditure, suggesting normal adaptation of the appetite regulating mechanisms).[2,34] The age-related loss of metabolically active skeletal muscle[35] can be modified by exercise.[36,37] As energy needs begin to decrease around age 40 along with physical activity levels, the contribution of a reduction in basal oxygen consumption due to age per se is difficult to determine.

Advancing age is associated with changes in body composition, including decreased lean body mass, increased fat mass, decreased total body water, and decreased bone density. Several studies have reported a decline in lean body mass with age, but an increase in body fat.[38-40] As muscle mass declines, increases in less metabolically active adipose tissue also lead to lowered caloric need.[41-44] A decline in lean body mass with aging has been reported from cross-sectional studies and, if significant, would have important implications for muscle strength, mobility, and respiratory function. Swerdloff et al.[45] have suggested that falling androgen levels may contribute to the decrease in muscle mass. By contrast, Durnin[46] showed that once men exceeded a Body Mass Index (BMI) of 23, their fat mass remained the same regardless of age — while in women, fat mass increased proportionately to the BMI. Slight increases in percentage of body fat measured by impedance analysis were recently reported between the ages of 20 to 39 years and 40 to 64 years, but no difference between ages 40 to 64, 65 to 74, and 75 to 84 for either males or females.[40] Over age 85, the percentage of body fat was significantly lower compared to all other age groups.

Chronic conditions common among the aged such as obesity, diabetes, and heart failure may affect dietary intake. One study, estimating an overall decline in energy intake of 19% between the ages of 70 and 80, suggests that disease and disability may be the most significant contributing factors.[47]

B. Decline in Activity

Older adults burn fewer calories because of lower activity levels. Mobility and the amount of physical activity is probably the most critical factor affecting nutritional intake and status among older adults.[46] Older laborers or physically active people can eat more without gaining weight than men in their thirties and forties with sedentary occupations. Two-thirds of the decline in nutrient intake in older populations is attributable to reduced physical activity.[34] Rural elderly French women consumed daily nearly 500 calories more than their urban counterparts, presumably because of their greater physical activity.[48] Two groups of Dutch women, aged 60 to 79 years, with different activity levels but similar nutrient intakes, differed significantly in body weight. Physically active women weighed on average 65 kg as compared with 77 kg in sedentary women, who had a higher percentage of body fat.[49,50] Increasing physical activity levels in elderly people does contribute significantly to increased energy expenditure and, hence, to improved nutritional status. A combination of pathological factors, life-long frailty,[51] immobility, a sedentary lifestyle, and the presence of acute and chronic disease in the elderly can result in muscle weakness or disuse atrophy.

C. Longitudinal Studies

In free-living elderly persons studied in the Aging Process Study of New Mexico,[52] nutrient intake, anthropometric parameters, and biochemical markers remained relatively constant over a 9-year period between 1980 and 1989. For men, body weight remained stable but their energy intake decreased, especially fat intake. The findings suggest either a change in body composition with an increase in fat mass or decreased activity levels. The small amount of weight loss in women could be accounted for by a progressive decrease in fat intake, roughly balanced by an increase in percent of energy from carbohydrate intake. These findings are similar to the Euronut Seneca Study,[9] where women showed a significant decrease in weight over time with little change in energy or protein intake.

In the New Mexico aging study, men showed no significant weight changes over time, whereas women lost 0.14 kg/year. Both men and women lost about the same in height, ~0.20 cm/year.[52] These findings suggest that temporal changes in body weight with age ought to be reported not only as actual weight in kilograms, but be standardized for height: kg/m^2 = body mass index (BMI).

Increasing awareness about the contribution of psychosocial conditions to good nutrition and metabolic homeostasis has resulted in the design of studies which give as much weight to living conditions and to the social context as to biological measures. The Euronut Investigators SENECA Project,[9] which began in 1988 to study aging in birth cohorts born between 1912 and 1919 from 12 participating countries, is an example of such a prospective study. More than 60% of the men were married or lived with a partner, whereas more than 50% of the women were widowed. Over 90% lived in private homes. More than 50% had a child who lived in the vicinity. About 50% of the men, but few women, smoked regularly. A third among men and slightly fewer among women had a drink every day.

In these studies, mean body weight ranged from 70.1 ± 15.4 to 78.2 ± 10.7 kg in men and from 56.8 ± 8.1 to 71.4 ± 11.4 kg in women, with subjects from Northern European towns being taller than subjects from Southern towns. Subjects born in 1917 to 1918 were on average 1.3 to 1.7 cm taller than those born in 1913 to 1914. More than 90% of the elderly ate at home and had a cooked meal daily. Specific diets were used by less than 25%, and were mostly low-fat, low-salt diets with no differences between the sexes. Vitamin B_6 deficiency, estimated from plasma levels, was observed in 23.3%, as opposed to 2.7% for vitamin B_{12} deficiency, and 5 to 25% for vitamin E deficiency. Folic acid and vitamin A plasma levels were found to be adequate. Mediterranean countries had on average lower serum lipid levels. Females had more subcutaneous fat than males when measured by triceps skinfold thickness, but women had a lower waist/hip ratio. Despite a high prevalence (59 to 92%) of chronic disease, most people judged their health to be good. Mean energy intake for men ranged from 8.2 MJ (IMJ = 240 Kcal.) in Switzerland to 12.7 MJ in Poland and, for women, 6.3 MJ in Switzerland and Portugal to 10.9 MJ in Poland, although women spent more hours per day on physically active tasks — 2.6 to 3.9 h/d vs. 0.7 to 2.3 h/d for men.

VI. METABOLIC REGULATION

Aging changes in thyroid function are discussed on Chapter 5 but a direct correlation between thyroid hormone levels and basal metabolism in not yet available. Reduction in growth hormone secretion resulting in lower serum insulin-like growth factor (IGF-I) levels may be involved in many of the catabolic changes[53] such as muscle atrophy, osteoporosis, and sleep disturbances (Chapter 3). It is likely that the reduction in other systems such as lowered sex steroids and changes in opioid mediated systems contributes to the changes seen with aging.[54,55] The functional consequences of hormonal decline are most apparent in women, in whom the reduction in sexual hormones associated with the menopause results in skin, body composition, and bone density changes (Chapters 7 and 8). Controversy exists whether a high calcium intake prevents osteoporosis, especially in fair-skinned and light women (Chapter 13). Hegsted has argued persuasively that the recommended RDA of 1500 mg Ca/day for elderly women to prevent osteoporosis is not supported by sound data, and that protein intake, exercise, and/or estrogens might be equally important in the prevention of osteoporosis as calcium supplementation.[27]

Overall, with good health, a nutritionally complete diet, and an active lifestyle, the aging process up to 75 to 80 years has minor consequences for body composition. Beyond 80 to 85 years, a decreased food intake and weight loss, even in the absence of physical illness, is commonly observed.[34] Nonetheless, Evans[56] has shown a lasting capacity of men and women up to 96 years to increase muscle strength and size by more than 200% through high-resistance exercise.

A. Weight Loss

Weight loss in ambulatory elderly is uncommon. In a family clinic setting, 45/10,000 cases were identified with weight loss exceeding 75% of baseline body weight in a 6-month period.[18] In a quarter of the cases, two-thirds of them male, the etiology remained unknown; 18% were suffering from depression and 16% from cancer, and 9% each from hyperthyroidism and medication side effects. Poor food intake and cholesterol phobia accounted for weight loss in 4% of the cases. In a series of 650 cases of benign gastric ulcer, 80% of the patients lost 10 pounds or more.[57] Inasmuch as it is uncommon, any significant weight loss in the elderly deserves careful investigation to determine its origin.

B. Excessive Weight and Obesity

In the U.S., older adults are more frequently overweight than underweight. McGandy et al.[34] observed in the late 1960s a rise in the Body Mass Index (BMI) for males and females between the ages of 40 to 64 years, from 26.5 to 28.6 and 24.4 to 27.2, respectively, and a slow decline between ages 75 to 84, with a significant loss after age 85 (to 20.4 and 21.6, respectively). One quarter of older men are obese, i.e., their weight exceeds 15% of standard weight for age and height, whereas 33% of white women and nearly double this percentage of elderly black women are obese.[58] Survival is highest in the moderately obese,[59] whereas a low normal weight is associated with mortality rates similar to those found in subjects who are more than 100% overweight. Obesity is associated with a high incidence of diabetes mellitus, hypertension, cardiovascular disease, and stroke, but a low incidence of osteopenia and osteoporosis in females, despite often significantly reduced activity levels.

Overfeeding during the growth period during early life may affect the severity and timing of cardiovascular disease and of tumors, in particular, breast cancer and brain pathology. Epidemiological studies have linked excessive weight and fat intake to colon, prostate, breast, and endometrial cancer.[60] Rates of colon cancer have risen sharply in Japan, paralleling a nearly threefold increase in fat intake, whereas breast cancer rates in Japanese women have risen only slightly. A decreased energy intake in early life may reduce the incidence of breast cancer rates, since in the U.S. and Europe a high correlation has been observed between women's adult height and national cancer rates.[61] Obesity and an excessive intake of nutrients decrease immunocompetence.[62] Hyperglycemia, hyperlipidemia, and altered levels of insulin, glucagon, cortisol, and ACTH may in part be responsible for the impaired immune response.

C. Caloric Restriction

In animals (rodents), the beneficial effects on longevity from restricted feeding have been known for a long time.[63,64] Despite the reproducibility of this effect, the precise mechanisms underlying increased survival rates and reduction in tumor rates are not known. Caloric restriction has profound effects — lowering core body temperature, slowing metabolic processes, and decreasing metabolic rate.[65] Significant changes in the hypothalamic-pituitary system result in an overall decline in hormones and probably are responsible for the reduction of metabolic processes,[66] the changes in temperature regulation, and the delay in maturation and reproduction.

In humans the effects of chronic underfeeding in relation to longevity have not been studied systematically and are unlikely to be studied soon. Aside from ethical problems of depriving an infant of food, the effects of chronic caloric deprivation on the growing infant might be quite different from the rodent. Furthermore, a prospective study would require data collection for up to 80 or 100 years. Since infant monkeys have growth characteristics similar to those of the human infant, the study of caloric deprivation in primates might be a first step towards evaluating differences in survival rates.

VII. ORAL AND GASTROINTESTINAL FACTORS AFFECTING NUTRITION AND AGING

A. Taste and Smell

Physical and physiological changes that impair food intake include loss of teeth and reduced taste or smell. Nearly a third of persons between 65 to 75 years, about 44% of those 75 to 85 years of age, and 55% of those older than 85 years have lost all teeth.[67] In the Boston Nutritional Survey, 18 to 19% of community-dwelling older persons and 36 to 40% of institutionalized men and women reported problems chewing, biting, and/or swallowing food.[68] In Pacific Polynesian countries, dental and visual impairments are the most common health problems reported by older people.[69] Both of these are likely to interfere with nutritional intake.

Several studies suggest that taste can be adversely affected by age.[70,71] However, the methodology used in studies on age-related olfactory and taste changes has been questioned since many did not control for nutritional status or gender.[72] Several kinds of taste changes have been reported with aging such as mild dysgeusia (i.e., perversion of the sense of taste), taste threshold elevations, and loss of taste sensitivity at high substrate concentrations.[70] Salty and bitter taste are more affected than the sweet taste. Interestingly, the taste for sweet is also preserved longest in undernutrition in young people.[73] Sucrose and NaCl solutions were rated as more pleasant by older people than by the young.[72] Since a significant number of the very old did not even perceive salt at low concentrations, problems in taste could result in overuse of sugar or salt. However, only small losses for strong concentrations were found. Subjects with natural teeth showed a higher threshold than those with upper and lower dentures. Natural dentition, therefore, seems to contribute to a background taste, suggesting that good dental hygiene could improve taste perception.[74]

The influence of plasma levels of trace elements on nutrition has been studied in a limited manner. Zinc supplementation for 3 months raised zinc hair levels in the elderly, with no improvement in sweet and salt detection thresholds.[75] In contrast, zinc supplementation in refeeding anorexia nervosa patients improved taste acuity.[73] Despite the documentation of structural changes, such as loss of taste buds or papillae in the elderly, the functional taste changes overall appear minor and these can easily be compensated for by spicing foods with herbs in addition to condiments.[76]

Advancing age reduces the perceived intensity of olfactory sensations, thereby reducing the ability to detect odors. Smell seems dulled more than taste sensations.[77] In young people, repeated presentations decreased the pleasant sensation for menthol. Failure of older people to show this decrease suggests a decline in suprathreshold perceptions of odorants.[71] Little is known about age-related changes in the sensations of warmth, pungency, or cold.

Saliva is affected by estrogenic activity. The decrease in estrogen associated with menopause may play an etiologic role in the decreased quantity and quality of saliva in Sjogren's Syndrome.[78] Since saliva is necessary for upper GI function, the decreased saliva may lead to poor buffering of acid or acid reflux.

B. Gastrointestinal Tract

Aging may be associated with changes in gut motility. Esophageal motility disorders may result in swallowing difficulties of both solids and liquids and lead to aspiration pneumonia. Gastric emptying may be delayed and the physiology of gastrointestinal peptides that regulate food intake and modulate energy metabolism (Chapters 6 and 10) may be altered.[79]

Distinguishing normal aging from degenerative changes or the effects of the gastrointestinal diseases may be difficult. In one study of asymptomatic subjects (mean age 83 years), oral abnormalities such as difficulty transferring and controlling the food bolus occurred in 63%, pharyngeal/esophageal retention of the bolus and cricopharyngeal dysfunction in 60%, and motor abnormalities of the esophagus in 39% of the subjects. Only 16% were judged to swallow normally.[80] Dysphagia (i.e., difficulty in swallowing) may lead to anxiety at meal times and reduction in food intake to avoid symptoms. Incidence of achalasia (i.e., failure to relax the smooth muscles of the gastrointestinal tract), increases with age; it presents more insidiously in older patients and less often with chest pain than in younger patients.[81,82] Older patients with gastroesophageal reflux disease (GERD) typically have less chest pain and heartburn than younger patients. GERD can lead to esophagitis and Barrett's Metaplasia which, in turn, is associated with the development of adenocarcinoma.

The incidence of achlorhydria (i.e., absence of hydrochloric acid from gastric secretions) increases with age.[83] Both *Helicobacter pylori* infection and nonsteroidal antiinflammatory drugs (NSAIDS) are now recognized as predisposing factors for peptic ulcer disease associated with more complications in older patients. This is particularly true in women taking NSAIDS, who are at risk for ulcer complications and death. In one series, 10% presented clinically with gastric outlet obstruction.[81] Peptic ulcer is the leading cause of hemorrhage in patients 80 years and older. In another study of older patients requiring surgery for peptic ulcer disease, 92% had emergency surgery, 85% had duodenal ulcer disease, 50% had ulcer perforations, and more than half had serious postoperative complications.[85] Peptic ulcer is the leading cause of hemorrhage in patients 80 years and older. Patients who died from hemorrhage were more likely to have bleeding peptic ulcers and significant comorbid disease.[86] NSAIDS may cause distal small bowel ulcerations which may present as occult blood in the stool, recurrent abdominal pain, or perforation. NSAIDS also produce a syndrome resembling inflammatory bowel disease presenting with proctitis, segmental colitis, or discrete ulcerations throughout the colon. Quiescent, preexisting inflammatory bowel disease can also be reactivated by NSAIDS.[84]

C. Diarrhea

Patients aged 70 and over account for 50% of deaths due to diarrhea. At particular risk are older white women living in long-term care facilities. About half of the nonambulatory institutionalized patients who present with fecal soiling actually have fecal impaction. Medications, both prescription and over-the-counter products, are the commonest reversible causes of diarrhea in older patients, e.g., antibiotics, anticholinergics, antiinflammatory agents, antacids, and cardiovascular chemotherapeutic agents.

Bacterial overgrowth occurs in patients with anatomic abnormalities of the small intestine, e.g., blind loop syndrome or jejunal diverticulosis, or impaired intestinal motility, e.g., scleroderma. Elderly patients may present with impaired fat absorption as a result of bacterial overgrowth.[83]

D. Abdominal Pain

Abdominal pain syndromes may differ in older patients, perhaps related to a decrease in endogenous opiates, impairment of nerve conduction, and/or decreased sensitivity to pain. The prevalence of underlying conditions also differs. For example, cholecystitis occurred in 20% of patients aged 50 and over presenting with acute abdominal pain compared to 5% inpatients under 50. Because acute appendicitis may present with muted abdominal signs, gangrene and perforation are more common in older patients. One study found that the preliminary diagnosis of the etiology of acute abdominal pain was incorrect in up to two-thirds of the cases. Acute mesenteric ischemia and intestinal obstruction are additional causes of abdominal pain in older adults. One-quarter of patients presenting with acute intestinal obstruction have incarcerated umbilical, inguinal, or femoral hernias. Other causes include adhesions, inflammation, gallstones, colonic volvulus, and tumors. Many older adults complain of excessive flatus, which can be caused by swallowed air, malabsorbed carbohydrates, and/or disordered colonic motility.[87]

Pancreatic cancer, whose prevalence increases with age, often presents with painless jaundice or unexplained weight loss. Chapters 10 and 11 address aging and the pancreatic influences on insulin metabolism, while Chapter 13 addresses osteoporosis and calcium metabolism.

VIII. MALNUTRITION

Protein-energy malnutrition among older patients consists of two subtypes: (1) primary, in which an otherwise well patient suffers from inadequate nutrient intake; and (2) secondary, in which a patient with acute or chronic illness becomes malnourished due to an interaction of nutrient intake, nutrient needs, and underlying illness.

The prevalence of malnutrition among older adults varies depending on the setting and definition and ranges from 0 to 15% of ambulatory outpatients, 5 to 12% of homebound patients, 35 to 65% of hospitalized patients, and 25 to 60% of institutionalized patients.[88] Epidemiologic studies of older adults report intake less than 60% of the recommended dietary allowances for iron, riboflavin, nicotinic acid, calcium, vitamins C and D, folate, potassium, zinc, and magnesium.[10,89]

Disorders of heart, lungs, kidney, and liver can lead to anorexia (i.e., lack or loss of appetite for food) and cachexia (i.e., general ill health and malnutrition), with consequent nutrient deficiency. Patients with signs of protein-energy malnutrition have higher rates of morbidity and mortality than those with normal nutritional parameters.[90-92]

A. Illness and Hospitalization Effects on Nutrition

Marginal nutritional states can be aggravated by comorbid (i.e., associated) illnesses. Although specific clinical syndromes may be absent, elderly patients may manifest subclinical and nonspecific signs of malnutrition. Because physicians have traditionally been poorly trained in nutrition, they may be unaware that protein-energy malnutrition and its associated apathy may be a classic presenting feature in treatable diseases among older adults.[93] In hospital patients not only did preexisting deficiencies go unrecognized and untreated but also, perhaps most disturbing, malnutrition worsened during hospitalization; of patients admitted with adequate nutritional status, 75% developed nutritional deficiencies during hospitalization.[91] Although protein-energy malnutrition is common, it is rarely recognized or treated.[94]

Malnutrition associated with acute illness produces physiologic stress with some of the following consequences:

- The relative insensitivity of fat and muscle cells to insulin leads to decreased glucose uptake and storage.
- Glucagon, corticosteroid, and catecholamine levels increase.
- Fatty acid mobilization inhibited by elevated insulin levels leads to accelerated protein catabolism for gluconeogenesis and nitrogen loss.
- Acute illness raises the demand for protein synthesis.
- Protein depletion in acutely ill patients demands increased intake of amino acids, glucose, electrolytes, and water.
- Fever, proliferation of fibroblasts and polymorphonuclear leukocytes, tumors, and protein synthesis increase glucose demand, while the central nervous system, red blood cells, and renal medulla continue their need for glucose.
- Prolonged disruption of the body's amino acid "pool" for gluconeogenesis accelerates protein waste production due to primary failure of protein synthesis.[95]

Although protein depletion demands increased intake of amino acids, glucose, electrolytes, and water, loss of appetite associated with illness and dietary limitations imposed by X-ray preparation and perioperative status may inhibit intake. Severe protein-energy malnutrition may rapidly follow acute illness, affecting virtually every organ system. Weight loss correlates with loss of organ mass and impaired organ function. Cardiac wasting and electrocardiographic changes may occur.[96] Respiratory muscular weakness and atrophy also occur, impairing clearance of secretions and decreasing vital capacity and minute ventilation.[97]

Malnourished inpatients who were older than the normal weight inpatients had higher resting energy expenditure (REE) calculated for lean body mass.[98] Patients with inflammations or after recent surgery who have higher REE suffer severe undernutrition without caloric replacement.

IX. DRUG-NUTRIENT INTERACTIONS

Drug-nutrient interactions may reduce the intended therapeutic response to a drug, cause acute or chronic drug toxicity, or impair the patient's nutritional status. The frequent presence of preexisting impairment of nutritional status places older persons at greater risk from the adverse nutritional impact of medications. Medications such as corticosteroids, immunosuppressants, hypocholesterolemics, and antihypertensive and antiseizure agents, often taken by the elderly, affect nutrition (Table 12-3). Nutritional supplements, e.g., calcium and magnesium, can inhibit tetracycline absorption, as can food. The acidity of urine, which is affected by diet, may affect the excretion of drugs: a high protein (high acid diet) may enhance the excretion of weak bases, whereas a low protein (high alkaline diet) may enhance excretion of weak acids. Renal failure that also deplete nutrients represents another risk for drug-induced deficiencies, particularly mineral depletions. Thiazides and loop diuretics deplete potassium as does laxative abuse.[99] Gastrointestinal disease may affect absorption of fat-soluble vitamins, folic acid, and B_{12}.

Another cause of increased risk for elderly patients is their high rate of multiple nonprescription and prescription drug use. Drug-drug interactions are caused by multiple drug use, often precipitated by multiple physicians who are unaware of all the medications being taken by the patient. Many medications in common use among older patients, both prescription and nonprescription, may cause xerostomia (i.e., dryness of the mouth) and GI side effects. Older persons may self-medicate with nonprescription and prescription medications. Not uncommonly, they may use medications saved from previous prescriptions or borrow pills from family or friends who have "the same" condition. Adverse drug reactions may lead to anorexia and nausea, which can impair nutritional intake. The serotonin re-uptake inhibitors (SRIs) are being widely prescribed now for the treatment of depression because they do not have anticholinergic side effects. However, a recent study of fluoxetine documented highly significant anorexia and weight loss and marginally significant increased mortality in geriatric medical patients taking fluoxetine compared to either depressed patients on no medications or on anticholinergic agents.[100] This study raises concern about the use of SRIs in medically compromised older adults, particularly those below "ideal" body weight.

X. NUTRITIONAL ASSESSMENT

A profile of food-related behavior (e.g., appetite, vomiting, elimination, food choices) is the cornerstone of the nutritional history. Psychosocial factors that may influence nutrition need to be addressed (e.g., depression, financial status, and living situation). The physician evaluates the impact of underlying disease (e.g., malignancy, weight changes, liver or renal failure) and impaired self-care abilities (e.g., difficulty in shopping or preparing food), and any changes in food intake, weight, and performance of activities of daily living are recorded. Evidence of deficient nutrition are identified in the physical examination (e.g., skin lesions, jaundice, muscle wasting, loss of fat stores, edema, ascites, cheilosis, glossitis) and checks for specific signs of vitamin and mineral deficiencies. Indexing body composition to knee height as an index of stature revealed loss of lean body mass more accurately than body height.[101] Quantification of albumin, transferrin, and total lymphocyte count helps determine the degree of metabolic compromise (e.g., albumin 3.5 to 3.2 g/dl (mild), 3.2 to 2.8 g/dl (moderate), <2.8 g/dl (severe)). Observation over time includes assessment of overall clinical status, nutrient intake, and weekly documentation of body weight, as in the Nutritional Risk Screening Scales, a mnemonic scale designed to identify older persons at risk for malnutrition.[93] This scale identifies the common indicators of nutritional deficiency: deficient intake, impaired self-care ability, depression, and abnormal laboratory values. A second mnemonis Meals-On-Wheels focuses on treatable causes of weight loss in older adults, socioeconomic factors and endocrine disorders, and psychiatric and gastrointestinal disorders.[93]

TABLE 12-3   Selected Drug-Nutrient Interactions[99,116-118]

A. Drugs which alter nutrient absorption

Drug	GI Side effects	Nutrient Loss
1. Antacids		
Aluminum hydroxide	Dysmotility symptoms	Phosphate, vitamin A, thiamin (?), calcium (?)
2. Laxatives		
Phenolphthalein	Dysmotility symptoms	Fat (?), vitamin D, calcium, potassium
Bisacodyl		
Serna		
Mineral oil	Dysmotility symptoms	Beta carotene, vitamins A, D, and K, calcium, phosphorus
3. Bile acid sequestrant		
Cholestyramine	Dysmotility symptoms Steatorrhea	Fat, iron, folacin, betacarotene Vitamins A and K
4. Antiinflammatory agents		
Colchicine	Pain, diarrhea	Sodium (?), potasium (?), fat, nitrogen (?), betacarotene, B12
Sulfasalazine	Dysmotility symptoms	Folacin
5. Alcohol		Thiamine, folacin, fat, nitrogen
6. Antibiotics		
Tetracycline		Calcium
Neomycin		Fat, calcium
Gertamicin (? newer agents)		Potassium, magnesium

B. Drugs which alter nutrient metabolism

Drug	GI Side Effects	Nutrient Loss
1. Anticonvulsants		
Phenobarbital	Nausea, vomiting	Inactivation of 25 OH vit. D (hepatic microsomal enzyme induction), folacin, vitamin B12, pyridoxine, calcium, magnesium
Phenytoin	Nausea, vomiting, constipation	Inactivation of 25 OH vitamin D (hepatic microsomal enzyme induction), folacin (other minerals and vitamins?)
2. Antihypertensives		
Triamterene	Dysmotility symptoms	Electrolyte imbalance (possible hyperkalemia)
Hydralazine	Dysmotility symptoms	Vitamin B6 (antagonism, sodium and water retention)
Newer agents (?)		
3. Antineoplastic	Dysmotility symptoms	Folacin antagonism
Methotrexate	Ulceration and bleeding	Folacine, fat, vitamin B_{12}

C. Drugs that cause mineral depletion

Drug	GI Side effects	Nutrient loss
1. Diuretics		
Thiazides	Dysmotility symptoms	Potassium, magnesium, sodium and water (decreases calcium excretion)
Furosemide	Dysmotility symptoms	Potassium, calcium, magnesium, sodium chloride and water
Spironolactone	Dysmotility symptoms	Sodium, chloride, water
2. Analgesics		
Aspirin	Pain	Iron
NSAIDS	Bleeding	

XI. TREATMENT AND RECOMMENDATIONS

With fairly good health, a nutritionally balanced diet, and an active, socially involved lifestyle, life can be enjoyable and satisfying in old age, even though some adjustment may be necessary. Healthy older adults living in the community have, for the most part, a good appetite and a normal nutritional status. When appetite or nutrient intake is impaired, a first approach is to explore recent events which have led to worries, anxiety, or depression. In the absence of depression, it is important to maintain activity levels, encourage social interaction at mealtimes, and decrease alcohol and medication use. Among older adults, caloric consumption often ranges between 1,000 and 1,800 calories per day. At this level of consumption, consistent selection of foods with high nutrient density is necessary to ensure adequate nutrition.[102] For older patients with significant factors predisposing to severe nutritional deficits, clinical intervention should be considered on an individual basis — weighing risks, costs, and benefits.

When nutritional intervention is indicated, nutrient intake should be based on basal energy expenditure and RDAs, with additional allowances for premorbid level of nutrition, disease state, current activity level, and acute physiologic insult.[102] Aggressive oral supplementation is the first line of treatment.[103] When oral intake is not possible, tube feedings and peripheral parenteral nutrition should be considered for hospitalized patients. Clinical observation suggests that marginal nutritional states can be aggravated by comorbid illnesses. Although specific clinical syndromes may be absent, elderly patients may manifest subclinical and nonspecific signs of malnutrition. Nutritional supplementation in sick elderly patients speeds recovery and prevents complications. Calories combined with protein supplementation (250 cal + 20 g protein daily) significantly improved clinical outcome and reduced the length of hospital stay in patients with femoral neck fractures.[104] Two randomized controlled trials of nutritional supplementation have documented improved outcomes in older patients.[105,106]

Treating specific diseases that adversely affect nutritional intake or treating common causes of malnutrition are also indicated, e.g., administration of broad-spectrum antibiotics to patients with bacterial overgrowth improves nutritional status. Medroxyprogesterone acetate may improve appetite in older cancer patients.[107]

Compliance with dietary regimens for elders may improve by presenting ethnically oriented options and understanding the role of the grandmother as food provider in some households. Offering culturally familiar food options for hospital, nursing home, and home populations, e.g., rice for Asian or Latino elders, may increase caloric intake.

To our knowledge, systematic studies have not tested the impact of nutritional precursors on neuroendocrine processes in the aging organism. For instance, giving supplements of the serotonin precursor tryptophan may enhance serotonergic transmission,[108] but this supplement has not been tested in older adults. The practice has been discouraged by the severe side effects, such as the eosinophilia and collagen disease reported with exogenous tryptophan administration, even if the 'inert' filler substance used in the preparation of capsules might have produced the side effects rather than the tryptophan itself.

Since GH secretion and insulin growth factor-I decrease dramatically with age in the malnourished elderly, GH replacement may reverse the aging changes in bone and muscle (Chapter 3).[109] In fit athletes, GH administered for 6 weeks under double-blind, placebo-controlled conditions resulted in increased lean body mass and decreased adiposity.[110] Small (8.8%) increases in lean and small decreases (14%) in adipose tissue mass were reported in 21 men (ages 21 to 81 years) given GH at a dose of 0.03 mg/kg three times a week for 6 months.[109] Significantly reduced urinary nitrogen excretion and lowered cholesterol plasma levels were also reported in healthy men and women aged 60 years and over who were given GH doses between 0.03 to 0.12 mg/kg for 7 days.[111] In these doses, GH significantly impaired glucose tolerance. Two studies in which GH was given to malnourished elder patients reported increased caloric intake and weight gain, but no hyperglycemia, suggesting that GH might be beneficial in underweight, malnourished, elderly patients.[112,113]

XII. CONCLUSION

No particular nutrients or kinds of nutrition have been identified as either promoting or retarding the process of aging. In the future, the role of nutrition in relation to aging might be useful for the prevention of health problems through diet changes in early life. An optimal nutrient intake may ameliorate conditions associated with malnutrition and age-related physiologic alterations, but at the present time scientific databases do not exist for estimating nutritional requirements of older persons. Nutritional assessment should be incorporated into routine clinical examinations. The increased prevalence of chronic and acute illness and the ensuing changes in body composition and metabolic function due to immobility combine to increase the risk of malnutrition among older persons. It is therefore important to supply the isolated and hospitalized older population with safe and high quality foods that correspond to individual preferences and life habits, and to provide nutritional support for elderly hospitalized patients with evidence of malnutrition. Given the high risk for depression and physical illness in the older population and the ensuing loss of appetite, disease-specific treatments will be more beneficial if Hippocrates' advice is remembered, "Thy food shall be thy remedy."[114]

REFERENCES

1. Carroll, K. K., Lipids and carcinogenesis, *J. Environ. Path. Toxicol.*, 3, 253, 1980.
2. Hallfrisch, J., Muller, D., Drinkwater, D., Tobin, J., Andres, R., Continuing diet trends in Men: the Baltimore Longitudinal Study of Aging (1961-1987), *J. Gerontol.*, 45, M186, 1990.
3. Roth, T., Sleep in the Elderly: A Clinical Challenge, in *Sleep Disorders and Insomnia in the Elderly., Facts and Research in Gerontology,* Springer Publ. Co., New York, Vol. 7, 1993, 7.
4. Bliwise, D. L., Normal Aging, in *Principles and Practice of Sleep Medicine*, Kryger, M. H., Roth, T., and Dement, W. C., Eds., W.B. Saunders, Philadelphia, 1994, Chap. 3.
5. Gaillard, J. M., Nicholson, A. N., Pascoe, P. A., Neurotransmitter systems, in *Principles and Practice of Sleep Medicine*, Kryger, M. H., Roth, T., and Dement, W. C., Eds., W.B. Saunders, Philadelphia, 1994, Chap. 28.
6. Morley, J. E., Flood, J. F., Silver, A. J., Opioid peptides and aging, *Ann. N. Y. Acad. Sci.*, 579, 123, 1990.
7. Silver, A. J., Flood, J., Morley, J. E., Effect of aging on the anorectic effect of gut peptides, *Fed. Proc.*, 46, 1339, 1987.
8. Vellas, B., Balas, D., Albarede, J. L., Effects of aging process on digestive functions, *Comprehensive Therapy,* 17, 46, 1991.
9. Euronut Seneca Investigators, *European Journal of Clinical Nutrition,* 45 (Suppl. 3), 5, 1991.
10. Ten-State Survey 1968-1970. Highlights. DHEW Publication No. (HSM) 72-8134. Washington, D.C., U.S. Dept. Health, Education and Welfare, 1972.
11. Casper, R. C., Redmond, D. E., Jr., Katz, M. M., Schaffer, C. B., Davis, J. M., Koslow, S. H., Somatic symptoms in primary affective disorder. Presence and relation to the classification of depression, *Arch. Gen. Psychiat.*, 42, 1098, 1985.
12. Phillips, P. A., Rolls, B. J., Ledingham, J. G. G., Forsling, M. L., Morton, J. J., Crowe, M. J., Wollner, L., Reduced thirst after water deprivation in healthy elderly men, *N. Engl. J. Med.*, 311, 753, 1984.
13. Winograd, C. H., Malnutrition, in *Geriatric Medicine Annual 1987*, Ham, J., Ed., Medical Economics Press, Oradell, NJ, 1987, 175.
14. Lamy, P. P., Nutrition, drugs and the elderly, *Clin. Nutr.*, 2, 9, 1983.
15. Fukuba, H., Meeting the challenges of an aging population: an overview, *Nutrition Reviews*, 50, 467, 1992.
16. Zung, W. W., Depression in the normal aged, *Psychosomatics*, 8, 287, 1967.
17. Samiy, A. H., Clinical manifestations of disease in the elderly, *Med. Clin. North Am.*, 67, 333, 1983.
18. Thompson, M. P., Morris, L. K., Unexplained weight loss in the ambulatory elderly, *J. Am. Geriatr. Soc.*, 39, 497, 1991.
19. Sheikh, J. I., Yesavage, J. A., Geriatric Depression Scale (GDS): Recent evidence and development of a shorter version, *Clinical Gerontologist*, 5, 165, 1986.

20. Goodwin, J. S., Goodwin, J. M., Garry, P. J., Association between nutritional status and cognitive function-ing in a healthy elderly population, *J.A.M.A.,* 249, 2917, 1983.

21. Tucker, D. M., Penland, J. G., Sandstead, H. H., Milne, D. B., Heck, D. G., Klevay, L. M., Nutritional status and brain function in aging, *Am. J. Clin. Nutr.,* 52, 93, 1990.

22. Folstein, M. F., Folstein, S. E., McHugh, P. R., "Mini-mental state" A practical method for grading the cognitive state of patients for the clinician, *J. Psychiat. Res.,* 12, 189, 1975.

23. Giacobini, E., Cholinergic receptors in human brain: effects of aging and Alzheimer disease, *J. Neuro-science. Res.,* 27, 548, 1990.

24. Bartus, R. T., Dean, R. L., III, Sherman, K. A., Friedman, E., and Beer, B., Profound effects of combining choline and piracetam on memory enhancement and cholinergic function in aged rats, *Neurobiol. Aging,* 2, 105, 1981.

25. Winograd, C. H., Jacobson, D. H., Butterfield, G. E., Cragen, E., Edler, L. A., Taylor, B. S., Yesavage, J. A., Nutritional intake in patients with senile dementia of the Alzheimer type, *Alzheimer Disease and Associated Disorders Journal,* 5, 173, 1991.

26. Niskanen, L., Piirainen, M., Koljonen M., Uusitupa, M., Resting energy expenditure in relation to energy intake in patients with Alzheimer's disease, multi-infarct dementia and in control women, *Age and Ageing,* 22, 132, 1993.

27. Hegsted, D. M., Recommended dietary intakes of elderly subjects, *Am. J. Clin. Nutr.,* 50, 1190, 1989.

28. Recommended Dietary Allowances, 9th rev. ed. Washington, D.C.: National Academy of Sciences,1980.

29. Brants, H. A., Lowik, M. R., Westenbrink, S., Hulshof, K. F., Kistemaker, C., Adequacy of a vegetarian diet at old age (Dutch Nutrition Surveillance System), *J. Am. Coll. Nutr.,* 9, 292, 1990.

30. Exton-Smith, A. N., Vitamins, in *Metabolic and Nutritional Disorders in the Elderly,* Exton-Smith, A. N., Caird, F. I., Eds., Wright, Bristol, 1980, 26.

31. McGandy, R. B., Russell, R. M., Hartz, S. C., Jacob, R. A., Tannenbaum, S., Peters, H., Sahyoun, N., Otradovec, C. L., Nutritional status survey of healthy noninstitutionalized elderly. Energy and nutrient intakes from three-day diet records and nutrient supplements, *Nutrition Research,* 6, 785, 1986.

32. Health and Nutrition Examination Survey No. 2, Hyattsville, MD: US PHS Div. Health Stat., 1981.

33. Munro, H. N., Suter, P. M., Russell, R. M., Nutritional requirements of the elderly, *Ann. Rev. Nutr.,* 7, 23, 1987.

34. McGandy, R. B., Barrows, C. H., Jr., Spanias, A., Meredith, A., Stone, J. L., Norris, A. H., Nutrient intakes and energy expenditure in men of different ages, *J. Gerontol.,* 21, 581, 1966.

35. Munro, H. N., McGandy, R. B., Hartz, S. C., Russell, R. M., Jacob, R. A., and Otradovec, C. L., Protein nutriture of a group of free living elderly, *Am. J. Clin. Nutr.,* 46, 586, 1987.

36. Sidney, K. H., Shephard, R. J., Harrison, J. E., Endurance training and body composition of the elderly, *Am. J. Clin. Nutr.,* 30, 326, 1977.

37. Fiatarone, M. A., O'Neill, E. F., Doyle, N., Clements, K. M., Roberts, S. B., Kehayias, J. J., Lipsitz, L. A., Evans, W. J., The Boston FICSIT study. The effect of resistance training and nutritional supplementation on physical frailty in the oldest old, *J. Am. Geriatr. Soc.,* 41, 333, 1993.

38. Forbes, G. B., Reina, J. C., Adult lean body mass declines with age: some longitudinal observations, *Metabolism,* 19, 653, 1970.

39. Tzankoff, S. P., Norris, A. H., Effect of muscle mass decrease on age-related BMR changes, *J. Appl. Physiol.,* 43, 1001, 1977.

40. Silver, A. J., Guillen, C. P., Kahl, M. J., Morley, J. E., Effect of aging on body fat, *J. Am. Geriatr. Soc.,* 41, 211 1993.

41. Forbes, G. B., Halloran, E., The adult decline in lean body mass, *Hum. Biol.,* 48, 16e, 1976.

42. Steen, B., Bruce, A., Isaksson, B., Lewin, T., and Svanborg, A., Body composition in 70 year old males and females in Gothenberg, Sweden. A population study, *Acta Med. Scand.,* 611, 87, 1977.

43. Steen, B., Isaksson, B., Svanborg, A., Body composition at 70 and 75 years of age. A longitudinal population study, *J. Clin. Exp. Gerontol.,* 1, 185, 1979.

44. Calloway, D. H., Zanni, E., Energy requirements and energy expenditure of elderly men, *Am. J. Clin. Nutr.,* 33, 2088, 1980.

45. Swerdloff, R. S., Wang, C., Hines, M., Gorski, R., Effect of androgens on the brain and other organs during development and aging, *Psychoneuroendocrinology,* 17, 375, 1992.

46. Durnin, J. V. G. A., Energy intake, energy expenditure, and body composition in the elderly, in *Nutrition, Immunity and Illness in the Elderly,* Chandra, R. K., Ed., Pergamon Press, New York, 1985, 19.

47. Exton-Smith, A. N., Nutritional status. Diagnosis and prevention of malnutrition, in *Metabolic and Nutri-tional Disorders in the Elderly,* Exton-Smith, A. N., Caird, F. I., Eds., Wright, Bristol, 1980, 66.

48. Debry, GM., Bleyer, R., Martin, J. M., Nutrition of the elderly, *J. Hum. Nutr.,* 31, 195, 1977.

49. Lowik, M. R., Westenbrink, S., Hulshof, K. F., Kistemaker, C., Hermus, R. J., Nutrition and aging:dietary intake of "apparently healthy" elderly (Dutch Nutrition Surveillance System), *J. Am. Coll. Nutr.,* 8, 347, 1989.

50. Lowik, M. R., Schrijver, J., Odink, J., van den Berg, H., Wedel, M., Hermus, R. J., Nutrition and aging: nutritional status of "apparently healthy" elderly (Dutch Nutrition Surveillance System), *J. Am .Coll. Nutr.*, 9, 18, 1990.

51. Buchner, D. M., Wagner, E. H., Preventing frail health, *Clin. Geriatr. Med.*, 8, 1, 1992.

52. Garry, P. J., Hunt, W. C., Koehler, K. M., VanderJagt, J. D., Vellas, B. J., Longitudinal study of dietary intakes and plasma lipids in healthy elderly men and women, *Am J Clin Nutr,* 55, 682, 1992.

53. Cohen, P., Ocrant, I., Fielder, P. J., Neely, E. K., Gargosky, S. E., Deal, C. I., Ceda, G. P., Youngman, O., Pham, H., Lamson, G., Giudice, L. C., Rosenfeld, R. G., Insulin-like growth factors (IGFs): implications for aging, *Psychoneuroendocrinology*, 17, 335, 1992.

54. Morley, J. E., Flood, J., Silver, A. J., Effects of peripheral hormones on memory and ingestive behaviors, *Psychoneuroendocrinology*, 17, 391, 1992.

55. Timiras, P. S., Cole, G., Croteau, M., Hudson, D. B., Miller, C., Segall, P. E., Changes in brain serotonin with aging and modification through precursor availability, in *Aging, Vol. 23, Aging Brain and Ergot Alkaloids*, Agnoli, A., Crepaldi, G., Spano, P. F., Trabuchi, M., Eds., Raven Press, New York, 1983, 25.

56. Evans, W. J., Exercise, nutrition and aging, *J. Nutr.,* 122, 796, 1992.

57. Palmer, E. D., Benign chronic gastric ulcer and weight loss, *Am. Fam. Physician*, 8, 109, 1973.

58. Van Itallie, T. B., Health implications of overweight and obesity in the United States, *Ann. Intern. Med.,* 103, 983, 1985.

59. Potter, J. F., Schafer, D. F., Bohi, R. L., In-hospital mortality as a function of body mass index: an age dependent variable, *J. Gerontol.,* 43, M59, 1988.

60. Trichopoulos, D., Nutritional etiology of human cancer: past and future of epidemiological research, *Europ. J. Clin. Nutrition,* 45, 16, 1991.

61. Willett, W. C., Diet and human cancer of the breast, colon and prostate, *Europ. J. Clin. Nutrition*, 45, 19, 1991.

62. Chandra, R. K., Nutritional regulation of immune function at the extremes of life in infants and the elderly, in *Malnutrition: Determinants and Consequences,* White, P .L., Selvey, N., Eds., Alan R. Liss, New York, 1984, pp. 245-251.

63. McCay, C. M., Maynard, L. A., Sperling, G., Barnes, L. L., Retarded growth, lifespan, ultimate body size and age changes in the albino rat after feeding diets restricted in calories, *J. Nutr.*, 18, 1, 1939.

64. Ross, M. H., Length of life and caloric intake, *Am. J. Clin. Nutr.*, 25, 834, 1972.

65. Casper, R. C., Neuroendocrine aspects of anorexia nervosa and bulimia nervosa, *Child Adol. Psychiatr. Clinics of North America*, 2, 161, 1993.

66. Meites, J., Aging: hypothalamic catecholamines, neuroendocrine-immune interactions, and dietary restriction, *Proceedings of the Society for Experimental Biology and Medicine,* 195, 304, 1990.

67. Jack, S. S., Bloom, B., Use of dental services and dental health: United States, 1986, Vital Health Stat., Series 10: Data from the National Health Survey, 165, 1, 1988.

68. Hartz, S. C., The NSS study population, in *Nutrition in the Elderly: The Boston Nutritional Status Survey*, Hartz, S. C., Russel, R. M, Rosenberg, I. H., Eds., Smith Gordon, London, 1992.

69. Andrews, G. P., Esterman, A. J., Braunack-Mayer, A. J., Rungie, C. M., Aging in the Western Pacific. Manila: World Health Organization Regional Office for the Western Pacific, 1986.

70. Bartoshuk, L. M., Rifkin, B., Marks, L. E., Bars, P., Taste and aging, *J. Gerontol.,* 41, 51, 1986.

71. Murphy, C., Nutrition and chemosensory perception in the elderly, *Critical Reviews in Food Science and Nutrition,* 33, 3, 1993.

72. Chauhan, J., Hawrysh, Z. J., Gee, M., Donald, E. A., Basu, T. K., Age-related olfactory and taste changes and interrelationships between taste and nutrition, *J. Am. Dietetic. Assoc.*, 87, 1543, 1987.

73. Casper, R. C., Kirschner, B., Sandstead, H. H., Jacob, R. A., Davis, J. M., An evaluation of trace metals, vitamins, and taste function in anorexia nervosa, *Am. J. Clin. Nutr.*, 33, 1801, 1980.

74. Hyde, R. J., Feller, R. P., Sharon, I. M., Tongue brushing, dentifrice, and age effects on taste and smell, *Journal of Dental Research*, 60, 1730, 1981.

75. Hutton, C. W., Hayes-Davis, R. B., Assessment of the zinc nutritional status of selected elderly subjects, *J. Am. Diet. Assoc.,* 82, 148, 1983.

76. Kimura, S., Taste and nutrition, *Nutrition Reviews,* 50, 427, 1992.

77. Stevens, J. C., Bartoshuk, L. M., Cain, W. S., Chemical senses and aging: taste versus smell, *Chem. Sens.*, 9, 167, 1984.

78. Navazesh, M., Salivary gland hypofunction in elderly patients, *Senior Care, Journal of the California Dental Association*, 22, 62, 1994.

79. Morley, J. E., Gastrointestinal peptides and aging, *Peptide Therapy Index & Reviews,* III, front/back cover, 1991.

80. Ekberg, O., Feinberg, M. J., Altered swallowing function in elderly patients without dysphagia: radiologic findings in 56 cases, *Am. J. Radiol.,* 156, 1181, 1991.

81. Richter, J. E., Bradley, L. A., Castell, D. O., Esophageal chest pain: current controversies in pathogenesis, diagnosis and therapy, *Ann. Intern. Med.,* 110, 66, 1988.

82. Castell, D. O., Esophageal disorders in the elderly, *Gastroenterol. Clin. North Am.*, 19, 235, 1990.

83. Holt, P. R., Rosenberg, I. H., Russell, R. M., Causes and consequences of hypochlorhydria in the elderly: proceedings of a workshop held at NIH 1987, *Dig. Dis. Sci.*, 34, 933, 1989.

84. Soll, A. H., Kurata, J., McGuigan, J. E., Ulcers, nonsteroidal antiinflammatory drugs and related matters, *Gastroenterology*, 96, 561, 1989.

85. Bardhan, K. D., Cust, G., Hinchliffe, R. F. C., Williamson, F. M., Lyon, C., and Bose, K., Changing pattern of admissions and operations for duodenal ulcer, *Br. J. Surg.*, 76, 230, 1989.

86. Cooper, B. T., Weston, C. F., Neumann, C. S., Acute gastrointestinal haemorrhage in patients aged 80 years or more, *Quarterly J. Med.*, 68, 765, 1988.

87. Oliver, N., Abdominal pain in the elderly, *Aust. Fam. Physician,* 13, 402, 1984.

88. Rudman, D., Feller, A. G., Protein-calorie undernutrition in the nursing home, *J. Am. Geriatr. Soc.*, 37, 173, 1989.

89. Stiedemann, M., Jansen, C., Harrill, I., Nutritional status of elderly men and women, *J. Am. Diet. Assoc.*, 73, 132, 1978.

90. Harvey, K. B., Bothe, A., Jr., Blackburn, G. L., Nutritional assessment and patient outcome during oncological therapy, *Cancer*, 43, 2065, 1979.

91. Weinsier, R. L., Hunker, E. M., Krumdieck, C. L., Butterfield, C. E., Jr., Hospital malnutrition. A prospective evaluation of general medical patients during the course of hospitalization, *Am. J. Clin. Nutr.*, 32, 418, 1979.

92. Jensen, J. E., Jensen, T. G., Smith, T. K., Johnston, D. A., Dudrick, S. J., Nutrition in orthopaedic surgery, *J. Bone Joint Surg.*, 64, 1263, 1982.

93. Morley, J. E., Why do physicians fail to recognize and treat malnutrition in older persons? (editorial), *J. Am. Geriatr. Soc.*, 39, 1139, 1991.

94. Mowé, M., Bohmer, T., The prevalence of undiagnosed protein-calorie undernutrition in a population of hospitalized elderly patients, *J Am. Geriatric. Soc.*, 39, 1089, 1991.

95. Zeman, F. J., *Clinical Nutrition and Dietetics,* Collamore Press, Lexington, MA, 1983.

96. Steffee, W. P., Malnutrition in hospitalized patients, *JAMA*, 244, 2630, 1980.

97. Keys, A., Brozek, J., Henschel, A., et al., *The Biology of Human Starvation,* University of Minnesota Press, Minneapolis, 1950.

98. Campillo, B., Bories, P. N., Devanlay, M., Pornin, P. N., Le Parco, J. C., Gaye-Bareyt, E., Fouet, P., Aging, energy expenditure and nutritional status: evidence of denutrition-related hypermetabolism, *Annals of Nutrition and Metabolism*, 36, 265, 1992.

99. Roe, D. A., Therapeutic significance of drug-nutrient interactions in the elderly, *Pharmacol. Rev.*, 36,109S, 1984.

100. Brymer, C., Winograd, C. H., Fluoxetine in elderly patients. Is there cause for concern?, *J. Am. Geriatr. Soc.*, 40, 902, 1992.

101. Roubenoff, R., Wilson, P. W., Advantage of knee height over height as an index of stature in expression of body composition in adults, *Am. J. Clin. Nutr.*, 57, 609, 1993.

102. Consensus Development Conference: diagnosis, prophylaxis and treatment of osteoporosis, *Am. J. Medicine*, 94, 646, 1993.

103. Winograd, C. H., Brown, E. M., Aggressive oral refeeding in hospitalized patients, *Am. J. Clin. Nutr.*, 52, 967, 1990.

104. Delmi, M., Rapin, C.-H., Bengoa, J. M., Delmas, P. D., Vasey, H., Bonjour, J.-P., Dietary supplementation in elderly patients with fractured neck of the femur, *Lancet*, 335, 1013, 1990.

105. Bastow, M. D., Rawlings, J., Allison, S. P., Benefits of supplementary tube feeding after fractured neck of femur: a randomized controlled trial, *Br. Med. J.,* 287, 1589, 1983.

106. Larsson, F., Unosson, M., Ek, A. C., Nilsson, L., Thorlund, E., Beer, B., Effect of dietary supplement on nutritional status and clinical outcome in 501 geriatric patients — a randomized study, *Clin. Nutr.*, 9, 179 1990.

107. Niiranen, A., Kajanti, M., Tammilehto, L., Mattson, K., The clinical effect of medroxyprogesterone in elderly patients with lung cancer, *Am. J. Clin. Oncol.*, 13, 113, 1990.

108. Wurtman, R. J., Nutrients affecting brain composition and behavior, *Integrative Psychiatry*, 5, 226, 1987.

109. Rudman, D., Feller, A. G., Nagraj, S. H., Gergans, G. A., Lalitha, P. Y., Goldberg, A. F., Chlenker, R. A., Cohn, L., Rudman, I. W., Mattson, D. E., Effects of human growth hormone in men over 60 years old, *N. Engl. J. Med.*, 323, 1, 1990.

110. Crist, D. M., Peake, G. T., Loftfield, R. B., Kraner, J. C., Egan, P. A., Supplemental growth hormone alters body composition, muscle protein metabolism, and serum lipids in fit adults: characterization of dose-dependent and response-recovery effects, *Mech. Ageing Dev.*, 58, 191, 1991.

111. Marcus, R., Butterfield, G., Holloway, L., Gilliland, L., Baylink, D. J., Hintz, R. L., Sherman, B. M., Effects of short term administration of recombinant human growth hormone to elderly people, *Journal of Clinical Endocrinology and Metabolism*, 70, 519, 1990.

112. Binnerts, A., Wilson, J. H., Lamberts, S. W., The effects of human growth hormone administration in elderly adults with recent weight loss, *J. Clin. Endocrinol. Metab.,* 67, 1312, 1988.
113. Kaiser, F. E., Aging and malnutrition: growth hormone therapy shows promise, *Geriatrics,* 47, 85, 1992.
114. Koretz, R. L., What supports nutritional support?, *Dig. Dis. Sci.,* 29, 577, 1984.
115. Koehler, K. M., Garry, P. J., Nutrition and aging, *Clinics in Laboratory Medicine,* 13, 433, 1993.
116. Roe, D. A., Drug-nutrient interactions in the elderly, *Geriatrics,* 41, 57, 1986.
117. Roe, D. A., Drug and food interactions as they affect the nutrition of older individuals, Aging, 5, 51, 1993.
118. Smith, C. H., Bidlack, W. R., Dietary concerns associated with the use of medications, *J. Am. Detetic Ass.,* 84, 901, 1984.

13

Osteoporosis: Pathogenesis, Diagnosis, and Treatment

Charles Y. C. Pak

CONTENTS

I. INTRODUCTION

Osteoporosis represents a major medical problem in the United States.[1] The annual incidence of vertebral crush fractures and of hip fractures due to this condition is estimated to be 0.77% and 0.2% of all Americans, respectively. Because of the predilection for the elderly, incidence of osteoporosis in the older age group is higher, 1.7% between 45 to 64 years and 2% among those 65 years or older. Approximately 20 million Americans suffer from osteoporosis, comprised mostly of elderly individuals, especially of the female sex.

The primary abnormality is the reduced amount of bone mass resulting from bone resorption which is proportionately greater than bone formation. The loss of bone affects bone mineral and matrix equally. Thus, the remaining bone is grossly normal. When the bone mass has decreased to a point where it is insufficient to support the normal structural integrity and weight-bearing function of the skeleton, fractures occur with minimum trauma. Common sites of fractures are the spine, hip, and wrist.

Recently, considerable progress has been made in the patho-physiology, diagnosis, and management of osteoporosis. This chapter will review this progress.

II. PATHOGENESIS

A. Cellular Basis For Osteoporosis

Bone undergoes continual breakdown and repair in discrete microscopic areas called basic multicellular units (BMU).[2] Each unit has areas of resorption and formation. The resorption is initiated by osteoclasts which destroy bone, forming a cavity of 50 to 250 μm in diameter. The osteoclasts are then replaced by osteoblasts which form osteoid rich in collagen. The mineralization of the osteoid completes the remodeling cycle. Normally, bone resorption initiated by osteoclasts is closely "coupled" to bone formation induced by osteoblasts. Thus, the amount of bone destroyed equals that restored, maintaining bone balance in each BMU.

In osteoporosis, the coupling of osteoblastic bone formation to osteoclastic resorption is impaired. Thus, the bone balance in each BMU is negative, because bone resorption is not fully compensated by bone formation. The precise mechanism for impaired coupling is not known. This defect may be related to deficiency of estrogen or of local skeletal growth factors, or it may represent a nonspecific manifestation of aging.

B. Causes of Osteoporosis

Osteoporosis may be broadly characterized into *primary and secondary forms* (Table 13-1). Primary osteoporosis is comprised of postmenopausal (Type I) and senile (Type II) types.[3] *Postmenopausal osteoporosis* is characterized by suppressed parathyroid function presumed to be secondary to estrogen lack, impaired 1,25-$(OH)_2$ vitamin D synthesis, reduced intestinal calcium absorption, involvement of trabecular bone, and clinical manifestation of crushed fractures of the spine. *Senile osteoporosis* affects both men and women of greater than 70 years of age. While serum 1,25-$(OH)_2$ vitamin D and intestinal calcium absorption are low, serum PTH is elevated. It affects cortical bone with a clinical manifestation of proximal femoral fracture. The distinction between Type I and Type II osteoporosis is not rigid, since both types could be present in the same patient.

Secondary osteoporosis depicts the disease process associated with certain hormonal disturbances (hyperadrenocorticism, thyrotoxicosis, and hyperparathyroidism), gastrointestinal diseases (malabsorption, resection, cirrhosis), immobilization and miscellaneous causes (renal tubular acidosis, multiple myeloma, renal failure, and idiopathic). In endogenous or exogenous steroid excess, osteoporosis develops from the direct impairment of osteoblastic activity, and from the indirect stimulation of osteoclastic resorption due to secondary

TABLE 13-1   Classification of Osteoporosis

Primary
   Type I (Postmenopausal)
   Type II (Elderly)
Secondary
   Hormonal disturbances (thyroid excess, steroid excess, hyperparathyroidism)
   Gastrointestinal diseases (malabsorption, resection, cirrhosis)
   Immobilization
   Miscellaneous causes (renal tubular acidosis, multiple myeloma, renal failure, idiopathic)

hyperparathyroidism.[4] The development of osteoporosis from long-standing thyrotoxicosis may be explained by the direct action of thyroid hormones (particularly thyroxin) in stimulating osteoclastic resorption.[5] Parathyroid hormone-excess is not associated with the loss of trabecular bone volume; rather, it causes excessive resorption of cortical bone. Thus, primary hyperparathyroidism is more likely to cause fractures of the appendicular skeleton rather than the spine.

The management of secondary osteoporosis should be directed at the detection and correction of the underlying disease or condition. Because of its common occurrence, this chapter will consider mainly primary osteoporosis.

C. Pathogenesis of Primary Osteoporosis

The etiology of primary osteoporosis is multifactorial, including genetic, nutritional-behavioral, and hormonal factors.

1. Genetic Factors

In postmenopausal women and elderly persons of both sexes, osteoporosis is more common in women of Northern European ethnic background than in black women, and in those who are of thin build. This predilection for thin white women may be partly due to their lower peak bone mass. Since their total bone mass at the crest of growth is reduced to begin with, the amount of bone loss that occurs normally with the postmenopausal state and aging may be sufficient to cause bone disease.

2. Nutritional-Behavioral Factors

An important nutritional factor is the amount of calcium intake required to maintain balance. There is considerable evidence that this requirement for calcium increases with advancing age because of the decline in serum $1,25\text{-}(OH)_2$ vitamin D and in intestinal calcium absorption.[6,7] Therefore, an intake of calcium below the calcium requirement could cause negative calcium balance and exaggerate bone loss. There is also recent evidence that calcium is critical for the optimum bone growth during teenage and premenopausal years in achieving peak bone mass.[8]

Other nutritional-behavioral factors include ethanol excess, smoking, high sodium intake, excessive physical exercise and dieting (leading to underweight status or menstrual irregularities),[9] and a sedentary lifestyle. A high alcohol consumption may produce bone loss from its direct impairment of osteoblastic activity and inhibition of intestinal calcium absorption.[10] Smoking may inactivate estrogens by stimulating 2-hydroxylation of estradiol.[11] The thin stature sometimes assumed by heavy smokers may further contribute to bone loss.

An excessive sodium intake may cause renal hypercalciuria by impairing renal calcium reabsorption, and produce secondary hyperparathyroidism. In young individuals and premenopausal women in whom the capacity for $1,25\text{-}(OH)_2$ vitamin D production is intact, the stimulation of intestinal calcium absorption ensues from sodium load consequent to the parathyroid hormone-dependent augmentation of $1,25\text{-}(OH)_2$ vitamin D synthesis.[12] Thus, calcium balance is maintained. However, in postmenopausal women, the compensatory rise in intestinal calcium absorption does not develop following sodium-induced calciuria, because of the disturbance in $1,25\text{-}(OH)_2$ vitamin D synthesis.[13] The postmenopausal women and elderly persons are therefore at risk theoretically for bone loss from habitual high sodium intake. This conclusion is supported by a study in experimental animals showing bone loss following excessive sodium intake.[14] However, more definitive evidence linking a high sodium diet to osteoporosis is lacking.

Extremes of physical activity may be harmful to skeletal health. Some degree of weight bearing is critical for assuring normal skeletal growth and attainment of peak bone mass. Moderate physical exercise may be useful in preventing bone loss which occurs in the postmenopausal state and with aging. However, strenuous physical exercise may cause dys- or amenorrhea by producing hypothalamic hypogonadism.[9] Significant loss of trabecular bone may occur. Habitual dieting and assumption of a thin stature may predispose subjects to osteoporosis in later life. Obese women have higher circulating estrogen levels, greater bone mass, and are less likely to develop symptomatic osteoporosis.

3.   Hormonal Factors

In Type I (postmenopausal) osteoporosis, estrogen lack plays a critical pathogenetic role.[3] Estrogen normally protects bone from PTH-induced bone resorption. Thus, the following scheme may operate during estrogen lack:

- Increased PTH-induced bone resorption, which leads to
- Increased skeletal mobilization of calcium, which leads to
- Reduced endogenous PTH secretion, which leads to
- Reduced $1,25\text{-}(OH)_2$ vitamin D synthesis, which leads to
- Reduced intestinal calcium absorption.

The validity of this scheme has been supported by the findings of reduced circulating concentrations of PTH and $1,25\text{-}(OH)_2$ vitamin D and a low intestinal calcium absorption in postmenopausal women. Moreover, a receptor for estrogen has been recently identified in osteoblasts.[15,16] The inhibition of bone resorption by estrogen could thus be explained by the osteoblastic elaboration upon estrogen activation of an inhibitor of osteoclasts.

4.   PTH Excess

In Type II (senile) osteoporosis,[3] serum PTH may be secondarily increased from the primary impairment in renal synthesis of $1,25\text{-}(OH)_2$ vitamin D or in intestinal absorption of calcium occurring as a part of the aging process. A minority of patients with postmenopausal osteoporosis may present with renal hypercalciuria with secondary hyperparathyroidism (Type Ib).[17] However, unlike patients with active renal stones, patients with Type Ib osteoporosis do not have high serum $1,25\text{-}(OH)_2$ vitamin D and lack compensatory intestinal hyperabsorption of calcium. Thiazide treatment restores normal parathyroid function and reduces osteoclastic bone resorption.

The cortical bone is destroyed preferentially in PTH excess. However, trabecular bone loss may also be apparent in many women with Type II osteoporosis, because of coexistent estrogen lack.

5.   Vitamin D Deficiency

In Type I osteoporosis, serum $1,25\text{-}(OH)_2$ vitamin D may be low due to parathyroid suppression as previously enumerated.[6] In Type II osteoporosis, renal synthesis of $1,25\text{-}(OH)_2$ vitamin D may be impaired, reflective of a generalized renal parenchymal loss associated with aging.

Some elderly subjects may have a reduced serum concentration of 25-hydroxyvitamin D probably due to inadequate exposure to sunlight or vitamin D consumption. Exogenous 25-hydroxyvitamin D may increase the circulating level of 1,25-$(OH)_2$ vitamin D, suggesting hypocalcitriolemia may partly have resulted from substrate deficiency.[18]

Vitamin D deficiency probably contributes to the development of osteoporosis by impairing intestinal absorption of calcium and causing negative calcium balance.

6. Other Factors

The pathogenetic role of calcitonin remains uncertain, although low circulating concentration of calcitonin and impaired secretory response to calcium infusion have been reported in the postmenopausal state.[19] Recently, a high content of interleukin-1 has been reported in osteoporotic patients with a high bone turnover.[20] The possibility that this local growth factor with bone resorbing capacity may play a pathogenetic role in osteoporosis is intriguing.

III. CLINICAL PRESENTATIONS

"Spontaneous" fractures, the hallmark of osteoporosis, represent fractures occurring from minimal trauma which could normally be sustained without incurring damage. Common sites of involvement are the vertebrae, ribs, proximal femur, and distal radius and ulna. Fractures may occur from a minor fall or bending to pick up an object.

Pain is the most common symptomatology of vertebral fracture. It is generally localized to the area of involvement, but may radiate laterally. It may be associated with paravertebral muscle spasm and localized tenderness. The severity and duration of pain vary considerably among patients. It may last for 1 to 2 months.

Skeletal deformity may develop from anterior wedging and collapse of vertebrae. "Dowager's hump" may occur from fractures of thoracic and lumbar vertebrae. Loss of height is common. Patients often complain of chronic back pain, occurring probably on a mechanical basis. When the spine becomes severely contracted by fractures, abdominal and pulmonary function may be embarrassed. Abdominal protuberance often accompanies Dowager's hump. The lower aspect of the rib cage may override the iliac crest in severe cases.

IV. LABORATORY FINDINGS IN PRIMARY OSTEOPOROSIS

Serum concentrations of calcium, phosphorus, and alkaline phosphatase are normal in patients with postmenopausal osteoporosis. The serum concentration of PTH is usually normal, but it may be high in a minority of patients. Serum 1,25-$(OH)_2$ vitamin D and intestinal calcium absorption are generally reduced. Urinary calcium is normal or low in most patients; it may be elevated in a minority of patients, particularly if they suffer from renal hypercalciuria. Fasting urinary calcium may be high in some patients, indicative of appropriately high bone resorption.[21] To be meaningful, it is best expressed as milligrams of calcium per deciliter of glomerular filtrate. When expressed relative to urinary creatinine it may give an exaggerated value because serum creatinine is often low in elderly osteoporotic patients. Urinary hydroxyproline may be high in some patients, indicative of high bone resorption. Serum osteocalcin has been reported to be increased in Type II osteoporosis, probably reflective of osteoblastic response to the parathyroid stimulation.[22]

Radiologically, early signs include loss of the trabecular pattern on vertebrae and the femoral neck. The trabecular bone which is not parallel to the line of weight-bearing is lost first by the osteoporotic process; this accounts for the prominence of vertical striations in the vertebrae, and serves as the basis for the trabecular pattern index for staging of osteoporosis. The cortical thickness of metacarpal bone or the radius may be reduced in osteoporosis. In the long bones there is an accelerated bone loss endosteally with menopause; however, the bone continues to be deposited externally (periosteally) although at a slower rate. Thus, the total width of bone may be greater, but the cortical bone thickness may be less than in the premenopausal state. Other roentgenologic signs include prominence of vertebral end-plates, Schmorl's nodes, vertebral collapse, fractures of rib and femoral neck, and kyphoscoliosis.

Bone histologic examination has revealed morphologic heterogeneity, including low and high remodeling activity.[23,24] Unfortunately, the exact histomorphometric picture cannot be accurately predicted from biochemical presentation.[24]

The skeletal roentgenologic examination is inadequate to measure the extent of bone loss in osteoporosis because up to 40% of bone mineral may be lost before it can be detected roentgenologically. A more sensitive measure of bone density may be obtained from photon absorptiometric analysis or computer tomography (CT). The single photon absorptiometry may disclose low bone density in radial diaphysis in Type II osteoporosis;[25] low vertebral bone mass has been shown by dual photon absorptiometry (DPA)[26] or by CT[27] in Type I osteoporosis. The advantage of CT resides in its capability for measuring the mass of the inner trabecular bone of the vertebra, unlike dual photon absorptiometry which measures density of the whole vertebra including cortex, spinal process, and transverse processes which are rich in cortical bone. However, the CT has a higher radiation exposure and a worse precision of measurement. Quantitative assessment of bone density is useful in assessing the severity of bone loss, evaluating skeletal status in those at risk, and in quantitative response to treatment. Recently, an X-Ray-based dual photon absorptiometry has been introduced, providing quicker, and greater stability and precision of measurement than DPA.

V. THERAPY OF PRIMARY OSTEOPOROSIS

Treatment modalities[28] for osteoporosis may be broadly categorized into those which are directed at the prevention of bone loss, and those which are aimed at the augmentation of bone mass (Table 13-2). Modalities directed at the prevention of bone loss should ideally be applied before a substantial amount of bone has been lost and before osteoporosis has developed. The primary goal of osteoporosis prevention is optimizing the attainment of peak bone mass. The secondary goal is to avert subsequent bone loss that occurs following menopause and advancing age.

The modalities aimed at augmentation of bone mass would be particularly useful in patients with established osteoporosis who have already lost much bone and sustained fractures.

A. Optimization of Peak Bone Mass

Bone tissue normally continues to grow well into adulthood. Growth ceases when the peak bone mass is attained at 25 to 35 years of age for the trabecular bone, and at 35 to 45 years for the cortical bone.

There is emerging evidence that the provision of adequate calcium intake in the diet or as a calcium supplement in the teenage period and in early adulthood is critical for the attainment of peak bone mass, particularly of cortical bone.[29] Thus, individuals who had been maintained on an adequate calcium intake are likely to have greater peak bone mass,[8] especially in the long bones, than those who had taken insufficient amount of calcium. Physical exercise program providing resistance against gravity, but which is not of such severity so as to cause underweight constitution or dys- or amenorrhea, may exert similar action as calcium in the attainment of peak bone mass.

B. Prevention of Bone Loss After Attainment of Peak Bone Mass

These treatment modalities should ideally be begun at the perimenopausal period or middle age and continued before a substantial amount of bone has been lost. These drugs may be called **antiresorptive** medications. They include currently available drugs:

TABLE 13-2   Therapy of Primary Osteoporosis

Prevention of Bone Loss (Before Osteoporosis Development)
  a. Optimization of peak bone mass
    i. Calcium
    ii. Exercise
  b. Prevention of postmenopausal bone loss
    i. Estrogen
    ii. Calcium
    iii. Calcitonin
Augmentation of Bone Mass (After Osteoporosis Development)
  a. PTH (parathyroid hormone)
  b. ADFR (activation-depression-free-repeat)
  c. Fluoride

- Estrogen,
- Calcitonin,
- Calcium supplements.

Their principal mode of action is the inhibition of osteoclastic resorption. There may be a transient increase in bone mass due to this action. With continued treatment, however, a compensatory decline in bone formation ensues due to coupling. Thus, bone mass stabilizes; it does not continue to increase.

1. Estrogen

There is now convincing evidence that estrogen therapy is capable of preventing the loss of cortical and trabecular bone mass in women deficient in estrogen from natural menopause or surgical castration.[30] The response may be less marked in late postmenopausal women. Disadvantages of estrogen treatment include potential complication of endometrial cancer, renin-dependent hypertension, thromboembolism, withdrawal uterine bleeding, and gallstones. In postmenopausal women with an intact uterus, an acceptable program is to provide a conjugated estrogen 0.625 mg/day for 25 days of each month and progesterone 10 mg/day for the last 10 days of estrogen treatment. Estrogen may be protective against the development of cardiovascular disease, increasing serum HDL, and reducing total serum cholesterol. These effects on lipids may be opposed by progesterone. In those with hysterectomy, conjugated estrogen alone may be provided on a continuing basis (see also Chapters 7 and 8).

A similar favorable response has been found with calcitonin.[31] Both drugs may cause an initial increase in bone mass during the first 6 to 24 months. Thereafter, the bone mass remains stable without a further increase.

2. Oral Calcium

The rationale for oral calcium supplementation is to overcome inadequate calcium absorption resulting from low calcium intake and defective intestinal calcium absorption often encountered in postmenopausal women and elderly subjects, as previously enumerated. The total amount of calcium absorbed may be increased substantially by higher calcium intake (probably by the operation of passive absorption), even though the fractional calcium absorption remains subnormal. By enhancing calcium absorption, oral calcium supplements may inhibit parathyroid function and thereby suppress PTH-dependent bone resorption.[32] The rate of bone remodeling or the birth rate of new basic multicellular units is therefore reduced. Thus, this form of therapy may retard loss but is not expected to augment bone mass.

There is conflicting literature regarding the efficacy of calcium supplementation in preventing bone loss in the postmenopausal and elderly state. However, the following general conclusions may be drawn:

1. Calcium supplementation may be more effective in preventing cortical bone loss than trabecular bone loss,[29,33]
2. The effectiveness of calcium in stabilizing bone mass varies among different calcium preparations, and depends on duration of the postmenopausal (hypoestrogenic) state.

Thus, general calcium supplementation stabilizes the bone mass of the skeleton rich in cortical bone (proximal femur and diaphysis of long bones) in early and late postmenopausal women and in elderly men. In late postmenopausal women, calcium carbonate may prevent vertebral (trabecular) bone loss. However, in early postmenopausal women (within 5 years of menopause), calcium carbonate has been reported to be ineffective in preventing the decline in spinal mass (by computer tomography).[34] A recent study, though uncontrolled, suggests that calcium citrate could avert spinal bone loss in such women.[35]

The relative ineffectiveness of calcium carbonate might be due to its dependence on gastric acid secretion for dissolution and subsequent absorption of calcium from the intestinal tract. Gastric acid secretion may become impaired with advancing age. Thus, an insufficient amount of absorbable calcium may be available to suppress PTH-dependent bone resorption in some postmenopausal women. It has been suggested that the ingestion of calcium carbonate with a meal might enhance its calcium absorption.[36] However, this effect probably depends on the type of food.

In contrast, calcium citrate is less dependent on acid for dissolution, since it has a modest solubility even in water.[35] It is more soluble than calcium carbonate in various states of acid secretion, except in a very high-acid secretory state, where it has an equivalent solubility. Moreover, the solubilized calcium citrate does not readily precipitate out of solution when the gastric effluent is neutralized by pancreatic bicarbonate secretion. The complexation of calcium by citrate may reduce the amount of ionic calcium, the principal species of calcium absorbed from the intestinal tract. However, there is recent evidence that calcium citrate complex may be absorbed via paracellular transport. Due probably to these factors, most available reports have shown a superior absorbability of calcium from calcium citrate than from calcium carbonate.[35] This finding may account for the apparent superiority of calcium citrate over calcium carbonate in preventing spinal bone loss of early postmenopausal women.

C. Augmentation of Bone Mass

The treatment modalities directed at the augmentation of bone mass may be called formation-stimulating drugs, since they are directed at promoting osteoblastic bone formation.[28] These drugs are ideally suited for the management of established osteoporosis. While no drugs have been approved for this purpose in the United States, several investigational approaches hold promise. They are

- Exogenous PTH,
- Coherence therapy (ADFR or activation-depression-free-repeat), and
- Sodium fluoride.

1. PTH

Parathyroid hormone could theoretically increase bone mass by raising the number of bone multicellular units and by creating a net positive balance of each BMU. Previous studies disclosed that the treatment with human PTH 1-34 peptide increased trabecular bone mass in osteoporotic women.[37] However, this beneficial effect may have occurred at the expense of cortical bone. There is some evidence that a sequential treatment with PTH followed by 1,25-$(OH)_2$ vitamin D may overcome this "steal" syndrome (redistribution of trabecular and cortical fractions). In male patients with idiopathic osteoporosis, this sequential treatment has been shown to significantly increase the mass of trabecular bone of the spine without altering radial (cortical) bone mass.[38] This approach has not been tested in postmenopausal osteoporosis.

2. ADFR

In this novel treatment approach,[39] a bone resorptive (**activating**) agent is applied first in order to initiate the bone remodeling cycle and increase the number of BMUs. An osteoclastic **depressive** agent is then applied to cause cessation of resorption. During the subsequent drug-**free** period, osteoblastic formation is allowed to continue. The sequence is then **repeated**. A form of coherence therapy involving phosphate treatment of 3-days duration for activation, diphosphonate treatment of 15 days for depression and 70 days of drug-free period, has been tested.[40] A preliminary report in five patients with osteoporosis disclosed a histological improvement; however, no improvement was shown in another study.[41] This treatment approach is undergoing a multiclinic trial. The main drawback to this approach resides in the reservation that three days of orthophosphate therapy could stimulate parathyroid function sufficiently to cause activation.

3. Fluoride

The principal action of fluoride on the skeleton is the promotion of appositional bone growth on existing surfaces from the stimulation of osteoblastic formation.[42] There is recent evidence, however, that fluoride may cause focal osteoclastic resorption. Thus, fluoride treatment could allow remodeling of bone and increase the number of BMUs.

There is extensive literature concerning the action of fluoride on the skeleton. The evidence that fluoride could augment bone mass, particularly of the trabecular bone, is convincing. Numerous studies indicate that fluoride treatment appropriately applied could augment bone mass and inhibit fractures in osteoporosis.[43,44] It has been proclaimed by some investigators as the "single most effective agent" for osteoporosis.[45] However, several problems have kept this drug from approval by the FDA; they include:

- Frequent gastrointestinal rheumatic complications,
- Nonresponsiveness in some patients, and
- The concern that it may cause the formation of a mechanically defective bone.[44]

There is emerging evidence that the above problems of sodium fluoride could be overcome. One approach undergoing multiclinic trial is intermittent slow-release sodium fluoride therapy (12-month treatment cycles separated by 1-month withdrawal periods) combined with continuous calcium citrate therapy (0.4 g calcium two to three times/day). The rationale for this approach is provided below.

D. Slow Release Sodium Fluoride

1. Pharmacokinetics

Fluoride is absorbed from the intestinal tract passively, largely in its undissociated form in the stomach.[46] Fluoride is also absorbed in its anionic form in the intestinal tract distal to the stomach, but to a lesser degree.[47]

When sodium fluoride is given orally as a plain preparation, fluoride is rapidly released into gastric lumen, and reacts with hydrochloric acid to form hydrofluoric acid. The rapid absorption of hydrofluoric acid accounts for a sharp rise and rapid decline in serum fluoride concentration. When it is given in a customary twice-daily schedule, two sharp peaks and valleys in serum fluoride levels are disclosed, with peaks exceeding the toxic threshold and valleys falling below the therapeutic threshold.[48] The high levels of fluoride reached in the circulation probably account for various rheumatic complications (to be enumerated). The corrosiveness of hydrofluoric acid leads to gastrointestinal complications (to be discussed).

In contrast, when sodium fluoride in a slow-release form is delivered orally, serum fluoride concentration rises more slowly, reaching a peak at about 4 to 5 h, reflecting absorption of fluoride anion distal to the stomach.[47] Thereafter, serum fluoride concentration declines slowly, maintaining a value above the basal level even at 12 h. Thus, twice-daily administration of slow-release sodium fluoride results in the maintenance of serum fluoride level within the "therapeutic window" (below the toxic threshold and above the therapeutic threshold), with only a modest circadian fluctuation.[47]

E. Bone Histomorphometry

The effect of fluoride on the histomorphometric picture of bone depends on the fluoride dosage and on whether it is given alone or with calcium. When fluoride is given, especially at a high dosage without calcium, osteomalacia may develop.[49,50] The newly formed matrix may be abnormal and may not undergo adequate mineralization. Thus, a typical histomorphometric picture is represented by a pronounced increased in osteoid (nonmineralized matrix) and a reduced calcification front. The formation of abnormal, fibrous, or mosaic bone may occur.

When sodium fluoride (enteric-coated) is given with an adequate calcium intake, the newly formed matrix may become adequately mineralized. Typical changes include an increase in trabecular bone volume without a substantial change in the osteoclastic resorption surface or calcification front.[51] A modest increase in total osteoid surface and osteoid seam has been demonstrated; however, these changes do not approach those encountered in osteomalacia. The impairment in mineralization may become less severe with continued therapy.[52] However, approximately 15% of patients may show mild osteomalacia and 25% of patients may not show any histological response.[51]

When slow-release sodium fluoride is given intermittently with calcium citrate, histomorphometric analysis of bone has disclosed an increased formation of normally appearing lamellar bone, without a defect in mineralization. The results suggest that the maintenance of serum fluoride within the therapeutic window, avoidance of toxic levels in blood, and provision of readily bioavailable calcium supplement assures formation of normally mineralized bone.

1. Bone Mass

In a review of 7 publications,[53-59] sodium fluoride given at a dosage of 30 to 80 mg/day to 209 patients with osteoporosis caused a rise in vertebral bone mass ranging from 2.9 to 23.5% per year, for a mean (corrected for the number of patients) of 7.3% per year. In contrast, the control group without fluoride therapy (available in three reports)[55,56,59] showed a slight decline or a slight increase. The effect of fluoride therapy on the bone mass of the appendicular skeleton is much less marked, with most reports showing only a slight change (less than 1% per year). Thus, it is apparent that fluoride treatment augments spinal bone mass without causing a loss of bone at other sites.

2. Fracture Rates

Six long-term trials with sodium fluoride, involving 164 patients with osteoporosis, have been reported.[51,54,58,60-62] The dose of sodium fluoride ranged from 40 to 110 mg/day, and the duration of treatment ranged from 1.5 to 4.11 years/patient. In these studies, the fracture rate of the vertebra during treatment ranged from 50 to 304 fractures per 1000 patient years, yielding an average fracture rate during fluoride treatment (corrected for number of patients) in combined trials of 207 fractures per 1000 patient years.

None of the above studies included a randomly allocated placebo-controlled group. However, there are four studies in which a control group or a group taking no medication had been included.[61-63] Among 108 patients followed from 2 to 4.5 years/patient, the vertebral fracture rate ranged from 250 to 834 per 1000 patient years for an adjusted mean rate of 554 per 1000 patient years.

The above higher figure in the control group (554 vs. 207) supported the contention that fluoride therapy reduces the vertebral fracture rate. The fracture rate on slow-release sodium fluoride treatment of 160 per 1000 patient years was equivalent to that of other preparations.[58] This conclusion needs validation by a randomized placebo-controlled trial.

3. Side Effects

Complications of plain or coated sodium fluoride therapy were reviewed from 9 published reports involving 413 patients with osteoporosis.[55,56,60,62,64-68] Gastrointestinal complications usually comprised minor adverse symptoms such as cramping, nausea, or diarrhea. Symptoms were sometimes more severe, involving gastrointestinal bleeding. These gastrointestinal complications ranged from 6 to 50% of patients among various series, with a mean figure of 23.5% (corrected for number of patients). Rheumatic complications included joint pain, plantar fascitis, and synovitis. They ranged from 15 to 37%, for a mean of 29.0%.

In contrast, in our study with slow-release sodium fluoride,[47] gastrointestinal and rheumatic complications were encountered in only 6.0 and 7.9%, respectively. These findings could be attributed to the limited formation of corrosive hydrofluoric acid in the gastric lumen due to the delayed release of fluoride, and to the possible avoidance of sharp peaks in the blood exceeding the toxic threshold due to a less efficient absorbability of fluoride in its anionic form.

It has been suggested that long-term fluoride therapy may exaggerate the risk of hip fractures.[69] In a recent study, however, compiled data from five sites did not disclose a higher rate of fracture of the proximal femur than in the untreated population.[70] It is noteworthy that patients who sustained femoral neck fracture were often those who took a high dose of sodium fluoride. The finding suggested the possibility that an inadequate mineralization of bone from a high fluoride dose may have contributed to femoral neck fracture. It is apparent that this complication could be obviated by avoiding a high dose of sodium fluoride and by taking calcium supplementation to assure adequate mineralization.

REFERENCES

1. Cummings, S. R., Epidemiology of osteoporotic fractures: selected topics, in Osteoporosis: Current Concepts: Report of the seventh Ross Conference on Medical Research, Roche, A. F., Gussler, J. D. and Redfern, D. E., Eds., Ross Laboratories, Columbus, 1987, 3.
2. Pak, C. Y. C., Postmenopausal osteoporosis, in *The Menopause,* Buschbaum, H. J., Ed., Springer-Verlag, New York, 1983, 35.
3. Riggs, B. L. and Melton, L. J., III, Involutional osteoporosis, *N. Engl. J. Med.,* 314, 1676, 1986.
4. Hahn, T. J., Halstead, L. R., Teitelbaum, S. L. and Hahn, B. H., Altered mineral metabolism in glucocorticoid-induced osteopenia, *J. Clin. Invest.,* 64, 655, 1979.
5. Mundy, G. R., Shapiro, J. L., Bandelin, J. G., Canalis, E. M. and Raisz, L. G., Direct stimulation of bone resorption by thyroid hormones, *J. Clin. Invest.,* 58, 529, 1976.
6. Gallagher, J. C., Riggs, B. L., Eisman, J., Hamstra, A., Arnaud, S. B. and DeLuca, H. F., Intestinal calcium absorption and serum vitamin D metabolites in normal subjects and osteoporotic patients: effect of age and dietary calcium, *J. Clin. Invest.,* 64, 729, 1979.
7. Heaney, R. P., Recker, R. R. and Saville, P. D., Menopausal changes in calcium balance performance, *J. Lab. Clin. Med.,* 92, 953, 1978.
8. Matkovic, V., Developing strong bones: the young adult female, *Proc. Clin. Disorders of Bone and Min. Metab.,* Detroit, MI, 1988.
9. Drinkwater, B. L., Nilson, K., Chesnut, C. H., III, Bremner, W. J., Shainholtz, S. and Southworth, M. B., Bone mineral content of amenorrheic and eumenorrheic athletes, *N. Engl. J. Med.,* 311, 277, 1984.

10. Turner, R. T., Greene, V. S. and Bell, N. H., Demonstration that ethanol inhibits bone matrix synthesis and mineralization in the rat, *J. Bone Min. Res.*, 2, 61, 1987.

11. Michnovicz, J. J., Hershcopf, R. J., Naganuma, H., Bradlow, H. L. and Fishman, J., Increased 2-hydroxylation of estradiol as a possible mechanism for the anti-estrogenic effect of cigarette smoking, *N. Engl. J. Med.*, 315, 1305, 1986.

12. Breslau, N. A., McGuire, J. L., Zerwekh, J. E. and Pak, C. Y. C., The role of dietary sodium on renal excretion and intestinal absorption of calcium and on vitamin D metabolism, *J. Clin. Endocrinol. Metab.*, 55, 369, 1982.

13. Breslau, N. A., Sakhaee, K. and Pak, C. Y. C., Impaired adaptation to salt-induced urinary calcium losses in postmenopausal osteoporosis., *Trans. Assoc. Amer. Phys.*, 98, 107, 1985.

14. Goulding, A., Effect of dietary NaCl supplements on parathyroid function, bone turnover and bone composition in rats taking restricted amounts of calcium, *Min. Elect. Metab.*, 4, 203, 1980.

15. Eriksen, E. F., Colvard, D. S., Berg, N. J., Graham, M. L., Mann, K. G., Spelsberg, T. C. and Riggs, B. L., Evidence of estrogen receptors in normal human osteoblast-like cells, *Science*, 241, 84, 1988.

16. Komm, B. S., Terpening, C. M., Benz, D. J., Graeme, K. A., Gallegos, A., Korc, M., Greene, G. L., O'Malley, B. W. and Haussler, M. R., Estrogen binding, receptor mRNA, and biologic response in osteoblast-like osteosarcoma cells, *Science*, 241, 81, 1988.

17. Sakhaee, K., Nicar, M. J., Glass, K. and Pak, C. Y. C., Postmenopausal osteoporosis as a manifestation of renal hypercalciuria with secondary hyperparathyroidism, *J. Clin. Endocrinol. Metab.*, 61, 368, 1985.

18. Zerwekh, J. E., Sakhaee, K., Glass, K. and Pak, C. Y. C., Long-term 25-hydroxyvitamin D_3 therapy in postmenopausal osteoporosis: demonstration of responsive and nonresponsive subgroups, *J. Clin. Endocrinol. Metab.*, 56, 410, 1983.

19. Deftos, L. J., Weisman, M. H., Williams, G. W., Karpf, D. B., Frumar, A. M., Davidson, B. J., Parthemore, J. C. and Judd, H. L., Influence of age and sex on plasma calcitonin in human beings, *N. Engl. J. Med.*, 302, 1351, 1980, 1984.

20. Pacifici, R., Rifas, K., Vered, I., McMurtry, C., McCracken, R., Avioli, L. V. and Peck, W. A., Interleukin-1 secretion from human blood monocytes in normal and osteoporotic women: effect of menopause and estrogen/progesterone treatment, in *Journal of Bone Mineral Research Program & Abstracts*, Tenth Annual Scientific Meeting, New Orleans, LA, S204, 1988.

21. Christiansen, C., Riis, B. J. and Rodbro, P., Prediction of rapid bone loss in postmenopausal women, *Lancet*, I, 1105, 1987.

22. Epstein, S., Poser, J., McClintock, R., Johnston, C. C., Jr., Bryce, G. and Hui, S., Differences in serum bone GLA protein with age and sex, *Lancet*, I, 307, 1984.

23. Meunier, P. J., Courpron, P., Edouard, C., et al., Bone histomorphometry in osteoporotic states, in *Osteoporosis II*, International symposium on osteoporosis, Barzel, U. S., Ed., Grune & Stratton, New York, 1979, 27.

24. Whyte, M. P., Bergfeld, M. A., Murphy, W. A., Avioli, L. V. and Teitelbaum, S. L., Postmenopausal osteoporosis. A heterogeneous disorder as assessed by histomorphometric analysis of iliac crest bone from untreated patients, *Am. J. Med.*, 72, 193, 1982.

25. Lawoyin, S., Sismilich, S., Browne, R. and Pak, C. Y. C., Bone mineral content in patients with calcium urolithiasis, *Metabolism*, 28, 1250, 1979.

26. Riggs, B. L., Wahner, H. W., Dunn, W. L., Mazess, R. B., Offord, K. P. and Melton, L. J., III, Differential changes in bone mineral density of the appendicular and axial skeleton with aging: relationship to spinal osteoporosis, *J. Clin. Invest.*, 67, 328, 1981.

27. Genant, H. K., Cann, C. E., Ettinger, B. and Gordan, G. S., Quantitative computed tomography of vertebral spongiosa: a sensitive method for detecting early bone loss after oophorectomy, *Ann. Intern. Med.*, 97, 699, 1982.

28. Eastell, R. and Riggs, B. L., Treatment of osteoporosis, *Obstet. Gyn. Clin. N. Am.*, 14, 77, 1987.

29. Matkovic, V., Kostial, K., Simonovic, I., Buzina, A., Brodarec, A. and Nordin, B. E., Bone status and fracture rates in two regions of Yugoslavia, *Am. J. Clin. Nutr.*, 32, 540, 1979.

30. Al-Azzawi, F., Hart, D. M. and Lindsay, R., Long term effect of oestrogen replacement therapy on bone mass as measured by dual photon absorptiometry, *Brit. Med. J.*, 294, 1261, 1987.

31. Gennari, C., Chierichetti, M. and Bigazzi, S., Comparative effects on bone mineral content of calcium and calcium plus salmon calcitonin given in two different regimens in postmenopausal osteoporosis, *Current Therap. Res.*, 38, 455, 1985.

32. Recker, R. R., Continuous treatment of osteoporosis: current status, *Orthop. Clin. N. Am.*, 12, 611, 1981.

33. Riis, B., Thomsen, K. and Christiansen, C., Does calcium supplementation prevent postmenopausal bone loss?, *N. Engl. J. Med.*, 316, 173, 1987.

34. Ettinger, B., Genant, H. K. and Cann, C. E., Postmenopausal bone loss is prevented by treatment with low-dosage estrogen with calcium, *Ann. Int. Med.*, 106, 40, 1987.

35. Pak, C. Y. C., Calcium bioavailability and clinical uses of calcium salts, *National Kidney Foundation's CRN Quarterly*, 12, 8, 1988.

36. Recker, R. R., Calcium absorption and achlorhydria, *N. Engl. J. Med.*, 313, 70, 1985.

37. Reeve, J., Meunier, P. J., Parsons, J. A., Bernat, M., Bijvoet, O. L. M., Courpron, P., Edouard, C., Klenerman, L., Neer, R. M. and Renier, J. C., Anabolic effect of human parathyroid hormone fragment on trabecular bone in involutional osteoporosis: a multicentre trial, *Brit. Med. J.,* 280, 1340, 1980.

38. Slovik, D. M., Rosenthal, D. I., Doppelt, S. H., Potts, J. T., Jr., Daly, M. A., Campbell, J. A. and Neer, R. M., Restoration of spinal bone in osteoporotic men by treatment with human parathyroid hormone (1-34) and 1,25-dihydroxyvitamin D, *J. Bone Min. Res.*, 1, 377, 1986.

39. Frost, H. M., Treatment of osteoporosis by manipulation of coherent bone cell populations, *Clin. Ortho. Rel. Res.*, 143, 227, 1979.

40. Anderson, C., Cape, R. D., Crilly, R. G., Hodsman, A. B. and Wolfe, B. M., Preliminary observations of a form of coherence therapy for osteoporosis, *Calc. Tiss. Int.*, 36, 341, 1984.

41. Pacifici, R., McMurtry, C., Vered, I., Rupich, R. and Avioli, L. V., Coherence therapy does not prevent axial bone loss in osteoporotic women: a preliminary comparative study, *J. Clin. Endocrinol. Metab.*, 66, 747, 1988.

42. Raisz, L. G. and Smith, J., Prevention and therapy of osteoporosis, *Rat. Drug Therap.*, 19, 1, 1985.

43. Bikle, D. D., Fluoride treatment of osteoporosis: a new look at an old drug, *Ann. Int. Med.*, 98, 1013, 1983.

44. Kanis, J. A. and Meunier, P. J., Should we use fluoride to treat osteoporosis? A review, *Quar. J. Med.*, 53, 145, 1984.

45. Farley, S. M., Wergedal, J. E., Smith, L. C., Lundy, M. W., Farley, J. R. and Baylink, D. J., Fluoride therapy for osteoporosis: characterization of the skeletal response by serial measurements of serum alkaline phosphatase activity, *Metabolism: Clin. Exp.*, 36, 211, 1987.

46. Whitford, G. M. and Pashley, D. H., Fluoride absorption: the influence of gastric acidity, *Calc. Tiss. Int.*, 36, 302, 1984.

47. Pak, C. Y. C., Sakhaee, K., Gallagher, C., Parcel, C., Peterson, R., Zerwekh, J. E., Lemke, M., Britton, F., Hsu, M. C. and Adams, B., Attainment of therapeutic fluoride levels in serum without major side effects using a slow-release preparation of sodium fluoride in postmenopausal osteoporosis, *J. Bone Min. Res.*, 1, 563, 1986.

48. Ekstrand, J., Alvan, G., Boreus, L. O. and Norlin, A., Pharmacokinetics of fluoride in man after single and multiple oral doses, *Eur. J. Clin. Pharm.*, 12, 311, 1977.

49. Compston, J. E., Chadha, S. and Merrett, A. L., Osteomalacia developing during treatment of osteoporosis with sodium fluoride and vitamin D, *Brit. Med. J.*, 281, 910, 1980.

50. Jowsey, J., Schenk, R. K. and Reutter, F. W., Some results of the effect of fluoride on bone tissue in osteoporosis, *J. Clin. Endocrinol. Metab.*, 28, 869, 1968.

51. Meunier, P. J., Galus, K., Briancon, D., Reeve, J., Podseb, R., Edouard, C., Arlot, M., Charhon, S., Delmas, P., Benev, B., Valentin, A. and Chapuy, M., Treatment of primary osteoporosis with drugs that increase bone formation: sodium fluoride, hPTH 1-34, ADFR concept, in *Osteoporosis: Copenhagen Int. Symp. Osteop.*, June 3-9, 1984, Christiansen, C., Arnaud, C. D., Nordin, B. E. C., et al., Eds., Dept. of Clinical Chemistry, Oylosbrun Hospital, Aalborg Stiftsbogtrykkeri, Copenhagen, Denmark, 1984, 595.

52. Lundy, M. W., Wergedal, J. E., Teubner, E., Burnell, J. and Baylink, D. J., The effect of prolonged fluoride therapy for osteoporosis: bone composition and histology, 34th Annual Meeting, Orthopaedic Research Society, Atlanta, Georgia, 1988.

53. Duursma, S. A., Glerum, J. H., van Dijk, A., Bosch, R., Kerkhoff, H., van Putten, J. and Raymakers, J. A., Responders and non-responders after fluoride therapy in osteoporosis, *Bone*, 8, 131, 1987.

54. Farley, S. M., Libanati, C. L., Odvina, C. V., Smith, L., Eliel, L., Wakley, G. K., Kilocoyne, R., Schulz, E. E. and Baylink, D. J., Efficacy of long-term fluoride and calcium therapy in to correcting the deficit of spinal bone density in osteoporosis, *J. Clin. Epidemiol.*, 42, 1067, 1989.

55. Hansson, T. and Roos, B., The effect of fluoride and calcium on spinal bone mineral content: a controlled, prospective (3 years) study, *Calc. Tiss. Int.*, 40, 315, 1987.

56. Harrison, J. E., McNeill, K. G., Sturtridge, W. C., Bayley, T. A., Murray, T. M., Williams, C., Tam, C. and Fornasier, V., Three-year changes in bone mineral mass of postmenopausal osteoporotic patients based on neutron activation analysis of the central third of the skeleton, *J. Clin. Endocrinol. Metab.*, 52, 751, 1981.

57. Juhn, A., Healey, J. H., Schneider, R., Lane, J. M. and Bansal, M., Reversal of femoral and vertebral osteoporotic bone loss, 34th Annual Meeting, Orthopaedic Research Society, Atlanta, Georgia, 1988.

58. Pak, C. Y. C., Fluoride and osteoporosis, *Proc. Soc. Exp. Biol. Med.*, 191, 278, 1989.

59. Raymakers, J. A., Van Dijke, C. F., Hoekstra, A. and Duursma, S. A., Monitoring fluoride therapy in osteoporosis by dual photon absorptiometry, *Bone*, 8, 143, 1987.

60. Lane, J. M., Healey, J. H., Schwartz, E., Vigorita, V. J., Schneider, R., Einhorn, T. A., Suda, M. and Robbins, W. C., Treatment of osteoporosis with sodium fluoride and calcium: effects on vertebral fracture incidence and bone histomorphometry, *Orthop. Clin. N. Am.*, 15, 729, 1984.

61. Power, G. R. and Gay, J. D., Sodium fluoride in the treatment of osteoporosis, *Clin. Invest. Med.*, 9, 41, 1986.

62. Riggs, B. L., Seeman, E., Hodgson, S. F., Taves, D. R. and O'Fallon, W. M., Effect of the fluoride/calcium regimen on vertebral fracture occurrence in postmenopausal osteoporosis: comparison with conventional therapy, *N. Engl. J. Med.*, 306, 446, 1982.

63. Dambacher, M.A., Ittner, J. and Ruegsegger, P., Long-term therapy of postmenopausal osteoporosis, *Bone*, 7, 199, 1986.

64. Briancon, D. and Meunier, P. J., Treatment of osteoporosis with fluoride, calcium and vitamin D, *Orthop. Clin. N. Am.*, 12, 629, 1981.

65. Franke, J., Rempel, H. and Franke, M., Three years' experience with sodium-fluoride therapy of osteoporosis, *Acta Orthop. Scand.*, 45, 1, 1974.

66. Hasling, C., Nielsen, H. E., Melsen, F. and Mosekilde, L., Safety of osteoporosis treatment with sodium fluoride, calcium phosphate and vitamin D., *Min. Elect. Metab.*, 13, 96, 1987.

67. Kuntz, D., Marie, P., Naveau, B., Maziere, B., Tubiana, M. and Ryckewaert, A., Extended treatment of primary osteoporosis by sodium fluoride combined with 25 hydroxycholecalciferol, *Clin. Rheum.*, 3, 145, 1984.

68. van Kesteren, R. G., Duursma, S. A., Visser, W. J., van der Sluys Veer, J. and Backer Dirks, O., Fluoride in serum and bone during treatment of osteoporosis with sodium fluoride, calcium and vitamin D, *Metab. Bone Dis. & Rel. Res.*, 4, 31, 1982.

69. Gutteridge, D. H., Price, R. I., Nicholson, G. C., Kent, G. N., Retallack, R. W., Devlin, R. D., Worth, G. K., Glancy, J. J., Michell, P. and Gruber, H., Fluoride in osteoporotic vertebral fractures — trabecular increase, vertebral protection, femoral fractures, Osteoporosis: Copenhagen Int. Symp. Osteop., June 3-9, 1984, Christiansen, C., Arnaud, C. D., Nordin, B. E. C., et al., Eds., Dept. of Clinical Chemistry, Oylosbrun Hospital, Aalborg Stiftsbogtrykkeri, Copenhagen, Denmark, 1984, 595.

70. Riggs, B. L., Baylink, D. J., Kleerekoper, M., Lane, J. M., Melton, L. J., III, and Meunier, P. J., Incidence of hip fractures in osteoporotic women treated with sodium fluoride, *J. Bone Min. Res.*, 2, 123, 1987.

14

Glucocorticoids, Stress, and Aging

Luis Goya, Francisco Rivero, and A. M. Pascual-Leone

CONTENTS

I. INTRODUCTION

Aging has been defined as a progressive decline in organ function associated with decreased capacity for adaptation to changes in the environment and for restoration of homeostasis (Chapter 1). Age-related cellular and molecular degenerative changes (see Chapter 15) impact dramatically on adaptation when integrative and homeostatic systems are affected. One of the key elements in the response of the organism to adaptive changes is the hypothalamic-pituitary-adrenal (HPA) system which utilizes diverse compounds such as amines, peptides, and corticosteroids to accomplish complex functions in order to maintain homeostasis. The glucocorticoids (GCs), a group of adrenocortical steroids, are secreted in response to numerous psychological or somatic stressors and they are essential for appropriate adaptation to stress.[1] The GCs trigger energy mobilization from the storage sites in the body, increase cardiovascular tone, and suppress anabolic processes such as growth and reproduction, which are deferred until the emergency situation is resolved.[2,3] An organism incapable of secreting GCs in response to stress is highly vulnerable.

Glucocorticoids, when secreted in excess, may be damaging because of their essentially catabolic nature. A number of degenerative changes characteristic of the aging process occur as a consequence of chronic hypersecretion of GCs (hypercorticism), including immunosuppression, muscle atrophy, osteoporosis, hyperglycemia, atherosclerosis, hypertension, reproductive suppression, and mental disturbances.[4] These pathologies are not due to the stressors themselves but to the defensive, damaging actions of GCs to stress.[2] Several early investigators found clear similarities between the pathologies typical of aging and those seen in pathological GC hypersecretion, such as Cushing's syndrome.[5] At least two different examples in nature are known where aging and subsequent death following mating are caused by a cascade of degenerative changes triggered by GCs: the Pacific salmon *Oncorhynkus nerka Kennerlyi*,[6,7] and the Australian marsupial *Antechinus swainsonii*.[8-10] With aging, organ responsiveness to hormones is diminished, and ACTH and GCs in plasma are often present in high levels. Hence, hypercorticism has been regarded over the years as an important factor in the aging process.

Considerable evidence is accumulating that GCs may be involved in neuronal cell death in the hippocampus (Chapter 16). This brain area is thought to play a role in the adrenocortical axis regulation, a role that has led several authors to formulate the "glucocorticoid cascade hypothesis" of aging involving the hypothalamus, the hippocampus, pituitary, and adrenal cortex (see below).

II. GLUCOCORTICOID SECRETION IN RESPONSE TO STRESS

A. Physiological Actions of Glucocorticoids (GCs)

GCs have numerous physiological actions and control several metabolic pathways (Chapter 2). These hormones stimulate gluconeogenesis and glycogen synthesis in the liver and reduce glucose uptake by adipose tissue cells, where they increase fatty acid mobilization. GCs act as immunosuppressors; they affect bone by decreasing calcium accumulation and depleting bone matrix, the cardiovascular system by increasing blood pressure, and development and differentiation of many tissues and organs, such as neural retina, lung (surfactant factor), and the mammary gland.[11]

B. Stress and Responses to Stress

Some of the actions mentioned above are operative in the physiological response of the body to an exogenous stress or alarm situation, since in these cases, adrenal cortex (mainly GCs) and adrenal medulla (catecholamines) secretions are increased, facilitating the "fight or flight" response of the body in that situation of emergency. The situation of stress can be defined as an environmental perturbation that leads to functional imbalance and triggers the stress response as a set of endocrine, neural, and metabolic adaptations that restore homeostasis. The alarm reaction can be provoked by stress conditions such as hypoxia, severe hypoglycemia, hunger, cold, heat, injury, evading a predator, or, in humans, psychological factors. Different stressors induce a similar and convergent stress response which was characterized and defined by Selye in his pioneering work as the "general adaptation syndrome".[12] One of the most consistent and important features of the response to a majority of stress situations is the secretion of GCs by the adrenal gland.

C. Role of the Hypothalamic-Pituitary-Adrenal (HPA) Axis in Response to Stress

Glucocorticoids are secreted in a final step of an endocrine axis beginning in the brain (Chapter 2). Adrenocortical steroids exert a wide array of effects throughout the body which are essential for successful adaptation to stress.[3] The HPA axis operates by coordinating the circadian (asleep-awake) cycle, and by mediating the animal's ability to cope with a stress situation. The presence or anticipation of an alarm situation stimulates, in the hypothalamus, the release of corticotropin releasing hormone (CRH) which is transported via the hypothalamic-hypophysial portal circulation to the pituitary where it stimulates the production and secretion of the adrenocorticotropic hormone (ACTH). Several other hormones and neurotransmitters can also enhance ACTH secretion from the pituitary, such as vasopressin (ADH), oxytocin, and catecholamines (Chapters 3 and 4).[13] ACTH released in the blood reaches the adrenal cortex where it stimulates the synthesis and secretion of corticosteroids, mainly GCs. In physiological conditions, peak levels of GCs after stress rising more than 40-fold are attained within 15 to 30 min and return to basal levels 60 to 90 min later.

The maintenance of GC concentration within the physiological range is accomplished through complex regulatory circuits.[14,15] Under basal conditions, GCs block or inhibit CRH and ACTH secretion via negative feedback loops; during stress, the GC-negative feedback is less effective in blocking release of ACTH. Under both basal and stress conditions, the secretion of the mineralocorticoids (MCs) is only slightly affected by ACTH (Chapter 2).[16]

In a stressful situation, catecholamines from the adrenal medulla, growth hormone (GH) from the pituitary, and glucagon from the pancreas are also secreted. Together with these hormones, GCs mobilize the stored energy, mainly glucose, and enhance the production of more fuel by stimulating gluconeogenesis, thereby supplying fast energy to muscles critical for the adaptive response. GCs, along with catecholamines, increase cardiovascular tone, facilitating the delivery of energy nutrients to the muscle. Simultaneously, GCs inhibit those processes such as digestion, growth, inflammation, and reproduction that are irrelevant to adaptation.[17,18]

The importance of GCs in the stress response is clearly demonstrated: in the absence of these hormones, adrenalectomized animals cannot survive severe stress. Yet, these same actions, critical for survival, can be highly deleterious if prolonged. The consequences are seen in many stress-related diseases. Thus, the catabolic effects of GCs, critical to face a transient stress, become damaging if such stress is repeated or extended. Among these consequences are adult-onset diabetes, hypertension, osteoporosis, reproductive dysfunctions, and immune suppression.[2,17]

The excessive secretion of GCs in response to a stressor could perhaps be mitigated by a negative feedback on the HPA axis. Primary sites of negative feedback action of GCs are the pituitary corticotropes and the parvocellular neurons in the paraventricular nucleus of the hypothalamus, where these steroids inhibit stress-induced activation of the HPA axis. The effectiveness of this feedback loop may be disrupted or reduced with aging by a number of factors, such as reduced sensitivity of the GC receptors (GCr) in brain cells, decreased number of receptors due to neuronal loss, or others.

D. Role of the Hippocampus in Response to Stress

Extensive literature points to the hippocampus as an additional site of control of HPA activity.[19,20] The hippocampus, with the amygdala and septal nuclei, is part of the limbic system. The limbic system is concerned with olfaction (a relatively minor function in humans) and feeding behavior. With the hypothalamus, it is also concerned with sexual behavior, the emotions of rage and fear, and motivation; the hippocampus has also been implicated in learning and memory. Studies of animals with lesions of the hippocampus or in which specific hippocampal areas have been stimulated, indicate that the hippocampus exerts an inhibitory influence over the HPA axis, probably as part of its involvement in rage, fear, and motivation control. Thus, the hippocampus would regulate the severity and the duration of the stress response.

III. HPA AXIS IN THE AGED ANIMAL

A. Glucocorticoid Secretion

A number of age-related changes occur in the HPA axis (Chapter 2). With aging, a rise in the blood GC concentration is observed in many different rat strains, more pronounced in males,[21-24] with increases ranging between 15 and 200% and high variability. Elevated concentrations of blood GCs have been also found during stress, as aged rats have a reduced ability to terminate their stress response by decreasing the GC levels to basal prestress values.[23,25,26] During stress itself, the response seems normal in aged, male animals compared with young adults, with the expected elevations of GCs in blood in response to different stressors such as immobilization, ether, cold, laparotomy, or histamine injection.[23] However, in females, stress may elicit a less severe response.[22,27,28] Estrogens increase GC levels by inducing transcortin (or cortico-steroid-binding globulin, CBG), thereby lowering free GC concentration during stress in the older females.[29] Half-life of radiolabeled GCs does not change with age, and blood volume substantially increases in old animals; therefore, increased circulating GC levels reflect a rise in adrenal cortex secretion rather than a diminished clearance of the hormones from the blood.[23]

B. ACTH Secretion

Plasma ACTH levels are elevated in aged Long-Evans rats during the afternoon period of the diurnal cycle,[30] and after an acute emotional response (rather than during exposure of the animals to a novelty stress) in the Brown Norway rat.[31] The data reported from studies with the Brown Norway rat demonstrate that the level of ACTH release is increased with aging after stress, with little change observed in the adrenocortical secretion of corticosterone. A reduced adrenal sensitivity to ACTH has been suggested.[32] As the most pronounced ACTH response occurs after the conditioned emotional response, changes in the central control of the pituitary ACTH release may have occurred.

The decline with age in adrenal responsiveness to ACTH may result from decreased delivery of cholesterol to the mitochondria for steroidogenesis.[33-35] If the aged adrenal cortex is less responsive to ACTH but continues to secrete more GCs, the adrenal must be receiving huge amounts of ACTH, and the problem may reside in the pituitary, where high concentrations of ACTH have been reported.[21] Moving along the HPA axis, the altered adrenal responsiveness to ACTH may be due to:

- Hypersensitivity of the pituitary to hypothalamic secretagogues, or
- Hypersecretion of secretagogues in the face of an hyposensitive pituitary, as occurs in the adrenals, or
- Failure of feedback inhibition.

C. Glucocorticoid Feedback

The efficiency with which GCs exert a feedback signal declines with aging in the rat. In the young adult, administration of a synthetic steroid such as dexamethasone is a strong negative feedback signal, and concentrations of ACTH and corticosterone (the most abundant GC in the rat, the species in which most of the experiments have been conducted) rapidly decline. In the aged rat, some component of the axis must have lost its sensitivity to the feedback regulation, for dexamethasone resistance occurs and endogenous corticosterone levels remain high for a longer time.[36,37] Thus, GC hypersecretion in the aged rat probably reflects the reduced sensitivity of the axis to the feedback regulation. The aged pituitary is hyporesponsive to CRH.[38] The inhibitory signal from the corticosteroids may be operative at the brain level. This fact is consistent with the observations that the brain is the most sensitive site of the HPA axis for the GC feedback inhibition.[39]

IV. HPA AXIS AND THE HIPPOCAMPUS

The hippocampus is the only brain site where a major loss of corticosteroid receptors has been observed — with a progressive depletion of approximately half the corticosteroid receptors with aging.[16,26,40,41] The two classes of corticosteroid receptors (GCr and MCr) in the brain include (Chapter 2):

- Type I receptors, primarily for mineralocorticoids (MCr). These also bind GCs such as corticosterone with high affinity but low capacity. The hippocampus is the main, and almost sole, site of steroid type I receptors (MCr) in the brain, and has as many type II receptors as other brain regions.
- Type II receptors primarily for GCs. These GCrs bind dexamethasone and corticosterone with lower affinity but higher capacity than type I.[42]

Both types of steroid receptors are found in the hippocampus, and regardless of the strain of rats studied, a reduction in hippocampal MCr binding capacity of 40 to 50% with aging is observed. GCr are found unaltered,[30] reduced,[30,43] or impaired in other binding properties, such as resistance to GC-induced down-regulation.[44] Changes in MCr and GCr with age are site-specific in the brain. In the Wistar rat, MCr are reduced by 50% and GCr by 28% in the aged hippocampus.[26] In the brown Norway rat, a 40% reduction in MCr occurs with age in the hippocampus without change in GCr. In the hypothalamus and anterior pituitary, GCr capacity is reduced but is associated with a pronounced increase in GCr affinity.[31] However, MCr mRNA measured by *in situ* hybridization is not altered in all hippocampal cell fields. Therefore, a differential effect of aging on translation, receptor processing, or posttranslational events cannot be excluded. Studies showing that the reduced MCr capacity of senescent rats may be stimulated by the administration of a potent neurotropic agent, the ACTH4-9 analog, support the view that MCr and GCr sensitivity is diminished with aging but that a neurotropic agent can enhance plasticity at least in the case of MCr.[26,31]

The dominant negative feedback action occurs primarily at the level of the corticotropes in the pituitary and the paraventricular nucleus in the hypothalamus. The decreased hippocampal MCr and decreased hypothalamic and pituitary GCr are consistent with the increased basal and stress-induced ACTH levels observed in aged Brown Norway rats.[31]

The hippocampus loses neurons with age,[45] and cell counting coupled with corticosteroid receptor high-resolution autoradiography reveal that the neurons with the highest concentrations of such receptors are the ones that are lost.[46] Thus receptor loss may be partially due to loss of the neurons themselves in the hippocampus.

Although the pituitary and the hypothalamus are the major sites for the regulation of the GC feedback signal, suprahypothalamic sites are also involved in the feedback response to GCs. In particular, the hippocampus has an inhibitory effect on the HPA axis.[27] As already mentioned, it is one of the most sensitive areas for GCs in the brain, and its involvement in the negative feedback signals is mediated, via the bed nucleus of the stria terminalis, on to the hypothalamic neurons containing the ACTH secretagogues.

Adrenocortical hyperactivity due to lesions in the entire hippocampus illustrates the "brake" effect of this area on the HPA axis. This effect is present at both the pituitary and adrenal levels, with ACTH and/or corticosterone hypersecretion during basal conditions,[47-50] stress,[27,49] and poststress period.[23,51] To further support the idea of the hippocampus as a brake for the HPA axis, electrical stimulation of this brain area inhibits the paraventricular nucleus activity and reduces adrenocortical secretion.[52,53]

Hippocampal lesions by experimental manipulation are massive, and a fornix cut completely isolates the structure. In contrast, the hippocampal neuronal loss observed with aging is diffuse and involves no more than 15% of neuronal loss. However, the corticosteroid receptor depletion in the aged hippocampus affects, as already mentioned, 50% of the total receptor capacity, and the extent of occupancy of the receptors determines the extent of the feedback response, thus, regardless of the neuron loss, the depletion of the receptors should desensitize the HPA axis.

Based on the phenomenon of receptor down-regulation, a regimen of stress or GC administration that reduces the amount of hippocampal receptors, without decreasing concentrations of receptors elsewhere in the brain, has been devised.[54] Rats so treated have shown similar defects in the HPA axis as aged animals, and the removal of the stressor has returned the situation to normality.[54]

A. Hippocampal Inhibition of the HPA Axis

Given the hippocampal inhibition on the HPA axis, the question raised is whether the mechanism of inhibition is intrinsic or represents a mediation of GC feedback. At least some inhibition seems to involve the feedback response: thus, dexamethasone resistance has been associated with hippocampal damage.[27,49,55] In addition, adrenalectomy, both in hippocampal damaged and intact rats, induces hypersecretion of ACTH similar to that which occurs in rats after hippocampal damage alone.[49] This suggests that the ACTH hypersecretion found in the adrenal-intact rat following hippocampal damage represents lack of sensitivity to the GC feedback signal. This signal, mediated by the extent of occupancy of corticosteroid receptors at the hippocampus, is the best predictor of the extent of secretion of CRH, vasopressin, and oxytocin prior to stress.

The hippocampal component of the corticosteroid feedback inhibition, however, is relatively small, and the majority of the feedback regulation is mediated at pituitary and hypothalamic levels. The strength of the hippocampal component varies over the circadian cycle, stronger at the circadian nadir and weaker at the circadian peak, when a hippocampal input may not be observed.[47-49] The hippocampus seems to have a role in the slow component of the feedback response.[56] Finally, the limbic system presents other putative regulators for the HPA axis and the strength of their inputs is variable, therefore, the endocrine consequences of the damage to the hippocampal area may not be permanent.[48] Thus, the hippocampus plays an important role, although limited, in the regulation of the GC feedback signal.

The fact that an adrenal hypersecretion results from aging of the hippocampus through receptor depletion and/or neuron loss seems to provide an explanation for the inability of aged organisms to cope with stress. Although the HPA axis is manifestly altered with aging, and the aged hippocampus apparently involved in this altered response, the question remains: are GCs involved in the process of aging of the hippocampus? The observations that chronic GC exposure is associated with neuronal loss in the hippocampus strongly implicate GCs in accelerating some aspects of aging.

V. GLUCOCORTICOIDS AND THE AGING HIPPOCAMPUS

Given the decisive role played by GCs in the loss of hippocampal neurons with age, the degree of GC hypersecretion is used as an index for hippocampal neuronal loss.[57] Adrenalectomized rats at mid-age and maintained GC-free for the rest of their lifespan, are protected from the neuropathology typical of the aging hippocampus, as well as from several of the cognitive deficits typical of aging and thought to be hippocampal dependent.[58] Other data demonstrate that some factor from the adrenals damages the hippocampus and that this is a normal, rather than pharmacological, part of the aging process. Sapolsky et al.[59] found that three months of exposure to corticosterone caused a pattern of hippocampal degeneration similar to that seen during aging. Major lesions included:

- A 25% loss of neurons in a specific area (CA3) but with little loss in another area (CA1 or dentate gyrus.) A similar distribution of neuron loss occurs during aging;[45,60]
- Preferential loss of neurons containing high concentration of corticosteroid receptors, the surviving neurons being those with the lowest concentration of receptors, the same as during aging;[46] and
- Neuron degeneration, compensatory glial hypertrophy and infiltration, as seen in the aging hippocampus.[61,62]

After a much shorter exposure of three weeks (rather than months), the same high corticosterone concentration[63] and exposure to prolonged stress[64] induce the loss of pyramidal neurons, loss of branching, and decreased length of apical dendrites. All these degenerative changes are most pronounced in the CA3 region of the hippocampus. When 18-month-old rats were exposed to a repeated footshock, which also induces considerable amounts of anxiety, and were examined at 2 years of age, they showed a 25% loss of pyramidal neurons compared to nonstressed controls of the same age. Immobilization or immersion into water of rats for 15 min/day for a month produced a significant loss of CA3 and CA4 pyramidal neurons.[65] The fact that only castrated animals showed this neuronal loss remains unexplained.

Thus, GC exposure appear to modulate the rate of hippocampal neuronal loss during aging: low GC levels spare hippocampal neurons, whereas high GC levels and stress accelerate neuronal loss.

A. Regulation of Hippocampal Sensitivity to GCs

The sensitivity of the hippocampus to GC levels was investigated to explore whether a behavioral manipulation which caused a long-term reduction in GC secretion would also delay some features of hippocampal aging.[66,67] Handling of neonatal rats, daily, for the first weeks of life, induces in adulthood long-lasting changes in adrenocortical function:[66,67]

- Basal GC levels are lower than in controls (nonhandled rats);
- Recovery to basal GC concentrations after stress is faster;
- Sensitivity to GCs negative feedback is greater;
- Type II corticosteroid receptors are increased in hippocampus;
- Hippocampal neuronal loss is decreased; and
- Hippocampal-dependent cognitive skills are improved.

Adrenalectomy (which eliminates other hormones besides GCs), GC treatment or stress exposure (where the animal has to cope with supraphysiological levels of GCs), or neonatal handling (which has other consequences than a reduced basal GC secretion) are very unphysiological situations. Nevertheless, studies utilizing these interventions clearly suggest that the duration and degree of GC exposure over the lifespan of the rat can be a crucial determinant for the severity of neuron loss in the hippocampus. Moreover, the hippocampus is sensitive to relatively small changes in patterns of GC exposure.

The hippocampus may be damaged by GCs and stress also in primates.[68] Trapped wild vervet monkeys living in captivity display a "dominance hierarchy". Many of the "oppressed" animals die of exposure to sustained "social stress". At autopsy, the dead animals show loss of neurons and, in the remaining cells, reduced and irregularly shaped perikarya, and atrophic or swollen dendrites. The damage is extensive in the hippocampus, relatively mild in the cerebral cortex, and absent in other brain areas such as the thalamus and hypothalamus. Overall, this distribution of damage closely resembles the pattern reported in rats exposed to sustained stress or GC treatment.

Is neuronal damage in primates submitted to social stress caused by GC hypersecretion? The answer is positive: vervet monkeys were implanted with GC-secreting pellets in one hippocampus, and cholesterol-secreting pellets, as control, in the contralateral hippocampus; after one year of treatment, post-mortem examination showed markers of hippocampal degeneration restricted to the CA3 region only in the GC-treated side.[69]

These studies suggest that in both the rodent and the primate, GC excess or prolonged stress can damage the hippocampus and worsen the functional consequences of hippocampal aging. Since the complete elimination of GCs via adrenalectomy also damages the hippocampus,[70] the maintenance of GC concentration within the physiological range throughout life becomes very important.

B. Glucocorticoid-Induced Neurotoxicity and/or Hippocampal Vulnerability

GCs may not be directly toxic to hippocampal neurons but may alter some aspects of their function and metabolism. In the latter case, a sublethal concentration of GCs not sufficient only by itself to damage the hippocampal neuron, could compromise its ability to withstand and survive other neurological insults. In other words, GC exposure would lower the threshold for other insults that damage the hippocampus.

That GCs, in nontoxic doses, may reduce viability of hippocampal neurons has been demonstrated in a variety of models:

- Repeated epileptic seizures, induced by the administration of kainic acid (binding to receptors of the excitatory amino acid glutamate) to rats, damage preferentially CA3 neurons in the hippocampus.[71] Surgical or chemical adrenalectomy will reduce the extent of this damage while GC treatment will increase it.[72-74] The short duration of GC treatment in this model, only a few days, was not sufficient for the GCs to destroy the hippocampal neurons, but was sufficient to increase their vulnerability to kainic acid.

- Severe hypoglycemia preferentially damages the neurons of the dentate gyrus in the hippocampus. A similar pattern of damage is achieved by the administration of the antimetabolite 3-acetylpyridine to rats, which produces a cell energy crisis by electron transport uncoupling. Adrenalectomy reduces and GC treatment increases the toxicity of this antimetabolite.[72,73]

- Hippocampal CA1 region neurons are primarily damaged by the hypoxia-ischemia that occurs during cardiac arrest. The four-vessel occlusion model in the rodent, in which vertebral arteries are cauterized and the carotids are reversibly occluded, closely models the neuronal damage of hypoxia-ischemia. Surgical or chemical adrenalectomy decreases, while GC treatment enhances the neurological damage.[75-77]

- Concussive trauma to the brain damages the hippocampus, and GC treatment increases the cognitive defects induced by such insult.[78]

- The cholinergic neurotoxin, ethylcholine aziridinium, preferentially damages hippocampal neurons. Again, GC treatment enhances toxicity.[79]

- The serotonergic neurotoxin 3,4-methylenedioxymethamphetamine damages neurons of the hippocampus and cortex. Adrenalectomy reduces its toxicity in the hippocampus, while GC treatment restores toxicity.[80]

Potentially, GCs endangerment may represent a side effect of the many primary actions that these hormones exert throughout the rest of the body. However, GCs appear to directly enhance excitotoxic, ischemic, and hypoglycemic damage to cultured hippocampal neurons and glia.[81-83] This specific, direct action of the GCs on the hippocampus is mediated by interaction with GCr, and hippocampal damage can be prevented by blocking the receptor.[84] Synthetic GCs such as dexamethasone also endanger the hippocampus,[76] whereas other steroids such as estrogens, progestins, and androgens do not.[83,84] It should not be surprising, therefore, that only the brain areas rich in GCr, such as the hippocampus, become endangered by the presence of these hormones.

The presence of high concentrations of GCs is necessary but not sufficient to compromise the ability of hippocampal neurons to respond to the challenge of a neurological insult. It is possible that these neurons are particularly sensitive to the insult itself.[16] The damage is more pronounced in the areas in which the neurons are more sensitive to the insult: CA3 for kainic acid, CA1 for hypoxia-ischemia, and the dentate gyrus for antimetabolite toxins.

Another interpretation of these observations is that GCs do not themselves endanger the hippocampus. Rather the increased vulnerability would be caused by the decreased ACTH levels following the negative feedback of high GCs levels. This view is based on the stimulatory effect of ACTH upon the brain, and the loss of this stimulatory effect when ACTH levels are low. Conversely, it would be the high levels of ACTH that follow adrenalectomy, rather than the absence of GCs, that would prevent hippocampal damage.[58] This interpretation seems to be valid only in the young adult animals, where the feedback regulation of the HPA axis is intact and high concentrations of GCs drive down the pituitary ACTH secretion. In the aged rat, the pituitary is not as sensitive to GCs, and ACTH concentrations are in fact elevated. Perhaps both ACTH and GCs influence the system at different levels.

C. Cellular Mechanisms of GC Toxicity

Cellular and molecular mechanisms of the relationship of GCs to aging are discussed in Chapter 15. The GC action in enhancing the toxicity of several neuron insults is relatively rapid: as little as 24 h of GC exposure *in vivo* or *in vitro* compromises cell survival. GCs would exacerbate the damaging effect of glutamate and calcium, producing necrotic neuronal death.

Glutamate, as well as aspartate, are excitatory amino acid (EAA) neurotransmitters, and are involved in many of the excitatory and plastic events regulated by the hippocampus, such as learning and memory. It is now well known that some neurological insults such as hypoxia-ischemia, seizures and hypoglycemia involve extracellular accumulation of EAAs at the synapse. This excess of EAAs mobilizes calcium in the postsynaptic neuron and leads to overactivation of calcium-dependent nucleases, proteases, lipases, and oxygen radical-producing cascades. Importantly, blockade of the binding of EAAs to their receptors and/or antagonism of calcium action protect neurons from these insults.[85]

Considerable evidence involves the EAA/calcium cascade in GC endangerment. Both stress and seizures increase metabolism in the hippocampus by activation of EAA cascade, and in both cases, adrenalectomy reduces or blocks this effect.[86] The specific mechanism of the GCs interaction with the EAA/calcium cascade involves different steps:

- GCs and stress increase the extracellular accumulation of EAAs in the hippocampus.[87] Excessive extracellular concentration of EAAs may arise from an impaired re-uptake of the neurotransmitter. GCs inhibit glutamate uptake in the hippocampal glia.[88]
- GCs and stress enhance calcium mobilization in the postsynaptic neurons by impairing removal of calcium from the cytosolic pool.[89,90]
- GCs, by mobilizing calcium, would exacerbate various degenerative events in neurons. GCs stimulate calcium-mediated cytoskeletal breakdown and microtubule degeneration after kainic acid-induced seizures in the rat hippocampus.[91]

The disruption of the various steps mentioned above by the GCs does not affect the glutamate uptake pump directly, but rather indirectly. Hypoxia-ischemia and hypoglycemia disrupt energy production, and seizures increase the demand for energy, placing the neurons on the brink of an energy crisis. In fact, the severity of these insults can be buffered by energy supplementation of the neuronal cell.[92] In this scenario, the presence of GCs, by further disrupting cell energetics, would make the neurons less likely to survive the insults.

GCs decrease glucose entry into different peripheral tissues such as fat cells and fibroblasts, resulting in the rerouting of the circulating glucose to the muscle. This catabolic action of the GCs is regarded as part of the overall strategy of energy mobilization and reorganization during an emergency.[1] In the brain, GCs decrease glucose utilization in the hippocampus[93] by inhibiting glucose entry into hippocampal neurons and glia.[88,94] Conversely, adrenalectomy increases local cerebral glucose utilization, the strongest effects occurring in the hippocampus.[93] The effect, specific of the GCs, is mediated through type II receptors. Although inhibition of glucose transport is lower in the hippocampus than in peripheral tissues, 20% vs. 70%, it is sufficient to impair the ability of these neurons to cope with an energy crisis induced by a neurological insult. As evidence of the important role of GC-induced energy depletion on the calcium/EAA cascade, energy supplementation of the brain will reverse all steps within the cascade compromised by the presence of GCs.[88,89,91,95] Thus, GCs may not directly destroy the neuron, even during the course of aging, but may endanger the neuron and impair its capacity to survive everyday insults.

VI. GLUCOCORTICOID ENDANGERMENT: ONLY A HYPOTHESIS?

Although most experiments seem to support the crucial role of GCs on the hippocampal degeneration observed during aging, the following observations among others are in conflict with the GC cascade hypothesis or present paradoxes:

- The GC cascade leading to hippocampal damage during aging has not been observed in all rat strains.
- Aged Brown Norway rats show a reduced expression of type II corticosteroid receptors in the hippocampus and hypersecretion of ACTH following a stressor, but these rats do not have elevated GC blood levels, either on the basal condition or after stress.[31]
- In aged rats, 34% within a single strain do not show impairment in learning capacity.[30] These same rats do not present the remainder of the degenerative features of the GC cascade.

Considerable individual variability within a strain can account for some of the differences in the physiological responses observed in aged animals. Undoubtedly, the environment plays a critical role in the animal's ability to cope with the process of aging. The quality of the environment at both neonatal and adult stages seems to regulate the GC-induced endangerment of the brain.

As mentioned earlier, handling of rats during the neonatal period has proved to be a remarkable example of the effects of the environment on the development of the adrenocortical function in adulthood. Adult rats, neonatally handled compared to nonhandled controls present a number of characteristics that suggest a more efficient adaptation.[96] Thus, the GC cascade of hippocampal damage can be prevented by interventions (e.g., handling) at the neonatal stages. During adulthood, environmental enrichment can also ameliorate neuroanatomical and cognitive changes observed during aging.[97]

If the GC endangerment hypothesis is correct, the chronic use of GCs in current medical practice would seem to border on "malpractice". A steady use of relatively high doses of GCs in humans would cause irreversible brain damage and accelerate the degenerating features of aging. But the reality is that millions of patients around the world have been treated with large doses of GCs for decades without any clinical evidence of hippocampal damage (as revealed by short-term memory impairment). The lack of reports concerning memory loss in many patients over many years would suggest that hippocampal damage is not occurring.[98] Perhaps the effect of GCs is limited to specific areas within the hippocampus, sparing other nuclei involved in the process of memory. Other explanations of the response to stress should also be considered.

A. Corticosteroid Receptor Balance Hypothesis

Another hypothesis proposes that both the GCr- and MCr-mediated effects at the hippocampus are of critical importance for homeostatic control.[16,31] GCr- and MCr-mediated effects are antagonistic in the regulation of cellular excitability and, therefore, any imbalance at the corticosteroid receptor level could alter neuron excitability and behavioral adaptation. Such a condition is met during the aging process.

Experimental data support this hypothesis. As pointed out earlier, hippocampal binding capacity of MCr is reduced by 40 to 50% during aging, whereas that of GCr is unaltered,[30] reduced,[30,43] or affinity for ligands enhanced.[31] Hippocampal MCr controls the sensitivity of the stress response mediating the negative feedback signal, whereas hippocampal GCrs have an opposite effect. The significant reduction in the number of the former during aging, would induce a corticosteroid receptor imbalance at the limbic region. The subsequent loss of MCr/GCr balance would damage the HPA axis regulation and thereby alter homeostatic control in aging.[16]

VII. CONCLUSION

The hypothesis of the GC cascade postulates that stress and GCs facilitate the aging process in a feed-forward manner.[37] It is based on the observation that a sustained period of stress induces down-regulation of corticosteroid receptors in the hippocampus. As a consequence, GC feedback on stress-induced HPA axis activation is impaired, resulting in elevated basal corticosterone levels (in rats) and extended GC secretion following stress (Figure 14-1). If the stressor is removed, the GC receptors number returns to basal levels, as does feedback sensitivity, but if stress is prolonged beyond a certain threshold period, actual damage to the neuron occurs, and the feedback response may be lost permanently. Chronically elevated levels of GCs are toxic,[72-76] and their catabolic effects would deprive the hippocampal neurons of substrates for energy metabolism and, therefore, increase cell vulnerability.[37,72-76]

The hippocampus may act as a brake on the neuroendocrine response to stress, and its stimulation would decrease HPA axis secretions. The unrestrained surge of GCs, along with the reduction in the hippocampal GCr (Figure 14-1), would lead to the progressive inability of the feedback mechanisms to terminate the response to stress.[46] The beneficial effects at adulthood observed in rats handled neonatally during the first weeks of life support this hypothesis.[96]

Other investigations, however, present results that are in conflict with the GC cascade hypothesis. Hypersecretion of GCs has not been observed in all studies and every strain; GCr-mediated effects at the hippocampal level may not be crucial in regulating the negative feedback on stress-induced HPA activity, and the GCr down-regulation claimed by the GC cascade hypothesis could not be responsible for the failure of the stress response to terminate.[16] The role of MCr cannot be disregarded. MCr-mediated effects are opposite to those from GCr. The MCr-mediated negative feedback signal, needed to terminate the response to stress, is counteracted in old age by an enhanced GCr-mediated positive feedback signal at the hippocampal level; this would diminish the capacity of the limbic system to inhibit HPA activity, with a subsequent hypersecretion of GCs (a feed-forward process would start the cascade cycle again).[16,58]

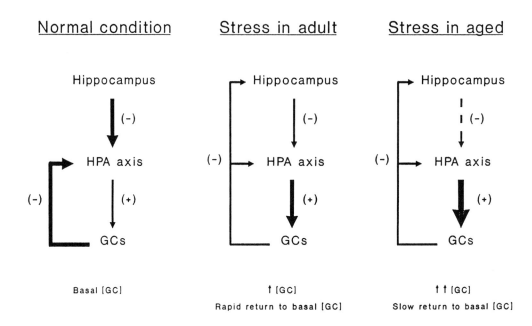

Figure 14-1   The glucocorticoid cascade hypothesis of hippocampal damage. **Normal condition**: lack of activation
of the HPA axis implies low secretion of ACTH from the pituitary and, therefore, serum GCs basal
levels. The hippocampus successfully helps to inhibit HPA axis activity. **Stress in adult**: activation
of HPA axis increases serum GCs to face emergency. Both feedback effect of GCs on HPA axis and
its inhibition by an undamaged hippocampus lead to a rapid return of GCs to basal concentrations.
Stress in aged: activation of HPA axis increases serum GCs to face emergency. A lifelong GC-
damaged hippocampus cannot exert its inhibition on HPA axis activity; the feedback effect of GCs
on the axis is not sufficient to ensure a rapid return to a basal condition. Concentrations of GCs remain
higher and longer in serum, thereby damaging the hippocampus.

Overall, studies on the role of corticoids in aging support the GC cascade hypothesis.
However, GC hypersecretion is not always found in old animals and hippocampal damage is
not reported in the large number of human subjects supported with exogenous GC therapy.
While experimental evidence reveals a relationship between stress and hippocampal degeneration, this link may not be intrinsic to the aging process. Rather, exposure to stress
throughout the lifespan would be one important factor, among several, involved in the
regulation of the process of aging. Perhaps, a "successful aging" is directly related to a correct
handling of the environment in the presence of mild to moderate stress (Chapter 1). In contrast,
exposure to severe, prolonged stress would impair homeostatic control, neuroendocrine
regulation, and behavioral adaptation, as frequently seen at senescence.

REFERENCES

1. Selye, H., Stress. *The Physiology and Pathology of Exposure to Stress*, Acta Medica Publ., Montreal,
   Quebec, 1950.
2. Krieger, D., Cushing's syndrome, *Monographs Endo.*, 22, 1, 1982.
3. Munck, A., Guyre, P. M. and Holbrook, N. J., Physiological functions of glucocorticoids in stress and their
   relation to pharmacological actions, *Endocrine Revs.*, 5, 25, 1984.
4. Selye, H. and Tuchweber, B., It is proposed that the effects of stress accumulate and ultimately lead to
   premature onset of pathological changes, in *Hypothalamus, Pituitary and Aging*, Everitt, A. F. and Burgess,
   J. A., Eds., Charles C Thomas, Springfield, IL, 1976, 553.
5. Solez, C., Aging and adrenal cortical hormones, *Geriatrics*, 7, 241, 1952.
6. Robertson, O. and Wexler, B., Pituitary degeneration and adrenal tissue hyperplasia in spawning Pacific
   salmon, *Science*, 125, 1295, 1957.

7. Robertson, O. and Wexler, B., Histological changes in the organs and tissues of migrating and spawning Pacific salmon, *Endocrinology,* 66, 222, 1960.

8. Lee, A. K. and Cockburn, A., *The Evolutionary Ecology of Marsupials,* Cambridge University Press, New York, 1985.

9. Lee, A. K. and McDonald, I., Stress and population regulation in small mammals, *Oxford Rev. Reprod. Biol.,* 7, 261, 1985.

10. McDonald I. R., Lee, A. K., Than, K. A. and Martin, R. W., Failure of glucocorticoid feedback in males of a population of small marsupials (*Antechinus swainsonii*) during the period of mating, *J. Endocrinol.,* 108, 63, 1986.

11. Beato, M. and Doenecke, D., Metabolic effects and modes of action of glucocorticoids, in *General Comparative and Clinical Endocrinology of the Adrenal Cortex,* Vol. 3, Jones, I. C. and Henderson, I. W., Eds., Academic Press, New York, 1980.

12. Selye, H., Confusion and controversy in the stress field, *J. Human Stress,* 1, 37, 1975.

13. Antoni, F., Hypothalamic control of adrenocorticotropin secretion: advances since the discovery of 41-residue corticotropin-releasing factor, *Endocrine Revs.,* 7, 351, 1986.

14. Dallman, M. F., Akana, S. F., Cascio, C., Darlington, D., Jacobson, L. and Levin, N., Regulation of ACTH secretion: variations on a theme of B., *Recent Prog. Horm. Res.,* 43, 113, 1987.

15. Dallman, M. F., Stress update, adaptation of the hypothalamic-pituitary-adrenal axis to chronic stress, *Trends Endocrinol. Metab.,* 4, 62, 1993.

16. De Kloet, E. R., Corticosteroids, stress and aging, *Ann. N.Y. Acad. Sci.,* 663, 357, 1992.

17. Sapolsky, R. M., Do glucocorticoid concentrations rise with age in the rat?, *Neurobiol. Aging,* 13, 171, 1992.

18. Sapolsky, R. M., Neuroendocrinology of the stress response, in *Behavioral Endocrinology,* Becker, J., Breedlove, S. M. and Crews, D., Eds., MIT Press, Cambridge, MA, 1992, 287.

19. Jacobson, L. and Sapolsky, R. M., The role of the hippocampus in feedback regulation of the hypothalamic-pituitary-adrenocortical axis, *Endocrine Rev.,* 12, 118, 1991.

20. Van Eekelen, J. A. and De Kloet, E. R., Co-localization of brain corticosteroid receptors in the rat hippocampus, *Prog. Histochem. Cytochem.,* 26, 250, 1992.

21. Tang, G. and Phillips, R., Some age-related changes in pituitary-adrenal function in the male laboratory rat, *J. Gerontol.,* 33, 377, 1978.

22. Brett, L. P., Chong, G., Coyle, S. and Levine, S., The pituitary-adrenal response to novel stimulation and ether stress in young adult and aged rats, *Neurobiol. Aging,* 4, 133, 1983.

23. Sapolsky, R. M., Krey, L. C. and McEwen, B. S., The adrenocortical stress-response in the aged male rat: impairment of recovery from stress, *Exp. Geront.,* 18, 55, 1983.

24. DeKosky, S., Scheff, S. and Cotman, C., Elevated corticosterone levels. A possible cause of reduced axon sprouting in aged animals, *Neuroendocrinology,* 38, 33, 1984.

25. Ida, Y, Tanaka, M., Tsuda, A., Kohmo, Y., Hoaki, Y., Nakagawa, R., Imori, K. and Nagasaki, N., Recovery of stress-induced increases in noradrenaline turnover is delayed in specific brain regions in the old rats, *Life Sci.,* 34, 2357, 1984.

26. Reul, J. M., Tonnaer, J. A. and de Kloet, E. R., Neurotrophic ACTH analogue promotes plasticity of type I corticosteroid receptor in brain of senescent male rats, *Neurobiol. Aging,* 9, 253, 1988.

27. Wilson, M., Hippocampal inhibition of the pituitary-adrenocortical response to stress, in *Psychological and Physiological Interactions in Response to Stress,* Birchfield, S., Ed., Academic Press, New York, 1985, 321.

28. Brett, L. P, Levine, R. and Levine, S., Bidirectional responsiveness of the pituitary-adrenal system in old and young male and female rats, *Neurobiol. Aging,* 7, 153, 1986.

29. Harmon, S. and Talbert, G., Reproductive aging, in *Handbook of the Biology of Aging,* 2nd ed., Finch, C. E. and Schneider, E. L., Eds.,Van Nostrand Reinhold, New York, 1985, 457.

30. Issa, A., Rowe, W., Gauthier, S. and Meaney, M. J., Hypothalamic-pituitary-adrenal activity in aged, cognitively impaired and cognitively unimpaired rats, *J. Neurosci.,* 10, 3247, 1990.

31. Van Eekelen, J. A. M., Rots, N. Y., Sutanto, W. and de Kloet, E. R., The effect of aging on stress responsiveness and central corticosteroid receptors in the brown Norway rat, *Neurobiol. Aging,* 13, 159, 1992.

32. Popplewell, P., Tsubokawa, M., Ramachandran, M. and Azhar, S., Differential effects of aging on ACTH receptors, adenosine 3′, 5′ monophosphate response, and corticosterone secretion in adrenocortical cells from Sprague-Dawley rats, *Endocrinology,* 119, 2206, 1986.

33. Malamed, S. and Carsia, R. V., Aging of the rat adrenocortical cell: response to ACTH and cyclic AMP in vitro, *J. Gerontol.,* 38, 130, 1983.

34. Popplewell, P. Y., Butte, J. and Azhar, S., The influence of age on steroidogenic enzyme activities of the rat adrenal gland: enhanced expression of cholesterol side-chain cleavage activity, *Endocrinology,* 120, 2521, 1987.

35. Popplewell, P.Y. and Azhar, S., Effects of aging on cholesterol content and cholesterol-metabolizing enzymes in the rat adrenal gland, *Endocrinology,* 121, 64, 1987.

36. Oxenkrug, G. F., McIntyre, I. M., Stanley, M. and Gershon, S., Dexamethasone suppression test: experimental model in rats, and effect of age, *Biol. Psychiatr.*, 19, 413, 1984.

37. Sapolsky, R., M., Krey, L. and McEwen, B. S., The adrenocortical axis in the aged rat: impaired sensitivity to both fast and delayed feedback inhibition, *Neurobiol. Aging* , 7, 331, 1986.

38. Hylka, V., Sonntag, W. and Meites, J., Reduced ability of old male rats to release ACTH and corticosterone in response to CRF administration, *Proc. Soc. Exp. Biol. Med.*, 175, 1, 1984.

39. Levin, N., Shinsako, J. and Dallman, M. F., Corticosterone acts on the brain to inhibit adrenalectomy-induced adrenocorticotropin (ACTH) secretion, *Endocrinology*, 122, 694, 1988.

40. Angelucci, L., Valeri, P. and Grossi, E., Involvement of hippocampal corticosterone receptors in behavioral phenomena, in *Progress in Psychoneuroendocrinology,* Brambilla, G., Rascagni, G. and de Wied, D., Eds., Elsevier, Amsterdam, 1980, 186.

41. Sapolsky, R. M., Krey, L. and McEwen, B. S., Corticosterone receptors decline in a site-specific manner in the aged rat brain, *Brain Res.*, 289, 235, 1983.

42. Reul, J. and de Kloet, R., Two receptor systems for corticosterone in rat brain: microdistribution and differential occupation, *Endocrinology*, 17, 2505, 1985.

43. Meaney, M. J., Viau, V., Bhatnagar, S., Betito, K., Iny, L., O´Donnell, D. and Mitchell, J. B., Cellular mechanisms underlying the development and expression of individual differences in the hypothalamic-pituitary-adrenal stress response, *J. Steroid Biochem. Molec. Biol.*, 39, 265, 1991.

44. Eldridge, J. C., Brodish, A., Kute, T. E. and Landfield, P. W., Apparent age-related resistance of type II hippocampal corticosteroid receptors to down-regulation during chronic escape training, *J. Neurosci.*, 9, 3237, 1989.

45. Coleman, P. and Flood, D., Neuron numbers and dendritic extent in normal aging and Alzheimer´s disease, *Neurobiol. Aging*, 8, 521, 1987.

46. Sapolsky, R. M., Krey, L. and McEwen, B. S., Stress down-regulates corticosterone receptors in a site-specific manner in the brain, *Endocrinology*, 114, 287, 1984.

47. Feldman, S. and Conforti, N., Participation of the dorsal hippocampus in the glucocorticoid feedback effect on adrenocortical activity, *Neuroendocrinology,* 30, 52, 1980.

48. Fishette, C., Komisaruk, B., Ediner, H., Feder, H. and Siegle, A., Differential fornix ablations and the circadian rhythmicity of adrenal corticosterone secretion, *Brain Res.*, 195, 373, 1980.

49. Wilson, M., Greer, M. and Roberts, L., Hippocampal inhibition of pituitary-adrenocortical function in female rats, *Brain Res.*, 197, 433, 1980.

50. Sapolsky, R. M., Zola-Morgan, S. and Squire, L., Inhibition of glucocorticoid secretion by the hippocampal formation in the primate, *J. Neurosci.*, 11, 3695, 1991.

51. Kant, G. J., Meyerhoff, J. L. and Jarrad, L. E., Biochemical indices of reactivity and habituation in rats with hippocampal lesions, *Phar. Biochem. Behav.*, 20, 793, 1984.

52. Dunn, J. and Orr, S., Differential plasma corticosterone responses to hippocampal stimulation, *Exp. Brain Res.*, 54, 1, 1984.

53. Saphier, D. and Feldman, S., Effects of septal and hippocampal stimuli on paraventricular nucleus neurons, *Neuroscience*, 20, 749, 1987.

54. Sapolsky, R. M., Krey, L. and McEwen, B. S., Glucocorticoid-sensitive hippocampal neurons are involved in terminating the adrenocortical stress response, *Proc. Nat. Acad. Sci. U.S.A.*, 81, 6174, 1984.

55. Feldman, S. and Conforti, N., Feedback effects of dexamethasone on adrenocortical responses of rats with fornix section, *Horm. Res.*, 7, 56, 1976.

56. De Kloet, E. R., de Kock, S., Schild, V. and Veldhuis, H., Antiglucocorticoid RU 38486 attenuates retention of a behaviour and disinhibits the hypothalamic-pituitary adrenal axis at different brain sites, *Neuroendocrinology,* 47, 109, 1988.

57. Landfield, P.W., Waymire, J. C. and Lynch, G., Hippocampal aging and adrenocorticoids: a quantitative correlations, *Science*, 202, 1098, 1978.

58. Landfield, P.W., Baskin, R. and Pitler, T., Brain-aging correlates: retardation by hormonal-pharmacological treatments, *Science*, 214, 581, 1981.

59. Sapolsky, R. M., Krey, L. and McEwen, B. S., Prolonged glucocorticoid exposure reduces hippocampal neuron number: implications for aging, *J. Neurosci.*, 5, 1222, 1985.

60. Landfield, P. W., Rose, G., Sandles, L., Wohlstadter, T. C. and Lynch, G., Patterns of astroglial hypertrophy and neuronal degeneration in the hippocampus of aged, memory-deficient rats, *J. Gerontol.*, 32, 3, 1977.

61. Ling, E. and Leblond, C., Investigation of glial cells in semi-thin sections. II. Variation with age in the number of the various glial cell types in rat cortex and corpus callosum, *J. Comp. Neurol.*, 149, 73, 1973.

62. Vaughan, D. and Peters, A., Neuroglial cells in the cerebral cortex of rats from young adulthood to old age: an electron microscope study, *J. Neurocytol.*, 3, 405, 1974.

63. Woolley, C., Gould, E. and McEwen, B. S., Exposure to excess glucocorticoids alters dendritic morphology of adult hippocampal pyramidal neurons, *Brain Res.*, 531, 225, 1990.

64. Kerr, D., Campbell, L., Applegate, M., Brodish, A. and Landfield, P. W., Chronic stress-induced accelera-tion of electrophysiologic and morphometric biomarkers of hippocampal aging, *J. Neurosci.*, 11, 1316, 1991.

65. Mizoguchi, K., Kunishita, T., Chui, D. H. and Tabira, T., Stress induces neuronal death in the hippocampus of castrated rats, *Neurosci. Lett.*, 138, 157, 1992.

66. Meaney, M. J., Aitken, D. H., van Berkel, C., Bhatnagar, S. and Sapolsky, R. M., Effect of neonatal handling on age-related impairments associated with the hippocampus, *Science*, 239, 766, 1988.

67. Meaney, M. J., Aitken, D. H., Bhatnagar, S. and Sapolsky, R. M., Postnatal handling attenuates certain neuroendocrine, anatomical and cognitive dysfunctions associated with aging in female rats, *Neurobiol. Aging*, 12, 31, 1991.

68. Uno, H., Tarara, R., Else, J. G., Suleman, M. A. and Sapolsky, R. M., Hippocampal damage associated with prolonged and fatal stress in primates, *J. Neurosci.*, 9, 1705, 1989.

69. Sapolsky, R. M., Uno, H., Rebert, C. S. and Finch, C. E., Hippocampal damage associated with prolonged glucocorticoid exposure in primates, *J. Neurosci.*, 10, 2897, 1990.

70. Sloviter, R. S., Valiquette, G., Abrams, G. M., Ronk, E. C., Sollas, A. L., Paul, L. A. and Neubort, S., Selective loss of hippocampal granule cells in the mature rat brain after adrenalectomy, *Science*, 243, 535, 1989.

71. Ben-Ari, Y., Limbic seizure and brain damage produced by kainic acid: mechanisms and relevance to human temporal lobe epilepsy, *Neuroscience*, 14, 375, 1985.

72. Sapolsky, R. M., A mechanism for glucocorticoid toxicity in the hippocampus: increased neuronal vulner-ability to metabolic insults, *J. Neurosci.*, 5, 1228, 1985.

73. Sapolsky, R. M., Glucocorticoid toxicity in the hippocampus: temporal aspects of neuronal vulnerability, *Brain Res.*, 359, 300, 1985.

74. Stein, B. A. and Sapolsky, R. M., Chemical adrenalectomy reduces hippocampal damage induced by kainic acid, *Brain Res.*, 473, 175, 1988.

75. Sapolsky, R. M. and Pulsinelli, W. A., Glucocorticoids potentiate ischemic injury to neurons: therapeutic implications, *Science*, 229, 1397, 1985.

76. Koide, T., Wieloch, T. and Siesjo, B., Chronic dexamethasone pretreatment aggravates ischemic neuronal necrosis, *J. Cereb. Blood Flow Metab.*, 6, 395, 1986.

77. Morse, J. K. and Davis, J. N., Regulation of ischemic hippocampal damage in the gerbil: adrenalectomy alters the rate of CA1 cell disappearance, *Exp. Neurol.*, 110, 86, 1990.

78. Gbadebo, D., Hamm, R., Lyeth, B., Jenkins, L., Stewart, J. and Porter, J., Corticosterone's mediation of traumatic brain injury, *Soc. Neurosci. Abstr.*, 17, 65.7, 1991.

79. Hortnagl, H., Berger M. L. and Hornykiewicz, O., Glucocorticoids aggravate the cholinergic deficit induced by ethylcholine aziridinium in rat hippocampus, *Soc. Neurosci. Abstr.*, 17, 285.1, 1991.

80. Johnson, M., Stone, D., Bush, L., Hanson, G. and Gibb, J., Glucocorticoids and 3,4-methylenedioxy-methamphetamine (MDMA)-induced neurotoxicity, *Eur. J. Pharmacol.*, 161, 181, 1989.

81. Sapolsky, R. M., Packan, D. R. and Vale, W. W., Glucocorticoid toxicity in the hippocampus: in vitro demonstration, *Brain Res.*, 453, 367, 1988.

82. Tombaugh, G. C., Yang, S. H., Swanson R.A. and Sapolsky, R. M., Glucocorticoids exacerbate hypoxic and hypoglycemic hippocampal injury in vitro: biochemical correlates and a role for astrocytes, *J. Neurochem.*, 59, 137, 1992.

83. Tombaugh, G. C. and Sapolsky, R. M., Endocrine features of glucocorticoid endangerment in hippocampal astrocytes, *Neuroendocrinology*, 57, 7, 1993.

84. Packan, D. and Sapolsky, R. M., Glucocorticoid endangerment of the hippocampus: tissue, steroid and receptor specificity, *Neuroendocrinology*, 51, 613, 1990.

85. Choi, D., Cerebral hypoxia: some new approaches and unanswered questions, *J. Neurosci.*, 10, 2493, 1990.

86. Krugers, H. J., Jaarsma, D. and Korf, J., Rat hippocampal lactate efflux during electroconvulsive shock or stress is differentially dependent on enthorinal cortex and adrenal integrity, *J. Neurochem.*, 58, 826, 1992.

87. Moghaddam, B., Stress preferentially increases extraneuronal levels of excitatory amino acids in the prefrontal cortex: comparison to hippocampus and basal ganglia, *J. Neurochem.*, 60, 1650, 1993.

88. Virgin, C. E., Jr., Ha, T. P., Packan, D. R., Tombaugh, G. C., Yang, S. H., Horner, H. C. and Sapolsky, R. M., Glucocorticoids inhibit glucose transport and glutamate uptake in hippocampal astrocytes: implications for glucocorticoid neurotoxicity, *J. Neurochem.*, 57, 1422, 1991.

89. Elliot, E. M. and Sapolsky, R. M., Corticosterone enhances kainic acid-induced calcium elevation in cultured hippocampal neurons, *J. Neurochem.*, 59, 1033, 1992.

90. Elliot, E. M. and Sapolsky, R. M., Corticosterone impairs hippocampal neuronal calcium regulation: possible mediating mechanisms, *Brain Res.*, 602, 84, 1993.

91. Elliot, E. M., Mattson, M. D., Vanderklish, P., Lynch, G., Chang, I. and Sapolsky, R. M., Corticosterone exacerbates kainate-induced alterations in hippocampal tau immunoreactivity and spectrin proteolysis in vivo, *J. Neurochem.*, 61, 57, 1993.

92. Sapolsky, R. M., *Stress, The Aging Brain and the Mechanisms of Neuron Death,* MIT Press, Cambridge, MA, 1992.

93. Kadekaro, M., Masanori, I. and Gross, P.I., Local cerebral glucose utilization is increased in acutely adrenalectomized rats, *Neuroendocrinology,* 47, 329, 1988.

94. Horner, H., Packan, D. and Sapolsky, R. M., Glucocorticoids inhibit glucose transport in cultured hippo-campal neurons and glia, *Neuroendocrinology,* 52, 57, 1990.

95. Stein-Behrens, B. A., Elliott, E. M., Miller, C. A., Schilling, J. W., Newcombe, R. and Sapolsky, R. M., Glucocorticoids exacerbate kainic acid-induced extracellular accumulation of excitatory amino acids in the rat hippocampus, *J. Neurochem.,* 58, 1730, 1992.

96. Meaney, M. J., Mitchell, J. B., Aitken, D. H., Bhatnagar, S., Bodnoff, S. R., Iny, L. J. and Sarrieau, A., The effects of neonatal handling on the development of the adrenocortical response to stress: implications for neuropathology and cognitive deficits in later life, *Psychoneuroendocrinology,* 16, 85, 1991.

97. Diamond, M. C., *Enriching Heredity: The Impact of the Environment on the Anatomy of the Brain,* Macmillan/Free Press, New York, 1988.

98. Sloviter, R. S., Endogenous Dangers (Book Review), *Science,* 259, 1630, 1993.

PART IV

Molecular Regulatory Mechanisms

15

Cellular and Molecular Basis of Aging

Suresh I. S. Rattan

CONTENTS

I. INTRODUCTION

Homeostasis is the property of living systems to maintain their stability and functional integrity while adjusting to internal and external sources of perturbation. There are many mechanisms of maintenance, also referred to as the longevity assurance processes,[1] employed by biological entities to prevail their homeostasis. These include the processes of cellular and subcellular repair, cell division, cell replacement, cellular responsiveness, immune response, detoxication, free-radical scavenging, macromolecular turnover, and maintaining the fidelity of genetic information transfer. When homeostatic regulation is successful, an equilibrium between stability and change is attained and life is sustained, whereas a loss of or deviation from homeostasis leads to the collapse of the system.

A senescing organism exhibits a broad spectrum of changes, manifested mainly as an overall decline in most of the body functions. Taken individually and in isolation, not all parts of the body become functionally exhausted, but it is the interactions between individual components that sustain the body and determine its survival. As a result of aging, the organism becomes increasingly vulnerable to intrinsic and extrinsic risk factors and the ability of the organism to survive diminishes. The highly complex nature of the process of aging, which implicates both genetic and epigenetic causative factors, makes the elucidation of the underlying mechanisms one of the most challenging tasks of modern biology. All species with repetitively reproducing (iteroparous) life history, experience aging after completing a period of reproductive fitness. The phenomenology of aging is rich in empirical data about age-related changes in numerous systems, many of which are highly specific for particular aging systems. While the process and the end result of aging are obvious, the causes and mechanisms remain elusive. The diversity of biological systems used in aging research, their widely varying rates in the progress of senescence, and the fact that almost all characteristics undergo alteration with age, make it very difficult to distinguish between "specific" changes and "universal" ones.

The aim of this article is to discuss the cellular and molecular basis of aging within the framework of aging as the failure of maintenance. Therefore, a critical overview of the major cellular and molecular mechanisms involved in the process of aging will be given with special reference to genomic instability, the regulation of transfer of genetic information, altered cellular responsiveness, and loss of cell proliferation.

II. INSTABILITY OF THE GENOME

The survival and continued existence of any life form depends upon the stability of its genome at least until its genetic information has been faithfully transmitted to the next generation. Therefore, the inability of organisms to live forever has often been linked to the possibility of progressive instability of their genome.[2-4] A large number of studies have been carried out on DNA damage and repair during aging using a wide range of aging systems, such as cells in culture and isolated cells and tissues from a diverse range of species.

A. DNA Damage and Repair

Various physical, chemical, and biological factors are continuously challenging the DNA in all cells of the body. At the same time, several DNA repair systems operate in the cell that counteract the effects of various DNA-damaging agents. Major DNA-damaging agents include solar UV radiation, background ionizing radiation, a wide range of chemicals in food and in the environment, and several endogenous agents such as aldehydes, active oxygen species, and other free radicals which are the result of metabolic pathways.[5-7] In addition to that, damage to DNA in a cell can also result from several spontaneous chemical changes in the DNA, such as those due to hydrolysis, deamination, methylation, demethylation, and glycation, along with the errors that can occur during DNA duplication and repair as a result of innate limits on the accuracy of any biochemical processes.[7]

The biological consequences of damage to DNA are generally very similar, irrespective of the nature of the damaging agent. For example, several DNA-damaging agents can be the cause of mutations, depurination, depyrimidation, dimers, strand breaks, cross-links, and epimutations. At present, there are no reliable methods available that can establish a cause-and-effect relationship between the origin of DNA damage and its consequences in a cell. Therefore, most studies measuring age-related changes in the levels of DNA damage have been unable to pinpoint the source of that damage — a factor that might be crucial in explaining differences in the type and rate of damage accumulation in different cell types, organs, and species.

A large number of studies have shown that some kinds of DNA damage do accumulate during aging. For example, single-strand breaks of DNA have been observed to increase in cultured cells of rodent and human origin and in the cells isolated from various rodent organs, including brain, heart, kidney, liver, spleen, and thymus, and in human lymphocytes and muscle tissue during aging.[8-11] An age-related increase in the number of alkali-labile sites in DNA occurred only in postmitotic rat liver parenchymal cells and not in actively dividing nonparenchymal cells in the same tissue.[12] Various other investigators have reported age-related increases in DNA cross-links, dicentric chromosomes, aneuploidy, polyploidy, loss of centromeric tandem repeats, and shorter linker regions between nucleosomes.[13,14] DNA adduct-like covalent modifications called indigenous (I)-compounds have been shown to increase during aging.[15]

An increase in the free-radical-induced oxidative damage, particularly the formation of 8-hydroxy-2'-deoxyguanosine in the nuclear and mitochondrial (mt) DNAs, has been reported to occur in various organs of aging rats and in human hearts.[16-19] Similarly, a fivefold increase in the frequency of deletions and additions was found in mtDNA isolated from livers of old mice as compared to those from young mice.[20] An age-related increase in a somatic deletion of mtDNA[49,77] in aging human nervous and muscle tissues has been reported.[21,22]

One of the most common results of DNA damage is the causation of mutations. An exponential increase in the number of rare variants with enhanced levels of glucose-6-phosphate dehydrogenase (G6PD) were reported in serially passaged cultures of human fibroblasts.[23,24] Similarly, a severalfold increase in the frequency of diphtheria toxin- and thioguanine-resistant mutants during cellular aging of human fibroblasts has been observed.[25] In human T lymphocytes isolated from blood obtained from donors of different ages, an exponential increase in the frequency of mutated cells at the HPRT locus was reported.[26,27] Using allele-specific PCR, occurrence of a point mutation by base substitution (from A to G) at nucleotide position 3243 on mtDNA has been demonstrated in several human tissues from old subjects as compared with infant tissues.[28]

Other kinds of DNA damage which have been studied in relation to aging are the so-called epimutations.[29] These include the presence of 5-methyl cytosine and 5-methyldeoxycytidine (5mC and 5mdC), and free radical-induced DNA damage products including thymine glycols, 5-hydroxymethyluracil and 8-hydroxyguanosine.[5,6,29-33] There is evidence that levels of 5mC and 5mdC decline during the aging of cells in culture[34] and in tissues and organs isolated from old rats, mice, and cattle.[35,36] Induction of this kind of DNA damage by treatment of cells with 5-azacytidine induces premature aging of human cells in culture.[37-39]

With respect to the repair of DNA damage during aging, only a few repair pathways have been studied until now. These include the reversal of damage through photoreactivation or through the removal of modifications from a base, excision repair of damaged bases and nucleotides, repair of single- and double-strand breaks, and repair of free-radical- and oxidation-induced damage. One of the most widely studied DNA repair pathways during aging is the repair by nucleotide excision. In this kind of DNA repair, recognition of the damaged site and the creation of a nick by an endonuclease enzyme is followed by its excision by an exonuclease.[40] In most cases, DNA repair during aging has been measured by the capacity of cells to repair DNA damage induced by a short, intense treatment with UV light, X-rays, γ-irradiation, mutagens, or free radicals. Although some investigators have reported some decline in the DNA repair capacity of very old cells in culture, or of cells isolated from old animals, the general consensus is that there is no age-related decline in the overall capacity of cells to repair DNA damage during aging.[4,41]

The notion that declining repair capacity may be the primary defect of aging is further undermined by the absence of a strong relationship between the extent of DNA repair and maximum lifespan. For example, cells from xeroderma pigmentosum patients do have severe DNA repair deficiency, but do not show either a reduced proliferative capacity or any other symptoms of accelerated aging.[42,43] Conversely, cells from patients with premature aging syndromes do not always have reduced DNA repair capacity,[44,45] and in some cases, such as lymphocytes from Down syndrome patients, the rate of DNA repair of γ-radiation-induced damage was much higher than in cells from normal individuals.[46]

In contrast to this, there is evidence that establishes a positive correlation between a species' lifespan and its capacity to repair certain kinds of DNA damage. Various lines of evidence in this regard include the repair of UV-induced damage in fibroblasts and lymphocytes,[47-49] the capacity of cells to metabolize 7,12-dimethylbenz(a)anthracene,[50,51] the activity of methyltransferase in removing the methyl group from damaged O^6-methylguanine in liver and in chondrocytes;[48,52] the activity of poly(ADP-ribose) polymerase involved in DNA repair,[53] the rate of loss of 5mC and 5mdC during aging;[34,36] and the extent of oxidative damage to DNA in various species.[54] Similarly, the extent of DNA repair measured by determining the rate of removal of benzo(a)pyrene-induced DNA adducts in the liver of three different congenic mice strains correlated well with their differences in longevity.[55]

Thus, although there is a correlation between the lifespan of a species and its capacity to repair DNA damage, there is no significant reduction in overall DNA repair capacity in old cells and tissues that could be considered to be the cause of aging. It must, however, be pointed out that the DNA repair capacity that has been studied until now gives only a gross overview of what might be happening in the genome as a whole, irrespective of the fact that only a small proportion of the genomic DNA is actually active and expressed in any cell type. Recent studies have shown that there is a strong intragenomic heterogeneity between the repair of active and inactive regions of the genome.[56,57] Furthermore, this phenomenon of preferential gene repair is extended to strand-specific repair in which the transcribed strand is repaired much more efficiently than the nontranscribed DNA strand.[56,58] Therefore, it is important to study the repair, maintenance, and functioning of individual genes, such as those involved in DNA repair, or the genes involved in genetic information transfer pathways, for example the genes for DNA/RNA polymerases, protein synthetic factors, and free-radical scavengers.

B. Stability of Gene Expression

Each cell type in an organism comes to acquire a unique pattern of gene expression through differentiation during development. It is obvious that this pattern of gene expression must be maintained for the normal functioning of cells and for the survival of the organism. Since aging is considered to be a result of failure of maintenance at all levels, attempts have been made to look for an age-related drifting away of cells from their proper state of differentiation, i.e., dysdifferentiation in terms of changes in the pattern of gene expression during aging.[59]

Several studies have been undertaken in order to determine the extent of expression of different genes during aging. In most cases, mRNA levels of different genes have been estimated by RNA-DNA hybridization, using cDNA or genomic probes for specific genes. The results obtained show that during aging the expression of some genes increases, of some it decreases, and of others it remains constant. In all such studies on measuring the levels of mRNA in young and old cells and tissues, it is assumed that this estimate is a direct measure of gene activity. This is a simplistic notion, because it is well known that posttranscriptional changes, such as the processing, transport, and turnover of RNA, change significantly the levels of mRNA.[60]

A better way to find out if the stability of the genome decreases and if the pattern of gene expression changes during aging is to study the expression of a cell-type-specific gene. For example, the globin gene is normally repressed in fibroblasts, and no globin-like RNA could be detected either in young or in old human fibroblasts, showing thereby that the stability of gene expression remains unchanged during aging.[61] Similar results have been reported for five tissue-specific genes (myelin basic protein in brain, atrial natriuretic factor in heart, albumin in liver, kappa immunoglobulin in spleen, and a skin-specific keratin), the fidelity of whose expressions were maintained during aging of Wistar rats.[62] In contrast to this, some relaxation of the expression of endogenous murine leukemia virus-related RNA and globin RNA was found in mouse brain and liver.[63,64] However, no reactivation of repressed α-fetoprotein genes was not observed in adult rat livers during aging.[65] More studies of a similar nature and with a wide range of cell-type-specific genes will be required in order to resolve this important issue of the stability of gene expression during aging.

Thus, it appears that at gross level the integrity of the genome is well maintained during the lifespan. However, it is also clear that several subtle changes in the organization and the functioning of the genome do occur that may be critical for cell survival. Several new developments in the methods of detecting low levels of specific DNA lesions, for example immunochemical methods, single-cell microgel electrophoresis, two-dimensional fingerprinting of DNA by denaturing electrophoresis, and methods for determining the extent of damage and repair at the level of a single strand of active and inactive genes will help to establish the role of genomic instability in aging.[56,58,66-68]

C. Organization of the Chromatin

The eukaryotic genome consists largely of the chromatin, which is a complex of DNA, histones, and nonhistone proteins that are arranged in a series of repeating units, termed nucleosomes. The stability of the structure and organization of chromatin is crucial both for the maintenance of the state of differentiation of a cell and for its function throughout the lifespan of the cell. In a large number of studies, the composition, structure, and function of the chromatin in young and old organisms, tissues, and cells have been compared. These include studies on age-related changes in DNA content, on DNA synthesis, on levels of histones and nonhistone proteins, on nucleosome spacing and linker regions, on protein-DNA interactions, and on physical properties of the chromatin, such as thermal denaturation and template activity. It is now well established that the chromatin becomes more condensed during aging, and this can have wide implications for DNA repair, DNA replication, and gene expression.[14,69,70-72] It has been suggested that the reorganization of chromatin structure is characterized by a succession of subtle changes through the lifespan and a final short stage with abrupt events. These changes include an increased fragility of the chromatin structure and an increase in sensitivity to strong detergents.[73]

At the gross level of chromosomal changes during aging, the failure of cells to maintain their diploid status has been observed in aging peripheral lymphocytes, bone marrow cells, fibroblasts and mouse kidney cells, and hepatocytes.[74,75] Other major chromosomal aberrations, such as deletions, rearrangements, endoreduplication, and sister chromatid exchange have not been observed in all aging systems without treatment with high doses of various DNA-damaging agents.[74,76,77]

Another line of research that indicates the possibility of decreased stability of chromatin is the reactivation of inactive X-chromosomes during aging. For example, in livers of old mice, a spontaneous 50-fold reactivation and expression of autosomal ornithine carbamoyl transferase (OCT) gene, which had been translocated to the inactive X-chromosome and had therefore become silent, was taken as a proof of instability of the genome during aging, possibly as a result of demethylation.[78] However, no such spontaneous reactivation of the human X-linked HPRT gene was observed in skin fibroblasts isolated from women with severe deficiency of this enzyme.[79] It is possible that the stability and maintenance of individual genes is a function of their cell-type- and species-specificity that is reflected in the great heterogeneity of the extent of DNA repair observed for various genes in the same genome.

At the level of genes, studies on age-related changes in the structural organization of genes are just beginning. For example, no difference in the restriction patterns of histone H3 and H4 genes in aging human fibroblasts has been observed.[80] Similarly, no sequence rearrangements of nine DNA regions, including genes for actin, dihydrofolate reductase, immunoglobulin μ constant region, and c-abl and c-ras proto-oncogenes, were detected in various tissues of young and old mice.[81] However, a decreased intensity of hybridization due to a possible loss of sequences of actin and globin genes, but not of the interferon gene, has been reported for senescent cultures of human fibroblasts.[82] Altered splicing of fibronectin mRNA during cellular aging[83] may be related to alterations in trans-acting factors that bind to cAMP-responsive elements (CRE) at the 5′ end of the fibronectin gene and regulate its expression.[84]

III. DISREGULATION OF GENETIC INFORMATION TRANSFER

The genome on its own is meaningless unless the information coded in it is accurately transcribed and translated into functional macromolecules. Two types of RNA, transfer (t) RNA and ribosomal (r) RNA, are themselves functional molecules. However, the genetic information transcribed into the third RNA, messenger (m) RNA, has to be generally translated to produce proteins which are functional gene products. Although proteins are the most common gene products through which the genetic instructions become materialized, the intermediary steps of the synthesis of RNA, its processing and transport, can be equally critical for the regulation of gene expression. However, accurate translation of genetic information from a language of nucleic acids into a language of amino acids and proteins has been considered a crucial regulatory step for growth, development, and aging. Not only the synthesis of proteins but also their posttranslational processing, including chemical modifications of amino acids, folding of the polypeptide chain, transport, and turnover are central to the process of aging.

A. Transcription and Processing

Studies on the synthesis of RNA and on its processing during aging have been few. There are three types of RNA in a cell, of which about 70 to 80% is rRNA, 10 to 15% is tRNA, and 5 to 7% is mRNA, and the proportion of these RNAs does not change significantly during aging.[85] However, for each type of RNA some age-related changes have been observed in various aging systems. For example, a significant decline in the content and synthesis of rRNAs has been reported in aging beagles, rodent organs, and cultured cells.[85] This decline in rRNAs was previously thought to be associated with the loss of ribosomal genes. However, no age-related decline in the gene copy number of rRNA has been observed in human fibroblasts or in mouse myocytes.[86] Furthermore, the number of rRNA genes in a cell is already in great excess (between 200 and 1000 copies), and a small loss with age may not have any serious consequences for cell function and survival.[85] However, whether there is a differential loss of various rRNA species during aging, and what effects such a loss might have, is not known.

The codon-restriction theory of aging[87,88] suggests that a random loss of more than 60 types of isoaccepting tRNAs will progressively restrict the readability of codons, resulting in an inefficiency and inaccuracy of protein synthesis. Several reports have been published showing both stable and unstable patterns of isoacceptors,[88-90] decreased or increased contents of tRNAs,[91] changed or unchanged composition of minor nucleosides in tRNAs,[92] and changed or unchanged capacity of tRNAs to accept various amino acids.[93,94] Similarly, in the case of aminoacyl-tRNA synthetases, an increase or decrease in the specific activities of almost all of them has been reported in various organs of aging mice without any apparent correlation with tissue or cell type and its protein synthetic activity.[95] It is, therefore, impossible to derive any general conclusions based on such contradictory data regarding qualitative and quantitative changes in tRNAs during aging.[96,97]

Another step in the transfer of genetic information that can be rate-limiting is the availability of mRNAs for translation. Posttranscriptional processing of eukaryotic mRNA is highly complex and is still not very well understood. However, a few reports are available on changes in various aspects of mRNA-processing during aging. For example, a decrease in the total poly(A+) mRNA has been reported in aging rat brain and liver, in rabbit liver, in the liver, heart, and oviduct of quails, and in the post-mortem brain tissues obtained from patients with Alzheimer´s disease.[85,98] This is thought to be due to both a decrease in the length of the poly(A) tail and the rate of polyadenylation of mRNA during aging. However, an application of more sensitive methods for measuring the age-related changes in the length of the poly(A) tail have shown no significant differences in rat hepatocytes[99] and in the liver, kidney, and brain samples obtained from calorie-restricted and freely-fed rats of different ages.[100] Similarly, no age-related differences in mRNA cap structure and its translatability *in vitro* have been observed.[99] Thus, although it appears that at a gross level there are no major alterations in mRNA characteristics, it is possible that individual mRNA species do undergo changes including their transport from nucleus to cytoplasm, binding to ribosomes, stability, and turnover during aging.

B. Regulation of Protein Synthesis

A decline in the rate of bulk protein synthesis is one of the most common age-associated biochemical changes that has been observed in a wide variety of cells, tissues, organs, and organisms, including human beings.[96,97,101-103] Although there is a considerable variability among different tissues and cell types in the extent of decline (varying from 20 to 80%), the fact remains that the overall protein synthesis slows down during aging. The consequences of slower rates of protein synthesis are manifold. They include (1) a decrease in the availability of enzymes for the maintenance, repair, and normal metabolic functioning of the cell; (2) an inefficient removal of intracellular damage due to free radicals or other damaging agents; (3) an accumulation of inactive, abnormal, and damaged macromolecules in the cell; (4) the inefficiency of the intracellular and intercellular signaling pathways including the receptors; and (5) a decrease in the production and secretion of various products, such as hormones, neurotransmitters, antibodies, and the components of the extracellular matrix including bone formation. Therefore, the regulation of protein synthesis occupies a central position in forming the biochemical basis of aging.

Eukaryotic protein synthesis is a highly complex process which requires almost 200 small and large components to function effectively and accurately in order to translate one mRNA molecule. Each of the several components of the protein synthetic machinery can be rate limiting for protein synthesis. These components include translatable mRNA, 40S small ribosomal subunits containing 18S rRNA and about 30 ribosomal proteins, 60S large subunits with 3 kinds of rRNAs, and about 50 ribosomal proteins, more than 60 tRNAs, at least 20 aminoacyl-tRNA synthetases, about 7 initiation factors (eIF) consisting of 24 different proteins, 4 elongation factor (eEF) proteins, one termination or release factor, and GTP as the energy source.[104,105]

There is an almost complete dearth of systematic studies on the regulation of protein synthesis during aging. Although several investigators have tried to study age-related changes in different components of protein synthesis, few general conclusions can be drawn because of the frequently contradictory results obtained. However, there is some consensus among the researchers regarding age-related changes in different steps in the protein synthesis. For example, most evidence points to an age-related slowing down of the elongation step of protein synthesis instead of its initiation and termination steps.[94,106] The overall elongation rates have been reported to decline more than twofold in the liver and brain of old rats.[107,108]

Although no major age-related changes in the rates of protein initiation have been reported, a few studies indicate that some changes may occur in various eIFs during aging. For example, the activity of eIF-2, which is required for the formation of the ternary complex of methionyl-tRNA, GTP, and eIF-2, has been reported to decrease in rat tissues during development and aging.[109-112] A decline in the amount (20 to 58%) and activity (30%) of GDP/GTP exchange factor eIF-2B has been reported in the brains and livers of 10-month-old Sprague-Dawley rats as compared with 1- and 4-month-old animals.[113] There is indirect evidence that the activity of eIF-3, the antiribosomal-association factor, may increase during aging, since an age-related decline in the polysomal fraction of the ribosomes has been reported.[114]

In the case of eEFs, the activity of eEF-1 declines with age and the drop parallels the decrease in protein synthesis in aging rat livers and *Drosophila*.[115,116] This decline in the activity of eEF-1 has been correlated only to eEF-1α as no changes were observed in the eEF-1βγ-mediated activity. Using more specific cell-free stoichiometric and catalytic assays, a 35 to 45% decrease in the activity and amounts of active eEF-1α have been reported for serially passaged senescent human fibroblasts and old mouse and rat livers and brains.[117-120] The reasons for the decline in the activity and amounts of active eEF-1α appear to be at multiple levels such as transcriptional, translational, and posttranslational. For example, in *Drosophila*, a decrease of more than 95% in the level of translatable mRNA for eEF-1 has been reported.[116] However, in the case of cultured human fibroblasts a 50-fold increase in RNA transcripts hybridizing to eEF-1α cDNA in quiescent and senescent cells has been reported.[121] It is also suggested that changes in the total amounts of eEF-1α and in the extent of its posttranslational modifications such as methylation and phosphorylation that modulate its activity can be the cause of age-related loss in activity.[122]

The second elongation factor eEF-2 is also a highly conserved monomeric protein that catalyzes the translocation of peptidyl-tRNA from the A site to the P site on the ribosome.[122] The translocation activity of eEF-2 is regulated by posttranslational modifications, such as ADP-ribosylation of its unique diphthamide residue and phosphorylation by a calcium- and calmodulin-dependent protein kinase III, also known as eEF-2 kinase.[123,124] Changes in the extent of phosphorylation of eEF-2 and the amounts of ADP-ribosylatable eEF-2 have been related to various phases of the human cell cycle.[125,126] However, no change in eEF-2-dependent translocational activity in *in vitro* assays is seen in *Drosophila*, or rat and mouse liver and kidney during aging.[116] Similarly, whereas the amount of ADP-ribosylatable active eEF-2 goes down by 60% in aging human fibroblasts in culture,[127] it does not decrease in aging rat livers.[128] Furthermore, although the proportion of heat labile eEF-2 increases during aging, the specific activity of purified eEF-2 does not differ in young and old rat and mouse livers.[129]

C. Posttranslational Events

1. Protein Modifications

Even when a protein is synthesized normally and accurately, several posttranslational events determine whether it can perform its function efficiently without being degraded immediately. More than 140 posttranslational modifications of proteins have been described that are involved in determining the biological activity, stability, folding, intra- and intercellular targeting, and the turnover of proteins.[130] Conformational changes in protein folding/unfolding have been suggested as an explanation for age-related loss in the activity of several enzymes, including enolase, phosphoglycerate kinase, aldolase, and 3-phosphoglyceraldehyde dehydrogenase.[131-134] Other posttranslational modifications considered to be involved in the inactivation of many enzymes during aging are the spontaneous deamidation of asparagine and glutamine residues in triose phosphate isomerase, racemization and isomerization of aspartyl residues, glycation, and oxidation by a mixed function oxidase (MFO) or metal catalyzed oxidation (MCO) system.[135]

Increased levels of carbonyl groups, which is a measure of oxidatively modified proteins, have been reported in a wide variety of aging systems including cultured cells, insects, and mammalian brain.[136-138] The oxidation and inactivation of several proteins including 6-phosphogluconate dehydrogenase, glyceraldehyde-3-phosphate dehydrogenase, collagen, lens crystallin, ornithine decarboxylase, and liver malic enzyme during aging have been reported.[139,140] Similarly, the formation of advanced glycosylation endproducts (AGE) as a result of glycation of various proteins including collagen, osteocalcin, lens crystallin, and hemoglobin has been considered as one of the age-related changes in protein structure and function.[141,142]

Phosphorylation and dephosphorylation of serine, threonine, and tyrosine residues of proteins are considered to be important regulators of protein activity during various biological processes such as cell division, signal transduction, growth, development, and aging. Among the phosphorylated proteins that may be of significance to the process of aging are DNA polymerase α, histones, protein synthetic factors, ribosomal proteins, cytoskeletal proteins, and various growth factor and hormone receptors.[143] Although there are a few reports on the age-related changes in the activities of various kinases[144,145] and in growth factor-induced phosphorylation of receptors,[146] information about changes in the extent of phosphorylation of individual proteins during aging is very scant.

In addition to the above types of posttranslational modifications, there are many other modifications that determine the structure and function of various proteins and may have a role to play during aging. For example, the incorporation of ethanolamine into protein synthetic factor eEF-1α may be involved in determining its stability and interaction with intracellular membranes.[147] Alterations in the extent of methylation of several proteins including histones, myosin, and ankyrin have been related to the changes in their characteristics during aging.[92,148,149]

2. Protein Degradation

Degradation of proteins is another posttranslational event that has been implicated in the regulation of enzyme activity, accumulation of abnormal molecules in old cells, and various other cellular characteristics during aging.[101,150] What determines the stability and half-life of a newly synthesized protein is beginning to be understood. The so-called PEST (proline, glutamic acid, serine, threonine) hypothesis and the N-terminal rule have been put forward to predict the half-life of a protein. For example, short-lived proteins appear to contain one or more regions rich in proline, glutamic acid, serine, and threonine PEST in single-letter amino acid code.[151] Similarly, changing amino acid residues at the N-terminal of β-galactosidase can increase its half-life from less than 3 min to more than 20 h, depending upon the nature of the amino acid at the N-terminal.[152]

Studies on bulk protein degradation during aging indicate a significant age-related decline in the degradation of proteins.[101,153-155] Estimations of the degradation rates of several proteins also show that, in general, protein turnover slows down with age. For example, microinjection of horseradish peroxidase in mouse hepatocyte cultures from young and old mice showed a slower degradation of the protein in the latter.[156] Similarly, 50% slower degradation of ovalbumin microinjected into liver parenchymal cells from old mice as compared with young mice was observed.[157]

Whether decreased protein turnover in old age is a result of decreased synthesis of proteolytic enzymes, of decreased efficiency of proteases in recognizing aged and abnormal proteins, of structural and conformational changes in proteins themselves making them poorer substrates for the degrading enzymes, or of a combination of all these factors is not known.[150,158] However, the fact remains that there is a decline in the rate of degradation of proteins and of other macromolecules during aging. This is also reflected in the frequently observed accumulation of the so-called age pigments and other abnormal macromolecules during aging.

IV. ALTERED CELLULAR RESPONSIVENESS

Altered cellular responsiveness is one of the critical aspects of the failure of homeostasis during aging.[159] It has been widely observed that the mitogenic and growth-stimulating effects of growth factors, hormones, and other agents are reduced significantly during cellular aging. For example, stimulation of protein synthesis and induction of several cell-cycle-related genes and DNA synthesis in response to extracellular serum, insulin, hydrocortisone, epidermal growth factor (EGF), fibroblast growth factor (FGF), platelet-derived growth factor (PDGF), and other hormones is reduced significantly in aging cells.[159-161] In contrast, the sensitivity of aging cells to toxic agents including antibiotics, phorbol esters, free-radical inducers, irradiation, and heat shock increases.[162]

The reasons for the age-related changes in the responsiveness of cells is a matter of continuing debate. Earlier studies generally attributed the decreasing response of old cells to hormones and other growth factors to a loss of cell surface receptors. However, later studies show that the diminished response of cells to externally supplied factors may be due not to any decrease in the number of receptors, but instead to defective pathways of signal transduction during aging. For example, no age-related changes in the binding characteristics and autophosphorylation of various growth factor receptor complexes during aging of human fibroblasts have been reported.[146,160,163,164]

Recently, some studies have shown the significance of postreceptor events during aging. It has been demonstrated that the ability of steroid receptor complexes to bind to nuclear acceptor sites is impaired and that changes in calcium mobilization occur during aging.[165] High calcium concentrations inside old cells may impede normal fluxes of free calcium, thus resulting in impaired responsiveness to hormones and neurotransmitters. However, it has been shown that the intracellular calcium concentration either stays the same[166,167] or decreases during aging and the defect may lie at the level of cellular capacity to mobilize calcium as a result of extracellular stimuli.[168]

The role of protein kinases as modulators of signal transduction is also well known.[169] In the case of calcium-dependent protein kinase C (PKC), no age-related changes have been observed in mice organs and human cells.[144,163,170] Furthermore, there is evidence that major pathways of signal transduction remain intact in old cells which can respond to extracellular stimuli. For example, several growth-regulated genes can be fully induced in senescent cells upon treatment with serum and other growth factors.[171-174] Similarly, phorbol esters can stimulate the synthesis of DNA, RNA, proteins, and protein elongation factors,[175,176] and induce c-fos expression and the translocation of PKC from the cytosol to the particulate compartment.[163] These studies underline a very important point in aging research by demonstrating that during cellular aging the integrity of the DNA-, RNA-, and protein-synthesizing machineries remain intact along with the structural and functional stability of the receptor system.

Therefore, the reasons for altered responsiveness and failure of homeostasis during aging may lie primarily in metabolic defects in the pathways of macromolecular synthesis. For example, a defect in the synthesis, fidelity, and efficiency of proteins can have implications ranging from impaired membrane function to inefficient signal transduction and a reduction in the synthesis and turnover of macromolecules. This would affect cellular homeostasis, and cells would not be able to maintain their responsiveness to external stimuli.[159]

The interactions of intracellular activities with the extracellular environment, including other cells, play a major role in the control of cell growth, differentiation, tissue morphogenesis, and pattern formation. The failure or impairment of such interactions has been suggested as part of the cellular basis of aging, particularly at the levels of neural and endocrine mechanisms,[177-179] autoimmunity,[180] and changes in ionic permeability of the plasma membrane and the colloid osmotic pressure.[181]

At the cellular level, cell surface receptors, pathways of signal transduction, and the cytoskeleton are the major components involved in inter- and intracellular communication. Several studies have been performed which document changes in the surface architecture of cells during aging along with the age-related changes in the ultrastructure, physiology, fluidity, permeability, surface antigens, extracellular matrix, and the biochemical composition of the plasma membrane, including gap junction proteins.[182-186] Similarly, the literature on changes in hormone receptors during development, adulthood, and aging is too large to be included here, and has been discussed separately in this book.

How the signals generated at the plasma membrane as a result of the binding of a ligand to its receptor reach their intracellular targets and elicit cellular responses, such as DNA synthesis, cell division, induction/suppression of genes, stimulation/inhibition of protein synthesis, and activation/inactivation of enzyme activities, is one of the most hotly pursued areas in modern biology. The discovery of several GTP-binding "G proteins" as intermediaries in a variety of transmembrane signaling processes, and of the role of inositol phosphates as second messengers, have significantly increased our understanding of the regulation of cell proliferation.[187] There is some evidence indicating that age-related changes in a variety of adrenergic responses may be due to a dysfunctioning of G proteins.[179,188] Thus, although it is clear that altered cellular responsiveness, decreased cell communication, and inefficient intracellular signal transduction are central to the progressive failure of homeostasis, the exact mechanisms behind these processes during aging are not known at present.

Recent understanding of the relationship between cytoskeleton and cytoplasmic organization, cell shape, spatial distribution of cellular organelles, intracellular communication, cell division, intracellular transport, gene expression, and protein synthesis has drawn attention to the role of the cytoskeleton in cellular aging. Since several studies have shown a disorganized cytoskeleton in continuously dividing transformed cells, age-related loss of proliferative capacity of normal cells is thought to be related to the integrity of the cytoskeleton.[189-191] It has also been reported that photo-aging of human skin cells induced by environmental wavelengths of UV light is related to disruption of the cytoskeletal microtubule complex.[192] Furthermore, observations that the aggregates of paired helical filaments (PHF) in the neurones of Alzheimer´s disease patients contain microtubule-associated proteins MAP2 and tau suggest a possible role of aberrant or modified cytoskeletal proteins in age-related pathology of the brain.[193] Thus it is becoming increasingly clear that the components of the cytoskeleton, their organization, stability, and integrity, along with their property of maintaining an equilibrium between their different structural and chemical forms, have far-reaching implications for the regulation of cell shape, cell motility, cell division, cell survival, and transformation.

V. LOSS OF CELL PROLIFERATION

In many organisms, several cell types retain the capacity to divide during most of the adult lifespan, and are required to divide repeatedly for various functions of the body such as immune response, blood formation, bone formation, and repair and regeneration of various tissues. For example, epithelial cells, epidermal basal cells, fibroblasts, bone marrow cells, lymphocytes, osteoblasts, myoblasts, and glial cells constitute some of the most crucial dividing cell compartments of an organism. It is not only their differentiated and specialized functions that are critical for the organism — their capacity to divide is an integral part of their role in organismic growth, development, maintenance, and survival. A loss of proliferative capacity of such cell types has global deteriorative impacts on the functioning and survival of the organism. A loss or slowing down of proliferation of cells (e.g., osteoblasts, myoblasts, epithelial, lymphocytes, and fibroblasts) can be the basis of the onset of many age-related diseases and impairments including osteoporosis, arthritis, immune deficiency, altered drug clearance, delayed wound healing, and altered functioning of the brain.[194]

On the basis of studies using a diverse range of cell types it has become well established that normal diploid cells with the ability to divide *in vivo* or *in vitro* can do so only a fixed number of times — a limit known as the Hayflick limit.[195-197] There are several lines of evidence in support of the view that the limited division potential of cells and other changes occurring during their limited lifespan are a genuine expression of the process of aging. These include the inverse relationship between the age of the cell donor and maximum division potential of cells in culture; the direct relationship between a species' maximum achievable lifespan and the proliferative capacity of its cells in culture; and the decreased proliferative capacity of cells from patients with premature aging syndromes.[196-199] In many ways, the aging of an organism can be regarded as a result of the limited proliferative capacity of its single-cell zygote from which the whole organism has developed by repeated cell division, growth, and differentiation.

A. Senescence-Specific Markers

A large number of studies have been undertaken to identify genes and gene products responsible for limiting and regulating cell proliferation. Based on studies performed by cell fusion and microinjection methods, there is evidence that senescence is dominant over unlimited proliferation and that negative growth effectors are involved in the pathway to cellular senescence.[200] Several potential markers of mortality have been identified by comparative studies on mortal, immortal, and hybrid cells. For example, tumor suppressor genes,[201,202] human chromosomes 1 and 4,[203-205] and a novel member of mouse hsp70 protein termed mortalin[206,207] have been associated with the mortal phenotype of normal and hybrid cells. Although a lot has been learnt about the biochemical nature of many of such gene products, it is not clear how they bring about the cellular changes associated with them.

A comparison of cDNA libraries made from young and senescent diploid cells have resulted in the isolation of differentially regulated gene products whose levels may be increased or decreased in old cells. Many of these mRNAs and proteins could be identified as well-known cellular products such as fibronectin,[208] procollagen, ferritin heavy chain, insulin-like growth factor binding protein-3, plasminogen activator inhibitor type 1, thrombospondin, crystallin,[209,210] cathapsin B,[211,212] and the mitochondrial genes for NADH dehydrogenase subunit 4 and for cytochrome *b* .[213] In other cases in which no similarities of the cDNA or the protein were found with any known gene products, new names were given to various gene products capable of inhibiting DNA synthesis, for example, statin,[214] terminin,[215] prohibitin,[216] SUSM-1 factor,[217] a growth inhibitory glycopeptide,[218] and a so-called senescence-associated gene SAG.[219] There are several other overexpressed gene products in normally senescent and prematurely aged Werner's syndrome fibroblasts whose identities have not been confirmed as yet.[220] What all such studies have shown is a quantitative change in the amounts of certain gene products during cellular aging without identifying any products unique to old cells. Furthermore, since the inhibitors of DNA synthesis are generally produced in cells that have already completed more than 90% of their lifespan *in vitro*, it is not clear whether these inhibitors are a cause of cellular aging or are a result of other age-related changes in gene expression, regulation, and metabolism during serial passaging of normal diploid cells.

B. Cell Division Counting Mechanisms

Since the proliferative capacity of normal diploid cells is related to the maximum lifespan of the species, the existence of some kind of counting mechanism has often been presumed. For example, a progressive loss of 5mC during serial passaging of cells has been considered as a counting mechanism for the number of completed cell divisions.[34,37,39] Recently, telomeres, which are the terminal repetitive sequences at the ends of the eukaryotic chromosomes, have been suggested to be a kind of determining mechanism for the number of divisions a cell can undergo.[221]

Shortening of telomeres may play a crucial role in cellular aging. A loss of terminal restriction fragment (TRF) telomeric DNA during aging has been reported for human fibroblasts,[222] peripheral blood leukocytes, colon mucosa epithelia,[223] skin,[224] and lymphocytes.[225] A strong relationship between telomere length, donor age, proliferative capacity of fibroblasts from normal donors and from patients with Hutchinson-Gilford premature aging syndrome has been established.[226] These studies have shown that in the case of fibroblasts an average loss of 50 ± 20 TRF base pairs (bp) per cell division *in vitro* and a decrease of 15 ± 6 TRF bp per year of life *in vivo* is a comparatively more accurate predictor of replicative lifespan than any other marker, for example, donor age.[226] Similarly, the rate of telomere loss in human lymphocytes was higher in subjects with Down´s syndrome (133 ± 15 bp) as compared with normal subjects (41 ± 7 bp) per year of life.[225]

Telomere length as a predictor of replicative lifespan of normal somatic cells and the rate of loss of telomeres as a molecular marker of aging is an attractive hypothesis. Furthermore, the observations that sperm telomeres are longer than somatic telomeres,[226,227] and that immortal cells with unlimited proliferative capacity have a shorter telomere but whose length is maintained during proliferation by virtue of telomerase activity,[228] have raised the possibilities of testing whether telomere loss and telomerase expression are coincidental or causal in cellular mortality and immortality.

VI. FUTURE PERSPECTIVES AND GERONTOGENES

The failure of maintenance at all levels of organization appears to be a universal characteristic of aging, and all attempts of slowing down aging and increasing the lifespan have been operative through one or more of these mechanisms of somatic maintenance.[229,230] However, apart from this very general characteristic, no other reliable biomarkers of age are available that can define aging in structural, functional, and physiological terms. Our failure to develop biomarkers of aging may be linked with the dominant reductionistic approach of contemporary scientific research. Although this approach has been very successful in establishing that the chemistry of diverse life forms is very similar, it is incapable of explaining the differences in the biology of different organisms and the ways in which they grow, develop, mature, reproduce, age, and die.[231] In many ways, the issue of the fundamental cellular and molecular basis of aging is a question of how one defines and measures biological time.

The functional definition of aging as the failure of maintenance postulates that the homeostatic mechanisms are implicated as the primary causes of senescence. Indeed, many of the theories of aging imply directly or indirectly that the progressive failure of homeostatic mechanisms is crucial for the process of aging.[232] However, the question of species-specific lifespan and the rates of aging and senescence can only be addressed by evolutionary theories of aging and longevity. Although arguments based on both the inadequacies of the available life tables[233] and experimental results of studies on large cohorts of insect populations[234, 235] have been put forward against the notion of a very rigid species-specific longevity, the fact remains that the lifespan of an individual is terminated within a limited period. For example, although studies with medflies *Ceratitis capitata* have shown that a highly extended lifespan of 170 days could be achieved for the last one in a million surviving medfly as compared with 20 days for 50% of the population, 64 days for 10% of the population, and 103 days for 1% of the population,[234] precisely these studies show that no fly could realistically attain longevity characteristics comparable to, say, mouse or man.

Therefore, even in the absence of all accidental causes of death, there are intrinsic processes that practically determine the limit to maximum achievable lifespan. This limit and its manifestation in death (either sudden and rapid or after a period of progressive aging and senescence) are linked with the life histories of various species.[236] For example, vegetative reproduction vs. sexual reproduction, and semelparous (single act of reproduction) life cycle vs. iteroparous (multiple reproduction) life cycle will dictate to what extent the lifespan of an individual within a population can be defined and whether aging and senescence can be clearly identified. However, once the view is held that the lifespan of an organism is intrinsically limited and is largely species-specific, it necessarily involves certain notions of genetic elements of regulation. In this context, the term gerontogenes[232,237] refers to any such genetic elements that are involved in the regulation of aging and lifespan.

A. Gerontogenes: Real or Virtual?

As to the nature of gerontogenes various suggestions have been made, and these range from aging genes per se that determine both the duration of lifespan and the time of death, to late-acting deleterious genes and pleiotropic trade-off genes with a beneficial early action at the expense of a later deleterious action. Of these, ideas regarding the existence of gerontogenes as genes for programmed self-destruction are largely discounted based on evolutionary grounds. For example, the theories based on the assumption of the adaptive nature of aging as being advantageous imply that selection for advantage for the species is stronger than that for individuals, and are not considered valid any more.[238-240] In contrast, the nonadaptive theories suggest that aging occurs either because natural selection is insufficient to prevent it, owing to its postreproductive nature, or that senescence is a byproduct of the expression of genes with early beneficial traits but deleterious and pleiotropic effects at later stages.

Two major schools of thought (whose ideas are not mutually exclusive) in the nonadaptive theories of the evolution of aging and lifespan are represented by antagonistic pleiotropy[241] and disposable soma theory.[238,239] According to both these theories, evolutionary forces have acted upon optimizing conditions for efficient and successful reproduction either by selecting for "good" early genes with later "bad" effects or selecting for efficient maintenance and repair of the germ cells at the cost of the somatic maintenance. The common element in these two theories is that, whatever the mechanisms, the central concept in the process of aging is a homeostatic balance retained until reproductive maturity, followed by the failure of homeostasis.

The ideas of late-acting deleterious genes or pleiotropic genes with early beneficial effects and late harmful effects both beg the question as to what constitutes "early" and "late" in life. Any genes whose expression or effect is dependent upon certain signals of passing biological time can at best be a consequence of the aging process rather than being its cause. Another view regarding the nature of gerontogenes can be derived from the disposable soma theory of the evolution of limited lifespan.[238,239] According to this theory, genes selected during evolution for the optimal maintenance of the soma until the continuation of the germ line is assured are the primary candidates qualifying as gerontogenes. Furthermore, this theory predicts that aging is due to an accumulation of unrepaired somatic defects and that aging rates can be modulated by changing the level of key homeostatic processes of maintenance and repair.

Therefore, the concept of gerontogenes is intimately linked with the idea of genes involved in the regulation of development and homeostasis. However, the term gerontogenes does not refer to a tangible physical reality but to a functional reality. For this purpose, the term virtual gerontogenes has been suggested[4,242] in which "virtual" is defined, as in the Shorter Oxford Dictionary, as something that "is so in essence or effect although not formally or actually; admitting of being called by the name so far as the effect or result is concerned." In science, the term "virtual" is used for entities that it is helpful to regard as being present, even though in terms of the theory applied they are known to be mere figments: the paradigm of such an entity is the "virtual image" of optics.

The concept of gerontogenes as being virtual implies that the DNA sequence of virtual gerontogenes cannot be identified, isolated, and cloned. This is because every time a potential aging gene is discovered it will, on sequencing and identification, turn out to be a familiar normal gene with a defined function. For example, several recent attempts at identifying senescence-specific genes in old cells and tissues have resulted in the isolation of genes, such as those of the components of the extracellular matrix, which are known to have other well-established functions apparently unrelated to their involvement in aging.[200,208,220,243] Similarly, *Drosophila* experiments on the addition of an extra copy of a protein elongation factor EF-1α gene resulting in the slowing down of aging[244] support the concept of virtual gerontogenes. The identification of the *age* genes in the nematode *Caenorhabditis elegans*, which affect both the longevity and the fecundity of these organisms,[245-247] may be another example of virtual gerontogenes. Other possibilities may be found in the complex regulatory mechanisms known to exist in connection with the end-replication problem of telomeres and the postreplicative processing of DNA, such as methylation.

At present, it is not possible to determine the number of real genes or set of genes that best qualify for being virtual gerontogenes. Obviously, not every gene is potentially a gerontogene. One could narrow down the possibilities to sets of genes involved in the maintenance and repair of the genome and the accuracy of the pathways of genetic information transfer as the primary candidates qualifying as virtual gerontogenes. Therefore the concept of virtual genes refers to the emergent property of several tightly coupled genes whose combined action and interaction resembled the effect of one gene. Treating it as a virtual gene is a useful conceptual tool while searching for the genetic elements of regulation of a complex biological process.

The notion of gerontogenes is not contradictory to the nonadaptive nature of aging and longevity discussed above. Rather, it reasserts the evolutionary optimization of the genetic mechanisms of somatic maintenance in order to assure germ line reproduction as visualized by both the antagonistic pleiotropy theory and disposable soma theory. On the other hand, the diversity of many different forms and variations in which aging is manifested throughout the living systems is indicative of its stochastic nature. In order to combine the genetic aspects of aging and longevity with the stochastic nature of age-related changes, we have attempted to discover links and relationships between them in a model presented in Figure 15-1.

According to this scheme, aging is seen as the ultimate failure of homeostasis due to interactions between genetic mechanisms of defense (longevity assurance processes) and stochastic causes of damage and perturbations. Mechanisms involved in maintaining the fidelity of genetic information transfer from genes to gene products, efficiency of inter- and intracellular communication, and the accuracy and efficiency of turnover of normal and

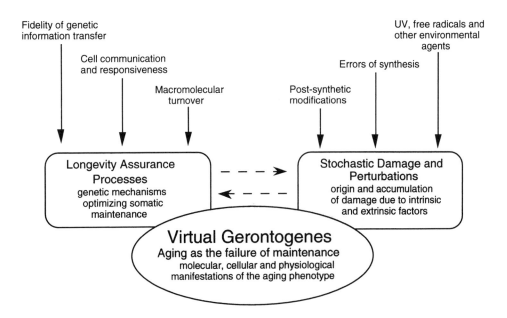

FIGURE 15-1 A simplified model suggesting interaction between the genetically determined capacity of somatic maintenance and the extent of stochastic damage resulting in the failure of maintenance.

abnormal macromolecules are the main longevity assurance processes. These processes have to work in the presence of extrinsic and intrinsic sources of damage, such as environmental and nutritional agents, spontaneous errors of macromolecular synthesis, postsynthetic modifications of macromolecules making them inactive or abnormal, and other defects occurring during the course of normal metabolism. Interactions between the causes of perturbations and the mechanisms of defense determine effectively the extent of damage and the state of homeostasis. The molecular, cellular, and physiological manifestations of the aging phenotype that includes the full range of age-related diseases is the result of such interactions. Elucidating the exact nature of such interactions resulting in a progressive failure of maintenance and homeostasis can be a useful framework for developing appropriate strategies for future gerontological research.

REFERENCES

1. Sacher, G. A., Evolutionary theory in gerontology, *Persp. Biol. Med.,* 25, 339, 1982.
2. Hart, R. W., D'Ambrosio, S. M., Ng, K. J. and Modak, S. P., Longevity, stability and DNA repair, *Mech. Ageing Dev.,* 9, 203, 1979.
3. Gensler, H. and Bernstein, H., DNA damage as the primary cause of aging, *Quart. Rev. Biol.,* 56, 279, 1981.
4. Rattan, S. I. S., DNA damage and repair during cellular aging, *Int. Rev. Cytol.,* 116, 47, 1989.
5. Ames, B. N., Saul, R. L., Schwiers, E., Adelman, R. and Cathcart, R., Oxidative DNA damage as related to cancer and aging: assay of thymine glycol, thymidine glycol and hydroxymethyluracil in human and rat urine., in *Molecular Biology of Aging: Gene Stability and Gene Expression*, Sohal, R. S., Birnbaum, L. S. and Cutler, R. G., Eds., Raven Press, New York, 1985, 137.
6. Ames, B. N. and Shigenaga, M. K., Oxidants are a major contributor to aging, *Ann. N.Y. Acad. Sci.,* 663, 85, 1992.
7. Lindahl, T., Instability and decay of the primary structure of DNA, *Nature,* 362, 709, 1993.
8. Beaupain, R., Icard, C. and Macieira-Coelho, A., Changes in DNA alkali-sensitive sites during senescence and establishment of fibroblasts in vitro, *Biochim. Biophys. Acta,* 606, 251, 1980.
9. Dell'Orco, R. T. and Whittle, W. L., Evidence for an increased level of DNA damage in high doubling level human diploid cells in culture, *Mech. Ageing Dev.,* 15, 141, 1981.
10. Tice, R. R. and Setlow, R. B., DNA repair and replication in aging organisms and cells, in *Handbook of the Biology of Aging*, Finch, C. E. and Schneider, E. L., Eds., Van Nostrand Reinhold, New York, 1985, 173.
11. Zahn, R. K., Reinmüller, J., Beyer, R. and Pondeljak, V., Age-correlated DNA damage in human muscle tissue, *Mech. Ageing Dev.,* 41, 73, 1987.
12. Mullaart, E., Boerrigter, M. E., Brouwer, A., Berends, F. and Vijg, J., Age-dependent accumulation of alkali-labile sites in DNA of post-mitotic but not in that of mitotic rat liver cells, *Mech. Ageing Dev.,* 45, 41, 1988.
13. Ishimi, Y., Kojima, M., Takeuchi, F., Miyamoto, T., Yamada, M. and Hanaoka, F., Changes in chromatin structure during aging of human skin fibroblasts, *Exp. Cell Res.,* 169, 458, 1987.
14. Macieira-Coelho, A., Chromatin reorganization during senescence of proliferating cells, *Mutat. Res.,* 256, 81, 1991.
15. Randerath, K., Li, D., Nath, R. and Randerath, E., Exogenous and endogeneous DNA modifications as monitored by ^{32}P-postlabelling: relationships to cancer and aging, *Exp. Gerontol.,* 27, 533, 1992.
16. Richter, C., Park, J. W. and Ames, B. N., Normal oxidative damage to mitochondrial and nuclear DNA is extensive, *Proc. Natl. Acad. Sci. U.S.A.,* 85, 6465, 1988.
17. Takasawa, M., Hayakawa, M., Sugiyama, S., Hattori, K., Ito, T. and Ozawa, T., Age-associated damage in mitochondrial function in rat hearts, *Exp. Gerontol.,* 28, 269, 1993.
18. Hayakawa, M., Hattori, K., Sugiyama, S. and Ozawa, T., Age-associated oxygen damage and mutations in mitochondrial DNA in human hearts, *Biochem. Biophys. Res. Commun.,* 189, 979, 1992.
19. Fraga, C. G., Shigenaga, M. K., Park, J. W., Degan, P. and Ames, B. N., Oxidative damage to DNA during aging: 8-hydroxy-2'-deoxyguanosine in rat organ DNA and urine, *Proc. Natl. Acad. Sci. U.S.A,* 87, 4533, 1990.
20. Pikó, L., Hougham, A. J. and Bulpitt, K. J., Studies of sequence heterogeneity of mitochondrial DNA from rat and mouse tissues: evidence for an increased frequency of deletions/additions with aging, *Mech. Ageing Dev.,* 43, 279, 1988.
21. Arnheim, N. and Cortopassi, G., Deleterious mitochondrial DNA mutations accumulate in aging human tissues, *Mutat. Res.,* 275, 157, 1992.
22. Cortopassi, G. A., Shibata, D., Soong, N. W. and Arnheim, N., A pattern of accumulation of a somatic deletion of mitochondrial DNA in aging human tissues, *Proc. Natl. Acad. Sci. U.S.A.,* 89, 7370, 1992.
23. Fulder, S. J. and Holliday, R., A rapid rise in cell variants during the senescence of populations of human fibroblasts, *Cell,* 6, 67, 1975.
24. Fulder, S. J., Evidence for an increase in presumed somatic mutation during the ageing of human cells in culture, *Mech. Ageing Dev.,* 10, 101, 1979.

25. Gupta, R. S., Senescence of cultured human diploid fibroblasts. Are mutations responsible?, *J. Cell. Physiol.*, 103, 209, 1980.

26. Morley, A. A., Trainor, K. J., Seshadri, R. and Ryall, R. G., Measurement of in vivo mutations in human lymphocytes, *Nature*, 302, 155, 1983.

27. Morley, A. A., Cox, S. and Holliday, R., Human lymphocytes resistant to 6-thioguanine increase with age, *Mech. Ageing Dev.*, 19, 21, 1982.

28. Zhang, C., Linnane, A. W. and Nagley, P., Occurrence of a particular base substitution (3243 A to G) in mitochondrial DNA of tissues of ageing humans, *Biochem. Biophys. Res. Commun.*, 195, 1104, 1993.

29. Holliday, R., The inheritance of epigenetic defects, *Science*, 238, 163, 1987.

30. Ames, B. N. and Gold, L. S., Endogenous mutagens and the causes of aging and cancer, *Mutat. Res.*, 250, 3, 1991.

31. Cathcart, R., Schwiers, E., Saul, R. L. and Ames, B. N., Thymine glycol and thymidine glycol in human and rat urine: a possible assay for oxidative DNA damage, *Proc. Natl. Acad. Sci. U.S.A.*, 81, 5633, 1984.

32. Kasai, H. and Nishimura, S., Hydroxylation of deoxyguanosine at the C-8 position by ascorbic acid and other reducing agents, *Nucl. Acids Res.*, 12, 2137, 1984.

33. Kasai, H., Nishimura, S., Kurokawa, Y. and Hayashi, Y., Oral administration of the renal carcinogen, potassium bromate, specifically produces 8-hydroxydeoxyguanosine in rat target organ DNA, *Carcinogenesis*, 8, 1959, 1987.

34. Wilson, V. L. and Jones, P. A., DNA methylation decreases in aging but not in immortal cells, *Science*, 220, 1055, 1983.

35. Singhal, R. P., Mays-Hoopes, L. L. and Eichhorn, G. L., DNA methylation in aging of mice, *Mech. Ageing Dev.*, 41, 199, 1987.

36. Wilson, V. L., Smith, R. A., Ma, S. and Cutler, R. G., Genomic 5-methyldeoxycytidine decreases with age, *J. Biol. Chem.*, 262, 9948, 1987.

37. Holliday, R., Strong effects of 5-azacytidine on the in vitro lifespan of human diploid fibroblasts, *Exp. Cell Res.*, 166, 543, 1986.

38. Fairweather, D. S., Fox, M. and Margison, G. P., The in vitro lifespan of MRC-5 cells is shortened by 5-azacytidine-induced demethylation, *Exp. Cell Res.*, 168, 153, 1987.

39. Catania, J. and Fairweather, D. S., DNA methylation and cellular ageing, *Mutat. Res.*, 256, 283, 1991.

40. Friedberg, E. C., The molecular biology of nucleotide excision repair of DNA: recent progress, *J. Cell Sci.*, Suppl. 6, 1, 1987.

41. Mullaart, E., Lohman, P. H., Berends, F. and Vijg, J., DNA damage metabolism and aging, *Mutat. Res.*, 237, 189, 1990.

42. Cleaver, J. E., DNA repair in human xeroderma pigmentosum group C cells involves a different distribution of damaged sites in confluent and growing cells, *Nucl. Acids Res.*, 14, 8155, 1986.

43. Lehmann, A. R., Ageing, DNA repair of radiation damage and carcinogenesis: fact and fiction, *IARC Sci. Pub.*, 58, 203, 1985.

44. Fujiwara, Y., Higashikawa, T. and Tatsumi, M., A retarded rate of DNA replication and normal level of DNA repair in Werner's syndrome fibroblasts in culture, *J. Cell. Physiol.*, 92, 365, 1977.

45. Stefanini, M., Orecchia, G, Rabbiosi, G. and Nuzzo, F., Altered cellular response to UV irradiation in a patient affected by premature ageing, *Hum. Genet.*, 73, 189, 1986.

46. Chiricolo, M., Musa, A. R., Monti, D., Zannotti, M. and Franceschi, C., Enhanced DNA repair in lymphocytes of Down syndrome patients: the influence of zinc nutritional supplementation, *Mutat. Res.*, 295, 105, 1993.

47. Francis, A. A., Lee, W. H. and Regan, J. D., The relationship of DNA excision repair of ultraviolet-induced lesions to the maximum lifespan of mammals, *Mech. Ageing Dev.*, 16, 181, 1981.

48. Hall, K. Y., Hart, R. W., Benirschke, A. K. and Walford, R. A., Correlation between ultraviolet-induced DNA repair in primate lymphocytes and fibroblasts and species maximum achievable life span, *Mech. Ageing Dev.*, 24, 163, 1984.

49. Hart, R. W. and Setlow, R. B., Correlation between deoxyribonucleic acid excision-repair and life span in a number of mammalian species, *Proc. Natl. Acad. Sci. U.S.A.*, 71, 2169, 1974.

50. Schwartz, A. G., Correlation between species life span and capacity to activate 7,12-dimethylbenz(a)anthracene to a form mutagenic to a mammalian cell, *Exp. Cell Res.*, 94, 445, 1975.

51. Schwartz, A. G. and Moore, C. J., Inverse correlation between species life span and capacity of cultured fibroblasts to bind 7,12-dimethylbenz(a)anthracene to DNA, *Exp. Cell Res.*, 109, 448, 1977.

52. Lipman, J. M., Sokoloff, L. and Setlow, R. B., DNA repair by articular chondrocytes. V. O6-methylguanine-acceptor protein activity in resting and cultured rabbit and human chondrocytes, *Mech. Ageing Dev.*, 40, 205, 1987.

53. Grube, K. and Bürkle, A., Poly(ADP-ribose) polymerase activity in mononuclear leukocytes of 13 mammalian species correlates with species-specific life span, *Proc. Natl. Acad. Sci. U.S.A.*, 89, 11759, 1992.

54. Adelman, R., Saul, R. L. and Ames, B. N., Oxidative damage to DNA: relation to species metabolic rate and life span, *Proc. Natl. Acad. Sci. U.S.A.,* 85, 2706, 1988.

55. Boerrigter, M. E., Yin, Y., Vijg, J. and Wei, J. Y., DNA repair in congenic mice: possible influence of chromosome 4 genetic region on the rate of benzo[a]pyrene-induced DNA adduct removal, *J. Gerontol.,* 48, B11, 1992.

56. Bohr, V., Gene specific DNA repair, *Carcinogenesis,* 12, 1983, 1991.

57. Hanawalt, P. C., Gee, P., Ho, L., Hsu, R. K. and Kane, C. J., Genomic heterogeneity of DNA repair. Role in aging?, *Ann. N.Y. Acad. Sci.,* 663, 17, 1992.

58. Link, C. J., Jr., Mitchell, D. L., Nairn, R. S. and Bohr, V. A., Preferential and strand-specific DNA repair of (6-4) photoproducts detected by a photochemical method in the hamster DHFR gene, *Carcinogenesis,* 13, 1975, 1992.

59. Cutler, R. G., Dysdifferentiation hypothesis of aging: a review, in *Molecular Biology of Aging: Gene Stability and Gene Expression,* Sohal, R. S., Birnbaum, L. S. and Cutler, R. G., Eds., Raven Press, New York, 1985, 307.

60. Ross, J., The turnover of messenger RNA, *Sci. Amer.,* 260, 48, 1989.

61. Kator, K., Cristofalo, V., Charpentier, R. and Cutler, R. G., Dysdifferentiative nature of aging: passage number dependency of globin gene expression in normal human diploid cells grown in tissue culture, *Gerontology,* 31, 355, 1985.

62. Sato, A. I., Schneider, E. L. and Danner, D. B., Aberrant gene expression and aging: examination of tissue-specific mRNAs in young and old rats, *Mech. Ageing Dev.,* 54, 1, 1990.

63. Ono, T., Dean, R. G., Chattopadhyay, S. K. and Cutler, R. G., Dysdifferentiative nature of aging: age-dependent expression of MuLV and globin genes in thymus, liver, and brain in the AKR mouse strain, *Gerontolology,* 31, 362, 1985.

64. Ono, T., Shinya, K., Uehara, Y. and Okada, S., Endogenous virus genomes become hypomethylated tissue-specifically during aging process of C57BL mice, *Mech. Ageing Dev.,* 50, 27, 1989.

65. Richardson, A., Rutherford, M. S., Birchenall-Sparks, M. C., Roberts, M. S., Wu, W. T. and Cheung, H. T., Levels of specific messenger RNA species as a function of age, in *Molecular Biology of Aging: Gene Stability and Gene Expression,* Sohal, R. S, Birnbaum, L. S. and Cutler, R. G., Eds., Raven Press, New York, 1985, 229.

66. Frankfurt, O. S., Detection of DNA damage in individual cells by flow cytometric analysis using anti-DNA monoclonal antibodies, *Exp. Cell Res.,* 170, 369, 1987.

67. Singh, N. P., McCoy, M. T., Tice, R. R. and Schneider, E. L., A simple technique for quantitation of low levels of DNA damage in individual cells, *Exp. Cell Res.,* 175, 184, 1988.

68. Uitterlinden, A. G., Slagboom, P. E., Knook, D. L. and Vijg, J., Two-dimensional DNA fingerprinting of human individuals, *Proc. Natl. Acad. Sci. U.S.A.,* 86, 2742, 1989.

69. Chaturvedi, M. M. and Kanungo, M. S., Analysis of conformation and function of the chromatin of the brain of young and old rats, *Mol. Biol. Rep.,* 10, 215, 1985.

70. Dell'Orco, R. T., Whittle, W. L. and Macieira-Coelho, A., Changes in the higher order organization of DNA during aging of human fibroblast-like cells, *Mech. Ageing Dev.,* 35, 199, 1986.

71. Medvedev, Z. A., Age changes of chromatin. A review, *Mech. Ageing Dev.,* 28, 139, 1984.

72. Thakur, M. K., Age-related changes in the structure and function of chromatin: a review, *Mech. Ageing Dev.,* 27, 263, 1984.

73. Macieira-Coelho, A., Genome organization through division: implications for aging of the mammalian organism, *Exp. Gerontol.,* 27, 369, 1992.

74. Martin, G. M., Fry, M. and Loeb, L. A., Somatic mutation and aging in mammalian cells, in *Molecular Biology of Aging: Gene Stability and Gene Expression,* Sohal, R. S., Birnbaum, L. S. and Cutler, R. G., Eds., Raven Press, New York, 1985, 7.

75. Medvedev, Z. A. and Medvedeva, M. N., Malignant polyploidization as a growth factor in the age-related spontaneous mouse hepatocarcinomas, *IRCS Med. Sci.,* 13, 699, 1985.

76. Medvedev, Z. A., DNA-information and aging: the balance between alteration and repair, in *Gerontology, 4th International Symposium: Present State and Research Perspectives in the Experimental and Clinical Gerontology,* Platt, D., Ed., Springer-Verlag, Berlin, 1989, 3.

77. Martin, G. M., Biological mechanisms of ageing, in *Oxford Textbook of Geriatric Medicine,* Evans, J. G. and Williams, T. F., Eds., Oxford University Press, Oxford, 1992, 41.

78. Wareham, K. A., Lyon, M. F., Glenister, P. H. and Williams, E. D., Age-related reactivation of an X-linked gene, *Nature,* 327, 725, 1987.

79. Migeon, B. R., Axelman, J. and Beggs, A. H., Effect of ageing on reactivation of the human X-linked HPRT locus, *Nature,* 335, 93, 1988.

80. Green, L., Whittle, W., Dell'Orco, R., Stein, G. and Stein, J., Histone gene stability during cellular senescence, *Mech. Ageing Dev.,* 36, 211, 1986.

81. Ono, T., Okada, S., Kawakami, T., Honjo, T. and Getz, M. J., Absence of gross change in primary DNA sequence during aging process of mice, *Mech. Ageing Dev.,* 32, 227, 1985.

82. Icard-Liepkalns, C., Doly, J. and Macieira-Coelho, A., Gene reorganization during serial divisions of normal human cells, *Biochem. Biophys. Res. Commun.*, 141, 112, 1986.

83. Burke, E. M. and Danner, D. B., Changes in fibronectin mRNA splicing with in vitro passage, *Biochem. Biophys. Res. Commun.*, 178, 620, 1991.

84. Singh, S. and Kanungo, M. S., Changes in expression and CRE binding proteins of the fibronectin gene during aging of the rat, *Biochem. Biophys. Res. Commun.*, 193, 440, 1993.

85. Medvedev, Z. A., Age-related changes of transcription and RNA processing, in *Drugs and Aging*, Platt, D., Ed., Springer-Verlag, Berlin, 1986, 1.

86. Adam, G., Simm, A. and Braun, F., Level of ribosomal RNA required for stimulation from quiescence increases during cellular aging in vitro of mammalian fibroblasts, *Exp. Cell Res.*, 169, 345, 1987.

87. Strehler, B. L., Hirsch, G., Gusseck, D., Johnson, R. and Bick, M., Codon restriction theory of ageing and development, *J. Theor. Biol.*, 33, 429, 1971.

88. Strehler, B. L., Ageing: concepts and theories, in *Lectures on Gerontology*, Viidik, A., Ed., Academic Press, London, 1982, 1.

89. Mays-Hoopes, L. L., Cleland, G., Bochantin, J., Kalunian, D., Miller, J., Wilson, W., Wong, M. K., Johnson, D. and Sharma, O. K., Function and fidelity of aging tRNA: in vivo acylation, analog discrimination, synthetase binding and in vitro translation, *Mech. Ageing Dev.*, 22, 135, 1983.

90. Vinayak, M., A comparison of tRNA populations of rat liver and skeletal muscle during aging, *Biochem. Int.*, 15, 279, 1987.

91. Neumeister, J. A. and Webster, G. C., Changes in the levels and the rate of synthesis of transfer RNA in tissues of mice of different ages, *Mech. Ageing Dev.*, 16, 319, 1981.

92. Mays-Hoopes, L. L., Macromolecular methylation during aging, *Rev. Biol. Res. Aging*, 2, 361, 1985.

93. Webster, G. C. and Webster, S. L., Aminoacylation of tRNA by cell-free preparations from aging *Drosophila melanogaster*, *Exp. Gerontol.*, 16, 487, 1981.

94. Webster, G. C., Protein synthesis in aging organisms., in *Molecular Biology of Aging: Gene Stability and Gene Expression*, Sohal, R. S., Birnbaum, L. S. and Cutler, R. G., Eds., Raven Press, New York, 1985, 263.

95. Takahashi, R., Mori, N. and Goto, S., Alteration of aminoacyl tRNA synthetases with age: accumulation of heat-labile enzyme molecules in rat liver, kidney and brain, *Mech. Ageing Dev.*, 33, 67, 1985.

96. Rattan, S. I. S., Regulation of protein synthesis during ageing, *Eur. J. Gerontol.*, 1, 128, 1992.

97. Johansen, L. B. and Rattan, S. I. S., Protein synthesis and aging, *Rev. Clin. Gerontol.*, 3, 3, 1993.

98. Bernd, A., Batke, E., Zahn, R. K. and Müller, W. E., Age-dependent gene induction in quail oviduct. XV. Alterations of the poly(A)-associated protein pattern and of the poly(A) chain length of mRNA, *Mech. Ageing Dev.*, 19, 361, 1982.

99. Birchenall-Sparks, M. C., Roberts, M. S., Rutherford, M. S. and Richardson, A., The effect of aging on the structure and function of liver messenger RNA, *Mech. Ageing Dev.*, 32, 99, 1985.

100. Kristal, B. S., Conrad, C. C., Richardson, A. and Yu, B. P., Is poly(A) tail length altered by aging or dietary restriction?, *Gerontol.*, 39, 152, 1993.

101. Makrides, S. C., Protein synthesis and degradation during aging and senescence, *Biol. Rev. Cambridge Philosophical Soc.*, 58, 343, 1983.

102. Rattan, S. I. S., Protein synthesis and the components of protein synthetic machinery, *Mutat. Res.*, 256, 115, 1991.

103. Ward, W. and Richardson, A., Effect of age on liver protein synthesis and degradation, *Hepatol.*, 14, 935, 1991.

104. Nygård, O. and Nilsson, L., Translational dynamics. Interactions between the translational factors, tRNA and ribosomes during eukaryotic protein synthesis, *Eur. J. Biochem.*, 191, 1, 1990.

105. Hershey, J. W., Translational control in mammalian cells, *Annu. Rev. Biochem.*, 60, 717, 1991.

106. Richardson, A. and Semsei, I., Effect of aging on translation and transcription, *Rev. Biol. Res. Aging*, 3, 467, 1987.

107. Khasigov, P. Z. and Nikolaev, A. Ya., Age-related changes in the rates of polypeptide chain elongation, *Biochem. Int.*, 15, 1171, 1987.

108. Merry, B. J. and Holehan, A. M., Effect of age and restricted feeding on polypeptide chain assembly kinetics in liver protein synthesis in vivo, *Mech. Ageing Dev.*, 58, 139, 1991.

109. Vargas, R. and Castaneda, M., Age-dependent decrease in the activity of protein-synthesis initiation factors in rat brain, *Mech. Ageing Dev.*, 21, 183, 1983.

110. Vargas, R. and Castaneda, M., Heterogeneity of protein-synthesis initiation factors in developing and aging rat brain, *Mech. Ageing Dev.*, 26, 371, 1984.

111. Cales, C., Fando, J. L., Azuara, C. and Salinas, M., Developmental studies of the first step of the initiation of brain protein synthesis, role for initiation factor 2, *Mech. Ageing Dev.*, 33, 147, 1986.

112. Castaneda, M., Vargas, R. and Galvan, S. C., Stagewise decline in the activity of brain protein synthesis factors and relationship between this decline and longevity in two rodent species, *Mech. Ageing Dev.*, 36, 197, 1986.

113. Kimball, S. R., Vary, T. C. and Jefferson, L. S., Age-dependent decrease in the amount of eukaryotic initiation factor 2 in various rat tissues, *Biochem. J.,* 286, 263, 1992.

114. Webster, G. C., Webster, S. L. and Landis, W. A., The effect of age on the initiation of protein synthesis in *Drosophila melanogaster, Mech. Ageing Dev.,* 16, 71, 1981.

115. Webster, G. C. and Webster, S. L., Specific disappearance of translatable messenger RNA for elongation factor one in aging *Drosophila melanogaster, Mech. Ageing Dev.,* 24, 335, 1984.

116. Webster, G. C., Effect of aging on the components of the protein synthesis system, in *Insect Aging,* Collatz, K. G. and Sohal, R. S., Eds., Springer-Verlag, Berlin, 1986, 207.

117. Cavallius, J., Rattan, S. I. S. and Clark, B. F., Changes in activity and amount of active elongation factor 1 α in aging and immortal human fibroblast cultures, *Exp. Gerontol.,* 21, 149, 1986.

118. Cavallius, J., Rattan, S. I. S. and Clark, B. F., A decrease in levels of mRNA for elongation factor 1 α accompanies the decline in its activity and the amounts of active enzyme in rat livers during ageing, *Topics Aging Res. Eur.,* 13, 125, 1989.

119. Rattan, S. I. S., Cavallius, J., Hartvigsen, G. and Clark, B. F. C., Amounts of active elongation factor 1 α and its activity in livers of mice during ageing, *Trends in Aging Research/Colloque INSERM,* 147, 135, 1986.

120. Rattan, S. I. S., Cavallius, J., Bhatia, P. and Clark, B. F. C., Protein elongation factor 1 α in ageing rodent brain, in *Aging — A Multifactorial Discussion,* Subba Rao, K. and Prabhakar, V., Eds., Association of Gerontology Publishers, India, 1987, 125.

121. Giordano, T., Kleinsek, D. and Foster, D. N., Increase in abundance of a transcript hybridizing to elongation factor 1 α during cellular senescence and quiescence, *Exp. Gerontol.,* 24, 501, 1989.

122. Riis, B., Rattan, S. I. S., Clark, B. F. C. and Merrick, W. C., Eukaryotic protein elongation factors, *Trends Biochem. Sci.,* 15, 420, 1990.

123. Nairn, A. C. and Palfrey, H. C., Identification of the major Mr 100,000 substrate for calmodulin-dependent protein kinase III in mammalian cells as elongation factor-2, *J. Biol. Chem.,* 262, 17299, 1987.

124. Carlberg, U., Nilsson, A., Skog, S., Palmquist, K. and Nygård, O., Increased activity of the eEF-2 specific, Ca2+ and calmodulin dependent protein kinase III during the S-phase in Ehrlich ascites cells, *Biochem. Biophys. Res. Commun.,* 180, 1372, 1991.

125. Celis, J. E., Madsen, P. and Ryazanov, A. G., Increased phosphorylation of elongation factor 2 during mitosis in transformed human amnion cells correlates with a decreased rate of protein synthesis, *Proc. Natl. Acad. Sci. U.S.A.,* 87, 4231, 1990.

126. Riis, B., Rattan, S. I. S., Cavallius, J. and Clark, B. F. C., ADP-ribosylatable content of elongation factor-2 changes during cell cycle of normal and cancerous human cells, *Biochem. Biophys. Res. Commun.,* 159, 1141, 1989.

127. Riis, B., Rattan, S. I. S., Derventzi, A. and Clark, B. F. C., Reduced levels of ADP-ribosylatable elongation factor-2 in aged and SV40-transformed human cell cultures, *FEBS Lett.,* 266, 45, 1990.

128. Riis, B., Rattan, S. I. S., Cavallius, J. and Clark, B. F. C., Levels of active elongation factor-2 in rat livers during ageing, *Topics Aging Res. Eur.,* 13, 117, 1989.

129. Takahashi, R., Mori, N. and Goto, S., Accumulation of heat-labile elongation factor 2 in the liver of mice and rats, *Exp. Gerontol.,* 20, 325, 1985.

130. Alix, J. H. and Hayes, D., Why are macromolecules modified postsynthetically?, *Biol. Cell.,* 47, 139, 1983.

131. Gafni, A., Age-related effects in enzyme metabolism and catalysis, *Rev. Biol. Res. Aging,* 4, 315, 1990.

132. Rothstein, M., The alteration of enzymes in aging animals, in *Molecular Biology of Aging,* Woodhead, A. D., Blackett, A. D. and Hollaender, A., Eds., Plenum Press, New York, 1985, 193.

133. Rothstein, M., Evidence for and against the error catastrophe hypothesis, in *Modern Biological Theories of Aging,* Warner, H. R., Butler, R. L., Sprott, R. L. and Schneider, E. L., Eds., Raven Press, New York, 1987, 139.

134. Zuniga, A. and Gafni, A., Age-related modifications in rat cardiac phosphoglycerate kinase. Rejuvenation of the old enzyme by unfolding-refolding, *Biochim. Biophys. Acta,* 955, 50, 1988.

135. Stadtman, E. R., Covalent modification reactions are marking steps in protein turnover, *Biochem.,* 29, 6323, 1990.

136. Oliver, C. N., Ahn, B. W., Moerman, E. J., Goldstein, S. and Stadtman, E. R., Age-related changes in oxidized proteins, *J. Biol. Chem.,* 262, 5488, 1987.

137. Carney, J. M., Starke-Reed, P. E., Oliver, C. N., Landum, R. W., Cheng, M. S., Wu, J. F. and Floyd, R. A., Reversal of age-related increase in brain protein oxidation, decrease in enzyme activity, and loss in temporal and spatial memory by chronic administration of the spin-trapping compound N-tert-butyl-α-phenylnitrone, *Proc. Natl. Acad. Sci. U.S.A.,* 88, 3633, 1991.

138. Sohal, R. S., Agarwal, S., Dubey, A. and Orr, W. C., Protein oxidative damage is associated with life expectancy of houseflies, *Proc. Natl. Acad. Sci. U.S.A.,* 90, 7255, 1993.

139. Stadtman, E. R., Biochemical markers of aging, *Exp. Gerontol.,* 23, 327, 1988.

140. Stadtman, E. R., Protein oxidation and aging, *Science,* 257, 1220, 1992.

141. Harding, J. J., Beswick, H. T., Ajiboye, R., Huby, R., Blakytny, R. and Rixon, K. C., Non-enzymic post-translational modification of proteins in aging: A review, *Mech. Ageing Dev.,* 50, 7, 1989.

142. Lee, A. T. and Cerami, A., Role of glycation in aging, *Ann. N.Y. Acad. Sci.,* 663, 63, 1992.

143. Rattan, S. I. S., Derventzi, A. and Clark, B. F. C., Protein synthesis, post-translational modifications, and aging, *Ann. N.Y. Acad. Sci.,* 663, 48, 1992.

144. Shigeoka, H. and Yang, H. C., Early kinase C dependent events in aging human diploid fibroblasts, *Mech. Ageing Dev.,* 55, 49, 1990.

145. Riis, B., Rattan, S. I. S., Palmquist, K., Nilsson, A., Nygard, O. and Clark, B. F. C., Elongation factor 2-specific calcium and calmodulin dependent protein kinase III activity in rat livers varies with age and calorie restriction, *Biochem. Biophys. Res. Commun.,* 192, 1210, 1993.

146. Gerhard, G. S., Phillips, P. D. and Cristofalo, V. J., EGF- and PDGF-stimulated phosphorylation in young and senescent WI-38 cells, *Exp. Cell Res.,* 193, 87, 1991.

147. Whiteheart, S. W., Shenbagamurthi, P., Chen, L., Cotter, R. J. and Hart, G. W., Murine elongation factor 1 alpha (EF-1α) is posttranslationally modified by novel amide-linked ethanolamine-phosphoglycerol moieties. Addition of ethanolamine-phosphoglycerol to specific glutamic acid residues on EF-1α, *J. Biol. Chem.,* 264, 14334, 1989.

148. McFadden, P. N. and Clarke, S., Protein carboxyl methyltransferase and methyl acceptor proteins in aging and cataractous tissue of the human eye lens, *Mech. Ageing Dev.,* 34, 91, 1986.

149. Sellinger, O. Z., Kramer, C. M., Conger, A. and Duboff, G. S., The carboxylmethylation of cerebral membrane-bound proteins increases with age, *Mech. Ageing Dev.,* 43, 161, 1988.

150. Rosenberger, R. F., Senescence and the accumulation of abnormal proteins, *Mutat. Res.,* 256, 255, 1991.

151. Rogers, S., Wells, R. and Rechsteiner, M., Amino acid sequences common to rapidly degraded proteins: the PEST hypothesis, *Science,* 234, 364, 1986.

152. Bachmair, A., Finley, D. and Varshavsky, A., In vivo half-life of a protein is a function of its amino-terminal residue, *Science,* 234, 179, 1986.

153. Gracy, R. W., Yüksel, K. Ü., Chapman, M. L., Cini, J. K., Jahani, M., Lu, H. S., Oray, B. and Talent, J. M., Impaired degradation may account for the accumulation of abnormal proteins in aging cells, in *Modification of Proteins During Aging,* Proc. Mini-Symposium Session "Impact of Aging on Biochemical Function," the 75th Annual Meeting Am. Soc. Biol. Chem., Adelman, R. C. and Dekker, E. E., Eds., Alan R. Liss, New York, 1985, 1.

154. Dice, J. F., Altered intracellular protein degradation in aging: a possible cause of proliferative arrest, *Exp. Gerontol.,* 24, 451, 1989.

155. Bergamini, E., Protein degradation and modification. Introduction and overview, *Ann. N.Y. Acad. Sci.,* 663, 43, 1992.

156. Ishigami, A. and Goto, S., Inactivation kinetics of horseradish peroxidase microinjected into hepatocytes from mice of various ages, *Mech. Ageing Dev.,* 46, 125, 1988.

157. Ishigami, A. and Goto, S., Age-related change in the degradation rate of ovalbumin microinjected into mouse liver parenchymal cells, *Arch. Biochem. Biophys.,* 277, 189, 1990.

158. Pan, J. X., Short, S. R., Goff, S. A. and Dice, J. F., Ubiquitin pools, ubiquitin mRNA levels, and ubiquitin-mediated proteolysis in aging human fibroblasts, *Exp. Gerontol.,* 28, 39, 1993.

159. Rattan, S. I. S. and Derventzi, A., Altered cellular responsiveness during ageing, *BioEssays,* 13, 601, 1991.

160. Cristofalo, V. J., Phillips, P. D., Sorger, T. and Gerhard, G., Alterations in the responsiveness of senescent cells to growth factors, *J. Gerontol.,* 44, B55, 1989.

161. Cristofalo, V. J., Pignolo, R. J. and Rotenberg, M. O., Molecular changes with in vitro cellular senescence, *Ann. N.Y. Acad. Sci.,* 663, 187, 1992.

162. Derventzi, A. and Rattan, S. I. S., Homeostatic imbalance during cellular ageing: altered responsiveness, *Mutat. Res.,* 256, 191, 1991.

163. De Tata, V., Ptasznik, A. and Cristofalo, V. J., Effect of tumor promoter phorbol 12-myristate 13-acetate (PMA) on proliferation of young and senescent WI-38 human diploid fibroblasts, *Exp. Cell Res.,* 205, 261, 1993.

164. Sell, C., Ptasznik, A., Chang, C. D., Swantek, J., Cristofalo, V. J. and Baserga, R., IGF-1 receptor levels and the proliferation of young and senescent human fibroblasts, *Biochem. Biophys. Res. Commun.,* 194, 259, 1993.

165. Roth, G. S., Receptors and post-receptor mechanisms in aging, *Trends Biomed. Gerontol.,* 1, 23, 1988.

166. Brooks-Frederich, K. M., Cianciarulo, F. L., Rittling, S. R. and Cristofalo, V. J., Cell cycle-dependent regulation of Ca2+ in young and senescent WI-38 cells, *Exp. Cell Res.,* 205, 412, 1993.

167. Takahashi, Y., Yoshida, T. and Takashima, S., The regulation of intracellular calcium ion and pH in young and old fibroblast cells (WI-38), *J. Gerontol.,* 47, B65, 1992.

168. Beit-Or, A., Nevo, Z., Kalina, M. and Eilam, Y., Decrease in the basal levels of cytosolic free calcium in chondrocytes during aging in culture: possible role as differentiation signal, *J. Cell. Physiol.,* 144, 197, 1990.

169. Hunter, T., A thousand and one protein kinases, *Cell,* 50, 823, 1987.

170. Blumenthal, E. J. and Malkinson, A. M., Age-dependent changes in murine protein kinase and protease enzymes, *Mech. Ageing Dev.,* 46, 201, 1988.

171. Rittling, S. R., Brooks, K. M., Cristofalo, V. J. and Baserga, R., Expression of cell cycle-dependent genes in young and senescent WI-38 fibroblasts, *Proc. Natl. Acad. Sci. U.S.A.,* 83, 3316, 1986.

172. Paulsson, Y., Bywater, M., Pfeifer-Ohlsson, R., Nilsson, S., Heldin, C. H., Westermark, B. and Betsholtz, C., Growth factors induce early pre-replicative changes in senescent human fibroblasts, *EMBO J.,* 5, 2157, 1986.

173. Kill, I. R. and Shall, S., Senescent human diploid fibroblasts are able to support DNA synthesis and to express markers associated with proliferation, *J. Cell Sci.,* 97, 473, 1990.

174. Seshadri, T. and Campisi, J., Repression of c-fos transcription and an altered genetic program in senescent human fibroblasts, *Science,* 247, 205, 1990.

175. Derventzi, A., Rattan, S. I. S. and Clark, B. F. C., Senescent human fibroblasts are more sensitive to the effects of a phorbol ester on macromolecular synthesis and growth characteristics, *Biochem. Int.,* 27, 903, 1992.

176. Derventzi, A., Rattan, S. I. S. and Clark, B. F. C., Phorbol ester PMA stimulates protein synthesis and increases the levels of active elongation factors EF-1 α and EF-2 in ageing human fibroblasts, *Mech. Ageing Dev.,* 69, 193, 1993.

177. Finch, C. E., Neural and endocrine determinants of senescence: investigation of casuality and reversibility by laboratory and clinical interventions, in *Modern Biological Theories of Aging,* Warner, H. R., Butler, R. N., Sprott, R. L. and Schneider, E. L., Eds., Raven Press, New York, 1987, 261.

178. Halter, J. B., Endocrine markers of aging, *Exp. Gerontol.,* 23, 377, 1988.

179. Insel, P. A., Adrenergic receptors, G proteins, and cell regulation: implications for aging research, *Exp. Gerontol.,* 28, 341, 1993.

180. Weksler, M. E. and Siskind, G. W., The cellular basis of immune senescence, *Monogr. Devel. Biol.,* 17, 110, 1984.

181. Zs-Nagy, I., Derecskei, B. and Lustyik, G., Age-dependent changes in the colloid osmotic pressure of rat brain and liver, *Trends Biomed. Gerontol.,* 1, 189, 1988.

182. Kay, M. M. B., Aging of cell membrane molecules leads to appearance of an aging antigen and removal of senescent cells, *Gerontology,* 31, 215, 1985.

183. Naeim, F. and Walford, R. L., Aging and cell membrane complexes: the lipid bilayer, integral proteins, and cytoskeleton, in *Handbook of the Biology of Aging,* Finch, C. E. and Schneider, E. L., Eds., Van Nostrand, New York, 1985, 272.

184. Yamamoto, K. and Yamamoto, M., Changes in cell surface of human diploid fibroblasts during cellular aging, *Mutat. Res.,* 256, 169, 1991.

185. Mann, P. L., Busse, S. C., Griffey, R. H. and Tellez, C. M., Cell surface oligosaccharide modulation during differentiation. V. Partial characterization of the regulated surface during substrate adhesion and spreading, *Mech. Ageing Dev.,* 62, 47, 1992.

186. Xie, H. Q., Huang, R. and Hu, V. W., Intercellular communication through gap junctions is reduced in senescent cells, *Biophys. J.,* 62, 45, 1992.

187. Bourne, H. R., Sanders, D. A. and McCormick, F., The GTPase superfamily: a conserved switch for diverse cell functions, *Nature,* 348, 125, 1991.

188. Ahmad, S. N., Alam, S. Q. and Alam, B. S., Effect of ageing on adenylate cyclase activity and G-proteins in rat submandibular salivary glands, *Arch. Oral Biol.,* 35, 885, 1990.

189. Namba, M., Karai, M. and Kimoto, T., Comparison of major cytoskeletons among normal human fibroblasts, immortal human fibroblasts transformed by exposure to Co-60 gamma rays, and the latter cells made tumorigenic by treatment with Harvey murine sarcoma virus, *Exp. Gerontol.,* 22, 179, 1987.

190. Raes, M., Involvement of microtubules in modifications associated with cellular aging, *Mutat. Res.,* 256, 149, 1991.

191. Rao, K. M. and Cohen, H. J., Actin cytoskeletal network in aging and cancer, *Mutat. Res.,* 256, 139, 1991.

192. Zamansky, G. B. and Chou, I. N., Environmental wavelengths of ultraviolet light induce cytoskeletal damage, *J. Invest. Dermatol.,* 89, 603, 1987.

193. Crawford, F. and Goate, A., Alzheimer's disease untangled, *BioEssays,* 14, 727, 1992.

194. Macieira-Coelho, A., Contributions made by the studies of cells in vitro for understanding of the mechanisms of aging, [Editorial], *Exp. Gerontol.,* 28, 1, 1993.

195. Hayflick, L., The limited in vitro lifetime of human diploid cell strains, *Exp. Cell Res.,* 37, 614, 1965.

196. Hayflick, L., Aging under glass, *Mutat. Res.,* 256, 69, 1991.

197. Stanulis-Praeger, B. M., Cellular senescence revisited: a review, *Mech. Ageing Dev.,* 38, 1, 1987.

198. Hayflick, L., Aging, longevity, and immortality in vitro, *Exp. Gerontol.,* 27, 363, 1992.

199. Macieira-Coelho, A., *Biology of Normal Proliferating Cells In Vitro. Relevance For In Vivo Aging,* Karger, Basel, 1988.

200. Smith, J. R., Inhibitors of DNA synthesis derived from senescent human diploid fibroblasts, *Exp. Gerontol.*, 27, 409, 1992.

201. Sager, R., Tumor suppressor genes: the puzzle and the promise, *Science*, 246, 1406, 1989.

202. Marshall, C. J., Tumor suppressor genes, *Cell*, 64, 313, 1991.

203. Sugawara, O., Oshimura, M., Koi, M., Annab, L. A. and Barrett, J. C., Induction of cellular senescence in immortalized cells by human chromosome 1, *Science*, 247, 707, 1990.

204. Ning, Y., Weber, J. L., Killary, A. M., Ledbetter, D. H., Smith, J. R. and Pereira-Smith, O. M., Genetic analyis of indefinite division in human cells: evidence for a cell senescence-related gene(s) on human chromosome 4, *Proc. Natl. Acad. Sci. U.S.A.*, 88, 5635, 1991.

205. Ning, Y., Shay, J. W., Lovell, M., Taylor, L., Ledbetter, D. H. and Pereira-Smith, O. M., Tumor suppression by chromosome 11 is not due to cellular senescence, *Exp. Cell Res.*, 192, 220, 1991.

206. Wadhwa, R., Kaul, S. C., Ikawa, Y. and Sugimoto, Y., Identification of a novel member of mouse hsp70 family. Its association with cellular mortal phenotype, *J. Biol. Chem.*, 268, 6615, 1993.

207. Wadhwa, R., Kaul, S. C., Mitsui, Y. and Sugimoto, Y., Differential subcellular distribution of mortalin in mortal and immortal mouse and human fibroblasts, *Exp. Cell Res.*, 207, 442, 1993.

208. Nuell, M. J., McClung, J. K., Smith, J. R. and Danner, D. B., Approach to the isolation of antiproliferative genes, *Exp. Gerontol.*, 24, 469, 1989.

209. Murano, S., Thweatt, R., Shmookler-Reis, R. J., Jones, R. A., Moerman, E. J. and Goldstein, S., Diverse gene sequences are overexpressed in Werner syndrome fibroblasts undergoing premature replicative senescence, *Mol. Cell. Biol.*, 11, 3905, 1991.

210. Moerman, E. J., Thweatt, R., Moerman, A. M., Jones, R. A. and Goldstein, S., Insulin-like growth factor binding protein-3 is overexpressed in senescent and quiescent human fibroblasts, *Exp. Gerontol.*, 28, 361, 1993.

211. DiPaolo, B. R., Pignolo, R. J. and Cristofalo, V. J., Overexpression of the two-chain form of cathepsin B in senescent WI-38 cells, *Exp. Cell Res.*, 201, 500, 1992.

212. Pignolo, R. J., Cristofalo, V. J. and Rotenberg, M. O., Senescent WI-38 cells fail to express EPC-1, a gene induced in young cells upon entry into the Go state, *J. Biol. Chem.*, 268, 8949, 1993.

213. Doggett, D. L., Rotenberg, M. O., Pignolo, R. J., Phillips, P. D. and Cristofalo, V. J., Differential gene expression between young and senescent, quiescent WI-38 cells, *Mech. Ageing Dev.*, 65, 239, 1992.

214. Wang, E., Statin, a nonproliferation-specific protein, is associated with the nuclear envelope and is heterogeneously distributed in cells leaving quiescent state, *J. Cell. Physiol.*, 140, 418, 1989.

215. Wang, E. and Tomaszewski, G., Granular presence of terminin is the marker to distinguish between the senescent and quiescent states, *J. Cell. Physiol.*, 147, 514, 1991.

216. McClung, J. K., King, R. L., Walker, L. S., Danner, D. B., Nuell, M. J., Stewart, C. A. and Dell'Orco, R. T., Expression of prohibitin, an antiproliferative protein, *Exp. Gerontol.*, 27, 413, 1992.

217. Spiering, A. L., Smith, J. R. and Pereira-Smith, O. M., A potent DNA synthesis inhibitor expressed by the immortal cell line SUSM-1, *Exp. Cell Res.*, 179, 159, 1988.

218. Macieira-Coelho, A. and Söderberg, A., Growth inhibitory activity in extracts from human fibroblasts, *J. Cell. Physiol.*, 154, 92, 1993.

219. Wistrom, C. and Villeponteau, B., Cloning and expression of SAG: a novel marker of cellular senescence, *Exp. Cell Res.*, 199, 355, 1992.

220. Thweatt, R., Murano, S., Fleischmann, R. D. and Goldstein, S., Isolation and characterization of gene sequences overexpressed in Werner syndrome fibroblasts during premature replicative senescence, *Exp. Gerontol.*, 27, 433, 1992.

221. Harley, C. B., Telomere loss: mitotic clock or genetic time bomb?, *Mutat. Res.*, 256, 271, 1991.

222. Harley, C. B., Futcher, A. B. and Greider, C. W., Telomeres shorten during ageing of human fibroblasts, *Nature*, 345, 458, 1990.

223. Hastie, N. D., Dempster, M., Dunlop, M. G., Thompson, A. M., Green, D. K. and Allshire, R. C., Telomere reduction in human colorectal carcinoma and with ageing, *Nature*, 346, 866, 1990.

224. Lindsey, J., McGill, N. I., Lindsey, L. A., Green, D. K. and Cooke, H. J., In vivo loss of telomeric repeats with age in humans, *Mutat. Res.*, 256, 45, 1991.

225. Vaziri, H., Schachter, F., Uchida, I., Wei, L., Zhu, X., Effros, R., Cohen, D. and Harley, C. B., Loss of telomeric DNA during aging of normal and trisomy 21 human lymphocytes, *Am. J. Hum. Genet.*, 52, 661, 1993.

226. Allsopp, R. C., Vaziri, H., Patterson, C., Goldstein, S., Younglai, E. V., Futcher, A. B., Greider, C. W. and Harley, C. B., Telomere length predicts replicative capacity of human fibroblasts, *Proc. Natl. Acad. Sci. U.S.A.*, 89, 10114, 1992.

227. de Lange, T., Shiue, L., Myers, R., Cox, D. R., Naylor, S. L., Killery, A. M. and Varmus, H. E., Structure and variability of human chromosome ends, *Mol. Cell Biol.*, 10, 518, 1990.

228. Counter, C. M., Avilion, A. A., LeFeuvre, C. E., Stewart, N. G., Greider, C. W., Harley, C. B. and Bacchetti, S., Telomere shortening associated with chromosome instability is arrested in immortal cells which express telomerase activity, *EMBO J.*, 11, 1921, 1992.

229. Holliday, R., Food, reproduction and longevity: is the extended lifespan of calorie-restricted animals an evolutionary adaptation?, *BioEssays,* 10, 125, 1989.

230. Yu, B. P., Food restriction research: past and present status, *Rev. Biol. Res. Aging,* 4, 349, 1990.

231. Rattan, S. I. S., Finding differences in biochemistry: the case of ageing, *Trends Biotech.,* 6, 267, 1988.

232. Rattan, S. I. S. and Clark, B. F. C., Ageing: a challenge for biotechnology, *Trends Biotech.,* 6, 58, 1988.

233. Gavrilov, L. A. and Gavrilova, N. S., *The Biology of Life Span: A Quantitative Approach,* Harwood Academic, New York, 1991.

234. Carey, J. R., Liedo, P., Orozco, D. and Vaupel, J. W., Slowing of mortality rates at older ages in large medfly cohorts, *Science,* 258, 457, 1992.

235. Curtsinger, J. W., Fukui, H. H., Townsend, D. R. and Vaupel, J. W., Demography of genotypes: failure of the limited life-span paradigm in Drosophila melanogaster, *Science,* 258, 461, 1992.

236. Finch, C. E., *Longevity, Senescence, and the Genome,* University of Chicago Press, Chicago, 1990.

237. Rattan, S. I. S., Beyond the present crisis in gerontology, *BioEssays,* 2, 226, 1985.

238. Kirkwood, T. B. L., Biological origins of ageing, in *Oxford Textbook of Geriatric Medicine,* Evans, J. G. and Williams, T. F., Eds., Oxford University Press, Oxford, 1992, 35.

239. Kirkwood, T. B. L., Comparative life spans of species: why do species have the life spans they do?, *Am. J. Clin. Nutr.,* 55, 1191S, 1992.

240. Partridge, L. and Barton, N. H., Optimality, mutation and the evolution of ageing, *Nature,* 362, 305, 1993.

241. Rose, M. R. and Graves, J. L., Evolution of aging, *Rev. Biol. Res. Aging,* 4, 3, 1990.

242. Rattan, S. I. S., Ageing and disease: proteins as the molecular link, *Persp. Biol. Med.,* 34, 526, 1991.

243. Friedman, V., Wagner, J. and Danner, D. B., Isolation and identification of aging-related cDNAs in the mouse, *Mech. Ageing Dev.,* 52, 27, 1990.

244. Shepherd, J. C., Walldorf, U., Hug, P. and Gehring, W. J., Fruit flies with additional expression of the elongation factor EF-1 α live longer, *Proc. Natl. Acad. Sci. U.S.A.,* 86, 7520, 1989.

245. Johnson, T. E., Genetic specification of life span: processes, problems, and potentials, *J. Gerontol.,* 43, B87, 1988.

246. Friedman, D. B. and Johnson, T. E., Three mutants that extend both mean and maximum life span of the nematode, *Caenorhabditis elegans,* define the age-1 gene, *J. Gerontol.,* 43, B102, 1988.

247. Friedman, D. B. and Johnson, T. E., A mutation in the age-1 gene in *Caenorhabditis elegans* lengthens life and reduces hermaphrodite fertility, *Genetics,* 118, 75, 1988.

16

Effects of Hormones on Neural Tissue: *In Vivo* and *In Vitro* Studies

Antonia Vernadakis

CONTENTS

I. INTRODUCTION

For many years, it was believed that memory and cognitive decline of the aged was simply the result of attrition of nerve cells, which are estimated to be lost at the rate of 50,000 to 100,000 cells per day. However, although neuronal loss must play a role in memory and cognitive decline in the aging, it is now clear that this is not the complete explanation. The neuron is only one component of the complex circuitry of the brain. Another significant cellular component is the neuroglia, the satellite cells of the central nervous system (CNS). Additionally, connective tissue cells such as endothelial cells, fibroblasts, and mesenchymal cells constitute another circuitry. All these cell components — neurons, neuroglia, connective

0-8493-2446-7/95/$0.00+$.50
© 1995 by CRC Press Inc.

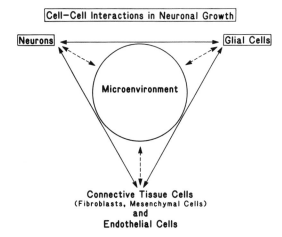

FIGURE 16-1   Schematic representation of cell-cell interactions in the central nervous system. (From Vernadakis, A. and Sakellaridis, N., *Progress in Neuroendocrinology,* Parvez, S., Parvez, H., and Gupta, G., Eds., VNU Science Press, The Netherlands, 1985. With permission.).

tissue — intercommunicate through their microenvironment and function as a unit (Figure 16-1). Age-related changes in any component of this cellular unit will shift the balance, interrupt intercellular relationships, and ultimately affect function.

Considerable evidence for our understanding of the influence of neuron-glia interactions in the maintenance of brain homeostasis has derived from neural culture systems, and the reader is referred to a recent review by this author.[1] The role of hormones, both as trophic factors and regulatory molecules in CNS function, has been the focus of numerous investigations.[2-4] However, the responsiveness of the CNS to hormones during aging awaits in-depth study. Again, *in vitro* models promise to provide basic information, both at the cellular and the molecular levels.

Because of the abundance of reviews of *in vivo* studies on CNS changes with aging,[5-7] this chapter will primarily focus on findings derived from *in vitro* studies with reference to *in vivo* findings when related. Emphasis will be placed on neurons and glial cells and their responsiveness to hormonal regulation in culture.

II. CENTRAL NERVOUS SYSTEM CHANGES WITH AGING: A BRIEF OVERVIEW

Changes in neurons, glial cells, synapse morphologic and electrophysiologic appearance and neurotransmission mechanisms during normal aging have been extensively reviewed by several authors in the last few years.[5-8] Thus, in this chapter only some key changes occurring with aging will be described to serve as reference points for discussions of *in vitro* findings.

Neuronal loss has been reported to occur in several species with normal aging, although only in discrete CNS structures.[9] In contrast, the number of glial cells increases with aging in most CNS areas. The increase in glial cells has received considerable attention and various speculations have been put forward for their functional role. More extensive discussion will be considered later in this chapter.

The neuronal loss observed in the aging brain cannot entirely account for the decline in brain function. There is now evidence that synaptic loss and decline in synaptic functions occur in the senescent brain and may play a role in the age-related decline in brain function.[5] However, despite the reported loss of dendritic spines with aging, evidence from Golgi studies reveals a potential for dendritic plasticity.[10-12] Several studies have attempted to explore the

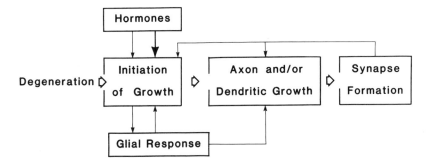

FIGURE 16-2   Model for reactive synaptogenesis. Partial denervation upsets normal trophic relationships between input and target neurons and induces a reactive growth response. The initiation of growth is dependent on trophic signals, hormones, and other growth-regulating factors. The glial cells prepare the neurophil for the growth of new synapses and may serve their own regulatory function. Once the growing fibers reach their targets, synapses rapidly form. As determined in the text, reactive synaptogenesis is slower in aged animals, presumably because of a less robust set of events in the initiation phase. Both hormonal and glial influences may act to suppress growth. (From Cotman, C. W. and Scheff, S. W., *Mech. Ageing Dev.,* 9, 103, 1979. With permission.)

possibility of compensation of neuronal loss by synapse growth in the aged brain. This process is referred to as "reactive synaptogenesis" or axon sprouting.[13-16] Of importance for this review is the proposal by Cotman and Scheff[16] that hormones and glial factors play an important role in "reactive synaptogenesis", as illustrated in Figure 16-2.

Associated with synaptic loss are changes in neurotransmitter function. Although decreases in levels of some neurotransmitters with aging have been reported, the changes are not consistent. Rather, it appears that with aging there is a neurotransmitter imbalance, with some neurotransmitters increasing (e.g., serotonin) and with others decreasing (e.g., norepinephrine and dopamine). Particular emphasis has been directed on changes in the cholinergic system and its implication in memory.[5]

In addition to neuronal loss and synapse decline, recent evidence has revealed that the function of remaining neurons may also be affected with aging, i.e., responsiveness to microenvironmental humoral stimuli and integration at the synapse. Electrophysiological studies have provided evidence for a decline in responsiveness of neurons to microenvironmental humoral stimuli, including neurotransmitters.[17-20] This decline in responsiveness can be partially attributed to the reported decrease in neurotransmitter receptors.[21-26] However, changes in membrane fluidity[27,28] and in second messenger intracellular mechanisms can also account for this decline.[29-31]

III. CHANGES IN HORMONE RECEPTORS IN THE CNS WITH AGING

In view of the extensive evidence (presented later in this chapter) that steroid and thyroid hormones are involved in neural growth, differentiation, and possibly aging, only studies on steroid and thyroid hormone receptors will be briefly reviewed here (see also Chapters 2 and 3), as they relate to hormonal *in vitro* findings discussed throughout this chapter.

A. Corticosteroid Receptors

The biological actions of corticosteroids are mediated by intracellular binding molecules, the corticosteroid receptors.[32-34] These receptors were initially identified by uptake and retention of radioactive steroids. In a study using neuron-enriched cultures from chick embryo cerebral hemispheres, ^{3}H-corticosteroid accumulation has been observed to be higher in cultures derived from 10-day-old chick embryos than from 6-day-old embryos.[35] In addition, after 30 days in culture, when almost all neuronal cells have disappeared and glial cells are the predominant cells, ^{3}H-corticosteroid accumulation is significantly higher than in the early neuronal-enriched cultures. These early studies implicated the presence of corticosteroid receptors both in neurons and in glial cells. The presence of a higher number of binding sites for the glucocorticoid type II receptor in astrocyte culture as compared with neuronal cultures has confirmed the early uptake studies.[36]

Two binding molecules for corticosteroids in the brain have been found: the mineralo-corticoid receptor, a high-affinity binding site with a preferential localization in the septo-hippocampal formation, and the glucocorticoid receptor, a lower affinity binding site with a widespread distribution in the brain,[37] (see Chapters 2 and 15). Both receptors have been recently reported to be present in rat hippocampal and neocortical brain cells in culture[38] and are very similar to those in tissue. The availability of highly specific synthetic steroids[39,40] has revealed the presence of at least two types of specific glucocorticoid receptors in the hippocampus.[37,41] The subpopulation referred to as type I has higher affinity for corticoste-rone than the type II subpopulation. It has been proposed that the type II receptor is the subtype that plays the important role in hippocampus contributions to negative feedback control of stress-induced ACTH release.[41]

The hippocampus of the rat progressively loses corticosterone receptors with age.[42,43] Some reports in the literature show that the depletion of corticosterone receptors in the aged hippocampus involves a loss of steroid-concentrating neurons.[44] However, recent studies measuring glucocorticoid receptor II and also mRNA levels in the hippocampus show a 40% decrease in binding capacity[45] and agree with the early findings.[46,47] In contrast, observations have been reported of both no change in the affinity[45] and an increased affinity of type II corticosteroid binding in aged rat hippocampus.[48] Moreover, in aged rats, type II corticoste-roid-binding receptors up-regulation occurs over a 10-day postadrenalectomy period.[49] These findings suggest an intrinsic deficit in corticosteroid binding receptor biosynthesis or lability that is independent of the acute endogenous adrenal steroid environment.[49] Of interest are observations of increased uptake of ^{3}H-thymidine in glial cells with age *in vivo,* reflecting the increase in glial cells with age.[50] In view of the fact that there is also a rise in basal corticosterone levels with age,[50-53] the role of glial cells becomes eminent in the response of the CNS to hormones with aging (see discussion later in this chapter). Type II glucocorticoid receptors are expressed in oligodendrocytes and astrocytes.[36,54]

B.　Thyroid Hormone Receptors

There is extensive research on thyroid hormone receptors in the CNS,[55-59] (see Chapter 5). The receptor density of triiodothyronine (T_3), the main form of thyroid hormone that regulates brain development, is high in the cerebral hemisphere of the newborn rats but declines to adult levels within the first two weeks of postnatal life. This age-related decline in the density of thyroid hormone nucleus receptors may underlie the well-known age-related decline in brain sensitivity to these hormones.[60] Studies at the molecular level have shown that protooncogene c-erbA and its analogues are genes which encode thyroid hormone receptors.[61] By hybridizing cDNA probes specific to various rat erbA-like transcripts with RNA extracted from develop-ing rat brain, changes in thyroid hormone receptor mRNA levels were found which correspond to changes in T_3-binding capacity in rat brain during postnatal development.[62]

Although most biochemical studies of thyroid hormone nuclear receptors suggest that the receptors in developing brain are similar to those in adult brain,[63] recent evidence in both humans[64] and in rats[61,65] indicates a genetic potential to produce at least two types of thyroid hormone nuclear receptors. Three thyroid hormone receptor genes are expressed in at least eight different human tissues including brain.[64] However, the significance of expression of multiple genes remains unclear.

IV. NEURAL CULTURE AS A MODEL

The methodology of neural tissue and cell culture has gained considerable importance during the last decade and has provided insights into cellular physiology as well as into factors in the "milieu interieur" regulating cell function. A brief description of the neural culture systems which will be discussed in this chapter will be presented here.[66-70]

Brain tissue explants maintained in organ and organotypic culture systems have been used to study biochemical, morphological, and electrophysiological changes induced by drug treatment. Harrison[71] pioneered the "hanging-drop" culture method for explants. Harrison placed fragments of embryonic tadpole tissue into a culture made with clotted lymph from adult frog. The cultures were viable for several weeks — long enough to observe the outgrowth of neuronal fibers from the bodies of individual cells. Murray and Stout in 1942[72] and in 1947[73] described the adaptation of the Maximow[74] double slip coverslip assembly for cultivating neural tissue. The characteristic advantage of this method over the organ culture is the longer time that the neural tissue can be maintained viable in culture.

Dissociated neural cell cultures obtained by disruption of immature central nervous system tissue using lytic enzymes or mechanical procedures have been used to address a variety of problems concerning the biochemical, physiological, and morphological organization of the central nervous system. Since dissociation procedures disrupt the original tissue organization and abolish the original cell-cell contacts, it is possible to examine cellular performance and characteristics that reflect inherent cell properties rather than those expressed by an organized tissue. Cells from different central nervous system regions and from a variety of species have been studied in culture since an attempt to dissociate and culture neural cells from chick embryo spinal cord was first reported.[75] Basically, two types of culture systems have been used to maintain dissociated neural cells for study: the aggregate culture system and the monolayer culture system.[75-77] Neuron-enriched and glia-enriched cultures can be obtained by using the appropriate animal age (fetal vs. postnatal) and plating substratum (e.g., plastic for glial cultures and polylysine-coated culture dishes for neuronal-enriched cultures).

The search for methods to obtain neurons and glial cells separately and in large quantities in order to do biochemical analyses has led investigators to use neoplastic tissue as a potential source of neuronal and glial elements. Most of the studies carried out thus far have involved principally two neoplastic sources: the mouse neuroblastoma C1300[78] and the C6 cell strain from a rat astrocytoma.[79]

Recently, several attempts have been made to culture adult CNS tissue. Culture and maintenance of sensory neurons prepared from 6-month-old and 12-month-old male CBA mice have been reported.[80] Cultures prepared from aged mice contain fewer neurons than those from adult mice. However, a higher neuronal number is retained in cultures receiving NGF (100 ng/ml) as compared to those not receiving NGF.

As will be discussed later in this chapter, glial cells derived from an aged mouse brain have been maintained in culture for several passages.[81,82]

A. Responsiveness of Neurons to Hormones

As discussed in other chapters in this book, it has been established that hormones regulate all systems including CNS function, both at the organismic and cellular levels (see Reference 83 for reviews).

The effects of steroid hormones on neural cells appear to be dependent on the brain area as the source of cells (i.e., cerebellum, spinal cord, hypothalamus, retina), age of the organism at the time of neural cell extirpation, and the culture system used. Both inhibitory and stimulatory hormonal effects have been found.[2] In cerebellar organ cultures from chick embryos, both cortisol and estradiol enhance cholinergic neuronal maturation as assessed by

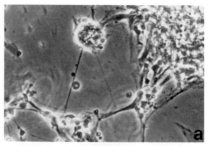
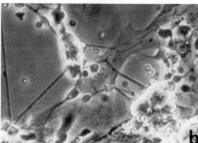
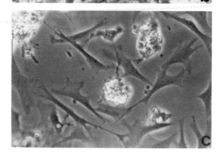

FIGURE 16-3   Retinal cultures at day 6 *in vitro.* a) Representative picture of control culture. The neuronal network is well developed and neuronal aggregates can be observed (520×). b) Serum-free cultures after 24 h of serum deprivation. Neuronal sprouting is more evident than in the controls (750×). c) Hormone-treated cultures 24 h after corticosterone treatment (10^{-7} *M*). The development of neuronal processes is minimal; flat cells are more numerous and not as confluent as in controls and serum-free cultures (520×). (From Gremo, F., Porru, S., and Vernadakis, A., *Dev. Brain Res.,* 15, 45, 1984. With permission.)

an increase in acetylcholinesterase activity.[4] Addition of estradiol to organotypic cultures of the fetal murine hypothalamus, preoptic area, and cerebral cortex elicits a striking enhancement of neurite growth.[84]

In contrast to the neurite-promoting effects of hormones in organ or organotypic cultures, in retina monolayer cell cultures from chick embryos corticosterone inhibits neuronal growth by affecting interactions between neurons and glial cells.[85] Inhibition of neuronal sprouting is detectable after 24 h of treatment (Figure 16-3). When higher doses of the hormone are used (10^{-7} *M*), process development is severely affected. Flat cells (presumptive glia) are fewer in number and are not confluent in the hormone-treated cultures, whereas in controls the flat cells form a 'carpet' over which neurons extend their processes. Neuronal sprouting can be directly inhibited by corticosterone, but it can also be a consequence of a hormone-induced interaction between the substratum and flat cells. The lack of flat cell confluency in hormone-treated cultures may be a result of lack of flat cell migration from the aggregates due to alteration in cell adhesiveness induced by the hormone. The number and orientation of flat cells can be due to a change in microtubule assembly, as has been previously shown in glial cell lines.[86] Also, cell surface modification could account for this phenomenon. Hydrocortisone alters the cell surface in several lines of rat, mouse, and human cells, as indicated by changes in cell morphology, rate of detachment from the dish, and pattern of surface proteins.[87] The peculiar behavior of flat cells, including their lack of confluency, may be partially responsible for the lack of neuronal sprouting. At present, it can only be speculated that absence of interaction between flat cells and neurons may interfere with neuronal growth.

Several recent reports[88-92] have implicated glucocorticoids in neuronal cell death as observed with neurotoxin, ischemia, and aging. However, neuronal loss is not anatomically homogeneous.[93] Adrenal steroid administration protects the dentate gyrus from destruction after adrenalectomy and potentiates cell loss in the Amon's horn. Although several mechanisms for these differential effects of glucocorticoids on neuronal loss have been advocated,[93] the role of glial cells should be considered in neuronal cell death (Figure 16-11 and also Section B of this section).

The view that peptides of the ACTH family can affect brain functions such as those involved in behavior, learning and memory, and motivation and pain perception[94-97] is widely accepted. Again, neural culture has provided some information on the influence of this hormonal peptide at the cellular level. ACTH promotes the survival and maturation of neurons from chick embryo cerebral hemispheres cultured in the absence of nonneural cells.[98] Also, ACTH and some of its N-terminal-related peptides influence deoxyglucose uptake in a time- and dose-dependent fashion.[99] These findings provide evidence of the neurotrophic action of ACTH independent of the hypophyseal system.

For lack, at the present time, of the ability to maintain adult neurons in culture conditions and, more desirably, neurons from aged brain, several investigators have been exploring tumor cell lines as models for neuronal aging and age-related pathologies. Cole and Timiras[100] have reported age-related human neuropathologies in a human teratocarcinoma cell line (NT2/D1) which differentiates to make neurons in response to retinoic acid (Figure 16-4A). They found that NT2/D1-derived neurons express three neurofilament proteins (Figure 16-4B) and generate cells that possess a surface marker, A4, present only in CNS. These investigators have used this cell model as a test system for agents capable of inducing Alzheimer's amyloid lesions. Moreover, they have proposed using this neuronal cell model to test responses to senile dementia of the Alzheimer type (SDAT). Thus, the possibility of using this cell model to test the role of hormones and growth factors in neuronal 'repair' mechanisms during aging is promising.

The use of invertebrate animal models for adult CNS may provide information on the role of hormones on adult neuronal function. Growth and synapse formation among major classes of adult salamander retinal neurons have been described *in vitro*.[101] As discussed earlier, the retinal cultures from embryonic tissue have provided information on neural growth and differentiation.[2] However, the success of adult retinal neurons to maintain their expected phenotype in culture is significant. Cell survival and synapse formation in adult retinal culture is an entirely different process from the well-known retinal regeneration that occurs in newt and salamander.[102] The regeneration by the adult retinal cells *in vitro* is probably related to the ability of lower vertebrate neurons to survive insult and reestablish functional connections.[102] This animal model promises to provide further information on the role of specific substrates, perhaps hormones, on regeneration and other aging phenomena.

B. Responsiveness of Glial Cells to Hormones

As stated previously, this chapter will only focus on studies concerned with the influence of thyroid hormones and steroid hormones on glial cells in culture. Table 16-1 summarizes some selected major *in vivo* effects of hormones on glial cells.[103] Most of these hormonal actions affect cell division, a major characteristic of glial cells responsiveness to a variety of stimuli.

1. Thyroid Hormones

As mentioned earlier in this chapter, extensive studies have established the importance of thyroid hormones in the developing organism.[6-8,60,104-113] Neural culture has provided information on the differential actions of thyroid hormones on neurons and glial cells.

Glioma and neuroblastoma cells have been used as models for glial cells and neurons, respectively, to study a variety of responses of thyroid hormone exposure in culture.[103,114,115] Of interest are the findings on nuclear T_3 receptors in C6 glioma and neuroblastoma (N2A and N18) cells; the number of T_3 receptors is significantly greater in the neuroblastoma than in the

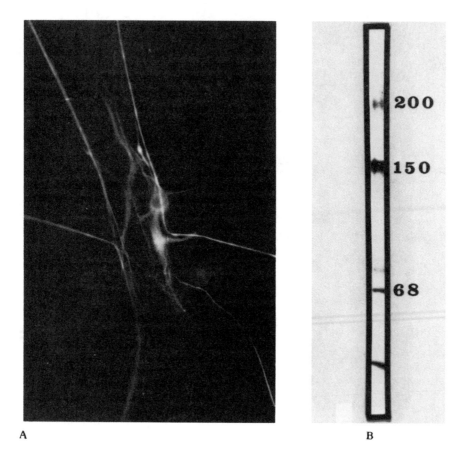

A   B

FIGURE 16-4   A) Retinoic acid-differentiated NT2/D1 human teratocarcinoma cells labelled with Anderton's
BF10 anti155k neurofilament antibody by indirect immunofluorescence show intense process
fluorescence. B) Western blot of Triton-insoluble cytoskeletal material developed with Dahl's
polyclonal antisera to neurofilament proteins shows band for all three neurofilament proteins as well
as several lower molecular weight bands that may represent degradation products. (From Cole
G. M. and Timiras, P. S., *Model System of Development and Aging of the Nervous System,*
Vernadakis, A., Privat, J. M., Lauder, P. S., Timiras, P. S., and Giacobini, E., Eds., Martinius
Nijhoff, Boston, 1987. With permission.)

glioma cells. When cells are cultured in medium containing calf serum from hypothyroid
calves, the number of receptors as well as binding capacity increase in both cell types (Table
16-2). Light and scanning electron microscopy studies on glioma cells have demonstrated
much less pronounced morphological alterations than those that occur in neuroblastoma cells
of the hypothyroid compared to the euthyroid state. While the neuroblastoma cells exhibit a
marked increase in neurite extension under hypothyroid conditions, the glioma cells are only
slightly altered (Figures 16-5 and 16-6). Consistent differences in polymerized tubulin are also
observed between glioma and neuroblastoma cells and between euthyroid and hypothyroid
states: total tubulin concentration, while similar in glioma and neuroblastoma cells, tends to
be higher in the euthyroid than hypothyroid condition. The percentage of polymerized tubulin
is significantly decreased in the glioma cells in the hypothyroid state, and a similar decrease
is also observed in neuroblastomas. In both control and hypothyroid conditions, glioma cells
have significantly less polymerized tubulin than either of the neuroblastoma cell lines. The
decrease in polymerized tubulin in hypothyroid glioma cells may contrast with the otherwise
demonstrated greater resistance of glial cells to alterations in thyroid hormones. However, the
level of significance of this reduction is less in glioma cells than in neuroblastoma. With

TABLE 16-1   Selected Hormonal Effects on Postnatal Glial Cell Development

Cerebrum	Cerebellum
Thyroid Hormones: Hypothyroidism	
No change in cell acquisition, age related decline of T3 receptors delayed, number remains high	Decreased mitoitic activity, indicating decreased acquisition; Bergmann astrocytes are increased (+33%); tendency to a glial hyperplasia in both the internal granular and the molecular layers; cell numbers become normal ultimately, but the cellular composition in the cerebellar cortex is far from normal; there is a substantial deficit in basket cells and an increase in glial cells
Thyroid Hormones: Hyperthyroidism	
Premature termination of cell proliferation leading to deficit of cells; excess thyroid hormone during the neonatal period affects the acquisition of glial cells; T3 receptors down regulated, reduced number	Selective increase in the rate of cell acquisition during the first postnatal week, the consequence of an increase in the number of germinal cells in the cerebellum; the change is not accompanied by alterations in cell cycle parameters; soon after the first week the rate of acquisition of new cells is reduced and this, together with premature emigration of cells from the germinal zone, explains the marked reduction in thickness of this zone; there is a reduction in astrocyte numbers, an effect that is opposite to that seen in hypothyroidism
Corticosteroids	
Corticosterone or cortisol treatment causes a cell deficit due mainly to suppression of postnatal DNA synthesis represents mainly glial formation; cytoplasmic and nuclear receptors present in limbic structures, hypothalamus, and pituitary probably in both neurons and glial cells	Deficit of cells as in the cerebrum with neonatal administration of corticosteroids; permanent deficit in the total DNA content greater than in the cerebrum

Growth Hormone

Administration of growth hormone during gestation reported to lead to increased number of cells in the brain; effect not consistent

Vasopressin

In vasopressin-deficient animals, DNA and incorporation of [³H]thymidine into DNA decreased in forebrain, cerebellum, and olfactory bulbs; effect greater in cerebellum than in forebrain; reversible with daily hormonal replacement

From Draves, D. J., Manley, N. B., and Timiras, P. S., *Astrocytes: Cell Biology & Pathology of Astrocytes,* Vol. 3, Fedoroff, S. and Vernadakis, A., Eds., Academic Press, New York, p. 186, 1986.

respect to the latter, light and scanning electron microscopic changes (e.g., dendritic abnormalities) in conjunction with decreased polymerized tubulin reflect alterations in microtubule (MT) distribution in the hypothyroid condition. The authors[103,114,115] suggest that while the neuroblastoma cells exhibit an increase in neurite extension, which seems at first to be indicative of greater MT assembly and increased polymerization of tubulin, the decreased levels of polymerized tubulin in these cells indicate that MTs are not increased, but rather, redistributed. It is further suggested that since MT assembly initiation sites determine where MT assembly will occur,[116] and that the number of these sites decreases in hypothyroidism,[117] lend further support to the redistribution of MTs as the cause of increased neurite extension in hypothyroid cells. In contrast, the glioma cells undergo fewer morphological alterations, measured by microscopic observations, despite the decrease in polymerized tubulin. From

TABLE 16-2   Comparison of Nuclear T3 Receptors in
Euthyroid and Hypothyroid Cell Cultures

Cell line	K_a ($\times 10^8$ M^{-1})	Binding capacity (ng T3 bound/mg DNA)
C6 (glioma)		
Euthyroid	70.0 ± 5.9[a]	0.039 ± 0.014
Hypothyroid	86.3 ± 16.0	0.084 ± 0.019
p value	<0.3[b]	<0.1
N18 (neuroblastoma)		
Euthyroid	1.12 ± 0.13	0.065 ± 0.01
Hypothyroid	2.50 ± 0.21	0.097 ± 0.08
p value	<0.001	<0.05
N2A (neuroblastoma)		
Euthyroid	1.45 ± 0.21	0.20 ± 0.004
Hypothyroid	1.51 ± 0.49	0.89 ± 0.018
p value	<0.9	<0.05

[a] Mean ± standard error of five determinations.

[b] Statistical analysis is by Student's *t* test.

From Draves, D. J., Manley, N. B., and Timiras, P. S., *Astrocytes: Cell Biology & Pathology of Astrocytes,* Vol. 3, Fedoroff, S. and Vernadakis, A., Eds., Academic Press, New York, p. 186, 1986.

these findings, it appears that glial cells are more stable or less plastic than neuronal cells in their responsiveness to this hormonal microenvironment. This differential responsiveness to the microenvironment further confirms the important role of glia cells in maintaining neuronal homeostasis.

In view of the fact that both hypothyroid and hyperthyroid states have been reported in the elderly (see Chapter 5; references 6 and 7 for reviews), the responsiveness of both neurons and glial cells to thyroid hormones and the balance between neurons and glial cells in the aging brain would be important factors in the behavioral and neurological manifestations associated with thyroid function.

2.   Glucocorticoid Hormones

The neuroregulatory role of steroid hormones, and more specifically, glucocorticoids, has been extensively investigated during brain development and in the adult (see References 2-4 for reviews). Again studies using neural culture systems have provided some clues into the actions of these hormones in neurons and glial cells, neuron-glia interactions, and neuronal homeostasis.

The effects of cortocosteroid hormones on glial cell proliferation in culture are dependent on the neural tissue or cell line studied. In cerebellar explant-organotypic cultures, cortisol, corticosterone, estradiol, and progesterone enhance glial cell proliferation.[118] In contrast, cortisol inhibits glial cell proliferation in monolayer retinal cultures. Furthermore, both inhibitory and stimulatory effects of steroids on cell proliferation have been reported, using various cell lines as experimental models. C6 glioma cells treated with cortisol during the log growth phase in culture first show proliferation, then cell proliferation ceases as growth in control cultures continues into a stationary phase.[119] A 2-day period of growth inhibition follows, then growth subsequently resumes.[119] It appears from these findings that the proliferative capacity of cortisol-treated cells is not irreparably damaged. A transient cell growth inhibitory effect by a synthetic steroid, dexamethasone, has also been observed in cell cultures of human glioblastomas.[120] Cortisol significantly increases the growth of primary monolayer cultures of lung cells from rabbit fetuses at 20 days of gestation; however, in cultures prepared from lung cells from fetuses at 28 days, the effect is reversed and cortisol reduces growth by a factor of 2.[121] Thus, the responsiveness of lung cells to cortisol appears to be age dependent.

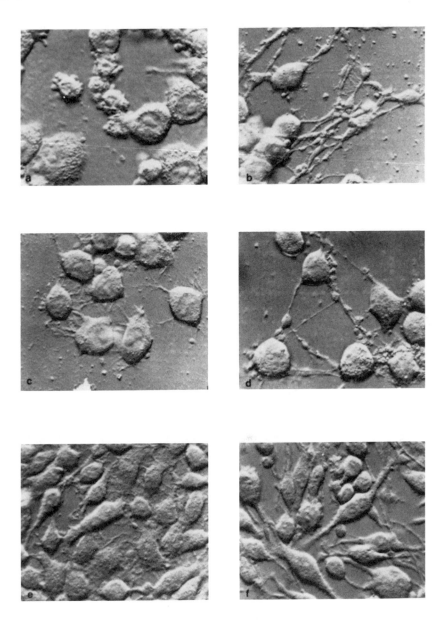

FIGURE 16-5 Light micrographs of neuroblastoma N18: a) euthyroid condition, and b) hypothyroid condition; neuroblastoma N2A: c) euthyroid condition, and d) hypothyroid condition; glioma C6: e) euthyroid condition, and f) hypothyroid condition. Cells were plated directly onto coverslips. The coverslips were harvested by inverting them onto clean glass microscope slides. The cells were then observed and photographed using Normarski optics on an Olympus B-03 microscope. (From Draves, D. J., Manley, N. B., and Timiras, P. S., *Astrocytes: Cell Biology and Pathology of Astrocytes,* Vol. 3, Fedoroff, S. and Vernadakis, A., Eds., Academic Press, New York, 1986. With permission.)

The possibility that steroid hormones may influence glial cell proliferation via an intracellular mechanism is supported by the findings discussed earlier in this chapter that these hormones accumulate in glial cells. A primary effect of corticoid hormones appears to be related to enzyme synthesis and induction. Glycerolphosphate dehydrogenase synthesis is reversibly induced by hydrocortisone.[122,123] Numerous reports have described the induction of glutamine synthetase in C6 glial cells,[124] primary astrocyte cultures,[125] rat glioma cells,[126] or retina Muller cells.[127] Glucocorticoid receptors have also been reported in C6 glioma cells.[128,129]

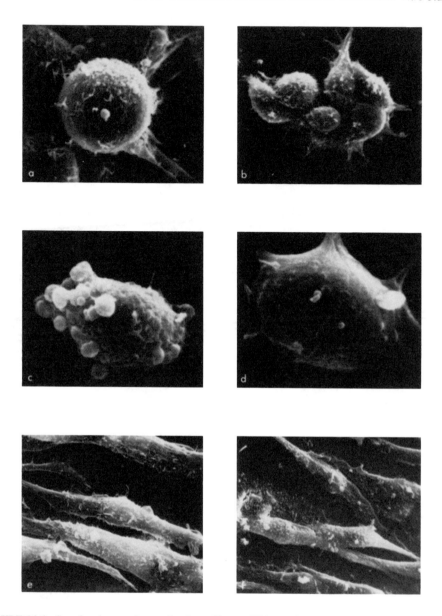

FIGURE 16-6   Scanning electron micrographs of neuroblastoma N18: a) euthyroid condition (×2208); b) hypothyroid condition (×1725); and neuroblastoma N2A; c) euthyroid condition (×2760). For further details, see Reference 103.

Early studies[130,131] have shown that cortisol treatment increases brain excitability in both adult and developing organisms, and this effect is mediated through the actions of steroids on Na and K ion transport. However, more recent studies in culture reveal that glial cells play a role in the effects of steroids on neurotransmission processes. Certain steroids are powerful inhibitors of extraneuronal uptake of norepinephrine (NE), uptake$_2$, in the peripheral nervous system.[132] Studies using cerebellar explants in organotypic culture have shown that cortisol inhibits low affinity ^{3}H-norepinephrine uptake.[133] It has been advocated that this uptake may represent uptake$_2$ glial uptake.[133] Uptake NE into astrocytes has also been reported.[134] The importance of extraneuronal, glial uptake of NE in the CNS is still to be elucidated. However, if the role of glial cells in neurotransmission is to provide a safety valve — i.e., to limit the possible build-up of neurotransmitter substances extracellularly — then inhibition of glial cell uptake by, for example, cortisol, could lead to an intracellular/extracellular imbalance resulting in excitation (see Reference 135 for review).

As discussed earlier, with aging there is an increased proliferation of glial cells. Therefore it would follow that with aging there would be a change in neurotransmitter compartmentation between neurons and glial cells. In addition, corticosteroid receptors decrease in several brain areas with aging (discussed previously). Thus, the low levels of some neurotransmitters reported with aging may partially be a result of a servomechanism attempting to balance the level of neurotransmitter at the synaptic cleft.

Evidence based on culture studies implicates the role of glial cells in glucocorticoid neuronal toxicity.[136,138] It appears that astrocytes may represent a distinct nonneuronal target for the damaging effects of glucocorticoids in the hippocampus and that metabolic derangements, i.e., glucose transport, in these cells during an energy crisis may become exacerbated by glucocorticoids.[136,138]

The role of glial cells in the response of the CNS to hormones is further substantiated by recent studies showing that glial cells in culture convert pregnenolone to progesterone and to 3-hydroxy-5-pregnane-20-one (3,5-TH PROG).[140,141] This is important since 3,5-TH PROG is a positive allosteric modulator of GABAergic neurotransmission.[142,143] Moreover, astrocytes in culture metabolize pregnenolone to dehydroepiandrosterone.[144] More importantly, astrocytes can also provide progesterone to neighboring neurons.[140] Therefore, by metabolizing pregnenolone to progesterone, astrocytes might intervene in the regulation of several brain functions. In addition to astrocytes, oligodendrocytes appear to also synthesize steroids from cholesterol.[145] It would be important to know if glial cells in the aging brain are capable of playing a role in the metabolism of neurosteroids.

V. CHANGES IN GLIAL CELLS WITH AGING

For several years we have been interested in the role of neuron-glia interrelations in CNS growth, development, and also aging.[1,5,146] The hypothesis has been that, in the aging brain, glial cells may not supply the required input in the microenvironment which is crucial for neuronal survival and function. It is only in the past decade that consideration has been given to glial cells in the aging process and the literature still contains very few specific studies. We have used late passages of primary glial cells derived from aged mouse (18-month-old) cerebral hemispheres and also C6 glial cells of early and late passages as models to study changes in glial cells with aging.

A. C6 Glial Cells as a Model

C6 glioma cells have provided a useful model to study glial cell properties, glial factors, and sensitivity of glial cells to various substances and conditions. C6 glioma cells, 2B clone, exhibit differential enzyme expression with cell passage:[147] the activity of cyclic nucleotide phosphohydrolase (CNP), an enzyme marker for oligodendrocytes,[148] is markedly high and that of glutamine synthetase (GS), an enzyme marker for astrocytes,[149] is low in early passages (up to passage 24). This relation is reversed in the late passages (beyond passage 70) (Figures 16-7 and 16-8). C6 glial cells of early passage can more easily be geared toward either astrocytic or oligodendrocytic expression while late passages are more committed to astrocytic expression.[150-152] Studies testing the responsiveness of early and late passage C6 glial cells to various culture conditions: substratum, comparing poly-L-lysine, collagen, and plastic; serum factors, using fetal bovine serum and inactivated fetal bovine serum; neuronal factors, using conditioned media from primary neuronal and neuroblastoma cell cultures;[150] platelet activating factor;[153] and muscle-derived factor[154] have led to the hypothesis that C6 glial cells of early passage have progenitor properties and can be geared towards either astrocytic or oligodendrocytic phenotypic expression, whereas the late passage C6 glial cells are more

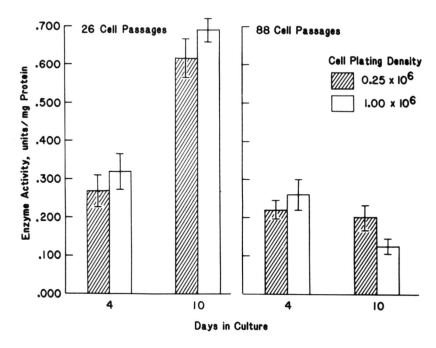

FIGURE 16-7 Changes in 2',3' cyclic nucleotide 3' phosphohydrolase activity in C6 glial cells of different cell passage. Cell plating densities were 0.25×10^6 cells (empty bars). Activity is expressed per mg protein. Units of activity represent µmol phosphate produced per minute derived from a standard phosphate curve produced from 2'adenosine monophosphate. Points with bracketed lines represent mean ± SE. (From Parker, K. P., Norenberg, M. D., and Vernadakis, A., *Science,* 208, 179, 1980. With permission.)

committed to astrocytic phenotype. C6 glial phenotypes from both early (20 to 24) and late (73 to 90) passages have also been immunocytochemically characterized[151] using double staining for glial fibrillary acidic protein (GFAP) and A2B5 antigen for type 1 and type 2 astrocytes or galactocerebroside (GalC) and A2B5 antigen for oligodendrocytes; cells positive for A2B5 antigen and negative for both GFAP and GalC are considered to be precursor glia cells. Early passage cells consist of both GFAP- and GalC-positive cells, whereas late passage cells exhibit predominantly GFAP-positive cells. Of importance is the fact that when early passage cells cultivated in the absence of serum appear differentiated, they express high GS activity, and also the predominant glia population is GFAP+ and A2B5+ positive, which indicates type 2 astrocytes. Based on these and previous studies, the hypothesis is put forward that early passage C6 glia cells are bipotential and can be geared to express either astrocytic or oligodendrocytic phenotype. In contrast, late passage C6 glia remain committed to their astrocytic phenotypic expression as shown by a high population of astrocytes type 1 and 2. Thus, the high GS activity expressed by late passage C6 glia (Figure 16-8) reflects the high population of type 1 and type 2 astrocytes.

B. Glial Cells Derived From Aged Mouse Cerebral Hemispheres

In 1984, the first report about glial cells prepared from 18-month-old mouse cerebral hemispheres was published.[81,82] Cells were cultured and subcultured for several passages and have been maintained frozen in liquid nitrogen at several passages. With increasing cell passage, GS activity increases, whereas CNP activity decreases during early passage and then remains at a low level (Figure 16-9). This increase in GS activity is interpreted to reflect an increase in the astrocyte population. As discussed earlier for the C6 glial cells, the glia phenotypes in

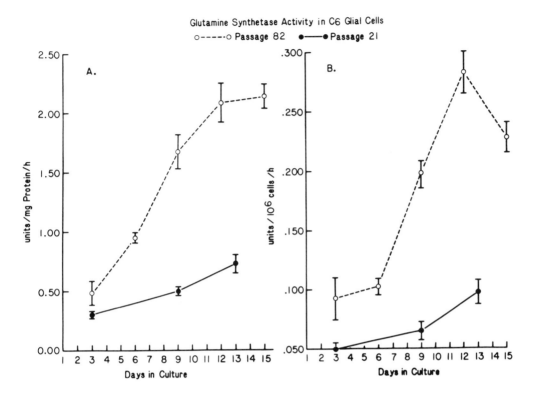

Glutamine Synthetase Activity in C6 Glial Cells

o- - - - -o Passage 82   •——• Passage 21

FIGURE 16-8   Changes in glutamine synthetase activity in C6 glial cells of different cell passages. A: activity expressed per mg protein. B: activity expressed per 10^6 cells. Units of activity represent μmoles of γ-glutamylhydroxamic acid formed. Points SE. Points with bracketed lines represent mean ± SE. (From Parker, K. P., Norenberg, M. D., and Vernadakis, A., *Science,* 208, 179, 1980. With permission.)

the aged cultures were characterized immunocytochemically using specific glial markers: glial fibrillary acidic protein (GFAP) for astrocytes, galactocerebroside (GalC) for oligodendro-cytes, and A2B5 for glial precursor cells.[151] Cultures from aged mouse cerebral hemisphere consist primarily of protoplasmic type 1 astrocytes, some differentiated type 2 astrocytes, and a few oligodendrocytes. Thus, the high GS activity in these glia cultures with passage reflects the high astrocyte population.

Although the increase in astrocytes with cell passage in culture cannot be equated with the astrogliosis occurring *in vivo* in the aging brain, it may be the equivalent of an *in vitro* astrogliosis as a response to a stressful environment. One of the most striking characteristics of astrocytes is the 'reactive hyperplasia' they exhibit in response to tissue injury (see Reference 1). This reactive response has been interpreted to express the involvement of these cells in the adaptive mechanisms leading to the restoration of tissue homeostasis. The above findings provide support that this function of the astrocyte is also expressed *in vitro*. Based on these parallel *in vivo* and *in vitro* phenomena, the astrocyte is a cell of great potential and adaptability and may be a key cell in the survival of the neuron during the aging process.

An increased activity in GS-containing astrocytes (Figure 16-9) would have further impli-cations in neuronal homeostasis. Hertz and Schousboe,[155] in an elegant series of experiments, have shown that astrocytes are intimately involved in the compartmentation of glutamic acid and the ultimate functional balance of GABAergic-glutamatergic neurons (Figure 16-10). Thus, it can be visualized that in the aging brain, a high number of GS-expressing astrocytes

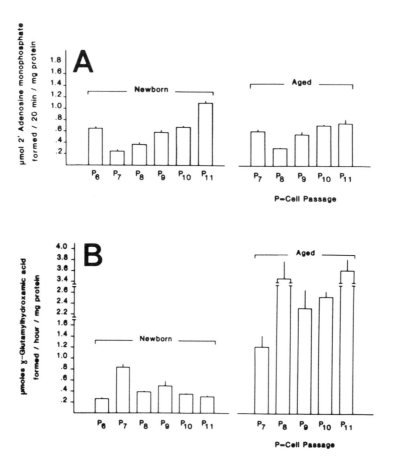

FIGURE 16-9   Cyclic nucleotide phosphohydrolase A and glutamine synthetase B activities in glial cells prepared from newborn and aged (18-month-old) mouse cerebral hemispheres. Cells were from passages 6 (P6) to 11 (P11). Points with lines represent means + SE of 3–5 cultures. Magnification: ×547. (From Vernadakis, A., Davies, D., Sakellaridis, N., and Mangoura, D., *J. Neurosci. Res.,* 15, 79, 1986. With permission.)

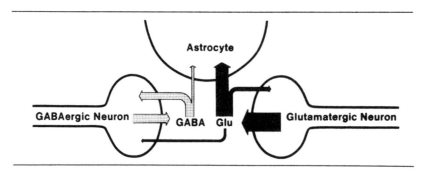

FIGURE 16-10   Schematic drawing of evoked release and uptake of glutamate and GABA in GABAergic or glutamatergic neurons and in astrocytes. The sizes of the arrows give an estimate of the relative magnitudes of the respective fluxes. It can be seen that neuronally released glutamate to a major extent is accumulated into astrocytes, whereas most of the released GABA is reaccumulated into neurons. (From Hertz, L. and Schousboe, A., *Model Systems of Development and Aging of the Nervous System,* Vernadakis, A., Privat, A., Lauder, J. L., Timaras, P. S., and Giacobini, E., Eds., Martinius Nijhoff, Boston, 1987. With permission.)

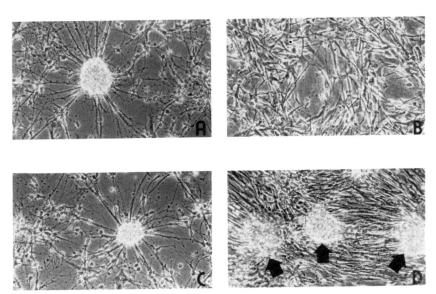

FIGURE 16-11 Photomicrographs of neuron-enriched cultures derived from 6-day-old cerebral hemispheres (E6CH) and grown in CDM/PS + 10% FBS (A) or in CDM supplemented with 20% conditioned medium from 5-day-old MACH cultures grown for 24 h in CDM (C). B. Glial cell culture derived from aged mouse cerebral hemispheres (MACH) passage 18, C11. *D.* Co-culture of brain cells derived from E6CH and plated onto a living glial cell substratum of MACH-P18 at C5. At time of photography, E6Ch culture and neuron-glia cultures were C6, whereas MACH cultures were C11. Note: (*D*, heavy arrows) that neuronal aggregates on the MACH substratum are devoid of any neuritic outgrowth. Magnification: ×147. (From Lee, K., Kentroti, S., and Vernadakis, A., *Brain Res. Bull.,* 28, 861, 1992. With permission.)

would provide a sink for elimination of any excessive glutamic acid, an excitatory amino acid which may contribute to the control of neuronal death.[156] Further evidence of the role of astrocytes in glucocorticoid neuronal toxicity are the findings by Virgin et al.,[137] showing that glucocorticoids inhibit glutamate uptake in hippocampal astrocytes. Thus, hippocampal neuronal cell death produced by an excess of glucocorticoids may be mediated by excessive glutamate in the synaptic cleft, as a result of astrocytic dysfunction.

VI. GLIA-NEURON INTERACTIONS IN CULTURE

Neuron-glia interactions during aging has only recently been considered. Using C6 glial cells (both early and late passage) and glial cells derived from aged mouse cerebral hemispheres, the glial influence on cholinergic neurons in culture has been reported.[152] The findings obtained from this study showed that immature glial cells enhanced cholinergic neuronal expression, whereas committed astrocytes or glial cells from aged mouse brain inhibit cholinergic neuronal expression. It is speculated that glial cells at certain maturational stages express adhesion molecules which can regulate the balance between stimulatory and inhibitory contact signals important for neuronal phenotypic expression. That neurons plated on glial cell substrata derived from aged glia do not exhibit the normal growth of neuronal aggregates with neurite outgrowth and neurite fasciculation (Figure 16-11) support the speculation that glial cells from aged brain may express cell surface molecules which inhibit neuronal growth. The inhibitory effect on neuronal phenotypic expression produced by aged glia substrata is reminiscent of the inhibitory influences of astroglia in the adult CNS scars. It is known that after a penetrating injury to the adult CNS, an astroglia-mesenchymal scar is formed and it is this structure that has traditionally been thought of as a major obstacle to axonal regeneration.[157]

VII. GENERAL CONCLUSIONS

Understanding the cellular and molecular mechanisms involved in aging in general and CNS aging in particular has become the focus of intensive research. The difficulty of investigating CNS aging has been the extreme cellular complexity and heterogeneity of the brain. In the last decade, considerable progress has been made in our knowledge from the use of culture models to assimilate some *in vivo* conditions. The information we have obtained thus far has been of cellular processes associated primarily with the growth of the nervous system. However, understanding growth has provided some clues into processes of regeneration, which may be the key to our understanding aging. Manipulation of the constituents of culture media and substrata has provided evidence that both neurons and glial cells can adapt to their microenvironment and that both cell populations exhibit considerable plasticity. Moreover, these *in vitro* models have solidified the view that interactions between neurons and glial cells are paramount for brain homeostasis.

Hormones have been primary components of the "milieu interieur" and their role in growth has been established. In this chapter, an attempt was made to review some findings which demonstrate that neurons and glial cells respond differentially to hormones and that hormones, as neuromodulators, have both stimulatory and inhibitory actions (see Chapter 18). Although the evidence on the responsiveness of CNS to hormones during aging *in vivo* is still meager, extrapolation of *in vitro* findings allows some conclusions and future directions. Neuronal aging in culture has not as yet been successfully modelled, and only by extrapolation of certain neuronal growth events, such as those related to neuronal sprouting, has some information been relevant to our further understanding neuronal regeneration and aging. However, *in vitro* cellular aging has been studied using other cells and, more specifically, fibroblasts and some basic mechanisms have been unravelled, e.g., DNA repair with aging. It is only with time that conditions will be further developed for a culture model to accurately represent neuronal aging.

The interdependence of neuronal and glial cells continues to be the key event in brain homeostasis. Differential aging in these cell populations creates shifts in the neuron-glia functional balance. It is only when we understand all the functional capabilities of these cells and the degree of their plasticity with age that we will be able to unravel the CNS aging process.

REFERENCES

1. Vernadakis, A., Neuron-glia interrelations. *Intl. Rev. Neurobiol.*, 30:149, 1988.
2. Gremo, F. and Vernadakis, A., Role of steroid hormones in neural growth and differentiation: *In vivo* and *in vitro* comparisons. In: *Model Systems of Development and Aging of the Nervous System.* Vernadakis, A., Privat, A., Lauder, J. M., Timiras, P. S., and Giacobini, E., Eds., Martinius Nijhoff, Boston. p. 321, 1987.
3. Vernadakis, A., Endocrine regulation of neural development: Physiological and biochemical aspects. In: *Hormones in Development and Aging.* Vernadakis, A. and Timiras, P. S., Eds., SP Medical & Scientific Books, New York. p. 207, 1982.
4. Vernadakis, A. and Culver, B., Neuroendocrine control systems in the adult. In: *Hormones in Development and Aging.* Vernadakis, A. and Timiras, P. S., Eds., SP Medical & Scientific Books, New York. p. 371, 1982.
5. Vernadakis, A., The aging brain. In: *Symposium on the Aging Process.* Geogas, M., Ed., Clinics in Geriatrics. Saunders, Philadelphia. p. 61, 1985.
6. Timiras, P. S., Aging of the nervous system: Functional changes. In: *Physiological Basis of Aging and Geriatrics.* 2nd ed., Timiras, P. S., Ed., CRC Press, Boca Raton, FL, p. 103, 1994.
7. Timiras, P. S., Aging of the nervous system: Structural and biochemical changes. In: *Physiological Basis of Aging and Geriatrics.* 2nd ed., Timiras, P. S., Ed., CRC Press, Boca Raton, FL, p. 89, 1994.
8. Meisami, E., Aging of the nervous system: Sensory changes. In: *Physiological Basis of Aging and Geriatrics.* 2nd ed., Timiras, P. S., Ed., CRC Press, Boca Raton, FL, p. 115, 1994.
9. Commentaries. Various authors. *Neurobiol. Aging*, 8:547, 1987.

10. Buell, S. J. and Colemann, P. D., Dendritic growth in the aged human brain and failure of growth in senile dementia. *Science,* 206:854, 1979.

11. Connor, J. R., Jr., Diamond, M. C., and Johnson, R. E., Occipital cortical morphology of the rat: Alterations with age and environment. *Exper. Neurobiol.,* 68:158, 1980.

12. Mervis, R. F., Cytomorphological alterations in the aging animal brain with emphasis of Golgi studies. In: *Aging and Cell Structure.* Johnson, J. E., Jr., Ed., Plenum Press, New York. p. 143, 1981.

13. Cotman, C. W., Ed., *Neuronal Plasticity.* Raven Press, New York. 1978.

14. Cotman, C. W. and Lynch, G. S., Reactive synaptogenesis in the adult nervous system. In: *Neuronal Recognition.* Barondes, S., Ed., Raven Press, New York. p. 227, 1976.

15. Cotman, C. W. and Nadler, J. V., Reactive synaptogenesis in the hippocampus. In: *Neuronal Plasticity.* Cotman, C. W., Ed., Raven Press, New York. p. 227, 1978.

16. Cotman, C. W. and Scheff, S. W., Compensatory synapse growth in aged animals after neuronal death. *Mech. Ageing Dev.,* 9:103, 1979.

17. Bickford, P. C., Hoffer, B. J., and Freedman, R., Interaction of norepinephrine with Purkinje cell responses to cerebellar afferent inputs in aged rats. *Neurobiol. Aging,* 6:89, 1985.

18. Bickford, P. C., Hoffer, B. J., and Freedman, R., Diminished interaction of norepinephrine with climbing fiber inputs to cerebellar Purkinje neurons in aged Fischer 344 rats. *Brain Res.,* 385:405, 1986.

19. Bickford-Wimer, P. C., Miller, J. A., Freedman, R., and Rose, G., Age-related reduction in responses of rat hippocampal neurons to locally applied monamines. *Neurobiol. Aging,* 9:173, 1988.

20. Hoffer, B. J,. Rose, G., Parfitt, K., Freedman, R., and Bickford-Wimer, P. C., Age-related changes in cerebellar noradrenergic function. *Ann. N.Y. Acad. Sci.,* 515:269, 1988.

21. Gurwitz, D., Egozi, Y., Henis, Y. I., Kloog, Y. , and Sokolorsky, M., Agonist and antagonist binding to rat brain muscarinic receptors: Influence of aging. *Neurobiol. Aging,* 8:115, 1987.

22. Kohno, A., Seeman, P., and Cinader, B., Age-related changes of beta-adrenoceptors in aging inbred mice. *J. Gerontol.,* 41:439, 1986.

23. Leprohon-Greenwood, C. E. and Cinader, B., Variations in age-related decline in striatal D_2-dopamine receptors in a variety of mouse strains. *Mech. Ageing Dev.,* 38:199, 1987.

24. Scarpace, P. J., Characterization of beta-adrenergic receptors throughout the replicative life span of IMR-90 cells. *J. Cell Physiol.,* 130:163, 1987.

25. Severson, J. A. and Randall, P. K., D_2-dopamine receptors in aging mouse striatum: Determination of high- and low-affinity agonist binding sites. *J. Pharmacol. Exp. Therap.,* 233:361, 1985.

26. Shenkman, L., Rabey, J. M., and Gilad, G. M., Cholinergic muscarinic binding by rat lymphocytes: Effects of antagonist treatment, strain and aging. *Brain Res.,* 380:303, 1986.

27. Cimino, M., Vantini, G., Algeri, S., Curatola, G., Pezzoli, C., and Stramentinole, G., Age-related modification of dopaminergic and beta-adrenergic receptor system: Restoration to normal activity by modifying membrane fluidity with S-adenosylmethionine. *Life Sci.,* 34:2029, 1984.

28. Von Hunger, K. and Banter, C. F., Are age-related changes in receptor activity or an expression of altered activity or an expression of altered membrane fluidity? In: *Model Systems of Development and Aging of the Nervous System.* Vernadakis, A., Privat, A., Lauder, J. M., Timiras, P. S., and Giacobini, E., Eds., Martinius Nijhoff, Boston. p. 375, 1984.

29. Kendall, M. J., Woods, K. L., Wilkins, M. R., and Worthington, D. J., Responsiveness of beta-adrenergic receptor stimulation: The effects of age are cardioselective. *Br. J. Clin. Pharmac.,* 14:821, 1982.

30. Scarpace, P. J., Decreased beta-adrenergic responsiveness during senescence. *Fed. Proc.,* 45:51, 1986.

31. Scarpace, P. J. and Abrass, I.. B., Alpha- and beta-adrenergic receptor function in the brain during senescence. *Neurobiol. Aging,* 9:53, 1988.

32. McEwen, B. S., Glucocorticoids and hippocampus: Receptors in search of a function. In: *Current Topics in Neuroendocrinology,* Vol 2. Ganten, P. and Pfaff, D., Eds., Springer-Verlag, Berlin. p. 23, 1982.

33. Beato, M., Gene regulation by steroid hormones. *Cell,* 56:335, 1989.

34. Evans, R. M., The steroid and thyroid hormone receptors superfamily. *Science,* 240:889, 1988.

35. Vernadakis, A., Culver, B., and Nidess, R., Actions of steroid hormones on neural growth in culture: Role of glial cells. *Psychoneuroendocrinology,* 3:47, 1978.

36. Chou, Y.-C., Luttage, W. G., and Sumners, C., Characterization of glucocorticoid type II receptors in neuronal and glial cultures from rat brain. *J. Neuroendocrinology,* 2:29, 1990.

37. Reul, J. M. H. M. and de Kloet, E. R., Two receptor systems for corticosterone in rat brain: Microdistribution an differential occupation. *Endocrinology,* 117:2505, 1985.

38. Vedder, H., Weiss, I., Holsboer, F., and Reul, J. M. H. M., Glucocorticoid and mineralocorticoid receptors in rat neocortical and hippocampal brain cells in culture: Characterization and regulatory studies. *Brain Res.,* 605:18, 1993.

39. Teutsch, G., Costerousse, G., Deraedt, R., Bonzoni, J., Fortin, M., and Philabert, D., 17-a-alkynyl-11β,-17-dihydroxyandrosase derivatives: A new class of potent glucocorticoids. *Steroids,* 38:651, 1981.

40. Raynaud, J. P., Ojasoo, J., Jouquey, A., Moguilewsky, M., and Teutsch, G., Probes for steroid receptors. In: *Endocrinology.* Labrie, F. and Prouix, L., Eds., Elsevier, New York. p. 533, 1984.

41. de Kloet, E. R. and Reul, J. M. H. M., Feedback action and toxic influence of corticosteroids on brain function: A concept arising from the heterogeneity of brain receptor systems. *Psychoneuroendocrinology,* 12:83, 1987.

42. Angelucci, L., Valeri, P., Grossi, L., Veldhuis, H., Bohus, B., and de Kloet, E., Involvement of hippocampal corticosterone receptors in behavioral phenomena. In: *Progress in Psychoneuroendocrinology.* Brambilla, F., Racagni, G., and de Wied, D., Eds., Elsevier, Amsterdam. p. 17, 1980.

43. Sapolsky, R., Krey, L., and McEwen, B. S., Prolonged glucocorticoid exposure reduces hippocampus neuron number: Implications for aging. *J. Neurosci.,* 5:1221, 1985.

44. Sapolsky, R., Krey, L., McEwen, B. S., and Rainbow, T. C., Do vasopressin-related peptides induce hippocampal corticosterone receptors? Implications for aging. *J. Neurosci.,* 4:1479, 1984.

45. Pfeiffer, A., Barden, N., and Meaney, M. J., Age-related changes in glucocorticoid receptor binding and mRNA levels in the rat brain and pituitary. *Neurobiol. Aging,* 12:475, 1991.

46. Roth, G. S., Reduced glucocorticoid binding site concentration in cortical neuronal perikarya from senescent rats. *Brain Res.,* 107:345, 1976.

47. Roth, G. S., Age-related changes in specific glucocorticoid binding by steroid-responsive tissues in rats. *Endocrinology,* 94:82, 1978.

48. Landfield, P. W. and Eldridge, J. C., Increased affinity of type II corticosteroid binding in aged rat hippocampus. *Exp. Neurobiol.,* 106:110, 1989.

49. Eldridge, J. C., Fleenor, D. G., Steven Kerr, D., and Landfield, P. W., Impaired up-regulation of type II corticosteroid receptors in hippocampus of aged rats. *Brain Res.,* 478:248, 1989.

50. Sapolsky, R., Krey, L., and McEwen, B. S., Corticosterone receptors decline in a site-specific manner in the aged rat brain. *Brain Res.,* 289:235, 1983.

51. Kerr, D. S., Campbell, L. W., Hao, S-Y, and Landfield, P. W., Corticosteroid modulation of hippocampal potentials: Increased effect with aging. *Science,* 245:1505, 1989.

52. Landfield, P. W., Waymire, J. C., and Lynch, G., Hippocampal aging and adrenocorticoids: Quantitative correlations. *Science,* 22:1098, 1978.

53. Sapolsky, R. M., Do glucocorticoid concentrations rise with age in the rat? *Neurobiol. Aging,* 13:171, 1991.

54. Vielkind, U., Walencewicz, A., Levine, J. M., and Churchill Bohn, M., Type II glucocorticoid receptors are expressed in oligodendrocytes and astrocytes. *J. Neurosci. Res.,* 27:360-373, 1990.

55. Valcana, T. and Timiras, P. S., Nuclear trisdothyronine receptors in the developing rat brain. *Mol. & Cell Endocrin.,* 11:31, 1978.

56. Eberhardt, N. L., Valcana, T., and Timiras, P. S., Triiodothyronine nuclear receptors: An *in vivo* comparison of the binding of triiodothyronine to nuclei of adult rat liver, cerebral hemispheres, and anterior pituitary. *Endocrinology,* 102:556, 1978.

57. Valcana, T., Conversion and binding of tetraiodothyroxine in developing rat brain. *Neurochem Res.,* 6:743, 1981.

58. Kastellakis, A. and Valcana, T., Characterization of thyroid hormone transport in synaptosomes from rat brain. *Mol. & Cell Endocrin.,* 67:231, 1989.

59. Margarity, M., Matsokis, N., and Valcana, T.. Characterization of nuclear triiodothyronine (T_3) and tetraiodothyronine (T_4) binding in developing brain tissue. *Mol. & Cell Endocrin.,* 31:333, 1983.

60. Valcana, T., Developmental changes in ionic composition of the brain in hypo and hyperthyroidism. In: *Advances in Behavioral Biology, Vol 9, Drugs & The Developing Brain.* Vernadakis, A. and Weiner, N., Eds., Plenum Press, New York. p. 289, 1974.

61. Murray, M. B., Zilz, N. D., McCreary, N. L., MacDonald, M. J., and Towle, H-C., Isolation and characterization of rat cDNA clones for two distinct thyroid hormone receptors. *J. Biol. Chem.,* 263:12770, 1988.

62. North, D. and Fisher, D. ,A., Thyroid hormone receptor and receptor-related RNA levels in developing rat brain. *Ped. Res.,* 28:622, 1990.

63. Oppenheimer, J. H., Schwartz, H. L., Mariask, C. N., Kinlaw, W. B., Wong, N. C., and Freake, H. C., Advances in our understanding of thyroid hormone action at the cellular level. *Endocrin. Res.,* 8:288, 1987.

64. Sakurai, A., Nakai, A., and DeGroot, J. L., Expression of three forms of thyroid hormone receptor in human tissues. *Mol. Endocrin.,* 3:392, 1989.

65. Thompson, C. C., Weinberger, C., Lebo, R., and Evans, R. M., Identification of a novel thyroid hormone receptor expressed in the mammalian central nervous system. *Science,* 237:1610, 1987.

66. Dimpfel, W., Rat nerve cell cultures in pharmacology and toxicology. *Arch. Toxicol.,* 4:55, 1980.

67. Murray, M. R., Nervous tissue *in vitro.* In: *Cells and Tissues in Culture.* Wiltmer, E. N,. Ed., Plenum Press, New York. p. 373, 1965.

68. Schrier, B. K., Nervous system cultures as toxicological test systems. In: *Nervous System Toxicology.* Mitchell, C. L., Ed., Raven Press, New York. p. 337, 1982.

69. Vernadakis, A. and Culver, B., Neural tissue culture: A biochemical tool. In: *Biochemistry of Brain.* Kumar, S., Ed., Pergamon Press, Oxford. p. 407, 1980.

70. Shahar, A., de Vellis, J., Vernadakis, A., and Haber, B., eds., *A dissection and culture manual of the nervous system*. Alan R. Liss, New York. 1989.

71. Harrison, R. G., Observations on the living developing nerve fiber. *Proc. Soc. Exp. Biol. Med.,* 4:140, 1907.

72. Murray, M. and Stout, A. P., Characteristics of human Schwann cells *in vitro. Anat. Rec.,* 84:275, 1942.

73. Murray, M. and Stout, A. P., Distinctive characteristics of the sympatheticoblastoma cultivated *in vitro*: A method for prompt diagnosis. *Am. J. Pathol.,* 23:429, 1947.

74. Maximow, A., Tissue cultures of young mammalian embryos. *Contrib. Embryol.,* 16:47, 1925.

75. Cavanaugh, M. W., Neuron development from trypsin-dissociated cells of differentiated spinal cord of the chick embryo. *Exp., Cell Res.,* 9:42, 1955.

76. Booher, H. and Sensenbrenner, M.. Growth and cultivation of dissociated neurons and glial cells from embryonic chick, rat and human brain in flask cultures. *Neurobiology,* 2:97, 1972.

77. Seeds, N. W., Biochemical differentiation in reaggregating brain cell culture. *Proc. Natl., Acad. Sci. U.S.A.,* 68:1858, 1971.

78. Augusti-Tocco, G. and Sato, G., Establishment of functional clonal lines of neurons from mouse neuroblastoma. *Proc. Natl. Acad. Sci. U.S.A.,* 64:311, 1969.

79. Benda, P. L., Lightbody, J., Sato, G., Levine, L., and Sweet, W., Differentiated rat glial strain in tissue culture. *Science,* 161:370, 1968.

80. Jiang, Z.-G. and Smith, R. A., Effects of nerve growth factor on the survival of primary cultured adult and aged mouse sensory neurons. *J. Neurosci. Res.,* 35:29-37, 1993.

81. Vernadakis, A., Mangoura, D., Sakellaridis, N., and Linderholm, S., Glial cells dissociated from newborn and aged mouse brain. *J. Neurosci. Res.,* 11:253, 1984.

82. Vernadakis, A., Davies, D., Sakellaridis, N., and Mangoura, D., Growth patterns of glial cells dissociated from newborn and aged mouse brain with cell passage. *J. Neurosci. Res.,* 15:79, 1986.

83. Vernadakis, A. and Timiras, P. S., Eds., *Hormones in Development and Aging*. SP Medical & Scientific, New York. 1982.

84. Toran-Allerand, C. D., Ellis, L., and Pfenninger, K., Estrogen and insulin synergism in neurite growth enhancement *in vitro*: Mediation of steroid effects by interactions with growth factors. *Dev. Brain Res.,* 41:87, 1988.

85. Gremo, F., Porru, S., and Vernadakis, A., Effects of corticosterone on chick embryonic retinal cells in culture. *Devel. Brain Res.,* 15:45, 1984.

86. Berliner, J. A., Bennett, K., and de Vellis, J., Effects of hydrocortisone on cell morphology in C6 cells. *J. Cell Physiol.,* 94:321, 1978.

87. Wu, R. and Sato, G. H., Replacement of serum in cell culture by hormones: A study of hormonal regulation of cell growth and specific gene expression. *J. Toxicol. Environ. Hlth.,* 4:427, 1978.

88. Sapolsky, R. M., Glucocorticoid toxicity in the hippocampus: Temporal aspects of neuronal vulnerability. *Brain Res.,* 359:300, 1985.

89. Sapolsky, R. M., A mechanism for glucocorticoid toxicity in the hippocampus: Increased neuronal vulnerability to metabolic insults. *J. Neurosci.,* 5:128, 1985.

90. Sapolsky, R. M. and Pulsinelli, W. A., Glucocorticoids potentiate ischemic injury to neurons: Therapeutic implications. *Science,* 229:1397, 1985.

91. Sapolsky, R. M., Packan, D., and Vale, W., Glucocorticoid toxicity in the hippocampus: *In vitro* demonstration. *Brain Res.,* 453:367, 1988.

92. Stein, B. A. and Sapolsky, R. M., Chemical adrenalectomy reduces hippocampal damage induced by kainic acid. *Brain Res.,* 473:175, 1988.

93. McEwen, B. S. and Gould, E., Adrenal steroid influences on the survival of hippocampal neurons. *Biochem. Pharmacol.,* 40:2393, 1990.

94. De Weid, D., Behavioral actions of neurohypophysial peptides. *Proc. R. Soc. Lond.,* 210:183, 1980.

95. De Weid, D. and Gispen, W. H., Behavioral effects of peptides. In: *Peptides in Neurobiology*. Grainer, H., Ed., Plenum Press, New York. p. 397, 1977.

96. Gispen, W. H., Zwiers, H., Wiegandt, V. M., Schotman, P., and Wilson, J. E., The behaviorally active neuropeptide ACTH as neurohormone and neuromodulator: The role of cyclic nucleotides and membrane phosphoproteins. In: *Modulators, Mediators, and Specifiers in Brain Function*. Erhlick, V. M., Volarka, J., Davis, L. G., and Brunngraber, E. D,, Eds., Plenum Press, New York. p. 19, 1979.

97. Kastin, A. J., Zadina, J. E., Coy, D. H., Schally, A. V., and Sandman, C. A., Hypothalamic peptides affect behavior after systemic injection. In: *Polypeptide Hormones*. Beers, R. J. and Basselt, E. G., Eds., Raven Press, New York. p. 223, 1980.

98. Daval, J. L., Louis, J. C., Gerard, M. J., and Vincendon, G., Influence of adrenocorticotropic hormone on the growth of isolated neurons in culture. *Neurosci. Ltr.,* 36:299, 1983.

99. Daval, J. L., Anglard, P., Gerard, M. J., Vincendon, G., and Louis, J. C., Regulation of deoxyglucose uptake by adrenocorticotropic hormone in cultured neurons. *J. Cell Physiol.,* 124:75, 1985.

100. Cole, G. M. and Timiras, P. S., Aging-related pathology in human neuroblastoma and teratocarcinoma cell lines. In: *Model System of Development and Aging of the Nervous System*. Vernadakis, A., Privat, J. M., Lauder, P. S., Timiras, P. S., and Giacobini, E., Martinius Nijhoff, Boston. p. 453, 1987.

101. MacLeich, P. R. and Townes-Anderson, E., Growth and synapse formation among major classes of adult salamander retinal neurons *in vitro. Neuron,* 1:751, 1988.

102. Stone, L. S., The role of retina pigment cells in regenerating neural retinae of adult Salamander eyes. *J. Exp. Zool.,* 113:9, 1950.

103. Draves, D. J., Manley, N. B., and Timiras, P. S., Glia hormone receptors: Thyroid hormones and microtubules in gliomas and neuroblastomas. In: *Astrocytes: Cell Biology & Pathology of Astrocytes,* Vol. 3. Fedoroff, S. and Vernadakis, A., Eds., Academic Press, New York. p. 186, 1986.

104. Geel, S. E. and Gonzales, L. W., Cerebral cortical ganglioside and glycoprotein metabolism in immature hypothyroidism. *Brain Res.,* 128:515, 1977.

105. Geel, S. E. and Timiras, P. S., The influence of neonatal hypothyroidism and thyroxine on the RNA and dRNA concentrations of rat cerebral cortex. *Brain Res.,* 4:135, 1967.

106. Valcana, T., Effect of neonatal hypothyroidism on the development of brain. In: *Influence of Hormones on the Nervous System.* Ford, D. H., Ed., Proc. Intl. Soc. Psychoneuroendocrin, Brooklyn. S Karger, Basel. pp. 174, 1971.

107. Valcana, T. and Eberhardt, N. L., Effects of neonatal hypothryoidism on protein synthesis in the developing rat brain: An open question. In: *Thyroid Hormones & Brain Development.* Group, G. D., Ed., Raven Press, New York. pp. 271, 1977.

108. Valcana, T. and Timiras, P. S., Effect of hypothyroidism on ionic metabolism and Na-K-activated ATP phosphohydrolase activity in the developing rat brain. *J. Neurochem* ., 16:935, 1969.

109. Valcana, T. and Timiras, P. S., Effect of thyroid hormones on ionic metabolism of the developing rat brain. In: *Hormones in Development.* Hamburgh, M. and Barrington, E. J. W., Eds., Appleton-Century-Crofts, New York. pp. 453, 1971.

110. Valcana, T., Einstein, E. M., Csegley, J., Dalal, K. R., and Timiras, P. S., Influence of thyroid hormones on myelin proteins in the developing rat brain. *J. Neurol. Sci.,* 25:19, 1975.

111. Meisami, E., Complete recovery of growth deficits after reversal of PTU-induced postnatal hypothyroidism in female rat: A model for catch-up growth. *Life Sci.,* 34:1487, 1984.

112. Tamasy, V., Meisami, E., Du, J. Z., and Timiras, P. S., Exploratory behavior, learning ability and thyroid hormonal responses to stress in female rats rehabilitating from postnatal hypothyroidism. *Devel. Psychobiol.,* 19:537, 1986.

113. Tamasy, V., Meisami, E., Du, J. Z., and Timiras, P. S., Rehabilitation from neonatal hyperthyroidism: Spontaneous motor activity, exploratory behavior, avoidance learning and responses of pituitary thyroid axis to stress in male rats. *Psychoneuroendocrinology* 11:91, 1986.

114. Draves, D. J. and Timiras, P. S., Differential effects of altered thyroid hormone state on nervous tumor cell lines. In: *Multidisciplinary Approach to Brain Development.* Benedetta, C. D., Balazs, R., Gombos, G., and Procellati, G., Eds., Elsevier, Amsterdam. pp. 313, 1980.

115. Draves, D. J. and Timiras, P. S., Thyroid hormone effects in neural (tumor) cell culture: Differential effects on triiodothyronine nuclear receptors, Na$^+$, K$^+$-ATPase activity, and intracellular electrolyte levels. In: *Tissue Culture in Neurobiology.* Giacobini, E., Shahar, A., and Vernadakis, A., Eds., Raven Press, New York. pp. 291, 1980.

116. Spiegelman, B. M., Lopata, M. S., and Kischner, M. W., Aggregation of microtubule initiation sites preceeding neurite outgrowth in mouse neuroblastoma cells. *Cell,* 16:253, 1979.

117. Nunez, J., Felous, A., Francon, J., and Lennon, A. M., Competitive inhibition of colchicine binding to tubulin by microtubule-associated proteins. *Proc. Natl. Acad. Sci. U.S.A.,* 76:86, 1979.

118. Vernadakis, A., Hormonal factors in the proliferation of glial cells in culture. In: *Influence of Hormones on the Nervous System.* Ford, D. H., Ed., S. Karger, Basel. pp. 42, 1971.

119. Grasso, K. J., Transient inhibition of cell proliferation in rat glioma monolayer cultures by cortisol. *Cancer Res.,* 36:2408, 1976.

120. Mealy, J. Jr., Chen, T. T., and Schanz, G. P., Effects of donamethasone and methylprednisolone on cell cultures of human glioblastomas. *J. Neurosur.,* 34:324-334, 1971.

121. Smith, B. J., Torday, J. S. and Giroud, C. J. P., Evidence for different gestation-dependent effects of cortisol on cultured fetal lung cells. *J. Clin. Invest.,* 53:1518, 1974.

122. Bennett, K., McGinnis, J. F., and de Vellis, J., Reversible inhibition of the hydrocortisone induction of glycerol phosphate dehydrogenase by cytochalasin B in rat glial C6 cells. *J, Cell Physiol.,* 86:523, 1977.

123. McGinnis, J. T. and de Vellis, J., Glucocorticoid regulation in rat cell cultures. *J. Biol. Chem.,* 253:8483, 1978.

124. Holbrook, N. J., Grasso, R. J., and Hackney, J. F., Glucocorticoid receptor properties and glucocorticoid regulation of glutamine synthetase activity in sensitive C6 and resistant C6H glial cells. *J. Neurosci. Res.,* 6:75, 1981.

125. Juurlink, B. H., Schousboe, A., Jorgensen, O. S., and Hertz, L., Induction of hydrocortisone of glutamine synthetase in mouse primary astrocyte cultures. *J. Neurochem.* 36:136, 1981.

126. Pisnak, M. R. and Phillips, A. T., Glucocorticoid stimulation of glutamine synthetase production in cultured rat glioma cells. *J. Neurochem;* 34:866, 1980.

127. Moscona, A. A., Mayerson, P., and Moscona, M., Induction of glutamine synthetase in the neural retina of the chick embryo: Localization of the enzyme in Müller fibers and effects of BrdU on cell separation. In: *Tissue Culture in Neurobiology.* Giacobini, E., Vernadakis, A., and Shahar, A., Eds., Raven Press, New York. p. 111, 1980.

128. Beaumont, K., Rat C6 glioma cells contain Type I as well as Type II corticosteroid receptors. *Brain Res.* 342:252, 1985.

129. Beaumont, K., Adrenocorticoid receptors in C6 glioma cells: Effects on cell growth. *Neurochem. Res.,* 12:701, 1987.

130. Vernadakis, A. and Woodbury, D. M., Effect of cortisol on the electroshock seizure thresholds in developing rats. *J, Pharmacol, Exp, Ther.,* 139:110-113, 1963.

131. Vernadakis, A. and Woodbury, D. M., Effects of cortisol on maturation of the central nervous system. In: *Influence of Hormones on the Nervous System.* Ford, D. H., Ed., S. Karger, Basel. p. 85-97, 1971.

132. Iversen, L. L. and Salt, P. J., Inhibition of catecholamine Uptake-2 by steroids in the isolated rat heart. *Br. J. Pharmacol.,* 40:528, 1970.

133. Vernadakis, A., Neurotransmission: A proposed mechanism of steroid hormones in the regulation of brain function. In: *Proc. Mie. Conf. Intl. Soc. Psychoneuroendocrin.,* Hatotani, N., Ed., S. Karger, Basel. p. 251-258, 1974.

134. Kimelberg, K. H., Catecholamine and serotonin uptake in astrocytes. In: *Astrocytes Vol 2: Biochemistry, Physiology, and Pharmacology of Astrocytes.* Federoff, S. and Vernadakis, A., Eds., Academic Press, New York. p. 107-131, 1986.

135. Vernadakis, A. and Sakellaridis, N., Role of glial cells in neurotransmission. In: *Progress in Neuroendocrinology.* Parvez, H., Parvez, S., and Gupta, G., Eds., VNU Science Press, The Netherlands. p. 17-44, 1985.

136. Horner, H. C., Packan, D. R., and Sapolsky, R. M., Glucocorticoids inhibit glucose transport in cultured hippocampal neurons and glia. *Neuroendocrinology,* 52:57-64, 1990.

137. Virgin, E. C., Jr., Ha, T. P.-I., Packan, D. R., Tombaugh, G. C., Pang, S. H., Horner, H. C., and Sapolsky, R. M., Glucocorticoids inhibit glucose transport and glutamate uptake in hippocampal astrocytes: Implications for glucocorticoid neurotoxicity. *J. Neurochem.,* 57:1422-1428, 1991.

138. Tombaugh, G. C., Yang, S. H., Swanson, R. A., and Sapolsky, R. M., Glucocorticoids exacerbate hypoxic and hypoglycemic hippocampal injury *in vitro*: Biochemical correlation and a role for astrocytes. *J. Neurochem.,* 59:137-146, 1992.

139. Tombaugh, G. C. and Sapolsky, R. M., Endocrine features of glucocorticoid endangerment in hippocampal astrocytes. *Neuroendocrinology,* 57:7-13, 1993.

140. Jung-Testas, I,. Hu, Z. Y., Baulieu, E. E., and Robel, P., Neurosteroids: Biosynthesis of pregnenolone and progesterone in primary cultures of rat glial cells. *Endocrinology,* 125:2083, 1989.

141. Kabbadj, K., El-Etr, M., Baulieu, E. E., and Robel, P., Pregnenolone metabolism in rodent embryonic neurons and astrocytes. *GLIA,* 7:170, 1993.

142. Majewska, M. D., Harrison, N. L., Schwartz, R. D., Barker, J., and Paul, S. M., Steroid hormone metabolites are barbiturate-like modulators of the GABA receptor. *Science,* 232:1004, 1986.

143. Paul, S. M. and Purdy, R. H., Neuroactive steroids. *FASEB J,* 6:2311, 1992.

144. Akwa, Y., Sahanes, N., Gouezou, M., Robel, P., Baulieu, E. E., and Le Goascogne, C.. Astrocytes and neurosteroids: Metabolism of pregnenolone and dehydroepiandrosterone. Regulation by cell density. *J. Cell Biol.,* 121:135, 1993.

145. Baulieu, E. E. and Robel, P., Neurosteroids: A new brain function? *J. Steroid Biochem. Mol. Biol.,* 37:395, 1990.

146. Vernadakis, A., Changes in astrocytes with aging. In: *Astrocytes, Biochemistry, Physiology, and Pharmacology of Astrocytes.* Fedoroff, S. and Vernadakis, A., Eds., Academic Press, New York. pp. 377, 1986.

147. Parker, K. P., Norenberg, M. D., and Vernadakis, A., Transdifferentiation of C6 glial cells in culture. *Science,* 208:179, 1980.

148. Poduslo, S. E. and Norton, W. T., Isolation and some chemical properties of oligodendroglia from calf brain. *J. Neurochem.,* 19:727, 1972.

149. Norenberg, M. D. and Martinez-Hernandez, A., Fine structural localization of glutamine synthetase in astrocytes of rat brain. *Brain Res.,* 161:303, 1979.

150. Mangoura, D., Sakellaridis, N., Jones, J., and Vernadakis, A., Early and late passage C6 glial cell growth: Similarities with primary glial cells in culture. *Neurochem. Res.,* 14:941, 1989.

151. Lee, K., Billie, H., Bruce, C., Kentroti, S., and Vernadakis, A., Comparative biochemical, morphological, and immunocytochemical studies between C6 glial cells of early and late passages and advanced passages of glial cells derived from aged mouse cerebral hemispheres. *GLIA,* 6:245, 1992.

152. Lee, K., Kentroti, S., and Vernadakis, A., Differences in neuronal and glial cell phenotypic expression in neuron-glia co-cultures: Influence of glia-conditioned media and living glia cell substrata. *Brain Res. Bull.,* 28:861, 1992.

153. Kentroti, S., Baker, R., Lee, K., Bruce, C., and Vernadakis, A., Platelet-activating factor increases glutamine synthetase in early and late passage C6 glia glioma cells. *J. Neurosci. Res.,* 28:497, 1991.

154. Brodie, C. and Vernadakis, A., Muscle-derived factors induce proliferation and astrocytic phenotypic expression in C6 glial cells. *GLIA,* 4:269, 1991.

155. Hertz, L. and Schousboe, A., Primary cultures of GABAergic and glutamatergic neurons as model systems to study neurotransmitter functions. I. Differentiated cells. In: *Model Systems of Development and Aging of the Nervous System.* Vernadakis, A., Privat, A., Lauder, J. L., Timiras, P. S., and Giacobini, E., Eds., Martinius Nijhoff, Boston, MA. p. 19, 1987.

156. Coyle, J. T., Bird, S. J., Evans, R. H., Gulley, R. L., Nadler, J. V., Nicklas, W. J., and Olney, J.W., Excitatory amino acid neurotoxins: Selectivity, specificity, and mechanisms of action. *Neurosci. Res. Prog. Bull.,* 19:331, 1981.

157. Reier, P. J., Gliosis following CNS injury: The anatomy of astrocytic scars and their influences on axonal elongation. In: *Astrocytes,* Vol. 3., Federoff, S. and Vernadakis, A., Eds. Academic Press, New York. p. 263, 1986.

17

Signal Transduction and Aging

James A. Joseph and Rafael Villalobos-Molina

CONTENTS

I. INTRODUCTION

As this book testifies, the manifestations of aging are multifactorial.[1,2] The frequency of decrements in central neural function is reflected in motor activity and certain types of memory[3] function is continuously increasing in the aging population (see Chapters 4, 16, and 21).

Unfortunately, very little is known about the mechanisms involved in these age-related deficits in memory and motor functions, and attempts to reverse or retard their decline have been, with very few exceptions, singularly unsuccessful. One promising avenue of research that we have been exploring involves the examination of the nature of the rather ubiquitous loss in neurotransmitter receptor sensitivity that occurs in aging. This age-related loss in receptor sensitivity is seen in several receptor systems including: cholinergic (see below), β-adrenergic (receptor-mediated relaxation of vasculature;[4,5] cardiovascular function;[6] inhibitory efficacy of norepinephrine on electrophysiological responses of cerebellar Purkinje cells[7]); and dopaminergic (e.g., reduced rotational behavioral responses to amphetamine in senescent rats[8]). In two of the most important of these systems which are involved in memory and motor function (dopaminergic and cholinergic), these alterations appear to be the result of decreases in the receptor number[9,10] and impairment in second messenger generation after receptor stimulation (see Chapter 19).[10,11]

In this chapter we will focus on a discussion of the nature of the decreased signal transduction (ST) in the aged brain and an outline of recent findings which may describe the mechanisms involved both in the ST decline and in the cell loss during aging. An emphasis also will be placed on other avenues of exploration that could be addressed in further research efforts.

II. SIGNAL TRANSDUCTION

There are few instances where the loss in receptor sensitvity during aging is more salient, behaviorally, than in decreased cognitive function. It has been postulated for a number of years that the age-related decreases in cognitive function are the result of alterations in the functioning of the central cholinergic systems. It is known that these systems (e.g., hippocampus and basal forebrain) play a major role in memory processing through the activation of muscarinic receptors (mAChR).[12,13] Loss of mAChR functioning may be at least partially responsible for this marked deterioration of cognitive function in normal aging, and more notably, Alzheimer's disease (AD). Previous work has shown virtually no success in improving performance in memory tasks in senescent animals or humans with cholinergic enhancing agents,[2,14-16] but these agents are quite effective in young animals with experimentally compromised cholinergic function.[17]

One reason that this replacement is not effective in senescent organisms may be that other systems are involved in the acquisition of memory (e.g., NMDA),[18,19] as well as in long-term potentiation (LTP).[20,21] However, cholinergic replacement for treatment of memory disorders also may involve either direct or indirect stimulation of mAChR, and, as stated above, it appears that there is a loss of sensitivity of these receptors in senescence.

Alteration during aging in second messenger generation after receptor occupancy has been well documented in recent years. The ST model for the generation of the second messenger 1,4,5-inositol trisphosphate (IP_3) (induced by M_1 and M_3 mAChR activation) is initiated by the binding of an agonist to a membrane receptor. The mAChR are part of a family of receptors that, structurally, contain seven membrane-spanning regions[22,24] (others include α_1 adrenergic; 5-HT_2 serotonergic; H_1 histaminergic; V_1 vasopressin, etc.) that are coupled to the phosphoinositide-calcium system through a G protein (α, β, and γ heterotrimer, the α subunit has an intrinsic GTPase activity) and to phospholipase C (PLC).[25]

Transduction is initiated once the ligand is bound to the receptor which, in turn, is coupled to the G protein. This configuration is called the **ternary complex (agonist-receptor-G protein)**. The formation of a ternary complex between the agonist (**A**), the receptor (**R**), and the **G** protein (**A-R-G**) as the functional unit in the transduction sequence was originally proposed by De Lean et al.;[26] the model involves the interaction between **A** and **R**, which can be present in two affinity states, low (L) and high (H), the latter affinity state (**A**R**H**) is thought to be associated to the **G** protein (see Figure 1 in Reference 30). Confirmation of this model has been accomplished by competitive binding techniques in which the use of nonhydrolizable GTP analogues [Gpp(NH)p; GTPγ(S)] shift the shape of the curve, indicating that the entire receptor population has conformationally changed to a low affinity state.[27-29] Until recently, only binding techniques were used to study the kinetics of this model, however, findings have been supported by using different approaches, such as the continuous spectrofluorometric measurement of the **A-R-G** that allows the temporal analysis of the coupling/uncoupling among the components of the complex;[30] the use of sucrose gradients, after receptor solubilization, to separate the complex by molecular weight;[31] the use of wheat germ agglutinin-agarose, after receptor solubilization, and binding or affinity labeling to define the G proteins involved in signal transduction;[32] and the use of antibodies against the receptor or the G protein to immunoprecipitate the complex.[33]

In the ternary complex, Gα uncouples from the G protein and binds GTP (guanosine triphosphate) displacing GDP (guanosine diphosphate) from the previous activation cycle, releases the $\beta\gamma$ complex and activates PLC, which hydrolizes phosphatidylinositol 4,5-bisphosphate (PIP_2) and produces IP_3 and diacylglycerol (DAG).[25] The activation cycle ends when Gα hydrolizes GTP and is able to reassociate with $\beta\gamma$ (see Figures 1 and 2 in Reference

**TABLE 17-1   Decrease in Second Messenger Generation/
Physiological Response During Aging in Rat Tissues**

Tissue	Second messengers/functions						
	IP	IP$_3$	Ca^{2+}	GTPase	Contr	cAMP	GP a
Liver	nc[36]					–[36,42]	–[42]
Brain	–[40]		–[39]	–[11,46,47]		–[57]	
	+[10]						
	nc[37]						
Parotids	–[51]	–[27,41]	–[27,41]	–[27]		nc[51,79]	
VSM					–[28,53]		
Heart					–[43,80]		

Note: nc, no change; +, increase; –, decrease of second messenger/response compared
to young rat tissues; IP, inositol phosphates; IP$_3$, inositol 1,4,5-trisphosphate;
Contr, contraction; GP a, glycogen phosphorylase a.

25). More recent studies have also ascribed a role to the βγ subunits as well as modulators per se of ionic channels (Ca^{2+}, K$^+$), PLCβ$_2$, and adenylyl cyclase II.[34,35]

It is obvious that decrements in any step of the ST pathway will result in decreases in the responsiveness of the system. In this regard, some researchers have reported decrements in the production of IP$_3$, while others have reported no changes in inositol phosphates (IP),[36] or even increases in IP,[10] (Table 17-1). It is important to note that the studies in which negative results were observed assessed the total accumulation of inositol phosphates in various regions of rat brain,[37,38] not IP$_3$ specifically. There have also been reports indicating decreases in the mobilization of intracellular Ca^{2+},[27,39-41] in cAMP levels and phosphorylase activity,[42] agonist-induced contraction,[43-45] and low Km GTPase activity[9-11] following receptor activation. This latter finding is of particular interest since it has been observed following mAChR activation both in striatum of the aged rat[46] and in AD.[47] Moreover, the degree of decrease of low Km GTPase activity appears to increase as a function of the duration of the disease.[47]

The suggested mechanism involved in these ST decrements appears to involve alterations in the coupling/uncoupling between the receptor and the G protein, since several studies have indicated that whenever the ligand-mAChR-G-protein interfaces are "bypassed", the age-related decrements in signal transduction are reduced, suggesting that the deficits occur early in the process. As examples, application of NaF (unpublished observations), IP$_3$, or the Ca^{2+} ionophore A23187 to the striatal slices to enhance oxotremorine-stimulation of K$^+$-evoked dopamine release (K$^+$-ERDA) from perifused slices of old (24 month) rats indicated no age differences in the enhancement.[48]

The exact nature of these putative changes in receptor-G protein coupling awaits further specification. It is possible that factors such as the composition of the membrane bilayer,[49-52] the phosphorylation state of the receptor,[53] the availability of G proteins,[54] and/or the activation/inactivation cycle of the G protein may be involved. The exact contribution of each of these components to the age-related ST changes awaits further research. However, it appears that some membrane parameters such as shape, permeability, and osmotic fragility are determined by membrane phospholipids — alterations in membrane structure may be a major factor contributing to these age-related ST declines. It is known that there are alterations in membrane fluidity,[50-52] cholesterol/phospholipid ratio,[50-52] and sphingomyelin[55] content with age. Moreover, recent research[56] indicates that both oxotremorine-enhanced K$^+$-ERDA and carbachol-stimulated low Km GTPase activity in striatal slices from old rats can be increased by preincubating the tissue with S-adenosyl-methionine, a membrane fluidizing agent. Conversely, treatment of striatal slices from young (6 month) rats with cholesterol reduces both of these indices.[56]

It appears, then, that alterations in ST during aging can have a profound effect on the receptor's ability to respond to stimulation and that one important factor mediating these

TABLE 17-2   Age Changes in Receptor Number in Different Species and Tissues

Species	Tissue/receptor	α	β	M	μ	D	5-HT
Rat	Brain	−[50]	−[57]	−[9,10,77]	−[60]	−[66-68,70]	
		nc[57]		nc[10,77]			
			+[57]				
	Heart	−[43]					
	Liver	−[42]	−[42]				
	VSM	nc[45]					
Human	Brain					−[58,78]	−[58]
Bovine	VSM	+[44]					

Note: α, β, adrenergic; M, muscarinic; μ, opioid; D, dopamine; 5-HT, serotonergic, receptors; VSM, vascular smooth muscle; nc, no change; +, increase; −, decrease in receptor number.

declines may be structural alterations in receptor-containing membranes.

III. RECEPTOR LOSS IN AGING

A decrease in the receptor number during aging has been described for adrenergic (α and β),[43,57] cholinergic,[9] dopaminergic and serotonergic,[58,59] and opioid[60] systems in different species and tissues (Table 17-2). However, there is controversy since some reports show no change in the number of some types of receptors with age,[10,57] or even an increase in their number.[44,57] One possible explanation for these results is that the methodology commonly used to assess the receptor number is binding, which only quantifies the specific sites in isolated membranes in a given moment, but gives no information about the dynamics to which the receptor is subjected throughout the life of the cell (i.e., turnover ratio, exposure in the membrane due to up- or down-regulation, sequestration inside the cell, etc.). Additionally, it is necessary to note that with so many receptor subtypes currently known[22] and the presence of spare receptors in many tissues,[61] it is possible to underestimate the receptor number.

However, some research attempts have been made to link receptor loss with more functional assessments of age-related neuronal and behavioral alterations. This has been done with respect to both the dopamine (DA) and mAChR receptors. In the case of DA receptors, investigators have identified, cloned, and sequenced several dopamine receptor subtypes (e.g., D_1,[59] D_{2S}, D_{2L}[62]) and identified them in the brain.[58,59] Only the D_1 and D_2 receptor subtypes have been examined in any great detail thus far in aging, and many of these determinations have focused on the striatum. Previous reviews[63-65] have indicated that there are profound declines in the concentrations of the D_2 receptors as a function of age. This loss is accompanied by decreases in D_2 mRNA levels[66] and synthesis.[67] In fact, D_2 receptor loss is one of the most consistent and widespread manifestations of brain aging.[58,68] Conversely, age-related D_1 receptor changes appear to be more variable and are highly strain and species dependent.[65,69,70] Although the pattern of loss may be different for the D_1 and D_2 subtypes, it is clear that the importance of the striatal D_1 and D_2 receptors in mediating motor behavioral control cannot be overestimated. A functional link was established with receptor number and motor behavior, since both experimental up- and down-regulation of these receptors can produce, respectively, deficits or improvements in motor behavioral performance.[63]

Similar functional links have also been established with mAChR number and the degree of oxotremorine-evoked DA release when Yamagami et al.[9] showed that there was a high positive significant correlation between oxotremorine-enhanced K^+-ERDA and overall mAChR concentration ($r = 0.60$). However, when two of the five[71] mAChR subtypes were assessed separately, the results indicated that the receptor concentration for m_2AChR was more highly correlated with the degree of oxotremorine enhancement of K^+-ERDA ($r = 0.71$) than m_1AChR

($r = 0.34$). Unfortunately, pharmacologic agents which would specify the role in oxotremorine-enhanced K^+-ERDA among the other various receptor subtypes are not available.

IV. PERSPECTIVES

Loss of sensitivity in neurotransmitter receptor signal transduction is one of the main problems occurring during aging that could lead to cognitive deficiency as well as decreased motor skills. Approaches such as the ones described above, which are directed toward understanding the nature of altered signal transduction in senescence, may be fruitful. One focus might be to more fully characterize the relationship between the receptor-G protein interface and to devise more specific measures of coupling/uncoupling between these entities. Our research has shown that although a binary complex is formed between a labeled antagonist (prazosin or QNB) and the receptor α_1-adrenergic or muscarinic, respectively [as detected by the sucrose gradient or the anti G(common α) methods[72]], the formation of the ternary complex was undetected by sucrose gradient when a labeled agonist was present. This was may be the result of to a dissociation between the agonist and the receptor; however, the use of specific G protein antibodies may help determine, quantitatively, age differences in ternary complex formation in several brain regions (e.g., cortex, striatum, and hippocampus[72]). The hypothesis being tested is that a lower number of ternary complexes will be found in tissues obtained from senescent rats as a result of phosphorylation of the receptor. A phosphorylated receptor cannot interact with its respective G protein and as a consequence a lower amount of second messengers are produced upon stimulation. Also important in this regard would be to characterize striatal and hippocampal neuronal membrane phospholipids (e.g., cholesterol/phospholipid ratios, sphingomyelin, phosphatidylserine, etc.), as well as membrane fluidity changes that may contribute to altered function of the ternary complex in aging.

A second approach might be to characterize the various effector-phospholipase C isoforms that ultimately initiate second messenger production. Their specification may give us a better understanding of the fine regulation in signal transduction. It also should be mentioned that further clarification is needed of how we might take advantage of "cross talk" among transduction systems to enhance signal transduction in senescence. This also might help explain how this dynamic process is kept active throughout the lifespan of cells, and if one or more of the macromolecules involved is (are) missing/altered during senescence.

While the further determinations of the nature of ST deficits during aging are imperative, equally important are studies directed toward elaborating the factors involved in receptor loss and cell death in aging. Research has suggested that these ST deficits and receptor loss may share a common mechanism that involves oxidative damage. If this is the case then it might be possible to retard or reverse these age-related changes through nutritional modification with antioxidants alone, or with agents that increase the availability of dopamine or acetylcholine. It might also be possible to retard age-related neuronal cell loss via reductions in glutamate and Ca^{2+} release. It has been shown, for example, that large increases in these agents (e.g., following application of neurotoxins such as kainic acid) ultimately results in oxidative stress and cell death.

However, although the "free radical hypothesis of aging" has been examined for more than 30 years,[73-76] it is only recently that the possible involvement of free radicals in neuronal dysfunction is beginning to be characterized. As examples:

1. Very little is known about locus and mechanism of oxidative damage in neuronal cell death in aging.
2. Virtually no information exists on the factors involved in selective vulnerability of neurons to oxidative damage.
3. The putative site of membrane damage and subsequent alterations in membrane-G protein interactions remain to be specified.

4. Determinations of interactions between decreased ability to reduce oxidative damage and increased membrane cholesterol that is seen in senescence have not been carried out.
5. Attempts to reduce neuronal "biomarkers of aging" with nitrone trapping agents or antioxidants are only now beginning to be addressed.

In this regard, it might be said that the majority of studies concerned with examining the effects of dietary antioxidants have focussed on tissues other than brain.

It should be evident from the above discussion that a multidisciplinary approach should be utilized to solve these deficits in neuronal function in senescence. If this is done, perhaps some of the alterations can be corrected or prevented and decrements in behavior reduced.

ACKNOWLEDGMENT

Research carried out in RVM's laboratory is partially supported by Grant LA-92-2-07 from the Sandoz Foundation for Gerontological Research.

REFERENCES

1. Global Aging: Comparative Indicators and Future Trends, CIR Population Studies, U.S. Department of Commerce, Washington, D.C., 1991.
2. Bartus, R. T., Drugs to treat age-related neurodegenerative problems. The final frontier of medical science?, *J. Amer. Ger. Soc.*, 38, 680, 1990.
3. Coleman, P., Personal communication, 1994.
4. Deisher, T. A., Mankani, S., and Hoffman, B. B., Role of cyclic AMP-dependent protein kinase in the diminished β adrenergic responsiveness of vascular smooth muscle with increasing age. *J. Pharmacol. Exptl. Ther.*, 249, 812, 1989.
5. Hiremath, A. N., Pershe, R. A., Hoffman, B. B., and Blaschke T. F., Comparison of age-related changes in prostaglandin E1 and β-adrenergic responsiveness of vascular smooth muscle in adult males. *J. Geront.*, 44, M13, 1989.
6. Lakatta, E. G., Diminished beta-adrenergic modulation of cardiovascular function in advanced age. *Cardiol. Clin.*, 4, 185, 1986.
7. Hoffer, B. J., Rose, G., Parfitt, K., Freedman, R., and Bickford-Wimer, P. C., Age-related changes in cerebellar noradrenergic function, in *Central Determinants of Age Related Declines in Motor Function*, Joseph, J. A., Ed., New York Academy of Sciences, 1988.
8. Joseph, J. A., Berger, R. E., Engel, B. T., and Roth, G. S., Age-related changes in the nigrostriatum. A behavioral and biochemical analysis. *J. Geront.*, 33, 64, 1978.
9. Yamagami, K., Joseph, J. A., and Roth, G. S., Muscarinic receptor concentrations and dopamine release in aged striata. *Neurobiol. Aging*, 13, 51, 1991.
10. Mundy, W., Tandon, P., Ali, S., and Tilson, H., Age-related changes in receptor-mediated phosphoinositide hydrolysis in various regions of rat brain. *Life Sci.*, 49, PL-97, 1991.
11. Villalobos-Molina, R., Joseph, J. A., and Roth, G. S., α_1 - Adrenergic stimulation of low K_M GTPase in rat striata is diminished with age. *Brain Res.*, 590, 303, 1992.
12. Bartus, R. T., Dean R. L., Beer, B., and Lippa, A. S., The cholinergic hypothesis of geriatric memory dysfunction. *Science*, 217, 408, 1982.
13. Fibiger, H. C., Cholinergic mechanisms in learning, memory and dementia: a review of recent evidence. *Trends in Neurosciences*, 14, 220, 1991.
14. Sherman, K. A., Kumar, V., Ashford, J. W., Murphy, J. W., Elble, R. J., and Giacobini, E., Effect of oral physostigmine in senile dementia patients. Utility of blood cholinesterase inhibition and neuroendocrine response to define pharmacokinetics and pharmacodynamics, in *Central Nervous System Disorders of Aging: Clinical Intervention and Research*, Strong, R., Wood, W. G., and Burke, W. J., Eds., Raven Press, New York, 1988, p. 71.
15. Flood, J. F. and Cherkin, A., Effect of acute arecoline, tacrine and arecoline + tacrine post-training administration on retention in old mice, *Neurobiol. Aging*, 9, 5, 1988.
16. Bartus, R. T. and Dean, R. L., Tetrahydroaminoacridine, 3, 4 diaminopyridine and physostigmine: direct comparison of effects on memory in aged primates. *Neurobiol. Aging*, 9, 351, 1988.
17. Haroutunian, V., Kanof, P., and Davis, K. L., Pharmacological alleviation of cholinergic lesion induced memory deficits in rats, *Life Sci.*, 37, 945, 1985.

18. Cotman, C. W. and Iversen, L. L., Excitatory amino acids in the brain-focus on NMDA receptors. *Trends Neurosci.*, 10, 263, 1987.

19. Gustafsson, B. and Wigstrom, H., Physiological mechanisms underlying LTP. *Trends Neurosci.*, 11, 156, 1988.

20. Collingridge, G. L. and Bliss, T. V. P., NMDA receptors. Their role in long-term potentiation. *Trends Neurosci.*, 10, 288, 1987.

21. Zolutsky, R. A. and Nicoll, R. A., Comparison of two forms of long-term potentiation in single hippocampal neurons. *Science,* 248, 1619, 1990.

22. Watson, S. and Abbott, A., Receptor nomenclature, *Trends Pharmacol. Sci.*, Supplement p,1, 1992.

23. Peralta, E. G., Winslow, J. W., Ashkenazi, A., Smith, D. H., Ramachandran, J., and Capon, D. J., Structural basis of muscarinic acetylcholine receptor subtype diversity, *Trends Pharmacol. Sci.*, Supplement: Subtypes of muscarinic receptors III, p. 6, 1988.

24. Wheatley, M., Hulme, E. C., Birdsall, N. J. M., Curtis, C. A. M., Eveleigh, P., Pedder, E. K., and Poyner, D., Peptide mapping on muscarinic receptors: receptor structure and location of the ligand binding site, *Trends Pharmacol. Sci.*, Supplement: Subtypes of muscarinic receptors III, p. 9, 1988.

25. Berridge, M. J., Inositol trisphosphate and calcium signalling, *Nature*, 361, 315, 1993.

26. De Lean, A., Stadel, J. M., and Lefkowitz, R. J., A ternary complex model explains the agonist-specific binding properties of the adenylate cyclase-coupled β-adrenergic receptor, *J. Biol. Chem.*, 255, 7108, 1980.

27. Miyamoto, A., Villalobos-Molina, R., Kowatch, M. A., and Roth, G. S., Altered coupling of α_1-adrenergic receptor-G protein in rat parotid during aging, *Amer. J. Physiol.*, 262, C1181, 1991.

28. Jagadeesh, G., Tian, W.-N., and Deth, R. C., Agonist-induced modulation of agonist binding to α_1-adrenoceptors in bovine aorta, *Eur. J. Pharmacol. MO.*, 208, 163, 1991.

29. Johansson, L.-H., Persson, H., and Rosengren, E., The role of Mg^{2+} on the formation of the ternary complex between agonist, β- adrenoceptor, and G_s-protein and an interpretation of high and low affinity binding of β-adrenoceptor agonists, *Pharmacol. Toxicol.*, 70, 192, 1992.

30. Posner, R. G., Fay, S. P., Domalewski, M. D., and Sklar, L. A., Continuous spectrofluorometric analysis of formyl peptide receptor ternary complex interactions, *Mol. Pharmacol.*, 45, 65, 1994.

31. Kimura, N. and Shimada, N., Evidence for complex formation between GTP binding protein (G_s) and membrane-associated nucleoside diphosphate kinase, *Biochem. Biophys. Res. Comm.*, 168, 99, 1990.

32. Im, M.-J. and Graham, R. M., A novel guanine nucleotide-binding protein coupled to the α_1-adrenergic receptor, *J. Biol. Chem.,* 265, 18944, 1990.

33. Matesic, D. F., Manning, D. R., Wolfe, B. B., and Luthin, G. R., Pharmacological and biochemical characterization of complexes of muscarinic acetylcholine receptor and guanine nucleotide-binding protein, *J. Biol. Chem.*, 264, 21368, 1989.

34. Iniguez-Lluhi, J., Kleuss, C., and Gilman, A. G., The importance of G-protein $\beta\gamma$ subunits, *Trends in Cell Biology,* 3, 230, 1993.

35. Taussig, R., Iniguez-Lluhi, J., and Gilman, A. G., Inhibition of adenylyl cyclase by $G_{i\alpha}$, *Science,* 261, 218, 1993.

36. Borst, S. E. and Scarpace, P. J., Alpha₁-adrenergic stimulation of inositide hydrolysis in liver of senescent rats, *Mechanisms of Ageing and Development*, 56, 275, 1990.

37. Surichamorn, W., Abdallah, E. A. M., and El-Fakahany, E. E., Aging does not alter brain muscarinic receptor-mediated phosphoinositide hydrolysis and its inhibition by phorbol esters, tetrodotoxin and receptor desensitization. *J. Pharmacol. Exp. Ther.*, 251, 543, 1989.

38. Crews, F. T., Gonzales, R. A., Polovcik R., Phillips, M. I., Theiss, C., and Raizada, M., Changes in receptor-stimulated phosphoinositide hydrolysis in brain during ethanol administration, aging and other pathological conditions. *Psychopharmacol. Bull.*, 22, 775, 1986.

39. Burnett, D. M., Daniell, L. C., and Zahniser, N. R., Decreased efficacy of inositol 1,4,5-trisphosphate to elicit calcium mobilization from cerebrocortical microsomes of aged rats, *Mol. Pharmacol.*, 37, 566, 1990.

40. Burnett, D. M., Bowyer, J. F., Masserano, J. M., and Zahniser, N. R., Effect of aging on alpha-1 adrenergic stimulation of phosphoinositide hydrolysis in various regions of rat brain, *J. Pharmacol. Exptl. Ther.*, 255, 1265, 1990.

41. Villalobos-Molina, R., Miyamoto, A., Kowatch, M. A., and Roth, G. S., α_1-adrenoceptors in parotid cells: age does not alter the ratio of α_{1A} and α_{1B} subtypes, *Eur. J. Pharmacol. MO*, 226, 129, 1992.

42. Tsujimoto, A., Tsujimoto, G., and Hoffman, B. B., Age-related change in adrenergic regulation of glycogen phosphorylase in rat hepatocytes, *Mech. Ageing Dev.*, 33, 167, 1986.

43. Kimball, K. A., Cornett, L. E., Seipun, E., and Kennedy, R. H., Aging: changes in cardiac α_1-adrenoceptor responsiveness and expression. *Eur. J. Pharmacol. MO.*, 208, 231, 1991.

44. Jagadeesh, G., Tian, W.-N., Gupta, S., and Deth, R. C., Developmental changes in α_1-adrenoceptor coupling to G-protein in bovine aorta, *Eur. J. Pharmacol. MO.*, 189, 11, 1990.

45. Docherty, J. R. and Hyland, L., α-Adrenoreceptor responsiveness in the aged rat, *Eur. J. Pharmacol.*, 126, 75, 1986.

46. Yamagami, K., Joseph, J. A., and Roth, G. S., Decrement of muscarinic receptor-stimulated low Km GTPase in striatum and hippocampus from the aged rat. *Brain Res.*, 576, 327, 1992.

47. Cutler, R., Joseph, J. A., Yamagami, K., Villalobos-Molina, R., and Roth, G. S., Area specific alterations in muscarinic stimulated low-Km GTPase activity in aging and Alzheimer's disease: implications for altered signal transduction, *Brain Res.*, 664, 54, 1994.

48. Joseph, J. A., Dalton, T. K., Roth, G. S., and Hunt, W. A., Alterations in muscarinic control of striatal dopamine autoreceptors in senescence: a deficit at the ligand-muscarinic receptor interface?, *Brain Res.*, 454, 149, 1988.

49. Sargent, D. F. and Schwyzer, R., Membrane lipid phase as catalyst for peptide-receptor interactions, *Proc. Natl. Acad. Sci. U.S.A.*, 83, 5774, 1986.

50. Miyamoto, A., Araiso, T., Koyama, T., and Ohshika, H., Membrane viscosity correlates with α_1-adrenergic signal transduction of the aged rat cerebral cortex, *J. Neurochem.*, 55, 70, 1990.

51. Miyamoto, A., Araiso, T., Koyama, T., and Ohshika, H., Adrenoceptor coupling mechanisms which regulate salivary secretion during aging, *Life Sci.*, 53, 1873, 1993.

52. Tacconi, M. T., Cizza, G., Fumagalli G, Sartori, P. S., and Salmona, M., Effect of hypothyroidism induced in adult rats on brain membrane fluidity and lipid content and composition, *Research Communications in Chemical Pathology and Pharmacology*, 71, 85, 1991.

53. Jagadeesh, G. and Deth, R. C., Phorbol ester-induced modulation of agonist binding to alpha-1 adrenergic receptors in bovine aortic membranes, *J. Pharmacol. Exptl. Ther.*, 247, 196, 1988.

54. Kimura, H., Miyamoto, A., Kawana, S., and Ohshika, H., Characterization of α_1-adrenoceptors which mediate chronotropy in neonatal rat cardiac myocytes, *Comp. Biochem. Physiol.*, 105C, 479, 1993.

55. Kelly, J. F., Joseph, J. A., Denisova, N., Erat, S., Mason, R. P., and Roth, G. S., Dissociation of striatal GTPase and dopamine release responses to muscarinic cholinergic agonists in F344 rats. Influence of age and dietary manipulation, *J. Neurochem.*, in press.

56. Joseph, J. A., Villalobos-Molina, R., Yamagami, K., Kelly, J. and Roth, G. S., Age specific alterations in muscarinic stimulation of K$^+$-evoked dopamine release from striated slices by cholesterol and 5-adenosyl-L-methionine, *Brain Res.*, in press.

57. Scarpace, P. J. and Abrass, I. B., α and β-adrenergic receptor function in the brain during senescence. *Neurobiol. Aging*, 9, 53, 1988.

58. Iyo, M. and Yamasaki, T., The detection of age-related decrease of dopamine D1, D2 and serotonin 5-HT2 receptors in living human brain. *Prog. Neuro-Psychopharmacol. Biol. Psychiat.*, 17, 415, 1993.

59. Gerfen, C. R., Engber, T. M., Mahan, L. C., Susel, Z., Chase, T. N., Monsma, F. J., Jr., and Sibley, D. R., D_1 and D_2 dopamine receptor-regulated gene expression of striatonigral and striatopallidal neurons. *Science*, 250, 1429, 1990.

60. Bem, W. T., Yeung, S. J., Belcheva, M., Barg, J., and Coscia, C. J., Age-dependent changes in the subcellular distribution of rat brain μ-opioid receptors and GTP binding regulatory proteins, *J. Neurochem.*, 57, 1470, 1991.

61. Hamilton, C. A., Reid, J. L., and Sumner, D. J., Acute effects of phenoxybenzamine of α-adrenoceptor responses *in vivo* and *in vitro* — relation of *in vivo* pressor responses to the number of specific adrenoceptor binding sites, *J. Cardiovasc. Pharmacol.*, 5, 868, 1983.

62. Montmayeur, J. P., Bausero, P., Amlaiky, N., Maroteaux, L., Hen, R., and Borrelli, E., Differential expression of the mouse D_2 dopamine receptor isoforms. *FEBS Lett.*, 278, 239, 1991.

63. Joseph, J. A. and Roth, G. S., Upregulation of striatal dopamine receptors and improvement of motor performance in senescence, in *Central Determinants of Age related Declines in Motor Function*, Joseph, J. A., Ed., New York Academy of Sciences, 1988, 355.

64. Joseph, J. A. and Roth, G. S., Loss of agonist receptor efficacy in senescence. Possible decrements in second messenger function and calcium mobilization, *Challenges in Aging: The 1990 Sandoz Lectures in Gerontology*, Bergener, M., Ermini, M., and Stahelin, H. B., Eds., Academic Press, New York, 1991, 167.

65. Morgan, D. G., The dopamine and serotonin systems during aging in human and rodent brain. A brief review. *Progr. Neuropsychopharmacol. Biol. Psychiatr.*, 11, 153, 1987.

66. Mesco, E. R., Joseph, J. A., Blake, M. J., and Roth, G. S., Loss of D_2 receptors during aging is partially due to decreased levels of mRNA. *Brain Res.*, 545, 355, 1991.

67. Mesco, E. R., Carlson, S. G., Joseph, J. A., and Roth, G. S., Synthetic rate of D_2-dopamine receptor mRNA is selectively reduced during aging. *Mol. Brain Res.*, 17, 160, 1993.

68. Han, Z., Kuyatt, B. L., Kochman, K. A., DeSouza, E. B., and Roth, G. S., Effect of aging on concentrations of D_2-receptor-containing neurons in the rat striatum. *Brain Res.*, 498, 299, 1989.

69. Henry, J. M., Joseph, J. A., Kochman, K., and Roth, G. S., Effect of aging on striatal dopamine receptor subtype recovery following N-ethoxycarbonyl-2-ethoxy-1,2-dihydroquinoline blockade and relation to motor function in Wistar rats. *Brain Res.*, 418, 334, 1987.

70. Hyttel, J., Age related decrease in the density of dopamine D_1 and D_2 receptors in corpus striatum of rats. *Pharmacol. Toxicol.*, 61, 126, 1987.

71. Bonner, T. I., The molecular basis of muscarinic receptor diversity, *Trends Neurosci.,* 12, 148, 1989.
72. Villalobos-Molina, R., Shock, D., Pineyro, M. A., Roth, G. S., Strain, J., and Joseph, J. A., Isolation of ternary complex during aging, unpublished results.
73. Halliwell, B. and Gutteridge, J. M. C., *Free Radicals in Biology and Medicine*, Clarendon Press, Oxford, England, 1989.
74. Harman, D., Aging: a theory based on free radical and radiation chemistry. *J. Gerontol.*, 11, 298, 1955.
75. Harman, D., Role of free radicals in mutation, cancer, aging and maintenance of life. *Rad. Res.*, 16, 753, 1962.
76. Harman, D., The aging process. *Proc. Natl. Acad. Sci. U.S.A.*, 78, 7124, 1981.
77. Araujo, D. M., Lapchak, P. A., Meaney, M. J., Collier, B., and Quirion, R., Effects of aging on nicotinic and muscarinic autoreceptor function in the rat brain: relationship to presynaptic cholinergic markers and binding sites, *J. Neuroscience,* 10, 3069, 1990.
78. Rinne, J. O., Lonnberg, P., and Marjamaki, P., Age-dependent decline in human brain dopamine D_1 and D_2 receptors, *Brain Res.*, 508, 349, 1990.
79. Miyamoto, A., Kimura, H., Kawana, S., and Ohshika, H., Desensitization of the myocardial β-adrenergic receptor system in aged rats, in *The Mechanism and New Approach on Drug Resistance of Cancer Cells,* Miyazaki, T., Takaku, F., and Sakurada, K., Eds., Excerpta Medica, New York, 1993, 237.
80. Miyamoto, A., Kawana, S., Kimura, H., and Ohshika, H., Impaired expression of $G_{s\alpha}$ protein mRNA in rat ventricular myocardium with aging, *Eur. J. Pharmacol. MO,* 266, 147, 1994.

18

Steroid and Protein Regulators of Normal and Abnormal Cell Proliferation

Gary L. Firestone, Anita C. Maiyar, and Ross A. Ramos

CONTENTS

0-8493-2446-7/95/$0.00+$.50
© 1995 by CRC Press Inc.

I. CELL CYCLE REGULATION IN NORMAL AND TRANSFORMED CELLS

Normal development, differentiation, and proliferation of specific tissues and cell types within multicellular organisms are stringently regulated by a complex combination of environmental cues that include systemic steroid and protein hormones, local acting growth factors, extracellular matrix components, and cell-cell interactions. In most tissues, cell differentiation is accompanied by a cessation of proliferation. Maintenance of the growth arrested state is controlled by specific hormonal signals which inhibit the expression or activity of growth stimulatory factors and/or induce growth suppressor gene products.[1-6] However, for certain physiological processes, cell proliferation is necessary to maintain populations of specific cell types. For example, stem cells in the bone marrow provide a continuous source of hematopoietic cells in animals.[7] Quiescent cells (such as hepatocytes in the liver) will proliferate during tissue regeneration in a damaged organ,[8] whereas, mammary epithelial cells are hormonally stimulated to proliferate during pregnancy and lactation.[9] The maintenance of these cells in the proliferative state, or the triggering of quiescent cells to proliferate, requires the selective regulation of growth stimulatory gene products and/or suppression of growth inhibitory gene products. However, uncontrolled cellular proliferation in higher eukaryotes is often detrimental to the survival of the organism and can lead to the growth of a hyperplastic tissue mass known as a tumor. Thus, in contrast to their normal cell counterparts, a distinguishing feature of tumor cells is the lack of responsiveness to specific extracellular and hormonal signals, which often can result in the loss of growth regulation and uncontrolled proliferation under conditions where nontransformed cells would be quiescent.[1,2,10,11]

Although steroid and protein growth regulators act through different classes of receptors, the final targets of their respective signal transduction pathways are components of the cell proliferation machinery which modulate or control the ability of a cell to divide. The cell cycle is a designation used to describe the discrete steps that cells go through as they proliferate and is composed of four phases: G1 (Gap 1), S (DNA synthesis), G2 (Gap 2), and M (Mitosis) as well as an "out of cycle" quiescent phase designated G0.[12,13] In recent years, several classes of proteins have been characterized which drive the cell through selective places within the cell cycle culminating in cell division. These cell cycle regulators include the various cyclins (cyclin A, cyclin B, cyclin C, cyclin D1, cyclin D2, cyclin D3, and cyclin E) and several cyclin dependent kinases (cdk2, cdk4, cdk5, and p34[cdc2]) which can form specific cyclin-cdk complexes depending on the phase of the cell cycle[14,15] (Figure 1). Several other components of the cell cycle have been identified by their ability to interact with specific cyclin-cdk complexes. For example, the proliferating cell nuclear antigen (PCNA), a subunit of DNA polymerase δ often associated with known cdk substrates present at DNA replication origins, interacts directly with cyclin-cdk complexes.[14,16] Recently, several of the cyclin-cdk complex-associated proteins have been shown to act as inhibitors of the kinase activity (such as INK4, cip1, cip2, and p27) which cause an arrest in cell cycle progression[17,18] (Figure 1).

In normal and nontransformed cells, it has been proposed that cellular proliferation is mediated by the concerted action of cell cycle regulated genes which drive the cells through G1 and the rest of the cell cycle. In contrast, dysregulation of the G1 phase of the cell cycle has been implicated in the uncontrolled proliferation observed in many types of neoplastically transformed cells.[1,10,11,19-21] By this view, proliferative changes associated with the transformed

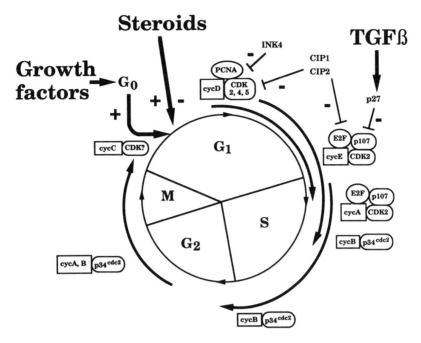

FIGURE 1   Cell cycle control by steroid and protein growth regulators. In mammalian cells, steroids and protein growth regulators exert most of their effects in the G1 phase of the cell cycle. Most growth factors and steroids act relatively early in G1, whereas, TGF-β inhibits cell cycle progression late in G1. The diagram shows the temporal appearance of cyclin complexes which form at specific steps within the cell cycle as well as the several recently discovered inhibitors of these complexes. cycA: cyclin A; cycB: cyclin B; cycC: cyclin C; cycD: cyclin D; cycE: cyclin E; CDK: cyclin dependent kinase; p34cdc2: cyclin dependent kinase-1; p107: Rb related protein; PCNA: proliferating cell nuclear antigen; E2F: E2F transcription factor; p27: TGF-β regulated cell cycle inhibitor; CIP: CDK-interacting protein; and INK4: 16,000-Da inhibitor of cyclin dependent kinase.

phenotype may result in part from the aberrant expression or activation of G1 associated genes, which selectively disrupt or overcome specific "check points" within the cell cycle.[1-3,10,11,21-24] For example, the development and proliferation of several types of tumors, such as breast cancers, have been associated with aberrant expression and/or amplification of cyclin D1 or cyclin E,[25-27] which function with their associated cdks (cyclin D1-cdk4 and cyclin E-cdk2) in the G1 phase of the cell cycle.[15,16,28] Alterations in mammalian G1 cyclin gene expression have been closely associated with changes in the proliferation rate of normal and tumor cells, not only following stimulation with peptide and steroid mitogens, but also upon growth arrest by steroid antagonists.[29-35] Various tumor cells can also inappropriately express normal or mutated G1 acting proto-oncogenes[36,37] as well as growth factors and/or their cognate receptors which stimulate progression through the G1 phase.[2,11,38,39] Furthermore, tumor cells can exhibit a loss in expression or function of certain growth suppressor genes (such as p53 and the retinablastoma tumor suppressor gene, Rb) which modulate cell cycle events late in the G1 phase.[3,23,40] Thus, a strong functional link has been established between hormone mediated disruptions in the regulation of G1 phase progression and the uncontrolled proliferation of cancer cells.

II. CELL CYCLE REGULATION BY STEROIDS, PROTEIN HORMONES, AND GROWTH FACTORS

In vitro and *in vivo* studies using many types of eukaryotic cells have uncovered different control points throughout the cell cycle.[11,22] In mammalian epithelial cells, control of the G1 phase by steroid hormones, protein growth factors, and other biological regulators appears to stringently control cell proliferation and differentiation.[11,31] The temporal location within G1 where extracellular signals act is dependent on the cell type, state of differentiation, and transformation, as well as the hormone and growth factor signals regulating the cell (Figure 1).

Steroid and steroid-like hormones which act through intracellular DNA binding receptors (see later section) have well-documented effects on the proliferation of a variety of normal and transformed cells, including those derived from the liver, pancreas, ovary, prostate, and mammary gland. Current evidence has shown that steroids and steroid antagonists exert their positive and negative growth effects relatively early in the G1 phase of the cell cycle[30-32,34,35] or, in some cases, by regulating entry into S phase.[41,42] For example, estrogens, which induce cell cycle progression early in G1, stimulate the proliferation of certain untransformed mammary cells as well as many breast cancer cells derived from hormone dependent tumors.[4,30-32,43] Progestins both stimulate and inhibit cell cycle progression in breast cancer cells. Intriguingly, in human T-47D breast cancer cells, the initial response to progestins is acceleration of the G1 phase, apparently due to stimulation of a rate limiting step in cell cycle progression.[44] However, following completion of a cell cycle, progestin treated cells are arrested in G1 phase. Antiprogestins arrest cells in the G1 phase with kinetics similar to those of growth arrested by antiestrogens.[33] Androgens can act as growth regulators of their respective target tissues; for example, treatment of human LNCaP prostatic cancer cells or hamster DDT-1 ductus deferens tumor cells with androgen accelerates progression to S phase.[42,45] Glucocorticoids block cell cycle progression of some hepatoma and mammary epithelial cell lines early in G1,[35,46-51] but stimulate the growth of certain pancreatic tumor cell lines and growth factor treated quiescent human WI-38 diploid fibroblasts.[52,53] Similarly, vitamin D3 prevents S phase entry in promyelocytic leukemia cells, as well as normal-like and malignant keratinocyte cell lines *in vitro*,[54,55] but accelerates S phase entry of rat liver cells *in vivo*.[56] Conceivably, steroid and steroid antagonists modulate the expression of a specific set of genes intimately involved in the control of cell cycle progression. Consistent with this notion, estrogens and progesterone stimulate cell cycle progression of the human T-47D breast cancer cell line with a concomitant stimulation of cyclin D1 expression,[32,44] whereas, antiestrogen treatment of T-47D mammary tumor cells coordinately reduce cyclin D1 expression and inhibit cell cycle progression.[30,32] In general, however, the molecular bases is unclear, in part because only a limited number of genes with potential cell cycle regulatory roles have been studied in hormone responsive cells.

The roles of protein growth factors in regulating progression through the cell cycle are well documented.[2,10,11,20] Growth factors generally act by inducing quiescent G0 cells to enter into and progress through G1 or by driving cells to cycle past a particular restriction point in G1. As part of the growth stimulatory mechanism, particular sets of cell cycle regulated G1 marker genes (such as the c-*fos* and c-*myc* proto-oncogenes) are temporally expressed in a specific pattern based on movement of the cells through G1 and into S phase.[11,20] Depending on the cell type, growth factors can either synergize with or override the effects of other growth regulatory hormones, or certain growth factor responses can be modulated by the presence of other environmental signals. For example, glucocorticoids can suppress the epidermal growth factor (EGF) mediated growth induction of adult rat hepatocytes *in vitro*,[57] whereas, EGF or transforming growth factor-α (TGF-α), which acts through the EGF receptor, can override the growth suppression effects of glucocorticoids in rat mammary tumor cells and in human submandibular salivary gland adenocarcinoma cells.[58-60] In addition, growth factors play an important role in conferring a proliferative advantage to tumors. For example, exogenous administration of EGF induces the proliferation of growth arrested rat H4IIE hepatoma cells and enhances the growth rate of hepatocellular carcinomas upon transplantation of liver cancer cell lines into athymic nude mice.[61,62] Moreover, many studies have documented that one mechanism by which transformed epithelial cells display a loss of environmental control is by the inappropriate production of growth factors and/or production or constitutive activation of their cognate receptors which can alter the way in which these cells function and respond to other extracellular signals.[2,10]

Transforming growth factor-β (TGF-β) is the most extensively characterized of the protein growth inhibitors.[63,64] TGF-β inhibits proliferation of a variety of epithelial cells by blocking cell cycle progression generally late in the G1 phase of the cell cycle (Figure 1). However, in certain epithelial cells, TGF-β appears to act somewhat earlier in G1 and, in rabbit articular chondrocytes, at the G2/M border.[65-67] In addition, depending on the cell type, TGF-β can override the growth stimulatory effects of growth factors, such as EGF in keratinocytes and ovarian cancer cells, as well as insulin-like growth factor-I (IGF-I) in Balb/c 3T3 fibroblasts.[68-71] In contrast, insulin can override the growth suppressive effects of TGF-β on human Hep3B hepatoma cells.[72] Contrary to its effects on epithelial cells, TGF-β exerts a stimulatory effect in early G1 and induces DNA synthesis in rat granulosa cells and some fibroblast derived cell lines *in vitro*, and in bovine blastocysts and vascular smooth muscle cells *in vivo*.[73-76] Interestingly, the *in vitro* treatment of rabbit articular chondrocytes with TGF-β stimulates the rate of entry into S phase in the presence of 10% fetal bovine serum, but is inhibitory in the presence of 2% serum.[65] The mechanistic differences between epithelial cells, in which TGF-β acts as a proliferation inhibitor, and other cell types that are growth stimulated by TGF-β, are not well understood.

Significantly less is known about the function of true protein hormones in cell cycle control. Prolactin induces cell cycle progression of pancreatic beta-islet cells *in vitro* and enhances the expression of G1 specific markers in cultured astrocytes.[77,78] Growth hormone administration to Snell dwarf mice results in a marked increase in DNA synthesis in the proximal tibial growth plate, primarily in chondrocytes.[79] Prolactin or growth hormone alone is sufficient to enhance the proliferation of rat Nb2-11C lymphoma cells.[80] Growth hormone apparently exerts its mitogenic effect in this system by increasing the G0/G1-to-S phase transition. Insulin stimulates cell cycle progression in certain breast cancer cells,[50,81] and following insulin treatment, cyclin D1 is induced early in G1 followed by the later inductions of cyclin D3, cyclin E, and cyclin A in late G1-early S phase.[32] Insulin promotes the growth of Swiss murine 3T3 fibroblasts, and similar to IGF-I, increases the rate of entry of isolated epiphyseal growth plate chondrocytes and human diploid fibroblasts into S phase.[52,82-87] Insulin can also override the growth suppressive effects of glucocorticoids or TGF-β in some hepatoma cell lines.[72,88] The development of defined *in vitro* culture conditions and establishment of new cell lines will provide important insights on the mechanism of how protein hormones regulate *in vivo* growth and function of specific target tissues and cell types.

III. POLYPEPTIDE GROWTH FACTORS, RECEPTORS, AND SIGNAL TRANSDUCTION PATHWAYS

Cellular responses orchestrated by polypeptide growth factors, differentiation factors, morphogens, and hormones primarily stem from a cascade of signals that emanate from the cell surface, are transduced within the cytoplasm, and eventually diffuse into the nucleus resulting in the expression of critical genes that dictate tissue and stimulus specific functions. The majority of growth factors, acting via autocrine and paracrine mechanisms, interact with tyrosine kinase cell surface receptors, which induce a wave of secondary messengers, protein-protein interactions, and activation of downstream serine/threonine protein kinases.[89] One of the final targets is the transcriptional machinery in the nucleus with the direct phosphorylation of sequence specific DNA binding proteins culminating in the induction/repression of particular sets of target genes.[90] Alterations in the program and rates of gene expression affect cell proliferation and differentiation. For example, in normal cells, growth factor mediated signalling can be viewed as a discrete series of steps regulated by dynamic and controlled interactions between positive and negative growth regulators. In contrast, in tumor cells, abnormal growth results from the dysregulation in any one of the steps in growth factor signalling pathways, which can have dramatic effects on the growth control machinery, cell proliferation, and/or differentiation programs. For example, overexpression of TGF-α in transgenic mice has been associated with a high incidence of mammary and liver neoplasias, suggesting the direct involvement of this growth factor in tumorigenesis.[91-94] Moreover, expression of many types of particular growth factors is highly prevalent in cells transformed by oncogenes, viruses, and chemical tumor promoters.[95]

A. Growth Factors and Protein Hormones

Protein hormones typically act in an endocrine manner in that the hormone is synthesized at one tissue site, secreted into the bloodstream, and is then transported to its site of action at the target tissue which expresses the appropriate receptor. In contrast, most growth factors function through autocrine and paracrine pathways. In an autocrine pathway, cells are endowed with the ability to both synthesize and respond (by production of the cognate receptor) to a specific growth factor. In a paracrine pathway, a growth factor is produced by one cell and acts upon a distal cell. In some cases, such as in wound healing, growth factors bind to extracellular matrix components after their secretion to be later utilized in either an autocrine or paracrine fashion.[96-98] As discussed below, several growth factors are initially synthesized in a membrane associated form and are then proteolytically cleaved from the plasma membrane into their secreted form.[99] Some evidence suggests that membrane forms of these growth factors are biologically active on adjacent cells and this mechanism of action has been termed juxtacrine. Certain growth factors, such as IGF-I, which is synthesized in the liver and enters the bloodstream to affect distal tissues, act in an endocrine fashion.[100] However, any aberration in autocrine, paracrine, or juxtacrine loops, such as overproduction of a growth factor or constitutive activation of a growth factor receptor, results in sustained autostimulated proliferation, as observed in many tumors.[101] Moreover, the biological processes involved in the synthesis and delivery of growth factors, local concentrations of ligands and their cognate receptors, and the integrity of downstream effector molecules can all potentially affect the growth regulation of normal and transformed cells.

An increasing list of polypeptide growth factors has been identified that not only regulate mitogenesis but also mediate a plethora of cellular functions such as cell differentiation, inflammatory responses, extracellular matrix composition, tissue repair, control of ion fluxes, and cell viability.[102] Some of the same signalling pathways and many of the same gene targets are induced by different classes of growth factors. This similarity may be due to the critical importance of certain genes, such as proto-oncogenes, in mediating cellular proliferation. Table 1 lists several of the better characterized growth factors and corresponding class of receptors which mediate their biological effects.

B. Membrane Anchored Growth Factors

A variety of growth factors such as EGF, TGF-α, amphiregulins, colony stimulating factor-1 (CSF-1), and tumor necrosis factor-α (TNF-α) are biologically active in the membrane imbedded precursor form acting in a nondiffusible manner.[99,103] For example, the glycoprotein precursors for EGF and TGF-α (which have a high degree of homology to each other and both act through the EGF receptor) contain growth factor domains in the extracellular region followed by a hydrophobic transmembrane region and a cytoplasmic domain. These precursors are relatively large transmembrane glycoproteins of approximately 140 to 170 kDa which can either remain membrane anchored or are proteolytically cleaved at the carboxyterminal domain to yield mature soluble growth factors.[99,103] The exact mechanism of proteolytic processing is not known, although in the case of the TGF-α precursor, the involvement of a specific membrane acting protease has been documented.[104]

TABLE 1   Classification of Growth Factor Receptors

Growth factor	Receptor class
Epidermal Growth Factor (EGF), Transforming Growth Factor-α (TGF-α), Amphiregulins	Transmembrane tyrosine kinase
Heparin Binding Growth Factors (HBGF), e.g., acidic and basic Fibroblast Growth Factor (FGF)	Transmembrane tyrosine kinase
Insulin, Insulin-Like Growth Factor-I (IGF-I)	Transmembrane tyrosine kinase
Platelet-Derived Growth Factor (PDGF)	Transmembrane tyrosine kinase
Colony Stimulating Growth Factor-I (CSF-I)	Transmembrane tyrosine kinase
Cytokines (Interleukins and Colony Stimulating Factors)	Transmembrane lacking a kinase domain
Growth Hormone	Transmembrane lacking a kinase domain
Prolactin	Transmembrane lacking a kinase domain
Neuropeptides, Neurotransmitters, Rhodopsin, Epinephrine, and Interleukin-8	Seven-Pass transmembrane receptors
Transforming Growth Factor-β (TGF-β), Activins, Inhibins and Bone Morphogenetic Factors	Transmembrane serine/threonine kinase

It has been proposed that membrane bound growth factors bind to and activate receptors on adjacent cells and thus may assist in controlling cell-cell contact and communication. Such accumulation and immobilization of growth factors on the cell surface may serve to locally concentrate the factors and prevent diffusion to distant cells. Besides mammalian cells, membrane anchored forms of growth factors exist in invertebrates and play important roles in development; examples include the *lin*-3 gene involved in epithelial cell fate in *Caenorhabditis elegans* and the *spitz* gene involved in dorsoventral axis formation in *Drosophila*.[105,106] In contrast to the membrane anchored growth factor precursors, certain growth factors, such as fibroblast growth factor (FGF) and TGF-β, are localized to the plasma membrane by binding to protoglycans present on the cell surface or in the extracellular matrix.[107] The membrane associated forms of these growth factors likely function to provide a prolonged autocrine growth signal and as a temporary confined source of growth factor for later paracrine function.

C. Growth Factor Receptors

Growth factors exert their pleiotropic actions by binding to cell surface receptor molecules. These receptors can be broadly categorized into three major functional groups: (1) seven-pass transmembrane receptors coupled to GTP binding proteins (G proteins) on the cytoplasmic side of the plasma membrane; (2) transmembrane receptors that lack protein kinase activity, but associate with cytoplasmic tyrosine kinases; and (3) cell surface spanning receptors which contain a tyrosine kinase domain (Figure 2). In addition, the TGF-β transmembrane receptor family contains a serine/threonine kinase domain on the cytoplasmic side (Figure 2, see discussion later in chapter). Each class of receptors uses distinct signal transduction pathways which effectively transmit and transduce the extracellular signal to the nuclear apparatus, resulting in the modulation of distinct sets of stimulus specific genes involved in cell growth, development, and differentiation.

1. Seven-Pass Transmembrane Receptors

Members of the seven-pass transmembrane subfamily of receptors are glycoproteins that bind ligands such as neurotransmitters, neuropeptides, and polypeptide hormones and growth factors.[108] The receptor structure contains an extracellular amino-terminal ligand binding domain, a central core composed of seven membrane spanning helices and connecting loops, and an intracellular carboxy-terminal domain that contains phosphorylation sites presumably important for receptor desensitization (Figure 2). The region containing the intracellular loops in the transmembrane region interacts with heterotrimeric G proteins. Upon receptor stimulation,

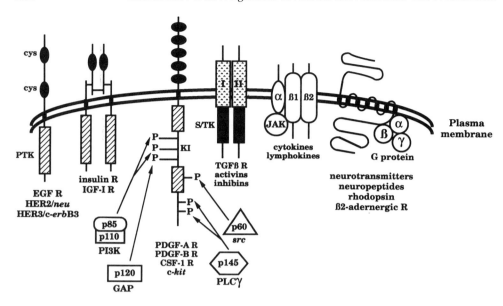

FIGURE 2   Structural organization and topology of growth factor receptor signalling molecules. Generalized structures are shown for transmembrane tyrosine protein kinase receptors (EGF receptor, insulin receptor, and PDGF receptor); transmembrane serine/threonine kinase receptors (TGFβ receptor); transmembrane receptors lacking a kinase domain (cytokines); and seven-pass transmembrane receptors (neurotransmitters). Extracellular domains of both monomeric (EGF receptor) and dimeric (insulin IGF receptor) receptors contain two cysteine rich regions (oval with dots), whereas, other transmembrane tyrosine kinases (PDGF receptor) have five immunoglobulin-like repeats (filled oval) in the extracellular domain. The cytoplasmic protein tyrosine kinase (PTK) domain (hatched bars) can be either interrupted by a kinase insert (KI) region (e.g., PDGF receptor), or remain uninterrupted. Phosphatidylinositol-3-kinase (PI3K), *ras*GTPase-activating protein (GAP), phospholipase lipase γ (PLCγ), and p60*src* are proteins containing SH2 domains (see Figure 3 for details) that interact with autophosphorylated tyrosine kinase receptors. Transmembrane serine/threonine kinase (S/TK) receptors (dark bars) contain Type I and Type II receptor components (e.g., TGFβ receptors). Receptors for cytokines, lymphokines, growth hormone and prolactin are transmembrane heteromeric complexes (α/β) lacking any protein kinase domain and are associated with cytoplasmic tyrosine kinases (e.g., JAK). The seven-pass transmembrane receptors interact with G proteins comprised of α, β, γ subunits (e.g., neurotransmitters).

the α subunit of the G protein, which has GTPase activity, dissociates from the membrane associated β-γ complex, and activates (Gαs) or inhibits (Gαi) specific enzymes, such as adenylate cyclase, to generate an array of second messengers including cAMP. In addition to adenylate cyclase, other targets of receptor activated G proteins are guanylate cyclase, and phospholipase C-β (PLC-β) which produce second messengers such as diacylglycerol (DAG) and inositol triphosphates (IP3) that alter calcium mobilization and activity of protein kinase C (PKC).[109,110] G proteins also couple cell surface receptors to specific ion channels.[109,110]

2.   Transmembrane Receptors Lacking Protein Kinase Activity

A second general class of transmembrane receptors bind ligands such as growth hormone, prolactin, and a variety of lymphokines and cytokines (Figure 2). These receptors do not possess any intrinsic tyrosine or serine/threonine protein kinase activity and are not associated with G proteins.[111] This class of receptors is comprised of a heterogeneous family of receptors. For example, in the case of some cytokine receptors, different ligand specific α subunits associate with common β subunits to form specific αβ heterodimers upon ligand binding.[112] Both long and short forms of prolactin receptors have been uncovered in which their cytoplasmic domains are of different lengths.[95] The precise mechanism of signal transduction by these receptors is not well characterized. Recent evidence has shown that rapid intracellular tyrosine phosphorylation occurs upon stimulation by cytokines and that the tyrosine kinase activity copurifies with cytokine-receptor complexes. Such studies have uncovered a family of cytoplasmic tyrosine kinases which include Tyk2, Jak1, and Jak2, all of which share the unusual feature of two kinase domains.[113] A variety of cytokines, including erythropoietin, growth hormone, interleukin-3, granulocyte-macrophage colony stimulating factor (GM-CSF), and γ-interferon, induce tyrosine phosphorylation of Jak2 that is directly associated with β-interferon receptor components, whereas, the Tyk2 tyrosine kinase is activated by α-interferons.[114,115] In essence, different combinations of cytoplasmic tyrosine kinases can be recruited by different cytokine receptor heterodimers, resulting in signal transduction pathway specificity.

3. Tyrosine Kinase Receptors

Many different growth factors, including EGF, IGF-I, and platelet-derived growth factor (PDGF) evoke cellular responses by binding to and activating cell surface receptors with intrinsic protein tyrosine kinase activity. Members within this family possess similar molecular topology in that the receptors contain an extracellular ligand binding domain, a single hydrophobic transmembrane domain, a juxtamembrane domain, and a cytoplasmic domain that contains tyrosine kinase catalytic activity (Figure 2). The tyrosine kinase domain transmits the extracellular signal intracellularly and thereby mediates the biological responses.[89] The tyrosine kinase receptors are the best characterized class of growth factor receptors and the following sections discuss in more detail their structure/function relationships.

a. Extracellular Growth Factor Ligand Binding Domain

Based on structural characteristics of their extracellular domains, tyrosine kinase receptors can be categorized into three major subclasses: (1) receptors with cysteine rich regions in the extracellular domain and an uninterrupted kinase domain [this group includes the EGF receptor and c-erb2/neu]; (2) receptors with disulfide-linked heterotetramers consisting of two α and two β subunits and contain a single cysteine rich region [insulin and IGF-I receptors, and hepatocyte-growth factor receptor c-met belong to this class of receptors]; and (3) receptors containing a variety of extracellular domain structural motifs,[89,116-119] (Figure 2). For example, certain receptors contain regularly spaced cysteines and β sheet rich repeats analogous to immunoglobulin (Ig) variable and constant regions.[120] The number of Ig-like domains vary between members of this subclass of receptors. PDGF, CSF-1, and c-kit receptors contain five Ig-like domains, whereas, three such motifs are present in the FGF receptor. These receptors also contain a kinase insert, a regulatory region found in the conserved kinase domain. Receptors for nerve growth factor (NGF or trk), constitute yet another category and lack both the cysteine rich region and the Ig-like motifs in the extracellular domain, but contain cysteines dispersed throughout the extracellular region.

Both monomeric (EGF and TGF-α) and dimeric (PDGF, CSF-I, NGF) growth factors activate their cognate receptors by inducing receptor oligomerization after binding to the extracellular domain.[120] Ligand binding is accompanied by a concomitant alteration in conformation of the extracellular domain, facilitating interactions between cytoplasmic domains of adjacent receptors. This process leads to activation of kinase function as assessed by autophosphorylation and phosphorylation of cellular substrates. A role for receptor protein dimerization in ligand dependent activation has been shown by DNA transfection of mutant receptor genes into cells which are incapable of heterodimerization.[121]

b. Transmembrane and Juxtamembrane Domains

The transmembrane domain primarily serves to anchor the receptor in the plane of plasma membrane, thereby connecting the ambient milieu with the interior of the cell. The transmembrane region appears to play a passive role in signal transduction as experiments with chimeric receptors consisting of combinations of extracellular, intracellular, and transmembrane domains of EGF, PDGF, and insulin receptors demonstrate that the identity of the transmembrane region has no influence on the signalling capacity of the cytoplasmic region.[122] In addition, kinase activity and various cellular responses to EGF were observed in EGF receptor mutants bearing alterations in the transmembrane region.

The juxtamembrane region constitutes that portion of the receptor that lies between the transmembrane domain and the cytoplasmic catalytic region. Juxtamembrane sequences are conserved between members of the same subclass of receptors but are divergent between receptor subclasses. These sequences appear to be involved in receptor transmodulation, providing negative feedback for receptor activity.[123] For example, phosphorylation of a critical residue, threonine-654, present in the juxtamembrane region of the EGF receptor by PKC, leads to loss of high affinity EGF binding sites and consequent inhibition of kinase activity.[117,123,124] Similar loss of insulin receptor kinase activity has been reported upon replacement of tyrosine-960 in the juxtamembrane region with phenylalanine, emphasizing the importance of the juxtamembrane region in receptor signalling.

c. Protein Kinase Domain

All receptor tyrosine kinases show strong conservation in the tyrosine kinase domain. The tyrosine kinase consensus glyXglyXXglyX(15-20)lys sequence functions as a part of the ATP binding site. Substitution of the lysine residue within the ATP binding site in EGF, insulin, and PDGF receptor completely abolishes kinase activity both in cell free assays and in intact cells.[120] Based on mutagenesis experiments, it has been unequivocally established that an intact kinase region is essential for receptor activity, signal transduction, and generation of both early and delayed cellular responses in both normal and tumor cells.[125] Activation of tyrosine kinase receptors leads to a variety of protein-protein interactions and phosphorylation of an array of cellular substrates. Signalling components bind to phosphorylated regions of this domain; this binding is dependent upon the appropriate autophosphorylation of the receptor at tyrosine residues (see later section). Apart from the role of tyrosine kinase function in signalling, an intact tyrosine kinase domain is also necessary for targeting of the EGF receptor to lysosomes upon ligand binding and receptor activation.[126]

The kinase domain of one of the subclasses of tyrosine kinase containing receptors (e.g., PDGF) is divided into two portions by insertions of up to 100 hydrophilic amino acids and are highly conserved between species, suggesting an important role for these sequences in receptor function. The evidence for the importance of this region, however, is conflicting. A deletion mutant lacking 82 amino acids of the PDGF kinase insert was shown to abrogate mitogenic signalling in CHO cells.[127] In contrast, other studies indicate that the kinase insert region is dispensable for kinase activity and mitogenesis.[128] Autophosphorylation of tyrosine-751 present in the kinase insert region triggers binding of activated PDGF receptors to cellular substrates, thereby identifying a role for this region in the interaction of receptors with substrates and effector molecules.

d. Carboxyterminal Tail

Sequences contained within the carboxyterminal region are the most poorly conserved between all known tyrosine kinases and may account for some of the diversity in substrate specificity between different types of receptors. Several tyrosine autophosphorylation sites have been mapped in this region of the EGF, *neu*/HER, and insulin receptors, and are quite conserved within members of a given receptor subclass. Although mutations in the carboxyterminal tail do not affect the tyrosine kinase activity and the biological properties of the receptor, it is believed that these sequences negatively regulate receptor function perhaps by modulating the ability of the kinase region to interact with exogenous substrates.[129]

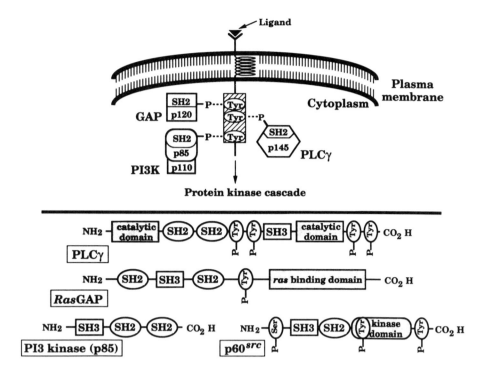

FIGURE 3 Receptor tyrosine kinase interactions with SH2-containing proteins. The top panel diagrams protein-protein interactions between phosphotyrosine containing tyrosine kinase receptors and SH2 (*src* homology) domains of *ras* GTPase-activating protein (GAP), phosphatidylinositol-3-kinase (PI3K), and phospholipase Cγ (PLCγ). The lower panel shows the structural domains in the SH2 containing proteins. The regions include the *src* homology regions 2 and 3 (SH2, SH3), catalytic domain (hatched bar), *ras* binding domain (straight bars), and kinase domain (empty bars).

D. Receptor Tyrosine Kinase Substrates

Upon ligand binding, growth factor receptors associate with specific sets of proteins which are substrates for the receptor kinase (Figure 3). These receptor associated proteins are critical components in growth factor induced signal transduction in both normal and cancerous cells. The tyrosine kinase receptor substrates are characterized by the presence of unique sequence motifs known as *src* homology or SH domains.[130] The *src* proto-oncogene family of cytoplasmic tyrosine kinases contained of three regions of distinct structural and functional modules: (1) the kinase catalytic domain termed as SH1; (2) an SH2 domain which is aminoterminal to the kinase domain and spans approximately 100 amino acids; and (3) an SH3 domain comprised of about 60 amino acids. SH2 motifs serve as docking sites for phosphotyrosine containing proteins, although in some cases (such as the product of the c-*abl* proto-oncogene) SH2 domains recognize phosphoserine sequences in the B cell receptor.[131] Thus, SH2 domains serve to recruit receptor substrates and other receptor binding proteins to specific autophosphorylated regions of growth factor receptor tyrosine kinases. SH3 motifs are believed to play a role in the interactions with cytoskeletal elements and/or downstream effectors and may not be required for interactions of SH2 domains with phosphotyrosine sequences.

Tyrosine phosphorylation creates high affinity sites for the binding of SH2 domain containing proteins such as *ras*GTPase Activating Protein (*ras*GAP), phosphatidyl inositide 3-kinase (PI3-kinase), phospholipase C γ (PLCγ), and pp60*src* (Figure 3). Such heteromeric complexes between SH2 containing proteins and an autophosphorylated region of growth factor receptors assemble at the plasma membrane where these substrates are tyrosine phosphorylated by growth factor receptors. The interactions between the SH2 containing proteins and growth factor receptors are specific and occur at distinct sites. For example, the p85 subunit of PI3-kinase binds to the kinase insert of the PDGF receptor, whereas, PLCγ binds to sequences C-terminal to the kinase insert of the PDGF receptor.[131] The exact nature of these receptor complexes and the factors regulating protein-protein interactions are not well understood.

Phospholipase C γ1 and γ2 (PLCγ1 and PLCγ2), as well as PI3-kinase, are direct substrates for tyrosine kinase containing receptors which are involved in inositol metabolism. Both PLCγ1 and PCLγ2 have SH2 domains which promote a specific interaction with the tyrosine kinase domain of the receptor (Figure 3). Tyrosine phosphorylation of PLCγ1 has been observed in response to several different mitogenic factors such as EGF, PDGF, FGF and NGF as well as the T cell receptor and the Ig receptor.[131] Phosphorylation of PLCγ1 leads to rapid hydrolysis of phosphoinositides, generating second messengers such as DAG and IP3, which then activate PKC and mobilize intracellular calcium. PKC activation in most cases then leads to phosphorylation of downstream targets that result in transcriptional activation and generation of biological responses. Purified PI3-kinase is composed of two polypeptides; a 85-kDa subunit that contains SH2 domains but lacks PI3-kinase activity, and a 110-kDa subunit that probably contains the catalytic activity.[131] In growth factor treated cells, increased amounts of PI3-kinase activity are recovered from antiphosphotyrosine precipitates, suggesting that PI3-kinase is tyrosine phosphorylated by growth factor addition (Figure 3). Insulin is known to activate PI3-kinase activity which associates with the tyrosine phosphorylated insulin receptor substrate (IRS-1 or pp185), as assessed by co-immunoprecipitation assays.[131]

Another important nonreceptor substrate for receptor tyrosine kinases is *ras*GAP, a molecule that modulates the GTPase activity of *ras* (Figure 3). *Ras* is a low molecular weight GTP binding protein that plays an important role in growth factor induced mitogenesis (see later section). In cells exposed to growth factors, GTP bound *ras* levels are enormously increased rendering it active and in turn leads to a cascade of protein phosphorylation events. Normal *ras* activity is modulated by *ras*GAP, although the role of *ras*GAP in modulating *ras* activity in tumor cells is not well understood. Growth factor treatment results in tyrosine phosphorylation of *ras*GAP, thereby decreasing its activity. Decreased *ras*GAP activity then leads to increased GTP loading of *ras*, thereby activating *ras* and propagating downstream signalling (see next section). In addition to the receptor tyrosine kinase substrates discussed above, several other protein substrates have been recently identified and include a phosphotyrosine phosphatase, a serine/threonine kinase, the p91 transcription factor, a cytoskeletal protein, and a growth factor receptor binding protein (Grb2).[131] The structural organization and interactions of several SH2-containing proteins with transmembrane receptors discussed above is depicted in Figure 3.

E. Growth Factor Receptor Signal Transduction Pathways

Binding of extracellular ligands to the cell surface tyrosine kinase receptors initiates signal transduction pathways which are then received and transduced within the cytoplasm by a variety of proteins. The signalling network governing the regulation of cell proliferation is controlled by various mechanisms involving protein phosphorylation cascades, protein-protein, protein-DNA interactions, ionic fluxes, gene expression changes, and cytoskeletal rearrangements. For example, signal transduction via growth factors leads to well-defined nuclear responses by inducing the expression of immediate "early" genes such as the c-*fos*, c-*jun*, and c-*myc* proto-oncogenes, which positively regulate cell cycle progression. Recent studies aimed at delineating the individual components of growth factor mediated intracellular signalling have unravelled at least two different cellular pathways that are either *ras*-dependent or independent (Figure 4).

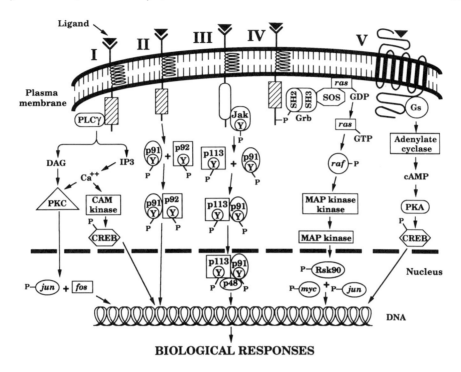

BIOLOGICAL RESPONSES

FIGURE 4   Signal transduction via *ras*-dependent and -independent mechanisms. Pathways I, II, III, and V represent *ras*-independent receptor signalling pathways, whereas, pathway IV constitutes a *ras*-dependent receptor signalling cascade. Phospholipase C γ (PLCγ); diacylglycerol (DAG); inositol triphosphate (IP3); protein kinase C (PKC); calmodulin kinases (CAM); cAMP response element binding protein (CREB); *Src* homology region 2 (SH2); growth factor receptor binding protein 2 (Grb2); son of sevenless (SOS); stimulatory subunit of G protein (Gs); adenylate cyclase (AC); protein kinase A (PKA).

1. Ras-Dependent Growth Factor Signalling

Intracellular amplification of extracellular growth factor signals (such as by EGF, PDGF, and insulin) is accomplished by ligand binding to specific receptor tyrosine kinases at the cell surface, leading to receptor dimerization and subsequent autophosphorylation of critical amino acid residues in the carboxyterminal tail of these receptors.[116] Following multiple tyrosine phosphorylation of the receptor, which serve as binding sites for SH2 containing proteins, significant increases in *ras*-guanine nucleotide exchange activity and the GTP bound fraction of *ras* is observed in growth factor stimulated cells (Figure 4: Receptor System IV). Recent studies have defined some of the key intermediates involved in the coupling of tyrosine kinase receptor with activation of *ras* proteins.[132-142] Two novel proteins designated as Grb2 (growth factor receptor binding protein) and SOS (son of sevenless), a nucleotide exchange factor, have been identified which play an important role in the *ras*-mediated growth stimulation pathway (Figure 4: Receptor System IV). Grb2 contains a single SH2 domain flanked by two SH3 domains and has been shown to couple receptor tyrosine kinases with SOS proteins. SOS proteins are mammalian homologs of yeast activities that stimulate GTP loading and activation of *ras*.[135,142] In EGF stimulated cells, the SH2 domain of Grb2 binds to the autophosphorylated receptor tyrosine kinase, and the SH3 domain mediates the interaction with the SOS protein, which in turn stimulates *ras* by promoting conversion of GDP bound *ras* to the active GTP bound form. However, it is not well understood how Grb2-SOS interactions regulate SOS activity, or how SOS-*ras* interactions modulate *ras* activity. It is speculated that binding of Grb2 to a phosphorylated receptor somehow facilitates the relocation of SOS towards the plasma membrane in the vicinity of *ras*, thereby activating *ras* function. Grb2 is not phosphorylated in response to EGF, whereas, SOS proteins have been found to be phosphorylated, although the implications of such modification are not clear.

In insulin stimulated cells, *ras* activation is also mediated by the Grb2 protein. However, in contrast to the EGF receptor that interacts directly with the Grb2-SOS complex, stimulation of insulin receptors leads to phosphorylation of two docking proteins, insulin receptor substrate-1 (IRS-1) and the *src*-homology and collagen protein (Shc). Subsequently, the Grb2-SOS complex then interacts with IRS-1 and Shc, providing an additional level of specificity in insulin receptor signalling. Binding of Grb2 to either IRS-1 or Shc or both, probably activates SOS by phosphorylation and recruits it to the membrane near *ras*, where it binds to *ras* and causes activation of *ras* GTPase exchange activity. Thus, Grb2 appears to be an important intermediate, acting as an adaptor and facilitating the coupling of tyrosine kinase with downstream protein substrates.

The remarkable conservation of Grb2 in yeast, insects, and mammals indicates that it is a critical element in the signalling pathways governing cell growth and differentiation. Activation of *ras* is an important step in the growth factor induced mitogenic pathway, as neutralizing anti-*ras* antibody and dominant negative *ras* mutants block growth factor induced DNA synthesis.[143] Although the immediate downstream target of the *ras* protein has not been firmly established, recent studies have characterized several serine/threonine protein kinases that appear to act downstream of *ras* in growth factor stimulated cells. Experiments with the yeast two-hybrid screen for interacting proteins has uncovered a direct interaction of *ras* with the c-*raf* proto-oncogene serine/threonine kinase [144] (Figure 4: Receptor System IV). In many signal transduction pathways, *raf* has been positioned downstream of *ras*, and in some cases, *raf* is activated by other regulators such as PKC (Figure 4: Receptor System I) or inhibited by protein kinase A (Figure 4: Receptor System V).

Another important kinase identified in growth factor stimulated cells is the Mitogen Activated Protein kinases (MAP kinase), also known as Extracellular Signal Regulated Kinases (ERK).[145] Upon activation of tyrosine kinase receptors, MAP kinases are activated by phosphorylation of critical tyrosine and threonine residues, presumably by *raf* kinase (Figure 4: Receptor System IV). Activation of MAP kinases has been documented during growth factor induced DNA synthesis and leads to either activation of other kinases such as p90[rsk] or the direct phosphorylation of transcription factors such as c-*myc* or c-*jun*[146,147] (Figure 4: Receptor System IV). In general, phosphorylation of transcription factors serves to propagate the signal transduced in the cytoplasm into the nucleus, enables the nuclear localization of latent cytoplasmic transcription factors, provides positive and negative regulation of their DNA binding activity, and allows interaction of the transactivation domain of transcription factors with the transcription apparatus. For example, MAP kinase dependent phosphorylation of c-*jun* and c-*myc* results in their activation and competence for transcriptional activity.[90]

2. *Ras*-Independent Pathways

Another important signalling network that links cell surface receptors (including receptors that either contain or lack an intrinsic tyrosine kinase activity) and nuclear events involves the "Direct Effector model" pathway [148-154] (Figure 4: Receptor Systems II and III). According to this model, latent cytoplasmic transcription factors, also known as Signal Transducers and Activators of Transcription (STAT) are directly phosphorylated at tyrosine residues by membrane receptor associated tyrosine kinases, upon binding of growth factors or cytokines. The inactive cytoplasmic transcription factors with SH2 domains appear to bind directly to ligand activated, receptor associated and autophosphorylated tyrosine kinase(s). This association between the kinase and the transcription factor leads to tyrosine phosphorylation and activation of the transcription factor, subsequent translocation to the nuclear compartment to form complexes with specific DNA binding factors, and stimulation of transcription of target genes. In the case of α-interferon signalling, treatment of cells with α-interferon results in tyrosine phosphorylation of two transcription factors (113-kDa and 91-kDa), by the Jak family of tyrosine kinases, resulting in the migration of the activated complex into the nucleus where it interacts with another 48-kDa subunit, to constitute the active DNA binding complex (Figure 4: Receptor System III). γ-Interferon preferentially activates only the p91 transcription factor by tyrosine phosphorylation, and causes it to translocate into the nucleus to activate transcription of γ-interferon activatable sequences (Figure 4: Receptor System II).

Growth factors, such as EGF and PDGF that signal via receptor tyrosine kinases, also utilize direct signalling pathways providing a specific link between receptor tyrosine kinases and gene transcription.[150] The SH2 domain of p91 directly interacts with growth factor receptors; after p91 is tyrosine phosphorylated, this regulatory subunit becomes competent for DNA binding and translocates into the nucleus. Disruption of this key SH2 domain by point mutations or deletion abrogates activation of p91, its tyrosine phosphorylation, nuclear translocation and transactivation.[150] Recently another new member of the STAT family of transcription factors, p92, has been implicated in EGF mediated signalling, probably forming a heterodimer with the p91 transcription factor[154] (Figure 4; Receptor System II). It is important to note that in cells expressing dominant negative mutations in *ras*, stimulation of cells with PDGF enhanced p91 transcriptional activity despite abundant mutant *ras* proteins, indicating that activation of p91 occurs by a *ras*-independent pathway.[151] Other *ras*-independent growth factor signalling pathways include the activation of PKC by second messengers such as DAG and IP3 generated by PDGF activation of tyrosine kinase receptors and PI3-kinase (Figure 4: Receptor System I). Activation of the PKC or the PKA pathway leads to phosphorylation of specific transcription factors, such as the AP-1 proteins (c-*fos* and c-*jun*) and CREB (cAMP response element binding) protein, which are closely linked to cell proliferation.

F.   Signal Transduction and Cancer

Constitutive activation of any of the components of growth factor signalling pathways can potentially affect the growth regulatory circuitry, resulting in unrestrained cell growth and neoplasia. For example, excessive signalling by receptor tyrosine kinases can lead to the subversion of molecular control mechanisms in response to extracellular signals. Unbridled production of growth factors, mutations in receptor tyrosine kinases, or their inappropriate expression due to gene amplification can mediate uncontrolled gene expression that is detrimental for cells. In a variety of tumors, aberrations in at least one or more components of the growth factor signal transduction pathways have been reported. For example, the v-*sis* viral oncogene encodes a protein highly similar to the B chain of PDGF, and uncontrolled production of this growth factor can result in the autocrine activation of cell proliferation.[21] Truncated forms of the EGF receptor, for example the c-*erb*B proto-oncogene product, or point mutations in the c-*fms* proto-oncogene receptor are constitutively activated leading to unregulated signalling.[21] Oncogenic versions of *ras* proteins, endowed with decreased GTPase activity and loss of negative regulation, can result in derangements in cell growth controls.[155] Other oncogenic mutations in downstream effectors of the pathway include mutations in the *raf* kinase that cause it to be constitutively active.[156] Dominant proto-oncogenes more distal in the signalling pathway are nuclear transcription factors. Overexpression of AP-1 family members driven by strong viral promoters leads to the constitutive expression of their target genes and oncogenesis.[157,158] The most common lesion in human cancers, however, involves autocrine activation of growth factors in conjunction with overproduction of receptor tyrosine kinases — 30% of human breast and ovarian carcinomas have amplified c-*erb*B2 genes due to gene amplification.[4] Many tumor cell lines produce excessive amounts of growth factors, such as TGF-α, PDGF, and FGF, and their cognate receptors. To summarize, inappropriate expression of growth factors their receptors, cytoplasmic tyrosine and serine/threonine protein kinases, GTP binding proteins, and mitogen activated nuclear transcription factors can impair the cell's ability to decipher cellular signals important for growth and differentiation.

IV. INHIBITION OF CELL GROWTH BY TRANSFORMING GROWTH FACTOR-β

Cellular responses to both positive and negative growth regulating environmental cues is a consequence of critical decisions made by the responding cell during the G1 phase of the cell cycle. As a result of environmental signalling, a cell can either multiply, differentiate, or exit from the cell cycle, depending upon the nature of the extracellular stimuli. As discussed earlier in this chapter, growth promoting agents, such as polypeptide growth factors, positively regulate cell proliferation by facilitating the progression of cells in G1 and driving entry into S phase, whereas, negative growth regulators can impede the G1 to S transition, thereby arresting the cells in the G1 phase of the cell cycle.

TGF-β represents a family of naturally occurring peptide growth inhibitors of epithelial cells that includes five members (TGF-β1 through TGF-β5), all of which demonstrate high amino acid sequence conservation.[64] In fact, the TGF-β gene family members are prototypic multifunctional cytokines that belong to a larger superfamily of peptide signalling molecules (such as Mullerian inhibiting substance, inhibins, activins, and bone morphogenetic factors) that are evolutionarily conserved between insects and vertebrates.[63] TGF-β exerts diverse effects on cellular functions including cell proliferation, differentiation, adhesion, migration, tissue repair, wound healing, and extracellular matrix formation.[64] For example, TGF-β stimulates the growth of rat kidney fibroblasts in soft agar in the presence of EGF, inhibits differentiation of certain cells of mesodermal origin, and inhibits the growth of various types of epithelial cells.[64] TGF-β also functions as a physiological regulator of mammary growth and function, modulates stromal-epithelial interactions, and specifically inhibits ductal growth causing ductal end bud involution and cessation of glandular growth under conditions where alveolar morphogenesis remains unaffected.[159]

A. TGF-β Receptors

Different isoforms of TGF-β typically form 25-kDa homodimers and mediate their biological effects by binding to cell surface associated heterodimeric receptor complexes, designated as Type I and Type II receptors[63] (Figure 2). A third nonreceptor component (Type III) is a proteoglycan known as betaglycan, that binds TGF-β via the protein core of the proteoglycan.[160] In contrast to receptor tyrosine kinases that mediate signalling by growth factors, receptors for TGF-β are transmembrane serine/threonine protein kinases.[63] The ectodomain of TGF-β receptors is small and cysteine rich, followed by a single transmembrane domain and a cytoplasmic region that comprises the intracellular serine/threonine kinase domain (Figure 2). These receptors appear to functionally discriminate between TGF-β isoforms in that they bind TGF-β1 and TGF-β3 more effectively than TGF-β2. The 53-kDa Type I receptor requires the presence of Type II receptors for both ligand binding and signalling and possesses intrinsic serine/threonine kinase activity necessary for signalling.[161] The Type II receptor is a 70-kDa transmembrane protein endowed with serine/threonine kinase activity, and functionally inter-acts with Type I receptors to mediate growth suppression as well as transcriptional regulation of TGF-β responsive genes.[162,163] Recent studies on such functional interdependency of the Type I and Type II receptors have demonstrated that in cells overexpressing dominant negative forms of the Type II receptor, which selectively block Type II receptor signalling, Type I receptor signalling was normal as evidenced by induction of extracellular matrix proteins (such as fibronectin) and increased c-*jun* expression.[164,165] The betaglycan Type III receptor is dispensable for TGF-β signalling and appears to recruit TGF-β to the plasma membrane and promote its access to either the Type I or Type II kinase containing receptors, forming a ternary complex.

B. Signal Transduction by TGF-β

The mechanisms of TGF-β induced growth inhibition and the signalling events that couple receptor binding to nuclear activation and growth control have not been resolved. Signalling by TGF-β does not appear to involve the known intracellular pathways such as modulation of cAMP levels, phosphoinositol breakdown, or tyrosine phosphorylation of latent cytoplasmic transcription factors. One of the primary determinants of TGF-β responsiveness may involve a signal transduction network that links the receptor to negative regulators of cell cycle progression. For example, in TGF-β growth arrested mink lung epithelial cells, phosphorylation of the Rb tumor suppressor is prevented, retaining Rb in its active hypophosphorylated form which blocks the G1 to S transition. The hypophosphorylation of Rb leads to an accumulation of cells in late G1 phase of the cell cycle.[166] This TGF-β mediated late G1 arrest of mink lung epithelial cells occurs with a concomitant suppression of cdk4 synthesis, a major catalytic subunit of mammalian D-type G1 cyclins (Figure 1), thus preventing cyclin D-cdk4 complex formation.[167] Since cdk4- and cdk2-associated cyclins can phosphorylate Rb,[168] rendering it inactive, their inactivation by TGF-β may explain the presence of hypophosphorylated Rb in cells which are growth suppressed by TGF-β. In addition to an inhibition of cdk4 synthesis, preexisting cyclin E-cdk2 complexes fail to exhibit kinase activity in TGF-β treated cells.[169] Recent studies have revealed that TGF-β induces the synthesis of an inhibitory protein, p27, that binds to cyclin E-cdk2 complexes (Figure 1), increasing the threshold level of cyclin E necessary to activate cdk2 and thereby inhibiting kinase activity.[170] Thus, TGF-β may negatively regulate growth by targeting critical components of the cell cycle machinery, and inducing novel growth inhibitory molecules which, by virtue of protein-protein interactions, effectively curtail cell cycle progression. In the absence of such growth regulatory devices, cells would escape the regulatory constraints and checkpoints and proliferate in an uncontrolled fashion, leading to tumorigenesis.

V. STEROID HORMONE REGULATION OF GROWTH

A. Steroid Receptor Mechanism of Action

Steroid and seco-steroid hormones are comprised of the estrogens, progestins, androgens, mineralocorticoids, glucocorticoids, and members of the vitamin D family. These hormones are derived from cholesterol and can be categorized into subfamilies based on their polycyclic structure.[171] Steroid and seco-steroid hormones have a wide range of biological activities which include the control of reproduction, stress, salt and water balance, metabolism, and development (see Chapter 2). Many studies have shown that steroid hormones are directly involved in the proliferative control of normal and cancerous cells. Steroid and seco-steroids, as well as retinoids (vitamin A derivatives synthesized in the skin), and thyroid hormones (tyrosine derivatives synthesized in the thyroid gland) have similar mechanisms of action in that they act through highly related intracellular receptors to regulate transcription of specific sets of target genes.[172-179]

Recent studies have uncovered key features of the molecular mechanism of steroid hormone action. After diffusion through the plasma membrane, steroids bind to and potentiate a functional change in their cognate receptor which results in either stimulated or repressed transcription of steroid regulated genes.[6,173-176] In the case of glucocorticoid receptors, ligand binding causes release of the 90-kDa heat shock protein from the inactive receptor complex in the cytoplasm which allows translocation into the nucleus. Other steroid receptors, such as

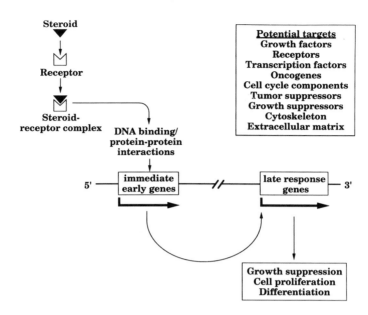

FIGURE 5   Cascade model for steroid regulation of cell proliferation. Activated steroid-receptor complexes interact with specific DNA binding sites and/or particular sets of transcription factors to regulate the expression of immediate "early" response genes. A subset of the immediate "early" response genes regulate the expression or activate a specific set of "late" response genes. A combination of steroid-regulated immediate "early" and "late" response genes mediate growth control and differentiation in normal and transformed cells. Potential target genes in a steroid regulated cascade include transcription factors, oncogenes, growth factors, growth factor receptors, cell cycle components, tumor and growth suppressors, cytoskeletal components, and extracellular matrix components.

the estrogen and androgen receptors, are localized in the nucleus prior to ligand binding. The potent effects of steroids on gene transcription can occur by specific binding of steroid-receptor complexes to DNA transcriptional enhancer elements known as hormone response elements (HREs) within promoters of steroid regulated genes[173,175-177] and/or by interfering or synergizing with the actions of other transcription factors.[173,175,176] For example, as discussed later in this chapter, glucocorticoid receptors modulate the transcriptional activity of the AP-1 transcription complex via direct protein-protein interactions.[180-184] In addition to these primary responses, glucocorticoids exert many of their actions by a cascade mechanism (Figure 5) in which the direct induction or repression of regulatory gene products influence the expression or activity of a wide variety of cellular components, such as those involved in cell proliferation and differentiation.[172] Potential "early" and "late" gene targets of steroids within a growth regulatory cascade include growth factors, growth factor receptors, transcription factors, oncogenes, cell cycle components, tumor and growth suppressors, as well as cytoskeletal and extracellular matrix components.

B.   Steroid Receptor Interactions With DNA and Transcription Factors

Steroid receptors are multifunctional proteins, and members of the steroid receptor gene family have the same general structure with at least three domains that are essential for normal receptor activity.[173,175,176] The carboxyterminus contains the ligand binding domain which, for most of the receptors, acts as a repressor of the DNA binding domain in the absence of steroid ligand. The aminoterminal region contains transcriptional activation domains and is the least conserved region between different classes of receptors. The central region encodes the "zinc finger" DNA binding domain which recognizes sequence specific motifs as well as mediates selective interactions with other receptors and transcription factors. The zinc finger DNA

TABLE 2 Consensus DNA Recognition Sequences
of the Steroid Hormone Receptor Gene
Family

Hormone receptor	Consensus DNA binding sites [a]
Glucocorticoid	AGAACAnnnTGTTCT
Androgen	AGAACAnnnTGTTCT
Mineralocorticoid	AGAACAnnnTGTTCT
Progestin	AGAACAnnnTGTTCT
Estrogen	AGGTCAnnnTGACCT
Thyroid	AGGTCA-TGACCT
	AGGTCAnnnnAGGTCA
Vitamin D family	GGGTGAnnnnnnGGGTCA
	AGGTCAnnnAGGTCA
Vitamin A family	
RAR	AGGTCAnnnnnAGGTCA
RXR	AGGTCAnAGGTCA

[a] The pairs of consensus DNA half sites of receptor binding can
be arranged either as palindromes or as direct repeats with
different spacing; n represents random base pairs between consensus half sites.

binding domain of steroid hormone receptors is the most conserved region between steroid
receptors and is a cysteine rich region which forms two zinc fingers typical of other transcription factors. This region is responsible for receptor binding to "simple" steroid response
elements independently of other cofactors. Surprisingly, the receptors for glucocorticoids,
progestins, mineralocorticoids, and androgens recognize the same steroid response element,
whereas, the receptors for estrogens, vitamin D, retinoids, and thyroid hormones recognize
similar DNA half sites which differ in their spacing and orientation. Table 2 shows consensus
DNA recognition sequences for various members of the steroid receptor gene family.

Recent evidence has demonstrated that steroid receptors mediate their transcriptional
effects by binding to the promoters of steroid regulated genes at a regulatory region designated
as a hormone response unit (HRU) which is comprised of simple steroid response elements
and specific binding sites for a variety of transcription factors.[173,185] The complex interactions
between steroid receptors and other transcriptional regulators via protein-DNA and/or protein-
protein binding defines the transcriptional capacity and regulation of the gene. As shown in
Figure 6, one well-characterized HRU is present within the promoter of the phosphoenol
pyruvate carboxykinase (PEPCK) gene, a rate limiting enzyme in gluconeogenesis.[185-192]
PEPCK expression correlates with hepatocytes entering the quiescent state. Evidence from
several laboratories has shown that glucocorticoids, retinoic acid, thyroid hormones, and
cAMP enhance PEPCK expression. Molecular dissection of the PEPCK HRU has identified
at least five regulatory domains: AF1, AF2, GRE1, GRE2, and CRE (Figure 6). The glucocorticoid receptor binds to both GRE1 and GRE2 and deletion of either AF site or either GRE
site abolishes glucocorticoid induction of PEPCK gene expression. The retinoic acid receptor
enhances PEPCK expression through binding the AF1 site which is inhibited by the unliganded
thyroid hormone (T3) receptor. The CRE site mediates both the cAMP induced responsiveness via DNA of the cAMP response element binding protein (CREB) as well as T3 induced
responsiveness. Moreover, the c-*jun* proto-oncoprotein and the CCAAT/Enhancer Binding
Protein (C/EBP) can enhance PEPCK expression through the CRE site, whereas, c-*fos*
represses expression from this regulatory element.[193-195] However, neither of these two transcription factors has been shown to physically interact with the CRE. In addition, PKA
activation by cAMP enhances the binding of the glucocorticoid receptor to the promoter of

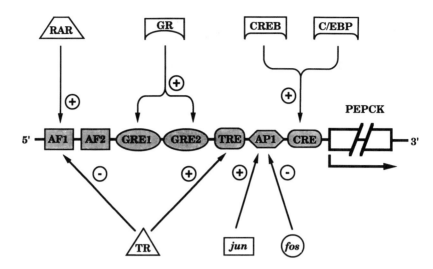

FIGURE 6   Structural features of the hormone response unit in the promoter region of the PEPCK gene. The hormone response unit of the upstream promoter region of the phosphoenolpyruvate carboxykinase (PEPCK) gene contains several regulatory regions which are responsible for the multihormonal regulation of transcription. These regulatory regions include the accessory factor site 1 (AF1), accessory factor site 2 (AF2), glucocorticoid response elements (GRE1 and GRE2), thyroid receptor response element (TRE), the AP1 transcription factor site, as well as a cAMP response element (CRE). Several transcriptional regulators interact with these DNA target sites and include the glucocorticoid receptor (GR), the retinoic acid receptor (RAR), the thyroid hormone receptor (TR), the cAMP response element binding protein (CREB), the CCAAT/enhancer binding protein (C/EBP), and the c-*jun* and c-*fos* components of the AP1 transcription complex.

PEPCK. This effect is likely to be mediated by CREB because *in vitro* analyses have demonstrated that there is a direct physical interaction between CREB and the glucocorticoid receptor. The PEPCK promoter, thus, provides a model for examining complex steroid receptor-transcription factor interactions involved in steroid regulated gene expression.

Steroid receptors can directly and reciprocally interact with certain transcription factors to inhibit transcription. For example, glucocorticoid receptors can prevent the activity of AP-1 transcription complexes (composed of c-*jun*/c-*fos* heterodimers or c-*jun* homodimers) by binding to the leucine zipper region of c-*jun*.[173,175,176,180-184] The glucocorticoid receptor/AP-1 complex interaction prevents binding of AP-1 proteins to their DNA binding site and thus reduces the transcriptional activity of the promoter. The zinc finger region in the DNA binding domain of the glucocorticoid receptor is essential for the functional inhibition of AP-1 activity, but the presence of a hormone response element or a direct physical interaction between the glucocorticoid receptor and DNA is not necessary for this inhibitory effect. Conversely, the presence of c-*jun* protein can prevent the glucocorticoid receptor from interacting with its DNA binding site in certain promoters through direct protein-protein interactions. Another example of reciprocal inhibition by a transcription factor complex and steroid hormone receptors is NFκB and the glucocorticoid receptor.[196] The NFκB transcription factor is a heterodimeric protein with a 50-kDa subunit (p50) and a 65-kDa subunit (p65).[197,198] Similar to the glucocorticoid receptor inhibition of AP-1 transcriptional activity, the glucocorticoid receptor prevents the binding of the p65 subunit to DNA. Conversely, overexpression of p65 inhibits glucocorticoid receptor mediated transcription from its glucocorticoid response element. The precise nature of the NFκB transcription factor and glucocorticoid receptor interaction has not been determined.

Recently, it has been shown that the thyroid hormone T3 receptor enhances AP-1 directed gene expression in the absence of T3, but inhibits AP-1 transcriptional activity in the presence of T3.[173,199] The DNA binding zinc finger domain in the T3 receptor is necessary for both the enhancement and the inhibition of transcription by the T3 receptor. It appears that the T3 receptor physically associates with the c-*jun* protein, but not the c-*fos* protein. Thus, an integral aspect of the cascade mechanism by which steroids regulate cell proliferation (Figure 5) is the selective interaction between steroid receptors and transcription factors which can positively or negatively regulate gene expression.[172,173]

C. Transcriptional Cascade of Growth Regulatory Genes by Steroid Hormones

Steroid hormones regulate the growth of cells by altering the expression and/or function of either stimulators or suppressors of cell proliferation. Thus, direct (early) or indirect (late) targets of the steroid receptor signalling cascade include a variety of growth regulatory molecules such as transcription factors, proto-oncogenes, growth factors and growth factor receptors, cell cycle components, and growth suppressors (Figure 5). The following sections describe in more detail some of these growth regulatory genes which are under steroid control in both normal and tumorigenic cells.

1. Steroid Regulation of Proto-Oncogenes

Proto-oncogenes have a variety of cellular functions and enhance the growth or are associated with proliferative signalling pathways of many different cell types.[1,21] Some proto-oncogenes encode modified growth factor receptors with tyrosine kinase activity (e.g., EGF receptor-like proto-oncogenes); others encode GTP binding proteins involved in signal transduction pathways (e.g., *ras*); and certain proto-oncogenes are transcription factors which regulate the expression of specific target genes (e.g., c-*myc*, c-*jun*, and c-*fos*). The positive and negative steroid regulation of proto-oncogene expression has been well documented.[200] For example, estrogen induces c-*myc* mRNA in certain hormone responsive mammary adenocarcinoma cell lines prior to the induction of DNA synthesis.[201] In fact, a steroid response element-like sequence has recently been uncovered in the c-*myc* promoter; however, the role of this potential DNA target site in mediating the transcriptional control of c-*myc* has not been determined.[202] Estrogen also increases c-*fos* mRNA levels in rat uterus, rat pituitary, and guinea pig endometrial cells[203-210] and c-*jun*, *jun*B, and *jun*D mRNA levels in the rat uterus.[203,206,211] In contrast, estrogen (as well as progesterone) down regulates the mRNA levels for c-*myc*, c-*fos*, and c-*jun* in the chick oviduct.[212,213] Progesterone stimulates the expression of c-*jun* and c-*myc* in human T-47D mammary tumor cells.[44,214,215]

Depending on the tissue type, glucocorticoids can either stimulate or suppress the growth of cells. As with estrogen, glucocorticoids can also affect the expression of proto-oncogenes.[200] For example, dexamethasone, a synthetic glucocorticoid, causes a rapid increase in c-*myc* mRNA levels in the chicken liver and a human osteoblastoid cell line, but down regulates c-*myc* expression in the chicken oviduct, a murine fibroblast cell line, and a T-lymphoma cell line.[202,216-218] The mRNA levels for c-*fos* are strongly enhanced in glucocorticoid treated chick embryo osteogenic cell cultures, and AtT-20/D-1 pituitary cells, but are significantly reduced in glucocorticoid treated C6 glioma cells, rat uterus cells, and U-937 leukemia cells.[219-223] Elevated levels of c-*jun* mRNA are detected in glucocorticoid treated NIH 3T3 cells, certain hepatoma and mammary cell lines, as well as in leukemia cells.[34,35,223,224] Other members of the steroid receptor family have similar regulatory effects on proto-oncogene expression in nontransformed and transformed cells under conditions in which cell proliferation is under hormonal control.

2. Regulation of Growth Factors and Growth Factor Receptors

Steroid hormones can regulate cell proliferation by modulating growth factor or growth factor receptor expression or function. For example, estrogen, which stimulates the growth of murine uterine cells, stimulates the expression of TGF-α in murine uterine epithelial cells and enhances TGF-α secretion into mouse uterine luminal fluid. It is likely that TGF-α is responsible for the estrogen induced uterine cell proliferation because anti-TGF-α antibodies block the growth response to estrogen.[225] In transfected mammary tumor cells, estrogen regulates transcriptional activity of the chloramphenicol acetyltransferase (CAT) reporter gene containing the TGF-α promoter.[226] Tamoxifen, an antiestrogen which blocks the proliferative effects of estrogen, was shown to inhibit estrogen inducible CAT activity in transfected cells. Interestingly, the estrogen stimulation of TGF-α promoter activity required a 24-h lag period suggesting that this growth factor is an indirect target of an estrogen receptor cascade. Estrogen has also been shown to decrease EGF binding in human endometrial cell cultures, but enhance EGF receptor levels and EGF binding in the uterus of ovariectomized mice.[227,228] Progesterone also enhances EGF receptor levels and EGF binding in the uterus of ovariectomized mice, as well as EGF and IGF-I receptor levels in human endometrial cell cultures.[227] This steroid has been shown to increase insulin receptor mRNA and protein levels in human T-47D breast cancer cells, but down-regulate IGF-I receptor levels in these cells.[229]

Dexamethasone increases EGF receptor levels in ovarian tumor cells with a concomitant suppression of growth.[230] Additionally, dexamethasone enhanced growth hormone binding to its cognate receptor in rat osteosarcoma cells and required *de novo* protein synthesis, suggesting that glucocorticoids stimulate growth hormone receptor levels.[231] Glucocorticoids coordinately suppress the growth and decrease PDGF A chain mRNA levels and secretion in rat hepatoma cells.[232] Moreover, glucocorticoids disrupt a TGF-α autocrine loop in a rat mammary tumor cell line by decreasing the level of secreted TGF-α.[58,59] Constitutive expression of TGF-α in this mammary tumor cell line by transfection of a TGF-α expression vector prevents glucocorticoids from suppressing cell proliferation.[59] Other studies have implicated the regulation of growth factors and their cognate receptors in proliferative control by other members of the steroid receptor gene family.

3. Steroid Regulation of Cell Cycle Components

The altered expression or amplification of cell cycle components has been observed in a variety of tumors and tumor cell lines. For example, cyclin D1 is amplified in approximately 15%, and overexpressed in up to 45% of breast tumors.[27] Moreover, overexpression of cyclin A, cyclin B, and p34[cdc2] were detected in some human primary mammary tumors and cyclin E was overexpressed in several mammary tumor cell lines.[26,27] These observations suggest that the dysregulated expression of cell cycle components may play a key role in the uncontrolled proliferation of cancer cells and may be targets of steroid induced proliferative cascades.[27,233] Consistent with this notion, the regulation of cellular proliferation by steroids and steroid antagonists occurs by cell cycle specific actions in the G1 phase of the cell cycle. For example, in rat Con8 mammary tumor cells and rat BDS1 hepatoma cells, the withdrawal of steroids after growth suppression is accompanied by transient regulation of cyclin D1 and cyclin D2 expression.[34,35] Moreover, TGF-α, which overrides the growth suppressive action of dexamethasone on mammary tumor cells, strongly stimulates the expression of cyclin D1 mRNA.[34,59]

Estrogen stimulates breast cancer cell cycle progression at a point in early G1, whereas, sensitivity to the growth inhibitory effects of antiestrogens is restricted to a limited time frame early in the G1 phase.[30,32,81,234] Antiestrogen treatment, but not antiprogestin treatment, reduces expression of cyclin D1, but both antagonists inhibit cell cycle progression.[32,33,235] The synthetic progestin ORG 2058 stimulates cell cycle progression by shortening the duration of G1 in insulin stimulated T-47D breast cancer cells and transiently induces the expression of cyclin D1.[32] The similarity between the patterns of cyclin gene expression in mitogen stimulated normal mammary epithelial cells and T-47D cells suggests that the G1 cyclins play a similar role in the regulation of proliferation in both normal and neoplastic mammary epithelium.

Thus, alterations in the steroid control of breast epithelial cell cycle progression and G1 cyclin expression is implicated in the aberrant growth control of some breast tumors.

4. Steroid Regulation of Putative Growth Suppressors

The *in vivo* expression of C/EBP is restricted to terminally differentiated adipose tissue, lung, liver, gastrointestinal tract, and placenta.[236] Because this transcription factor is a known growth suppressor of adipocytes *in vitro* and its expression is restricted to terminally differentiated cells *in vivo*, C/EBP may function in the growth arrest of some tissue types. Expression of C/EBP is low in growing hepatoma cells, elevated in mitotically quiescent hepatocytes, and is reduced in regenerating liver.[237,238] Within 1 h of steroid treatment, glucocorticoids maximally stimulate the expression of C/EBP transcripts in rat BDS1 hepatoma cells, at a time frame which is approximately 20 h prior to complete growth arrest.[239] Thus, the regulation of C/EBP transcripts presents a relatively early and perhaps important response to the glucocorticoid mediated growth suppression cascade in hepatoma cells. Consistent with a role for this transcription factor in the suppression of cell proliferation, C/EBP transcripts or protein were not detected in hepatoma cells resistant to the growth suppression effects of glucocorticoids.[239] Thus, the regulated expression of the C/EBP transcription factor is likely to play a role in the glucocorticoid mediated growth suppression of rat hepatoma cells. Recently, it was demonstrated that estrogen, which is involved in the differentiation of ovarian follicles, markedly induced the transcription of C/EBP in the *corpus lutea*.[240] However, the precise functional role of this regulatory molecule in mediating hepatoma cell or ovarian growth is unknown.

Recently, several recessive genes have been identified which, when both alleles are disrupted, correlate with the development of certain types of cancers.[3,23,241] Mutations which ablate the function of the Rb gene product have been shown to be responsible for the development of the pediatric cancer, retinoblastoma. This growth suppressing protein is undetectable in 47% of human breast cancers.[242] Regulation of Rb by steroid hormones is not well understood. However, in one report, dexamethasone inhibited the proliferation of T lymphocytes with a concomitant decrease in the levels of Rb phosphorylation which activates this growth suppressor.[243] Another growth suppressor gene implicated in several different cancer types is p53.[3,23,241] The presence of aberrations in p53 strongly correlates with primary breast cancers and aggressive mammary ductal carcinoma *in situ*.[244-247] Estrogen receptor status inversely correlates with p53 expression in human mammary tumors.[248-250] An inverse correlation between steroid hormone receptor status and p53 expression has also been documented in endometrial carcinomas.[251,252] Of 30 endometrial tumors, 5 expressed p53; none of these tumors expressed estrogen or progesterone receptors. Furthermore, 25 of the 30 endometrial tumors failed to express p53, but expressed both estrogen and progesterone receptors.[251] One study demonstrated that retinoids suppress the *in vitro* invasion of human A549 lung carcinoma cells while inducing the expression of p53.[253] Currently, evidence that steroid hormones regulate p53 expression or function is scant.

VI. COMBINATORIAL GROWTH EFFECTS OF STEROIDS AND GROWTH FACTORS

Growth suppression and growth induction are regulated by an intricate network of communication between cells through cell-cell contacts, cell-stroma interactions, the extracellular matrix, and the secretion and response to soluble factors such as steroid and protein growth regulators. In a variety of cell types, there is strong evidence for cross talk between steroid receptor and growth factor signalling. For example, steroids modulate growth factor and growth factor receptor expression in many different cell types[5] and recently, a novel serine/threonine protein kinase was shown to be a direct target of glucocorticoid receptors in that a glucocorticoid response element has been uncovered in the upstream promoter sequences of the kinase gene.[254,255] The mammary gland provides a useful model to discuss the complexities of combinatorial effects of steroids and growth factors. The reciprocal communication between the mammary epithelium and mesenchymal fibroblasts, and the presence of specific steroid and protein growth regulators, cause the differential development of the breast in males and females.[4,256,257] During mammary gland morphogenesis, epithelial cells trigger the expression of androgen receptors in the surrounding mesenchyme.[258,259] In the male breast, the presence of male sex hormones (e.g., androgens) induces mesenchymal cell condensation around and destruction of the mammary epithelial buds. However, the mere absence of androgen in the female is insufficient to allow for the growth and morphogenesis of the mammary gland. *In vivo* ablation experiments have demonstrated that a combination of estrogen and progesterone induced ductal growth and branching and a combination of these two steroid hormones plus prolactin or growth hormone caused lobuloalveolar development typical of late pregnancy.[260] Moreover, insulin enhances the effect of prolactin on lobuloalveolar development. Neither prolactin, growth hormone, estrogen, nor progesterone alone are sufficient to induce mammary gland development. Furthermore, the addition of both EGF and hydrocortisone were required to maintain the growth of mammary gland explants *in vitro* and a combination of prolactin, insulin, and hydrocortisone is necessary for the growth of normal mammary epithelial cells *in vitro*. In contrast, the *in vitro* growth of mammary tumor derived epithelial cells on plastic requires only prolactin. In some cases, the addition of FGF to serum free medium caused a significant increase in the *in vitro* growth of human T-47D breast cancer cells.[29] However, the effect of FGF on the growth of these cells was less dramatic when the medium was also supplemented with fetal bovine serum.

Interestingly, the *in vitro* growth of some transformed and normal-like mammary epithelial cells is suppressed by the addition of dexamethasone to serum supplemented medium. The growth suppressive effect of dexamethasone can be overridden by the addition of TGF-α or EGF.[34,58,59] Another growth regulator with suppressive activity is TGF-β. Synthetic copolymers containing TGF-β block the *in vivo* growth of mammary end buds without affecting the growth of the surrounding stroma.[261] Additionally, estrogen withdrawal or the addition of antiestrogens to the estrogen dependent MCF-7 mammary epithelial tumor cell line results in the concomitant growth suppression and secretion of TGF-β.[262,263] Furthermore, the estrogen unresponsive MDA-MB 231 mammary tumor cell line is growth suppressed by treatment with TGF-β.[264] The role of retinoids in mammary growth is less clear. It has been reported that vitamin A stimulated mammary duct formation and alveolar growth in the mouse, but inhibited duct formation and alveolar growth in the rat.[258,259] However, there is some evidence that vitamin A enhances the binding of EGF to its cognate receptor in mammary epithelial cells.[265] The complex interactions involved in the growth regulation of the mammary gland clearly have provided a model for understanding the intricacy of growth control that is likely to occur in other tissues and cell types.

In this chapter we have focused on only a few of the many systems for growth control of normal and abnormal cells by steroid and protein hormones and polypeptide growth factors. The signal transduction cascades and activation of transcription factors by these growth regulators are emerging as a common theme throughout the animal kingdom and in almost all cell and tissue types, emphasizing the importance of these mechanisms in cell proliferation and differentiation. We have shown by citing several examples how perturbation at any point within growth regulatory pathways leads to abnormal growth. Continued investigations into growth regulatory mechanisms are likely to provide us with new insights into antiproliferative strategies for combating cancer, an understanding of cell senescence, and perhaps, uncover novel growth regulatory schemes.

ACKNOWLEDGMENTS

We thank Jerry Kapler for his skillful photography and members of our laboratory for their interesting discussions during the preparation of this chapter.

REFERENCES

1. Bishop, J. M., Molecular themes in oncogenesis, *Cell*, 64, 235, 1991.
2. Aaronson, S. A., Growth factors and cancer, *Science*, 254, 1146, 1991.
3. Marshall, C. J., Tumor suppressor genes, *Cell*, 64, 313, 1991.
4. Lippman, M. E. and Dickson, R. B., Mechanisms of growth control in normal and malignant breast epithelium, *Recent Prog. Horm. Res.*, 45, 383, 1989.
5. Dickson, R. B. and Lippman, M. E., Estrogenic regulation of growth and polypeptide growth factor secretion in human breast carcinoma, *Endocr. Rev.*, 8, 29, 1987.
6. Cato, A. C., Konig, H., Ponta, H. and Herrlich, P., Steroids and growth promoting factors in the regulation of expression of genes and gene networks, *J. Steroid Biochem. Mol. Biol.*, 43, 63, 1992.
7. Zipori, D., The renewal and differentiation of hematopoietic stem cells, *FASEB. J.*, 6, 2691, 1992.
8. Fausto, N. and Webber, E. M., Mechanisms of growth regulation in liver regeneration and hepatic carcinogenesis, *Progress in Liver Diseases*, 11, 115, 1993.
9. Ceriani, R. C., Proceedings: hormones and other factors controlling growth in the mammary gland: a review, *J. Invest. Derm.*, 63, 93, 1974.
10. Goustin, A. S., Leof, E. B., Shipley, G. D. and Moses, H. L., Growth factors and cancer, *Cancer Res.*, 46, 1015, 1986.
11. Pardee, A. B., G1 events and regulation of cell proliferation, *Science*, 246, 603, 1989.
12. Howard, A. and Pelc, S. R., Synthesis of desoxyribonucleic acid in normal and irradiated cells and its relationship to chromosome breakage, *Heredity*, Suppl. 6, 261, 1953.
13. Fridovich, K. J., Hansen, L. J., Keyomarsi, K. and Pardee, A. B., Progression through the cell cycle: an overview, *Am. Rev. Respir. Dis.*, S3, 1990.
14. Pines, J., Cyclins and cyclin-dependent kinases: take your partners, *Trends Biochem. Sci.*, 18, 195, 1993.
15. Sherr, C. J., Mammalian G1 cyclins, *Cell*, 73, 1059, 1993.
16. Xiong, Y., Zhang, H. and Beach, D., D type cyclins associate with multiple protein kinases and the DNA replication and repair factor PCNA, *Cell*, 71, 505, 1992.
17. Pines, J., Arresting developments in cell-cycle control, *Trends Biochem. Sci.*, 19, 143, 1994.
18. Hunter, T., Braking the cycle, *Cell*, 75, 839, 1993.
19. Denhardt, D. T., Edwards, D. R. and Parfett, C. L., Gene expression during the mammalian cell cycle, *Biochim. Biophys. Acta*, 865, 83, 1986.
20. Herschman, H. R., Primary response genes induced by growth factors and tumor promoters, *Annu. Rev. Biochem.*, 60, 281, 1991.
21. Hunter, T., Cooperation between oncogenes, *Cell*, 64, 249, 1991.
22. Hartwell, L. H. and Weinert, T. A., Checkpoints: controls that ensure the order of cell cycle events, *Science*, 246, 629, 1989.
23. Weinberg, R. A., Tumor suppressor genes, *Science*, 254, 1138, 1991.
24. Dou, Q. P., Levin, A. H., Zhao, S. and Pardee, A. B., Cyclin E and cyclin A as candidates for the restriction point protein, *Cancer Res.*, 53, 1493, 1993.
25. Lammie, G. A., Fantl, V., Smith, R., Schuuring, E., Brookes, S., Michalides, R., Dickson, C., Arnold, A. and Peters, G., D11S287, a putative oncogene on chromosome 11q13, is amplified and expressed in squamous cell and mammary carcinomas and linked to BCL-1, *Oncogene*, 6, 439, 1991.
26. Keyomarsi, K. and Pardee, A. B., Redundant cyclin overexpression and gene amplification in breast cancer cells, *Proc. Natl. Acad. Sci. U.S.A.*, 90, 1112, 1993.
27. Buckley, M. F., Sweeney, K. J., Hamilton, J. A., Sini, R. L., Manning, D. L., Nicholson, R. I., deFazio, A., Watts, C. K., Musgrove, E. A. and Sutherland, R. L., Expression and amplification of cyclin genes in human breast cancer, *Oncogene*, 8, 2127, 1993.
28. Matsushime, H., Ewen, M. E., Strom, D. K., Kato, J. Y., Hanks, S. K., Roussel, M. F. and Sherr, C. J., Identification and properties of an atypical catalytic subunit (p34PSK-J3/cdk4) for mammalian D type G1 cyclins, *Cell*, 71, 323, 1992.
29. Sutherland, R. L., Lee, C. S., Feldman, R. S. and Musgrove, E. A., Regulation of breast cancer cell cycle progression by growth factors, steroids and steroid antagonists, *J. Steroid Biochem. Mol. Biol.*, 41, 315, 1992.

30. Musgrove, E. A., Wakeling, A. E. and Sutherland, R. L., Points of action of estrogen antagonists and a calmodulin antagonist within the MCF-7 human breast cancer cell cycle, *Cancer Res.*, 49, 2398, 1989.

31. Musgrove, E. A. and Sutherland, R. L., Steroids, growth factors, and cell cycle controls in breast cancer, *Cancer Treat Res.*, 53, 305, 1991.

32. Musgrove, E. A., Hamilton, J., Lee, C. S., Sweeney, K., Watts, C. and Sutherland, R. L., Growth factor, steroid, and steroid antagonist regulation of cyclin gene expression associated with changes in T-47D human breast cancer cell cycle progression, *Mol. Cell. Biol.*, 13, 3577, 1993.

33. Musgrove, E. A. and Sutherland, R. L., Effects of the progestin antagonist RU 486 on T-47D breast cancer cell cycle kinetics and cell cycle regulatory genes, *Biochem. Biophys. Res. Commun.*, 195, 1184, 1993.

34. Goya, L., Maiyar, A. C., Ge, Y. and Firestone, G. L., Glucocorticoids induce a G1/G0 cell cycle arrest of Con8 rat mammary tumor cells that is synchronously reversed by steroid withdrawal or addition of transforming growth factor-alpha, *Mol. Endocrinol.*, 7, 1121, 1993.

35. Sanchez, I., Goya, L., Vallerga, A. K. and Firestone, G. L., Glucocorticoids reversibly arrest rat hepatoma cell growth by inducing an early G1 block in cell cycle progression, *Cell Growth Differ.*, 4, 215, 1993.

36. Kreipe, H., Feist, H., Fischer, L., Felgner, J., Heidorn, K., Mettler, L. and Parwaresch, R., Amplification of c-myc but not of c-erbB-2 is associated with high proliferative capacity in breast cancer, *Cancer Res.*, 53, 1956, 1993.

37. Miyamoto, S., Sukumar, S., Guzman, R. C., Osborn, R. C. and Nandi, S., Transforming c-Ki-ras mutation is a preneoplastic event in mouse mammary carcinogenesis induced in vitro by N-methyl-N-nitrosourea, *Mol. Cell. Biol.*, 10, 1593, 1990.

38. Madsen, M. W., Lykkesfeldt, A. E., Laursen, I., Nielsen, K. V. and Briand, P., Altered gene expression of c-myc, epidermal growth factor receptor, transforming growth factor-alpha, and c-erb-B2 in an immortalized human breast epithelial cell line, HMT-3522, is associated with decreased growth factor requirements, *Cancer Res*, 52, 1210, 1992.

39. Klijn, J. G., Berns, P. M., Schmitz, P. I. and Foekens, J. A., The clinical significance of epidermal growth factor receptor (EGF-R) in human breast cancer: a review on 5232 patients, *Endocr. Rev.*, 13, 3, 1992.

40. Ozbun, M. A., Jerry, D. J., Kittrell, F. S., Medina, D. and Butel, J. S., p53 Mutations selected in vivo when mouse mammary epithelial cells form hyperplastic outgrowths are not necessary for establishment of mammary cell lines in vitro, *Cancer Res.*, 53, 1646, 1993.

41. Argiles, A., Kraft, N. E., Hutchinson, P., Senes, F. S. and Atkins, R. C., Retinoic acid affects the cell cycle and increases total protein content in epithelial cells, *Kidney Int.*, 36, 954, 1989.

42. Berns, E. M., Schuurmans, A. L., Bolt, J., Lamb, D. J., Foekens, J. A. and Mulder, E., Antiproliferative effects of suramin on androgen responsive tumour cells, *Eur. J. Cancer*, 26, 470, 1990.

43. Lippman, M., Bolan, G. and Huff, K., The effects of estrogens and antiestrogens on hormone-responsive human breast cancer in long-term tissue culture, *Cancer Res.*, 36, 4595, 1976.

44. Musgrove, E. A., Lee, C. S. and Sutherland, R. L., Progestins both stimulate and inhibit breast cancer cell cycle progression while increasing expression of transforming growth factor alpha, epidermal growth factor receptor, c-fos, and c-myc genes, *Mol. Cell. Biol.*, 11, 5032, 1991.

45. de Launoit, Y., Veilleux, R., Dufour, M., Simard, J. and Labrie, F., Characteristics of the biphasic action of androgens and of the potent antiproliferative effects of the new pure antiestrogen EM-139 on cell cycle kinetic parameters in LNCaP human prostatic cancer cells, *Cancer Res.*, 51, 5165, 1991.

46. Goya, L., Edwards, C. P., Glennemeier, K. A. and Firestone, G. L., In vivo effects of dexamethasone on the tumor growth of glucocorticoid-sensitive Fu5-derived rat hepatoma cells, *Cancer Lett.*, 58, 211, 1991.

47. Webster, M. K., Guthrie, J. and Firestone, G. L., Suppression of rat mammary tumor cell growth in vitro by glucocorticoids requires serum proteins. Characterization of wild type and glucocorticoid-resistant epithelial tumor cells, *J. Biol. Chem.*, 265, 4831, 1990.

48. Poulin, R., Baker, D., Poirier, D. and Labrie, F., Androgen and glucocorticoid receptor-mediated inhibition of cell proliferation by medroxyprogesterone acetate in ZR-75-1 human breast cancer cells, *Breast Cancer Res. Treat.*, 13, 161, 1989.

49. Cook, P. W., Swanson, K. T., Edwards, C. P. and Firestone, G. L., Glucocorticoid receptor-dependent inhibition of cellular proliferation in dexamethasone-resistant and hypersensitive rat hepatoma cell variants, *Mol. Cell. Biol.*, 8, 1449, 1988.

50. Osborne, C. K., Monaco, M. E., Kahn, C. R., Huff, K., Bronzert, D. and Lippman, M. E., Direct inhibition of growth and antagonism of insulin action by glucocorticoids in human breast cancer cells in culture, *Cancer Res.*, 39, 2422, 1979.

51. Castellano, T. J., Schiffman, R. L., Jacob, M. C. and Loeb, J. N., Suppression of liver cell proliferation by glucocorticoid hormone: a comparison of normally growing and regenerating tissue in the immature rat, *Endocrinology*, 102, 1107, 1978.

52. Owen, T. A., Soprano, D. R. and Soprano, K. J., Analysis of the growth factor requirements for stimulation of WI-38 cells after extended periods of density-dependent growth arrest, *J. Cell. Physiol.*, 139, 424, 1989.

53. Benz, C., Hollander, C. and Miller, B., Endocrine-responsive pancreatic carcinoma: steroid binding and cytotoxicity studies in human tumor cell lines, *Cancer Res.*, 46, 2276, 1986.

54. Daniel, C. P., Parreira, A., Goldman, J. M. and McCarthy, D. M., The effect of 1,25-dihydroxyvitamin D3 on the relationship between growth and differentiation in HL-60 cells, *Leuk. Res.*, 11, 191, 1987.

55. Sebag, M., Henderson, J., Rhim, J. and Kremer, R., Relative resistance to 1,25-dihydroxyvitamin D3 in a keratinocyte model of tumor progression, *J. Biol. Chem.*, 267, 12162, 1992.

56. Ethier, C., Goupil, D. and Gascon, B. M., Influence of the calcium and vitamin D endocrine system on the "priming" of the liver for compensatory growth, *Endocr. Res.*, 17, 421, 1991.

57. Vintermyr, O. K. and Doskeland, S. O., Characterization of the inhibitory effect of glucocorticoids on the DNA replication of adult rat hepatocytes growing at various cell densities, *J. Cell. Physiol.*, 138, 29, 1989.

58. Alexander, D. B., Goya, L., Webster, M. K., Haraguchi, T. and Firestone, G. L., Glucocorticoids coordinately disrupt a transforming growth factor alpha autocrine loop and suppress the growth of 13762NF-derived Con8 rat mammary adenocarcinoma cells, *Cancer Res.*, 53, 1808, 1993.

59. Goya, L., Alexander, D. B., Webster, M. K., Kern, F. G., Guzman, R. C., Nandi, S. and Firestone, G. L., Overexpression of transforming growth factor alpha overrides the glucocorticoid-mediated suppression of Con8 mammary tumor cell growth in vitro and in vivo, *Cancer Res.*, 53, 1816, 1993.

60. Hatakeyama, S., Suzuki, A., Yoshizumi, N., Sato, M. and Nishiya, I., Glucocorticoid-induced G1 arrest and the release effect of epidermal growth factor on the human salivary gland adenocarcinoma cell, *Cell. Biol. Int. Rep.*, 15, 55, 1991.

61. Squinto, S. P., Block, A. L. and Doucet, J. P., Epidermal growth factor induction of cellular proliferation and protooncogene expression in growth-arrested rat H4IIE hepatoma cells: role of cyclic adenosine monophosphate, *Mol. Endocrinol.*, 3, 433, 1989.

62. Hata, Y., Igarashi, M., Takada, N., Namieno, T., Sasaki, F., Une, Y., Uchino, J. and Kajiwara, M., [Development of a new therapeutic method in hepatocellular carcinoma using a culture system — the intensifying effect of human epidermal growth factor (hEGF) on the antitumor action of antitumor agents], *Gan To Kagaku Ryoho*, 16, 1874, 1989.

63. Massague, J., Receptors for the TGF-beta family, *Cell*, 69, 1067, 1992.

64. Sporn, M. B. and Roberts, A. B., Transforming growth factor-beta: recent progress and new challenges, *J. Cell. Biol.*, 119, 1017, 1992.

65. Vivien, D., Galera, P., Lebrun, E., Loyau, G. and Pujol, J. P., Differential effects of transforming growth factor-beta and epidermal growth factor on the cell cycle of cultured rabbit articular chondrocytes, *J. Cell. Physiol.*, 143, 534, 1990.

66. Vivien, D., Galera, P., Lebrun, E., Daireaux, M., Loyau, G. and Pujol, J. P., TGF-beta-induced G2/M delay in proliferating rabbit articular chondrocytes is associated with an enhancement of replication rate and a cAMP decrease: possible involvement of pertussis toxin-sensitive pathway, *J. Cell. Physiol.*, 150, 291, 1992.

67. Vivien, D., Boumedienne, K., Galera, P., Lebrun, E. and Pujol, J. P., Flow cytometric detection of transforming growth factor-beta expression in rabbit articular chondrocytes (RAC) in culture — association with S-phase traverse, *Exp. Cell. Res.*, 203, 56, 1992.

68. Zendegui, J. G., Inman, W. H. and Carpenter, G., Modulation of the mitogenic response of an epidermal growth factor-dependent keratinocyte cell line by dexamethasone, insulin, and transforming growth factor-beta, *J. Cell. Physiol.*, 136, 257, 1988.

69. Zhou, L. and Leung, B. S., Growth regulation of ovarian cancer cells by epidermal growth factor and transforming growth factors alpha and beta 1, *Biochim. Biophys. Acta.*, 1180, 130, 1992.

70. Reiss, M. and Dibble, C. L., Reinitiation of DNA synthesis in quiescent mouse keratinocytes; regulation by polypeptide hormones, cholera toxin, dexamethasone, and retinoic acid, *In Vitro Cell. Dev. Biol.*, 24, 537, 1988.

71. Jozan, S., Guerrin, M., Mazars, P., Dutaur, M., Monsarrat, B., Cheutin, F., Bugat, R., Martel, P. and Valette, A., Transforming growth factor beta 1 (TGF-beta 1) inhibits growth of a human ovarian carcinoma cell line (OVCCR1) and is expressed in human ovarian tumors, *Int. J. Cancer*, 52, 766, 1992.

72. Hung, W. C., Chuang, L. Y., Tsai, J. H. and Chang, C. C., Effects of insulin on TGF-beta 1-induced cell growth inhibition in the human hepatoma cell lines, *Biochem. Mol. Biol. Int.*, 30, 655, 1993.

73. Saltis, J., Agrotis, A. and Bobik, A., TGF-beta 1 potentiates growth factor-stimulated proliferation of vascular smooth muscle cells in genetic hypertension, *Am. J. Physiol.*, 263, C420, 1992.

74. Khan, S. A., Shum, L. W., Teerds, K. and Dorrington, J. H., Steroidogenesis-inducing protein interacts with transforming growth factor-beta to stimulate DNA synthesis in rat granulosa cells, *Mol. Cell. Endocrinol.*, 89, 97, 1992.

75. Larson, R. C., Ignotz, G. G. and Currie, W. B., Transforming growth factor beta and basic fibroblast growth factor synergistically promote early bovine embryo development during the fourth cell cycle, *Mol. Reprod. Dev.*, 33, 432, 1992.

76. Han, E. K., Guadagno, T. M., Dalton, S. L. and Assoian, R. K., A cell cycle and mutational analysis of anchorage-independent growth: cell adhesion and TGF-beta 1 control G1/S transit specifically, *J. Cell. Biol.*, 122, 461, 1993.

77. Brelje, T. C., Parsons, J. A. and Sorenson, R. L., Regulation of islet beta-cell proliferation by prolactin in rat islets, *Diabetes*, 43, 263, 1994.

78. DeVito, W. J., Okulicz, W. C., Stone, S. and Avakian, C., Prolactin-stimulated mitogenesis of cultured astrocytes, *Endocrinology*, 130, 2549, 1992.

79. Smeets, T. and van Buul-Offers, S., Influence of growth hormone and thyroxine on cell kinetics in the proximal tibial growth plate of Snell dwarf mice, *Cell Tissue Kinet.*, 19, 161, 1986.

80. Gertler, A., Walker, A. and Friesen, H. G., Enhancement of human growth hormone-stimulated mitogenesis of Nb2 node lymphoma cells by 12-O-tetradecanoyl-phorbol-13-acetate, *Endocrinology*, 116, 1636, 1985.

81. van der Burg, B., Rutteman, G. R., Blankenstein, M. A., de Laat, S. and van Zoelen, E., Mitogenic stimulation of human breast cancer cells in a growth factor-defined medium: synergistic action of insulin and estrogen, *J. Cell. Physiol.*, 134, 101, 1988.

82. Chen, Y. Y. and Rabinovitch, P. S., Mitogen response and cell cycle kinetics of Swiss 3T3 cells in defined medium: differences from human fibroblasts and effects of cell density, *Exp. Cell Res.*, 190, 145, 1990.

83. Larsson, O., Zetterberg, A. and Engstrom, W., Cell-cycle-specific induction of quiescence achieved by limited inhibition of protein synthesis: counteractive effect of addition of purified growth factors, *J. Cell Sci.*, 73, 375, 1985.

84. Lu, K. and Campisi, J., Ras proteins are essential and selective for the action of insulin-like growth factor 1 late in the G1 phase of the cell cycle in BALB/c murine fibroblasts, *Proc. Natl. Acad. Sci. U.S.A.*, 89, 3889, 1992.

85. Chen, Y. and Rabinovitch, P. S., Platelet-derived growth factor, epidermal growth factor, and insulin-like growth factor I regulate specific cell-cycle parameters of human diploid fibroblasts in serum-free culture, *J. Cell. Physiol.*, 140, 59, 1989.

86. Chen, Y. Y. and Rabinovitch, P. S., Altered cell cycle responses to insulin-like growth factor I, but not platelet-derived growth factor and epidermal growth factor, in senescing human fibroblasts, *J. Cell. Physiol.*, 144, 18, 1990.

87. Hill, D. J. and de Sousa, D., Insulin is a mitogen for isolated epiphyseal growth plate chondrocytes from the fetal lamb, *Endocrinology*, 126, 2661, 1990.

88. Spydevold, O., Sorensen, H., Clausen, O. P. and Gautvik, K. M., Dexamethasone inhibition of rat hepatoma cell growth and cell cycle traverse is reversed by insulin, *Biochim. Biophys. Acta.*, 1052, 221, 1990.

89. Ullrich, A. and Schlessinger, J., Signal transduction by receptors with tyrosine kinase activity, *Cell*, 61, 203, 1990.

90. Hunter, T. and Karin, M., The regulation of transcription by phosphorylation, *Cell*, 70, 375, 1992.

91. Sandgren, E. P., Luetteke, N. C., Qiu, T. H., Palmiter, R. D., Brinster, R. L. and Lee, D. C., Transforming growth factor alpha dramatically enhances oncogene-induced carcinogenesis in transgenic mouse pancreas and liver, *Mo. Cell Biol.*, 13, 320, 1993.

92. Lee, G. H., Merlino, G. and Fausto, N., Development of liver tumors in transforming growth factor alpha transgenic mice, *Cancer Res.*, 52, 5162, 1992.

93. Takagi, H., Sharp, R., Hammermeister, C., Goodrow, T., Bradley, M. O., Fausto, N. and Merlino, G., Molecular and genetic analysis of liver oncogenesis in transforming growth factor alpha transgenic mice, *Cancer Res.*, 52, 5171, 1992.

94. Matsui, Y., Halter, S. A., Holt, J. T., Hogan, B. L. and Coffey, R. J., Development of mammary hyperplasia and neoplasia in MMTV-TGF alpha transgenic mice, *Cell*, 61, 1147, 1990.

95. Cross, M. and Dexter, T. M., Growth factors in development, transformation, and tumorigenesis, *Cell*, 64, 271, 1991.

96. Taipale, J., Miyazono, K., Heldin, C. H. and Keski, O. J., Latent transforming growth factor-beta 1 associates to fibroblast extracellular matrix via latent TGF-beta binding protein, *J. Cell. Biol.*, 124, 171, 1994.

97. Alon, R., Cahalon, L., Hershkoviz, R., Elbaz, D., Reizis, B., Wallach, D., Akiyama, S. K., Yamada, K. M. and Lider, O., TNF-alpha binds to the N-terminal domain of fibronectin and augments the beta 1-integrin-mediated adhesion of CD4+ T lymphocytes to the glycoprotein, *J. Immunol.*, 152, 1304, 1994.

98. Murono, E. P., Washburn, A. L., Goforth, D. P. and Wu, N., Evidence that both receptor- and heparin sulfate proteoglycan-bound basic fibroblast growth factor are internalized by cultured immature Leydig cells, *Mol. Cell. Endocrinol.*, 98, 81, 1993.

99. Massague, J. and Pandiella, A., Membrane-anchored growth factors, *Annu. Rev. Biochem.*, 62, 515, 1993.

100. Schalch, D. S., Heinrich, U. E., Draznin, B., Johnson, C. J. and Miller, L. L., Role of the liver in regulating somatomedin activity: hormonal effects on the synthesis and release of insulin-like growth factor and its carrier protein by the isolated perfused rat liver, *Endocrinology*, 104, 1143, 1979.

101. Sporn, M. B. and Todaro, G. J., Autocrine secretion and malignant transformation of cells, *N. Engl. J. Med.*, 303, 878, 1980.

102. Deuel, T. F., Polypeptide growth factors: roles in normal and abnormal cell growth, *Annu. Rev. Cell Biol.*, 3, 443, 1987.

103. Luetteke, N. C. and Lee, D. C., Transforming growth factor alpha: expression, regulation and biological action of its integral membrane precursor, *Semin. Cancer Biol.*, 1, 265, 1990.

104. Pandiella, A., Bosenberg, M. W., Huang, E. J., Besmer, P. and Massague, J., Cleavage of membrane-anchored growth factors involves distinct protease activities regulated through common mechanisms, *J. Biol. Chem.*, 267, 24028, 1992.

105. Hill, R. J. and Sternberg, P. W., The gene lin-3 encodes an inductive signal for vulval development in C. elegans [see comments], *Nature*, 358, 470, 1992.

106. Rutledge, B. J., Zhang, K., Bier, E., Jan, Y. N. and Perrimon, N., The Drosophila spitz gene encodes a putative EGF-like growth factor involved in dorsal-ventral axis formation and neurogenesis, *Genes Dev.*, 6, 1503, 1992.

107. Ruoslahti, E. and Yamaguchi, Y., Proteoglycans as modulators of growth factor activities, *Cell*, 64, 867, 1991.

108. Dohlman, H. G., Thorner, J., Caron, M. G. and Lefkowitz, R. J., Model systems for the study of seven-transmembrane-segment receptors, *Annu. Rev. Biochem.*, 60, 653, 1991.

109. Gilman, A. G., G proteins: transducers of receptor-generated signals, *Annu. Rev. Biochem.*, 56, 615, 1987.

110. Simon, M. I., Strathmann, M. P. and Gautam, N., Diversity of G proteins in signal transduction, *Science*, 252, 802, 1991.

111. Bazan, J. F., A novel family of growth factor receptors: a common binding domain in the growth hormone, prolactin, erythropoietin and IL-6 receptors, and the p75 IL-2 receptor beta-chain, *Biochem. Biophys. Res. Commun.*, 164, 788, 1989.

112. Taga, T. and Kishimoto, T., Cytokine receptors and signal transduction, *FASEB J.*, 6, 3387, 1992.

113. Stahl, N. and Yancopoulos, G. D., The alphas, betas, and kinases of cytokine receptor complexes, *Cell*, 74, 587, 1993.

114. Witthuhn, B. A., Quelle, F. W., Silvennoinen, O., Yi, T., Tang, B., Miura, O. and Ihle, J. N., JAK2 associates with the erythropoietin receptor and is tyrosine phosphorylated and activated following stimulation with erythropoietin, *Cell*, 74, 227, 1993.

115. Velazquez, L., Fellous, M., Stark, G. R. and Pellegrini, S., A protein tyrosine kinase in the interferon alpha/beta signaling pathway, *Cell*, 70, 313, 1992.

116. Cadena, D. L. and Gill, G. N., Receptor tyrosine kinases, *FASEB. J.*, 6, 2332, 1992.

117. Yarden, Y. and Ullrich, A., Growth factor receptor tyrosine kinases, *Annu. Rev. Biochem.*, 57, 443, 1988.

118. Kraus, M. H., Issing, W., Miki, T., Popescu, N. C. and Aaronson, S. A., Isolation and characterization of ERBB3, a third member of the ERBB/epidermal growth factor receptor family: evidence for overexpression in a subset of human mammary tumors, *Proc. Natl. Acad. Sci. U.S.A.*, 86, 9193, 1989.

119. Pawson, T. and Bernstein, A., Receptor tyrosine kinases: genetic evidence for their role in Drosophila and mouse development, *Trends Genet.*, 6, 350, 1990.

120. Williams, L. T., Signal transduction by the platelet-derived growth factor receptor, *Science*, 243, 1564, 1989.

121. Ueno, H., Colbert, H., Escobedo, J. A. and Williams, L. T., Inhibition of PDGF beta receptor signal transduction by coexpression of a truncated receptor, *Science*, 252, 844, 1991.

122. Lee, J., Dull, T. J., Lax, I., Schlessinger, J. and Ullrich, A., HER2 cytoplasmic domain generates normal mitogenic and transforming signals in a chimeric receptor, *EMBO J.*, 8, 167, 1989.

123. Lin, C. R., Chen, W. S., Lazar, C. S., Carpenter, C. D., Gill, G. N., Evans, R. M. and Rosenfeld, M. G., Protein kinase C phosphorylation at Thr 654 of the unoccupied EGF receptor and EGF binding regulate functional receptor loss by independent mechanisms, *Cell*, 44, 839, 1986.

124. Davis, R. J., Independent mechanisms account for the regulation by protein kinase C of the epidermal growth factor receptor affinity and tyrosine-protein kinase activity, *J. Biol. Chem.*, 263, 9462, 1988.

125. Moolenaar, W. H., Bierman, A. J., Tilly, B. C., Verlaan, I., Defize, L. H., Honegger, A. M., Ullrich, A. and Schlessinger, J., A point mutation at the ATP-binding site of the EGF-receptor abolishes signal transduction, *EMBO J.*, 7, 707, 1988.

126. Felder, S., Miller, K., Moehren, G., Ullrich, A., Schlessinger, J. and Hopkins, C. R., Kinase activity controls the sorting of the epidermal growth factor receptor within the multivesicular body, *Cell*, 61, 623, 1990.

127. Escobedo, J. A. and Williams, L. T., A PDGF receptor domain essential for mitogenesis but not for many other responses to PDGF, *Nature*, 335, 85, 1988.

128. Taylor, G. R., Reedijk, M., Rothwell, V., Rohrschneider, L. and Pawson, T., The unique insert of cellular and viral fms protein tyrosine kinase domains is dispensable for enzymatic and transforming activities, *EMBO J.*, 8, 2029, 1989.

129. Roussel, M. F., Dull, T. J., Rettenmier, C. W., Ralph, P., Ullrich, A. and Sherr, C. J., Transforming potential of the c-fms proto-oncogene (CSF-1 receptor), *Nature*, 325, 549, 1987.

130. Koch, C. A., Anderson, D., Moran, M. F., Ellis, C. and Pawson, T., SH2 and SH3 domains: elements that control interactions of cytoplasmic signaling proteins, *Science*, 252, 668, 1991.

131. Carpenter, G., Receptor tyrosine kinase substrates: src homology domains and signal transduction, *FASEB J.*, 6, 3283, 1992.

132. McCormick, F., Signal transduction. How receptors turn Ras on [news; comment], *Nature*, 363, 15, 1993.

133. Egan, S. E., Giddings, B. W., Brooks, M. W., Buday, L., Sizeland, A. M. and Weinberg, R. A., Association of Sos Ras exchange protein with Grb2 is implicated in tyrosine kinase signal transduction and transformation [see comments], *Nature*, 363, 45, 1993.

134. Rozakis, A. M., Fernley, R., Wade, J., Pawson, T. and Bowtell, D., The SH2 and SH3 domains of mammalian Grb2 couple the EGF receptor to the Ras activator mSos1 [see comments], *Nature*, 363, 83, 1993.

135. Li, N., Batzer, A., Daly, R., Yajnik, V., Skolnik, E., Chardin, P., Bar-Sagi, D., Margolis, B. and Schlessinger, J., Guanine-nucleotide-releasing factor hSos1 binds to Grb2 and links receptor tyrosine kinases to Ras signalling [see comments], *Nature*, 363, 85, 1993.

136. Gale, N. W., Kaplan, S., Lowenstein, E. J., Schlessinger, J. and Bar, S. D., Grb2 mediates the EGF-dependent activation of guanine nucleotide exchange on Ras [see comments], *Nature*, 363, 88, 1993.

137. Simon, M. A., Dodson, G. S. and Rubin, G. M., An SH3-SH2-SH3 protein is required for p21Ras1 activation and binds to sevenless and Sos proteins in vitro, *Cell*, 73, 169, 1993.

138. Olivier, J. P., Raabe, T., Henkemeyer, M., Dickson, B., Mbamalu, G., Margolis, B., Schlessinger, J., Hafen, E. and Pawson, T., A Drosophila SH2-SH3 adaptor protein implicated in coupling the sevenless tyrosine kinase to an activator of Ras guanine nucleotide exchange, Sos, *Cell*, 73, 179, 1993.

139. Buday, L. and Downward, J., Epidermal growth factor regulates p21ras through the formation of a complex of receptor, Grb2 adapter protein, and Sos nucleotide exchange factor, *Cell*, 73, 611, 1993.

140. Baltensperger, K., Kozma, L. M., Cherniack, A. D., Klarlund, J. K., Chawla, A., Banerjee, U. and Czech, M. P., Binding of the Ras activator son of sevenless to insulin receptor substrate-1 signaling complexes, *Science*, 260, 1950, 1993.

141. Skolnik, E. Y., Batzer, A., Li, N., Lee, C. H., Lowenstein, E., Mohammadi, M., Margolis, B. and Schlessinger, J., The function of GRB2 in linking the insulin receptor to Ras signaling pathways, *Science*, 260, 1953, 1993.

142. Chardin, P., Camonis, J. H., Gale, N. W., van Aelst, L., Schlessinger, J., Wigler, M. H. and Bar Saqi, D., Human Sos1: a guanine nucleotide exchange factor for Ras that binds to GRB2, *Science*, 260, 1338, 1993.

143. Cantley, L. C., Auger, K. R., Carpenter, C., Duckworth, B., Graziani, A., Kapeller, R. and Soltoff, S., Oncogenes and signal transduction [published erratum appears in *Cell*, 65, following 914, 1991], *Cell*, 64, 281, 1991.

144. Vojtek, A. B., Hollenberg, S. M. and Cooper, J. A., Mammalian Ras interacts directly with the serine/threonine kinase Raf, *Cell*, 74, 205, 1993.

145. Thomas, G., MAP kinase by any other name smells just as sweet, *Cell*, 68, 3, 1992.

146. Crews, C. M., Alessandrini, A. and Erikson, R. L., Erks: their fifteen minutes has arrived, *Cell Growth Differ.*, 3, 135, 1992.

147. Howe, L. R., Leevers, S. J., Gomez, N., Nakielny, S., Cohen, P. and Marshall, C. J., Activation of the MAP kinase pathway by the protein kinase raf, *Cell*, 71, 335, 1992.

148. Ruff-Jamison, S., Chen, K. and Cohen, S., Induction by EGF and interferon-gamma of tyrosine phosphorylated DNA binding proteins in mouse liver nuclei [see comments], *Science*, 261, 1733, 1993.

149. Larner, A. C., David, M., Feldman, G. M., Igarashi, K., Hackett, R. H., Webb, D. S., Sweitzer, S. M., Petricoin, E. and Finbloom, D. S., Tyrosine phosphorylation of DNA binding proteins by multiple cytokines [see comments], *Science*, 261, 1730, 1993.

150. Fu, X. Y. and Zhang, J. J., Transcription factor p91 interacts with the epidermal growth factor receptor and mediates activation of the c-fos gene promoter, *Cell*, 74, 1135, 1993.

151. Silvennoinen, O., Schindler, C., Schlessinger, J. and Levy, D. E., Ras-independent growth factor signaling by transcription factor tyrosine phosphorylation [see comments], *Science*, 261, 1736, 1993.

152. Sadowski, H. B., Shuai, K., Darnell, J. J. and Gilman, M. Z., A common nuclear signal transduction pathway activated by growth factor and cytokine receptors [see comments], *Science*, 261, 1739, 1993.

153. Shuai, K., Stark, G. R., Kerr, I. M. and Darnell, J. J., A single phosphotyrosine residue of Stat91 required for gene activation by interferon-gamma [see comments], *Science*, 261, 1744, 1993.

154. Zhong, Z., Wen, Z. and Darnell, J. J., Stat3: a STAT family member activated by tyrosine phosphorylation in response to epidermal growth factor and interleukin-6, *Science*, 264, 95, 1994.

155. Bourne, H. R., Sanders, D. A. and McCormick, F., The GTPase superfamily: conserved structure and molecular mechanism, *Nature*, 349, 117, 1991.

156. Li, P., Wood, K., Mamon, H., Haser, W. and Roberts, T., Raf-1: a kinase currently without a cause but not lacking in effects, *Cell*, 64, 479, 1991.

157. Meijlink, F., Curran, T., Miller, A. D. and Verma, I. M., Removal of a 67-base-pair sequence in the noncoding region of protooncogene fos converts it to a transforming gene, *Proc. Natl. Acad. Sci. U.S.A.*, 82, 4987, 1985.

158. Bos, T. J., Monteclaro, F. S., Mitsunobu, F., Ball, A. J., Chang, C. H., Nishimura, T. and Vogt, P. K., Efficient transformation of chicken embryo fibroblasts by c-Jun requires structural modification in coding and noncoding sequences, *Genes Dev.*, 4, 1677, 1990.

159. Daniel, C. W. and Robinson, S. D., Regulation of mammary growth and function by TGF-beta, *Mol. Reprod. Dev.*, 32, 145, 1992.

160. Lopez-Casillas, F., Wrana, J. L. and Massague, J., Betaglycan presents ligand to the TGF beta signaling receptor, *Cell*, 73, 1435, 1993.

161. Bassing, C. H., Yingling, J. M., Howe, D. J., Wang, T., He, W. W., Gustafson, M. L., Shah, P., Donahoe, P. K. and Wang, X. F., A transforming growth factor beta type I receptor that signals to activate gene expression, *Science*, 263, 87, 1994.

162. Wrana, J. L., Attisano, L., Carcamo, J., Zentella, A., Doody, J., Laiho, M., Wang, X. F. and Massague, J., TGF beta signals through a heteromeric protein kinase receptor complex, *Cell*, 71, 1003, 1992.

163. Lin, H. Y., Wang, X. F., Ng, E. E., Weinberg, R. A. and Lodish, H. F., Expression cloning of the TGF-beta type II receptor, a functional transmembrane serine/threonine kinase [published erratum appears in *Cell*, 70, following 1068, 1992], *Cell*, 68, 775, 1992.

164. Chen, R. H., Ebner, R. and Derynck, R., Inactivation of the type II receptor reveals two receptor pathways for the diverse TGF-beta activities, *Science*, 260, 1335, 1993.

165. Ebner, R., Chen, R. H., Lawler, S., Zioncheck, T. and Derynck, R., Determination of type I receptor specificity by the type II receptors for TGF-beta or activin, *Science*, 262, 900, 1993.

166. Laiho, M., DeCaprio, J. A., Ludlow, J. W., Livingston, D. M. and Massague, J., Growth inhibition by TGF-beta linked to suppression of retinoblastoma protein phosphorylation, *Cell*, 62, 175, 1990.

167. Ewen, M. E., Sluss, H. K., Whitehouse, L. L. and Livingston, D. M., TGF beta inhibition of Cdk4 synthesis is linked to cell cycle arrest, *Cell*, 74, 1009, 1993.

168. Matsushime, H., Quelle, D. E., Shurtleff, S. A., Shibuya, M., Sherr, C. J. and Kato, J. Y., D-type cyclin-dependent kinase activity in mammalian cells, *Mol. Cell. Biol.*, 14, 2066, 1994.

169. Koff, A., Ohtsuki, M., Polyak, K., Roberts, J. M. and Massague, J., Negative regulation of G1 in mammalian cells: inhibition of cyclin E-dependent kinase by TGF-beta, *Science*, 260, 536, 1993.

170. Polyak, K., Kato, J. Y., Solomon, M. J., Sherr, C. J., Massague, J., Roberts, J. M. and Koff, A., p27Kip1, a cyclin-Cdk inhibitor, links transforming growth factor-beta and contact inhibition to cell cycle arrest, *Genes Dev.*, 8, 9, 1994.

171. Simpson, E. R., Cholesterol side-chain cleavage, cytochrome P-450, and the control of steroidogenesis, *Mol. Cell. Endocrinol.*, 13, 213, 1979.

172. Landers, J. P. and Spelsberg, T. C., New concepts in steroid hormone action: transcription factors, proto-oncogenes, and the cascade model for steroid regulation of gene expression, *Crit. Rev. Eukaryot. Gene Expr.*, 2, 19, 1992.

173. Truss, M. and Beato, M., Steroid hormone receptors: interaction with deoxyribonucleic acid and transcription factors, *Endocr. Rev.*, 14, 459, 1993.

174. Gronemeyer, H., Control of transcription activation by steroid hormone receptors, *FASEB J.*, 6, 2524, 1992.

175. Wahli, W. and Martinez, E., Superfamily of steroid nuclear receptors: positive and negative regulators of gene expression, *FASEB J.*, 5, 2243, 1991.

176. Fuller, P. J., The steroid receptor superfamily: mechanisms of diversity, *FASEB J.*, 5, 3092, 1991.

177. Beato, M., Transcriptional control by nuclear receptors, *FASEB J.*, 5, 2044, 1991.

178. Evans, R. M., The steroid and thyroid hormone receptor superfamily, *Science*, 240, 889, 1988.

179. Yamamoto, K. R., Steroid receptor regulated transcription of specific genes and gene networks, *Annu. Rev. Genet.*, 19, 209, 1985.

180. Diamond, M. I., Miner, J. N., Yoshinaga, S. K. and Yamamoto, K. R., Transcription factor interactions: selectors of positive or negative regulation from a single DNA element, *Science*, 249, 1266, 1990.

181. Jonat, C., Rahmsdorf, H. J., Park, K. K., Cato, A. C., Gebel, S., Ponta, H. and Herrlich, P., Antitumor promotion and antiinflammation: down-modulation of AP-1 (Fos/Jun) activity by glucocorticoid hormone, *Cell*, 62, 1189, 1990.

182. Schule, R., Rangarajan, P., Kliewer, S., Ransone, L., Bolado, J., Yang, N., Verma, I. and Evans, R., Functional antagonism between oncoprotein c-Jun and the glucocorticoid receptor, *Cell*, 62, 1217, 1990.

183. Schule, R. and Evans, R., Functional antagonism between oncoprotein c-Jun and steroid hormone receptors, *Cold Spring Harb. Symp. Quant. Biol.*, 56, 119, 1991.

184. Yang, Y. H., Chambard, J. C., Sun, Y. L., Smeal, T., Schmidt, T. J., Drouin, J. and Karin, M., Transcriptional interference between c-Jun and the glucocorticoid receptor: mutual inhibition of DNA binding due to direct protein-protein interaction, *Cell*, 62, 1205, 1990.

185. Lucas, P. C. and Granner, D. K., Hormone response domains in gene transcription, *Annu. Rev. Biochem.*, 61, 1131, 1992.

186. Cheyette, T. E., Ip, T., Faber, S., Matsui, Y. and Chalkley, R., Characterization of the factors binding to a PEPCK gene upstream hypersensitive site with LCR activity, *Nucleic Acids Res.*, 20, 3427, 1992.

187. Giralt, M., Park, E. A., Gurney, A. L., Liu, J. S., Hakimi, P. and Hanson, R. W., Identification of a thyroid hormone response element in the phosphoenolpyruvate carboxykinase (GTP) gene. Evidence for synergistic interaction between thyroid hormone and cAMP cis-regulatory elements, *J. Biol. Chem.*, 266, 21991, 1991.

188. Girard, J., Perdereau, D., Narkewicz, M., Coupe, C., Ferre, P., Decaux, J. F. and Bossard, P., Hormonal regulation of liver phosphoenolpyruvate carboxykinase and glucokinase gene expression at weaning in the rat, *Biochimie*, 73, 71, 1991.

189. Lucas, P. C., Forman, B. M., Samuels, H. H. and Granner, D. K., Specificity of a retinoic acid response element in the phosphoenolpyruvate carboxykinase gene promoter: consequences of both retinoic acid and thyroid hormone receptor binding [published erratum appears in *Mol. Cell. Biol.*, 11, 6343, 1991], *Mol. Cell. Biol.*, 11, 5164, 1991.

190. Lucas, P. C., O'Brien, R. M., Mitchell, J. A., Davis, C. M., Imai, E., Forman, B. M., Samuels, H. H. and Granner, D. K., A retinoic acid response element is part of a pleiotropic domain in the phosphoenolpyruvate carboxykinase gene, *Proc. Natl. Acad. Sci. U.S.A.*, 88, 2184, 1991.

191. Milland, J. and Schreiber, G., Transcriptional activity of the phosphoenolpyruvate carboxykinase gene decreases in regenerating rat liver, *FEBS Lett.*, 279, 184, 1991.

192. Schafer, A. J. and Fournier, R. E., Multiple elements regulate phosphoenolpyruvate carboxykinase gene expression in hepatoma hybrid cells, *Somat. Cell. Mol. Genet.*, 18, 571, 1992.

193. Park, E. A., Roesler, W. J., Liu, J., Klemm, D. J., Gurney, A. L., Thatcher, J. D., Shuman, J., Friedman, A. and Hanson, R. W., The role of the CCAAT/enhancer-binding protein in the transcriptional regulation of the gene for phosphoenolpyruvate carboxykinase (GTP), *Mol. Cell. Biol.*, 10, 6264, 1990.

194. Park, E. A., Gurney, A. L., Nizielski, S. E., Hakimi, P., Cao, Z., Moorman, A. and Hanson, R. W., Relative roles of CCAAT/enhancer-binding protein beta and cAMP regulatory element-binding protein in controlling transcription of the gene for phosphoenolpyruvate carboxykinase (GTP), *J. Biol. Chem.*, 268, 613, 1993.

195. Gurney, A. L., Park, E. A., Giralt, M., Liu, J. and Hanson, R. W., Opposing actions of Fos and Jun on transcription of the phosphoenolpyruvate carboxykinase (GTP) gene. Dominant negative regulation by Fos, *J. Biol. Chem.*, 267, 18133, 1992.

196. Ray, A. and Prefontaine, K. E., Physical association and functional antagonism between the p65 subunit of transcription factor NF-kappa B and the glucocorticoid receptor, *Proc. Natl. Acad. Sci. U.S.A.*, 91, 752, 1994.

197. Grimm, S. and Baeuerle, P. A., The inducible transcription factor NF-kappa B: structure-function relationship of its protein subunits, *Biochemical Journal*, 290, 297, 1993.

198. Liou, H. C. and Baltimore, D., Regulation of the NF-kappa B/rel transcription factor and I kappa B inhibitor system, *Current Opinion in Cell Biology*, 5, 477, 1993.

199. Zhang, X. K., Wills, K. N., Husmann, M., Hermann, T. and Pfahl, M., Novel pathway for thyroid hormone receptor action through interaction with jun and fos oncogene activities, *Mol. Cell. Biol.*, 11, 6016, 1991.

200. Schuchard, M., Landers, J. P., Sandhu, N. P. and Spelsberg, T. C., Steroid hormone regulation of nuclear proto-oncogenes, *Endocr. Rev.*, 14, 659, 1993.

201. Dubik, D., Dembinski, T. C. and Shiu, R. P., Stimulation of c-myc oncogene expression associated with estrogen-induced proliferation of human breast cancer cells, *Cancer Res.*, 47, 6517, 1987.

202. Ma, T., Mahajan, P. B. and Thompson, E. A., Glucocorticoid regulation of c-myc promoter utilization in P1798 T-lymphoma cells, *Mol. Endocrinol.*, 6, 960, 1992.

203. Persico, E., Scalona, M., Cicatiello, L., Sica, V., Bresciani, F. and Weisz, A., Activation of 'immediate-early' genes by estrogen is not sufficient to achieve stimulation of DNA synthesis in rat uterus, *Biochem. Biophys. Res. Commun.*, 171, 287, 1990.

204. Loose, M. D., Chiappetta, C. and Stancel, G. M., Estrogen regulation of c-fos messenger ribonucleic acid, *Mol. Endocrinol.*, 2, 946, 1988.

205. Weisz, A. and Bresciani, F., Estrogen induces expression of c-fos and c-myc protooncogenes in rat uterus, *Mol. Endocrinol.*, 2, 816, 1988.

206. Cicatiello, L., Sica, V., Bresciani, F. and Weisz, A., Identification of a specific pattern of "immediate-early" gene activation induced by estrogen during mitogenic stimulation of rat uterine cells, *Receptor*, 3, 17, 1993.

207. Cicatiello, L., Ambrosino, C., Coletta, B., Scalona, M., Sica, V., Bresciani, F. and Weisz, A., Transcriptional activation of jun and actin genes by estrogen during mitogenic stimulation of rat uterine cells, *J. Steroid Biochem. Mol. Biol.*, 41, 523, 1992.

208. Szijan, I., Parma, D. L. and Engel, N. I., Expression of c-myc and c-fos protooncogenes in the anterior pituitary gland of the rat. Effect of estrogen, *Horm. Metab. Res.*, 24, 154, 1992.

209. Pellerin, I., Vuillermoz, C., Jouvenot, M., Royez, M., Ordener, C., Marechal, G. and Adessi, G., Superinduction of c-fos gene expression by estrogen in cultured guinea-pig endometrial cells requires priming by a cycloheximide-dependent mechanism, *Endocrinology*, 131, 1094, 1992.

210. Jouvenot, M., Pellerin, I., Alkhalaf, M., Marechal, G., Royez, M. and Adessi, G. L., Effects of 17 beta-estradiol and growth factors on c-fos gene expression in endometrial epithelial cells in primary culture, *Mol. Cell. Endocrinol.*, 72, 149, 1990.

211. Weisz, A., Cicatiello, L., Persico, E., Scalona, M. and Bresciani, F., Estrogen stimulates transcription of c-jun protooncogene, *Mol. Endocrinol.*, 4, 1041, 1990.

212. Cohrs, R. J., Goswami, B. B. and Sharma, O. K., Down regulation of c-myc, c-fos and erb-B during estrogen induced proliferation of the chick oviduct, *Biochem. Biophys. Res. Commun.*, 150, 82, 1988.

213. Lau, C. K., Subramaniam, M., Rasmussen, K. and Spelsberg, T. C., Rapid inhibition of the c-jun proto-oncogene expression in avian oviduct by estrogen, *Endocrinology*, 127, 2595, 1990.

214. Alkhalaf, M. and Murphy, L. C., Regulation of c-jun and jun-B by progestins in T-47D human breast cancer cells, *Mol. Endocrinol.*, 6, 1625, 1992.

215. Wong, M. S. and Murphy, L. C., Differential regulation of c-myc by progestins and antiestrogens in T-47D human breast cancer cells, *J. Steroid Biochem. Mol. Biol.*, 39, 39, 1991.

216. Rories, C., Lau, C. K., Fink, K. and Spelsberg, T. C., Rapid inhibition of c-myc gene expression by a glucocorticoid in the avian oviduct, *Mol. Endocrinol.*, 3, 991, 1989.

217. O'Banion, M. K., Levenson, R. M., Brinckmann, U. G. and Young, D. A., Glucocorticoid modulation of transformed cell proliferation is oncogene specific and correlates with effects on c-myc levels, *Mol. Endocrinol.*, 6, 1371, 1992.

218. Forsthoefel, A. M. and Thompson, E. A., Glucocorticoid regulation of transcription of the c-myc cellular protooncogene in P1798 cells, *Mol. Endocrinol.*, 1, 899, 1987.

219. Birek, C., Huang, H. Z., Birek, P. and Tenenbaum, H. C., c-fos Oncogene expression in dexamethasone stimulated osteogenic cells in chick embryo periosteal cultures, *Bone Miner.*, 15, 193, 1991.

220. Lin, S. C., MacLeod, S. and Hardin, J. W., Effects of glucocorticoids on expression of the fos protooncogene in AtT-20 cells, *Endocrinology*, 130, 257, 1992.

221. Yin, J. and Howells, R. D., Glucocorticoid-mediated down regulation of c-fos mRNA in C6 glioma cells: lack of correlation with proenkephalin mRNA, *Mol. Brain Res.*, 12, 187, 1992.

222. Kirkland, J. L., Murthy, L. and Stancel, G. M., Progesterone inhibits the estrogen-induced expression of c-fos messenger ribonucleic acid in the uterus, *Endocrinology*, 130, 3223, 1992.

223. Hass, R., Brach, M., Kharbanda, S., Giese, G., Traub, P. and Kufe, D., Inhibition of phorbol ester-induced monocytic differentiation by dexamethasone is associated with down-regulation of c-fos and c-jun (AP-1), *J. Cell. Physiol.*, 149, 125, 1991.

224. Lee, H., Shaw, Y. T., Chiou, S. T., Chang, W. C. and Lai, M. D., The effects of glucocorticoid hormone on the expression of c-jun, *FEBS Lett.*, 280, 134, 1991.

225. Nelson, K. G., Takahashi, T., Lee, D. C., Luetteke, N. C., Bossert, N. L., Ross, K., Eitzman, B. E. and McLachlan, J. A., Transforming growth factor-alpha is a potential mediator of estrogen action in the mouse uterus, *Endocrinology*, 131, 1657, 1992.

226. Saeki, T., Cristiano, A., Lynch, M. J., Brittain, M., Kim, N., Mormanno, N., Kenney, N., Ciardiello, F. and Salomon, D. S., Regulation by estrogen through the 5'-flanking region of the transforming growth factor alpha gene, *Mol. Endocrinol.*, 5, 1955, 1991.

227. Reynolds, R. K., Talavera, F., Roberts, J. A., Hopkins, M. P. and Menon, K. M., Regulation of epidermal growth factor and insulin-like growth factor I receptors by estradiol and progesterone in normal and neoplastic endometrial cell cultures, *Gynecol. Oncol.*, 38, 396, 1990.

228. Das, S. K., Tsukamura, H., Paria, B. C., Andrews, G. K. and Dey, S. K., Differential expression of epidermal growth factor receptor (EGF-R) gene and regulation of EGF-R bioactivity by progesterone and estrogen in the adult mouse uterus, *Endocrinology*, 134, 971, 1994.

229. Goldfine, I. D., Papa, V., Vigneri, R., Siiteri, P. and Rosenthal, S., Progestin regulation of insulin and insulin-like growth factor I receptors in cultured human breast cancer cells, *Breast Cancer Res. Treat.*, 22, 69, 1992.

230. Ferrandina, G., Scambia, G., Benedetti, P. P., Bonanno, G., De, V. R., Rumi, C., Bussa, S., Genuardi, M., Spica, R. V. and Mancuso, S., Effects of dexamethasone on the growth and epidermal growth factor receptor expression of the OVCA 433 ovarian cancer cells, *Mol. Cell. Endocrinol.*, 83, 183, 1992.

231. Salles, J. P., De, V. C., Netelenbos, J. C. and Slootweg, M. C., Dexamethasone increases and serum decreases growth hormone receptor binding to UMR-106.01 rat osteosarcoma cells, *Endocrinology*, 134, 1455, 1994.

232. Haraguchi, T., Alexander, D. B., King, D. S., Edwards, C. P. and Firestone, G. L., Identification of the glucocorticoid suppressible mitogen from rat hepatoma cells as an angiogenic platelet-derived growth factor A-chain homodimer, *J. Biol. Chem.*, 266, 18299, 1991.

233. Keyomarsi, K., O'Leary, N., Molnar, G., Lees, E., Fingert, H. J. and Pardee, A. B., Cyclin E, a potential prognostic marker for breast cancer, *Cancer Res.*, 54, 380, 1994.

234. Spuzic, I., Nikolic, D., Sami, I. and Brankovic, M., [The effect of hormones on tumor growth], *Glas. Srp. Akad. Nauka [Med]*, 1990, 105, 1990.

235. Dong, X. F., Berthois, Y., Colomb, E. and Martin, P. M., Cell cycle phase dependence of estrogen and epidermal growth factor (EGF) receptor expression in MCF-7 cells: implications in antiestrogen and EGF cell responsiveness, *Endocrinology*, 129, 2719, 1991.

236. Umek, R. M., Friedman, A. D. and McKnight, S. L., CCAAT-enhancer binding protein: a component of a differentiation switch, *Science*, 251, 288, 1991.

237. Xanthopoulos, K. G. and Mirkovitch, J., Gene regulation in rodent hepatocytes during development, differentiation and disease, *Eur. J. Biochem.*, 216, 353, 1993.

238. Mischoulon, D., Rana, B., Bucher, N. L. and Farmer, S. R., Growth-dependent inhibition of CCAAT enhancer-binding protein (C/EBP alpha) gene expression during hepatocyte proliferation in the regenerating liver and in culture, *Mol. Cell. Biol.*, 12, 2553, 1992.

239. Ramos, R. A., Maiyar, A. C., Simon, K., Ridder, C. C. and Firestone, G. L., CCAAT/enhancer binding protein is associated with the glucocorticoid-mediated growth suppression of rat hepatoma cells, *Mol. Biol. Cell*, 4, 13a, 1993.

240. Piontkewitz, Y., Enerback, S. and Hedin, L., Expression and hormonal regulation of the CCAAT enhancer binding protein-alpha during differentiation of rat ovarian follicles, *Endocrinology*, 133, 2327, 1993.

241. Levine, A. J., The tumor suppressor genes, *Annu. Rev. Biochem.*, 62, 623, 1993.

242. Trudel, M., Mulligan, L., Cavenee, W., Margolese, R., Cote, J. and Gariepy, G., Retinoblastoma and p53 gene product expression in breast carcinoma: immunohistochemical analysis and clinicopathologic correlation, *Hum. Pathol.*, 23, 1388, 1992.

243. Paliogianni, F., Ahuja, S. S., Balow, J. P., Balow, J. E. and Boumpas, D. T., Novel mechanism for inhibition of human T cells by glucocorticoids. Glucocorticoids inhibit signal transduction through IL-2 receptor, *J. Immunol.*, 151, 4081, 1993.

244. Poller, D. N., Roberts, E. C., Bell, J. A., Elston, C. W., Blamey, R. W. and Ellis, I. O., p53 Protein expression in mammary ductal carcinoma in situ: relationship to immunohistochemical expression of estrogen receptor and c-erbB-2 protein, *Hum. Pathol.*, 24, 463, 1993.

245. Elledge, R. M., Fuqua, S. A., Clark, G. M., Pujol, P. and Allred, D. C., William L. McGuire Memorial Symposium. The role and prognostic significance of p53 gene alterations in breast cancer, *Breast Cancer Res. Treat.*, 27, 95, 1993.

246. Domagala, W., Markiewski, M., Kubiak, R., Bartkowiak, J. and Osborn, M., Immunohistochemical profile of invasive lobular carcinoma of the breast: predominantly vimentin and p53 protein negative, cathepsin D and oestrogen receptor positive, *Virchows Arch. Pathol. Anat. Histopathol.*, 423, 497, 1993.

247. Tsuda, H., Iwaya, K., Fukutomi, T. and Hirohashi, S., p53 Mutations and c-erbB-2 amplification in intraductal and invasive breast carcinomas of high histologic grade, *Jpn. J. Cancer Res.*, 84, 394, 1993.

248. Martinazzi, M., Crivelli, F., Zampatti, C. and Martinazzi, S., Relationship between p53 expression and other prognostic factors in human breast carcinoma. An immunohistochemical study, *Am. J. Clin. Pathol.*, 100, 213, 1993.

249. Mazars, R., Spinardi, L., BenCheikh, M., Simony Lafontaine, J., Jeanteur, P. and Theillet, C., p53 Mutations occur in aggressive breast cancer, *Cancer Res.*, 52, 3918, 1992.

250. Thompson, A. M., Anderson, T. J., Condie, A., Prosser, J., Chetty, U., Carter, D. C., Evans, H. J. and Steel, C. M., p53 Allele losses, mutations and expression in breast cancer and their relationship to clinico-pathological parameters, *Int. J. Cancer*, 50, 528, 1992.

251. Koshiyama, M., Konishi, I., Wang, D. P., Mandai, M., Komatsu, T., Yamamoto, S., Nanbu, K., Naito, M. F. and Mori, T., Immunohistochemical analysis of p53 protein over-expression in endometrial carcinomas: inverse correlation with sex steroid receptor status, *Virchows Arch. Pathol. Anat. Histopathol.*, 423, 265, 1993.

252. Kohler, M. F., Berchuck, A., Davidoff, A. M., Humphrey, P. A., Dodge, R. K., Iglehart, J. D., Soper, J. T. L., Clarke-Pearson, D. L., Bast, R. C., Jr. and Marks, J. R., Overexpression and mutation of p53 in endometrial carcinoma, *Cancer Res.*, 52, 1622, 1992.

253. Ledinko, N. and Costantino, R. L., Modulation of p53 gene expression and cytokeratin 18 in retinoid-mediated invasion suppressed lung carcinoma cells, *Anticancer Res.*, 10, 1335, 1990.

254. Webster, M. K., Goya, L. and Firestone, G. L., Immediate-early transcriptional regulation and rapid mRNA turnover of a putative serine/threonine protein kinase, *J. Biol. Chem.*, 268, 11482, 1993.

255. Webster, M. K., Goya, L., Ge, Y., Maiyar, A. C. and Firestone, G. L., Characterization of sgk, a novel member of the serine/threonine protein kinase gene family which is transcriptionally induced by glucocorticoids and serum, *Mol. Cell. Biol.*, 13, 2031, 1993.

256. Imagawa, W., Bandyopadhyay, G. K. and Nandi, S., Regulation of mammary epithelial cell growth in mice and rats, *Endocr. Rev.*, 11, 494, 1990.

257. Vonderhaar, B. K., Regulation of development of the normal mammary gland by hormones and growth factors, *Cancer Treat. Res.*, 40, 251, 1988.

258. Moon, R. C., Thompson, H. J., Becci, P. J., Grubbs, C. J., Gander, R. J., Newton, D. L., Smith, J. M., Phillips, S. L., Henderson, W. R., Mullen, L. T., Brown, C. C. and Sporn, M. B., N-(4-Hydroxyphenyl)retinamide, a new retinoid for prevention of breast cancer in the rat, *Cancer Res.*, 39, 1339, 1979.

259. Maiorana, A. and Gullino, P. M., Effect of retinyl acetate on the incidence of mammary carcinomas and hepatomas in mice, *J. Natl. Cancer Inst.*, 64, 655, 1980.

260. Topper, Y. J. and Freeman, C. S., Multiple hormone interactions in the developmental biology of the mammary gland, *Physiol. Rev.*, 60, 1049, 1980.

261. Robinson, S. D., Silberstein, G. B., Roberts, A. B., Flanders, K. C. and Daniel, C. W., Regulated expression and growth inhibitory effects of transforming growth factor-beta isoforms in mouse mammary gland development, *Development*, 113, 867, 1991.

262. Jeng, M. H. P., ten Dijke, P., Iwata, K. K. and Jordan, V. C., Regulation of the levels of three transforming growth factor beta mRNAs by estrogen and their effects on the proliferation of human breast cancer cells, *Mol. Cell. Endocrinol.*, 97, 115, 1993.

263. Knabbe, C., Zugmaier, G., Schmahl, M., Dietel, M., Lippman, M. E. and Dickson, R. B., Induction of transforming growth factor beta by the antiestrogens droloxifene, tamoxifen, and toremifene in MCF-7 cells, *Am. J. Clin. Oncol.*, S15, 1991.

264. Zugmaier, G., Ennis, B. W., Deschauer, B., Katz, D., Knabbe, C., Wilding, G., Daly, P., Lippman, M. E. and Dickson, R. B., Transforming growth factors type beta 1 and beta 2 are equipotent growth inhibitors of human breast cancer cell lines, *J. Cell. Physiol.*, 141, 353, 1989.

265. Komura, H., Wakimoto, H., Chen, C. F., Terakawa, N., Aono, T., Tanizawa, O. and Matsumoto, K., Retinoic acid enhances cell responses to epidermal growth factor in mouse mammary gland in culture, *Endocrinology*, 118, 1530, 1986.

19

Mechanisms of Altered Target Cell Response With Particular Reference to Adrenergic Response

Tamàs Fülöp, Jr. and Elizabeth M. Dax

CONTENTS

I. INTRODUCTION

Target cells are cells capable of responding to chemical stimuli that are generated extracellularly. They possess receptors to decipher these stimuli. Receptors, as they interact with other proteins, initiate particular intracellular responses, depending upon the biochemical pathways to which they are coupled.

Most cells respond to a large variety of stimulators. The specific stimuli to which a particular target cell responds depend on which receptor it expresses at any given time. Different stimuli may cause a variety of responses mediated through a variety of mechanisms in any given cell.[1-3] Alternatively, the same stimulus in a particular cell may cause multiple effects.[4] Furthermore, responses may be multiphasic. The complexities of these interactions present an infinite variety of mechanisms by which target cell responsiveness may be altered by age or, for that matter, by any alteration in homeostasis.

II. BIOCHEMICAL PATHWAYS IN TARGET CELL RESPONSES

The targets for hormones and neurotransmitters in cells are known as "receptors". These macromolecular proteins are either situated within the cell membrane's bilayer (membrane receptors) or situated within the cytoplasm (intracellular receptors) or in the nucleus (nuclear receptors). Receptors belong to "superfamilies" that fall into categories depending on their structure and function. That is, receptors of individual superfamilies tend to have similar biochemical characteristics (see Chapters 2, 4, 5, 16, and 18). They may activate different cellular biochemical pathways (i.e., couple with different second messenger systems) to transmit an extracellular stimulus into the target cell. For example:

- β-Adrenergic receptors stimulate adenylyl cyclase via G_s protein,
- $α_2$-Adrenergic receptors inhibit adenylyl cyclase via pertussis toxin substrates G_i and G_o proteins, and
- $α_1$-Adrenergic receptors are coupled by a G protein (probably the G_q/G_{q11} protein) to phospholipase C (PLC),[5,6] even though these individual receptors retain similar secondary and tertiary structures with highly conserved regions of sequence.[7]

Increasing numbers of biochemical steps are being defined in the mechanisms of target cell responses. To be defined as a chemical stimulator or ligand, hormones, neurotransmitters, or drugs must react with a specific receptor on or in a target cell. Membrane receptors are closely associated with other membrane proteins. A large family of cell surface receptors conforming with the predicted topography of seven transmembrane-spanning proteins elicit their physiological effect by first coupling to and activating a population of heterotrimeric GTP-binding proteins that then mediate the responses via a plethora of cellular effectors, including enzymes and ion channels (Figure 1).

The adrenergic receptors which bind and mediate the actions of adrenaline and noradrenaline are the prototypic members of the extended superfamily of receptors which couple to guanylnucleotide regulatory proteins.[8,9] The regions of receptor involved in coupling to the G proteins appear to be located on the cytoplasmic surface of the receptor, generally in close apposition to the plasma membrane. Thus, sequences in the second cytoplasmic loop, the amino and carboxyl termini of the third cytoplasmic loop, as well as sequences in the proximal portion of the carboxy terminal cytoplasmic tail all appear to be crucially involved in forming a binding surface for interaction with G proteins.[9,10] The most studied of these modulating guanine nucleotide sensitive-proteins (the G proteins) which activate second messengers are those coupled to adenylyl cyclase, phosphatidyl inositol bisphosphate, phospholipase (PLC), and ion channels (Ca^{2+} or K^+) systems.[11]

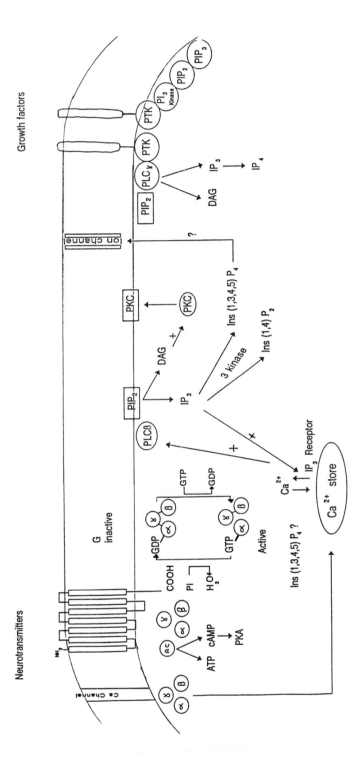

FIGURE 1 Possible intracellular signalling pathways occurring under various surface receptor stimulations. Neurotransmitter receptors act through various guanine nucleotide binding proteins (G proteins) to stimulate either phospholipase C, ion channels or the adenylyl cylase complex. The receptor is composed of seven membrane-spanning domains. The G protein is associated with the cytoplasmic surface of the membrane. The G protein may be in its activate (GTP-bound) or inactivate form (GDP-bound). This is regulated by the G protein GTPase cycle. Growth factor receptors act through protein tyrosine kinase activation (PTK). PTK is phosphorylating the PLCγ, being thus part of the phosphatidyl hydrolysis. PKC: protein kinase C; Ins(1,4,5)P3: inositol trisphosphate; Ins(1,3,4,5)P4: inositol tetrakisphosphate; PIP2: phosphatidylinositol 4,5-bisphosphate; PLC: phospholipase C; DAG: diacylglycerol; PTK: protein tyrosine kinase; αβγ: G protein subunits; AC: adenylyl cyclase.

The family of heterotrimeric G proteins, a subset of the superfamily of proteins that bind GTP (guanosine triphosphate) with high affinity and specificity, is now recognized to play a critical role in signal transduction by coupling diverse receptors to effectors.[12,13] Each G protein is composed of three distinct subunits, designated α, γ, and β. Receptor activation of the G protein leads to release of bound GDP (guanosine diphosphate) from the α subunit, binding of GTP, and dissociation of the β γ complex from the α subunit. The α subunit interacts with and modulates the activity of effectors such as adenylyl cyclase and other enzymes of second messenger metabolism, as well as ion channels. At least 16 distinct α subunit genes have been identified. α subunit interaction with the effector is terminated by an intrinsic GTPase activity that hydrolyzes the terminal phosphate of GTP, leaving the α subunit in its inactive GDP bound state.

When the G protein is activated by the receptor, the G protein dissociates into α and $\beta\gamma$ components.[14] The γ subunit has been shown to be geronylgeronylated. The $\beta\gamma$ subunit interacts with βARK and binds tightly to it. This interaction serves to facilitate and enhance the interaction of the enzyme with the lipid bylayer and its receptor substrate.[15] Because $\beta\gamma$ subunits are only released from G proteins upon receptor stimulation, this mechanism seems to provide another way of tightly coupling receptor activation to receptor desensitization. Rapid desensitization appears to involve primarily the phosphorylation of the receptor. Two distinct types of Ser/Thr protein kinases seem to be involved: the second messenger activated PKA and PKC and the second messenger independent G protein coupled receptor kinases (GRKs). GRKs are unique in their specificity for agonist-occupied or activated receptors.[16,17]

Other membrane receptors, such as those for insulin and growth factors, activate intracellular mechanisms initially by agonist-induced protein tyrosine kinase autophosphorylation of the receptor.[18]

If a ligand acts as an antagonist it binds to the receptor, but induces no further cellular responses. An agonist, however, will induce a cascade of biochemical events which initially result in a macromolecular complex of the receptor, the G protein, and the enzyme generating the second messenger, and which culminates in cellular responses. The specificity of this cascade depends upon the particular receptor which a ligand activates. Ligands bind to receptors in a concentration dependent manner, but because the number of receptors on a target cell is finite, binding is saturable and therefore may be quantitated.

When membrane receptors are occupied by appropriate agonists, second messenger systems are activated via coupling G proteins. Binding results in the activation of the receptor so that ternary macromolecular complexes of these membrane proteins are formed. The result is activation of enzymes that generate second messengers which amplify the binding signal. The activation of the second messenger systems are modified through both stimulatory and inhibitory guanine nucleotide dependent proteins (Gs or Gi proteins, respectively). The intracellular components of the responses are effected through protein kinases.[19]

Following interaction of adrenergic and cholinergic agents with their receptors on the plasma membrane, activation of phospholipase C results in the production of diacylglycerol (DAG) and inositol trisphosphate (IP$_3$). While the former activates the PKC, resulting in various phosphorylation dependent cellular effects, the latter elicits release of calcium from intracellular storage sites.[20]

Responses to ligands occupying intracellular receptors, for example steroid molecules, operate by entirely different mechanisms. Ligands enter the cell to bind to appropriate receptors. A translocation of the hormone:receptor complex to the cell nucleus occurs where there follows a modification of protein synthesis.[21,22] Reviews on alterations of these mechanisms with aging have been published recently[23,24] and will not be detailed in this chapter.

A. Definition of Target Cell Response

A target cell response is the outcome of the binding of a ligand to a receptor on, or in, the cell. The response may be measured as a change in a consequent biochemical step distal to the binding event. Responses may depend to some extent on the cell previous exposure to the ligand. If levels of chemical stimulators to which the cell is exposed are chronically altered, the characteristic of the receptors may be altered, thereby modifying cell responsiveness. This is known as either down-regulation (decrease in receptor number/cell) and occurs in response to a chronic elevation of ligand, or up-regulation (increase in receptor number/cell) following chronic ligand depletion. The alteration may be manifest as an alteration in receptor number or in the ability of the receptor to couple through G proteins to second messenger systems.

In many situations the G proteins that are activated by agonist-occupied receptors are down-regulated, while in some cases a G protein that opposes the generation of the second messenger produced in response to the agonist is up-regulated.[25]

However, mutations of the β_2-adreno-receptors that impair coupling to G_s interfere with agonist-induced down-regulation of the receptor.[26] Such observations indicate that functional interactions between the receptor and G protein are required to produce effective agonist-induced regulation of receptors.

Responses in the isolated target cell may be quite different from those seen *in vivo* under similar stimulating conditions. The reason appears to be that the ligand cannot act in isolation, i.e., the response may be modified through distant feedback loops or separate local mechanisms. For example, catecholamine released at a nerve terminal may stimulate adenylate cyclase activity through the β-adrenergic receptors, but simultaneously these stimulatory responses may be counterbalanced through adenylate cyclase-inhibiting α-adrenergic receptors. At the same time, blood flow to the cell and the release of other local transmitters may be altered, indirectly modifying the cellular response. Therefore, an altered response seen in particular target cells may be compensated for in other systems, thus maintaining homeostasis in the whole animal.

B. Role of Altered Target Cell Responsiveness in Aging

The aged animal has often been defined as having lost the ability to maintain homeostasis, particularly in the face of stress.[23,27-31] This may be due in part to the failure of target cells to respond appropriately or completely to chemical stimuli such as hormones or neurotransmitters. On the other hand, alterations in function of one target cell may be compensated by modifications in another function and homeostasis maintained. Because of the compensatory mechanisms, alterations in target cell function need to be defined as primary or secondary, and with increasing age, aspects of physiological function may deteriorate, show an alteration, or may even improve.[32-35]

In a large body of age-related research, questions have been raised as to whether changes in target tissue responses can explain age-related alterations in physiological functions. These studies have attempted to define common mechanisms of these alterations.[30] Usually, the approach has been to attempt to dissect out the mechanisms of alterations by examining the biochemical steps involved in a target tissue response to an appropriate chemical stimulator. The aim has been to determine the point at which the pathway is altered, in the hope of finding common points of age-related alterations.[30,36,37]

1. Importance of Age Selection in Studies on Aging

A cautionary note is indicated here, and reiterates the concerns of these authors[33,37,38] and echos those of others[39,40] concerning the interpretation of reports of alterations in age-related, target cell reponses. Many studies on aging have employed limited age-groups of animals or subjects. Often young (immature) groups are compared with a senescent group (old) and conclusions are drawn that alterations observed between the groups are related to senescence. This may or may not be the case depending at which stage of the life span it occurs. For example, Greenberg and Weiss[41] have reported that cyclical up-regulation of β-adrenergic receptors in rat pineal glands was lost during aging. However a more extensive comparison between multiple age groups demonstrated that this ability to up-regulate receptors on a diurnal basis was lost during maturation.[34] Further, it should be remembered that alterations of old age may be superimposed on those secondary to disease.[32,39-41] Although this may account for a wide variability in responses sometimes observed in aged subjects, the variability itself may be important in interpreting the importance of age-related alterations.[42]

III. CHANGES IN LEVELS OF TARGET CELL STIMULATORS

Circulating ligands are classified as hormones whereas local stimulators are termed transmitters. The distinction between the two is somewhat arbitrary,[40] but has been made.[43] (Altered response to exogenous stimulators such as drugs are a result of altered mechanisms of responses to endogenous stimulators since these substances act through the same pathways.) The reason that concentrations of stimulators are relevant to response mechanisms is that they can exert a control over receptor density or number per cell.[3] Although the basal and stimulated [29,44] levels of hormones and some neurotransmitters[29,40] are amazingly stable over the lifespan, there are notable exceptions. Further, baseline levels may not vary, whereas responses to stimulation tests may. This points out the necessity of dynamic assessments in all aging studies. The stable stimulator levels may be particularly pertinent with regard to maintaining homeostasis.[29] It is evident that other features of secretion besides circulating levels, such as modification by disease, altered diurnal rhythm, or altered secretogogues, may be of greater consequence in modifying responses with age.[39,40,45-48]

IV. ALTERATIONS IN RECEPTORS WITH AGING

A. Methodology

Receptors are quantified by radioactive ligand binding studies in suitable tissue preparations which may be either tissue particulates or slices of tissue. The advantage of binding in tissue slices is that the distribution of receptors, as well as their quantification, is achieved.[49] However, the methodology is more complicated and requires sophisticated interpretation.[50] More usually, tissue particulates are incubated with selected radiolabeled ligand in the absence and in the presence of appropriate unlabeled ligand to define total and nonspecific radiolabel binding, respectively. Specific binding is the difference between the two. Among parameters that may be examined are receptor number/cell and affinity for radioactive ligands. Competition studies using fixed concentrations of labeled ligand with a range of concentrations of appropriate unlabeled ligands may be used to assess affinities of these ligands and hence their pharmacological specificities. To examine aspects of macromolecular complex formation between receptor and G proteins, the affinity of receptors for agonists is examined in the presence and absence of guanine nucleotide. The ratio of agonist-induced high affinity sites compared with those of lower affinity occurring in the presence of guanine nucleotides is one means of assessing this complex formation. The difference between the affinity in the presence of nucleotide and in its absence is a measure of the efficacy of this agonist. The methodological pitfalls in aging studies are numerous, but have been previously discussed.[35,40] In terms of defining altered target cell responses in aging, these types of experiments have been usually performed in tissue particulates.

B. The Adrenergic Receptors

The adrenergic, cholinergic, and serotoninergic membrane receptors constitute part of a superfamily which is one of the most extensively studied membrane receptor superfamilies.[51] A wide range of pharmacological agents are available for study. This has facilitated purification studies which have led to the elucidation of molecular structures. These consist of seven transmembrane regions with extracellular and intracellular amino acid chains. For α- and β-adrenergic receptors, their subtype specificity resides in the amino acid sequence of specific transmembrane regions. The β-adrenergic receptors stimulated by appropriate agonists form high affinity states of the receptor, and ternary molecular complexes with one of a series of G proteins and the adenylyl cyclase catalytic unit. The catalytic unit catalyzes the formation of cAMP from ATP.

α-Adrenergic receptors modify adenylyl cyclase through an inhibitory G-protein-mediated mechanism, or act through phosphatidyl bisphosphate phospholipase, another second messenger sytem. This complex series of events transmits and amplifies receptor-stimulated signals across cell membranes.

C. Receptor Number Per Cell

Representative and more recent reports of receptor binding studies for catecholaminergic receptors during aging are listed in Table 1. Despite the many reports of changed receptor number/cell during aging, there are few explanations for the change. It is noteworthy to remark that the changes are far from being uniform. Certainly, no uniform hypothesis has been advanced and proven. As with other age-related alterations, an observed change is usually the result of a variety of factors that come to bear on a given target tissue. In order to maintain homeostasis, when the level of a stimulator such as epinephrine is elevated chronically at the target site, the target cell may respond by down-regulating the specific receptors on which epinephrine acts.[2] Conversely a decrease in the stimulator may result in an up-regulation.

Systemic catecholamines generally rise with age in humans and rodents,[52-55] so a uniform decrease in adrenergic receptors in all appropriate target tissues might be expected with aging. However, examination of Table 1 shows that this expectation is not always fulfilled, suggesting that an extracellular influence (such as a circulating concentration of ligands) is not the principal regulator during aging.

A need to look beyond the receptor quantitation for altered responsiveness with aging has been suggested.[35,56,57] In his commentary, Bloom[56] points out that:

1. "Ligand binding sites are but one component of the macromolecular complex that underlies 'receptor' function,
2. Target cells use pharmacologically defined subtypes for a given transmitter collectively and not separately (underscoring the importance of not making interpretations in single receptor systems), and
3. Interactions between receptor subtypes of one pharmacologically defined system and other transmitters converging on a common target cell represent an untapped form of pathophysiological change in transmitter function of the aging process."

Although these more general approaches of Bloom's have often been discussed, it has not been until recently that they are being used as guidelines to addressing mechanisms of altered age-related responses. Given the present literature on mechanisms of target cell responses in aging that overwhelmingly reports investigations in single receptor systems, and the absence of concomitant data on any other components of the responsiveness, the question remains open of how a multifactorial approach might direct receptor studies to more useful conclusions. We

TABLE 1   Changes in Adrenergic and Cholinergic Receptors From the Recent Literature that Have Been Noted Between Animals of at Least Two Age Groups

Receptor type	Increase ($\uparrow$) decrease ($\downarrow$) no change ($\leftrightarrow$)	Species	Tissue	Ref.
α-Adrenergic receptors				
1 & 2	$\downarrow$	Rabbit	Forebrain Midbrain	2
1	$\leftrightarrow$	Rat	Heart	90
2	$\leftrightarrow$	Human	Platelets	61[a]
2	$\leftrightarrow$	Rabbit	Platelets Fore-hind brain	120
2	$\downarrow$	Rat	Pineal	7[a]
Muscarinic cholinergic				
	$\downarrow$	Rat	Corpus striatum Frontal cortex Hypothalamus	89[a,b]
	$\leftrightarrow$		Hippocampus	
	$\uparrow$	Human	Lymphocytes	121[a]
	$\downarrow$	Rat	Lymphocytes	40
	$\downarrow$		Cerebral cortex Hippocampus Striatum Olfactory bulb	160
	$\downarrow$		Hippocampus	161[b]
	$\uparrow$		Brainstem	132
	$\leftrightarrow$?		Heart	
Dopamine (D_1,D_2)				
	$\downarrow, \downarrow$	Rhesus monkey	Caudate, putamen	96
	$\downarrow, \downarrow$	Rat	Caudate, putamen	153
	$\downarrow,$	Rabbit	Renal artery	154
	$\downarrow, \downarrow$	Human	Caudate, putamen	155[a]
	$\downarrow,$		Frontal cortex	
D1	$\uparrow$	Human	Caudate, putamen	101
D2	$\downarrow$	Human	Caudate	101
	$\downarrow$	Mouse	Striatum	156
	$\downarrow$	Rat	Striatum	21
	$\downarrow$		Striatum	157
β-Adrenergic receptors				
	$\downarrow$	Mouse	Spleen, cortex	158
	$\uparrow$		Lymphocytes	
	$\downarrow$		Lymphocytes (B&T)	
	$\uparrow$	Human	Lymphocytes (B&T)	89
	$\leftrightarrow$		Lymphocytes	81[a]
	$\leftrightarrow$		Lymphocytes	24[a]
	$\leftrightarrow$		Lymphocytes	53[a,b]
	$\leftrightarrow$		Lymphocytes	83[a]
	$\downarrow$		Platelets	54
	$\leftrightarrow$	Rat	Mononuclear cells	159
	$\uparrow$		Liver	35[a,b]
	$\uparrow$		Liver	150[a,b]
	$\uparrow$		Liver	149[a,b]
	$\leftrightarrow$		Pineal	34
	$\downarrow$		Thalamus, cerebellum, brainstem	49
	$\leftrightarrow$		Cortex, hippocampus	49

[a] Based on research done with only an immature and a senescent group.

[b] Observations paired with measurement of at least one other parameter.

will attempt to answer some of the questions raised above, although the available information is still quite sparse.

V. BEYOND RECEPTOR QUANTITATION IN STUDYING AGE-RELATED ALTERATIONS IN TARGET CELL RESPONSES

A. Membrane Receptors as Macromolecular Complexes in Aging

Membrane receptors, but also ion channels, transport proteins, G proteins, and second messenger generating proteins are integral components of plasma membranes. The methodologies to examine the complexing of receptors with their second messengers are sophisticated and are particularly well developed for adrenergic receptors. Basically, along with the quantitation of receptors, second messengers and mediating function need to be considered.[11] Membrane protein functions in producing target cell responses depend on (1) their ability to complex with each other, (2) with other proteins, and (3) possibly to move within the membrane.[3] Evidence suggests that the composition and fluidity of membranes may influence the ability of the macromolecular complex to function.[58-60]

1. Effects of Membrane Alterations on the Macromolecular Complex

Membranes undergo marked alterations during aging.[61-63] Membranes readily take up fatty acids and other lipid-soluble molecules such as steroids from the extracellular environment. Many of the lipid-soluble components of plasma membrane (e.g., cholesterol) alter during aging. In human platelets, both fluorescence polarization and plasma cholesterol increase with age.[61]

An age-related increase in free cholesterol is associated with a decrease in the phospholipid content. These changes lead to an increment in the molar ratio of cholesterol/phospholipid with age.[64] The molar ratio of cholesterol/phospholipid is considered to be a main determinant of lipid fluidity of both artificial and biological membranes.

Decreased fluidity or increased structural order in plasma membrane has been observed and proposed as an explanation of age-related alterations in tissues of humans[61] and animals.[65,66] The lipid composition of membranes in aged rats differs from that of young rats in a number of tissues including heart mitochondrial membranes, where negatively charged phospholipids and polyunsaturated fatty acids are reduced between 3 and 30 months of age.[67] The saturated:unsaturated fatty acid ratio increases in rat liver plasma membranes between 3 and 30 months of age.[68] Such alterations favoring decreased membrane fluidity occur in a wide range of tissues during aging.

Changes in membrane fluidity and composition may lead to functional alterations. For example, movement of receptors within plasma membranes may be demonstrated by the redistribution of membrane receptors to one pole of cells. In human lymphocytes, "capping" of Concanavalin A receptors decreased in aged (84 ± 1 years) compared to young (23 ± 2 years) subjects.[69] The capping phenomenon has relevance in the response to some ligands: reduced capping ability implies a reduced functional ability of the macromolecular complex. Furthermore, the coupling between the receptor and G protein is a diffusion limited process,[70] hence all conditions affecting membrane fluidity might influence receptor-G protein coupling.[71,72]

Studies in forebrain synaptic membrane demonstrated that an age-associated decrease in [^{3}H] serotonin binding could be restored to levels of young mice by feeding the old mice a diet of membrane fluidizing lipids.[65] Further systematic studies of membrane composition or fluidity and of macromolecular complex functions are needed.

2. Age-Related Alterations in Macromolecular Complex Function

Most studies examining receptor functions with age have concentrated on assessing receptor number/cell because earlier it was assumed that this was the parameter that dictated the magnitude of the response. An increasing body of information suggests that receptor number/cell is not always the principal regulator of membrane receptor mediated responses. For example, G protein complexing is the rate limiting step in the formation of the macromolecular complex. Examination of Table 1 and its footnote demonstrates that receptors are seldom quantitated with other parameters, and macromolecular complex function with aging has been investigated in a single study. Currently, these studies are becoming more frequent in aging research.[73-79]

In general, aging is correlated with reduction in responsiveness to adrenergic stimulation, but the effects of age on the number of β receptors in human lymphocytes is still being questioned.[2,80] Most often in human lymphocytes, the number/cell of β-adrenergic receptors does not change with aging,[81-84] but receptor affinity (Bmax) is significantly increased in the aged when compared to young groups. However, cAMP production in response to β-adrenergic agonist is compromised in lymphocytes from aged subjects,[2,86] but not in all cases.[87] The reported trend toward decreases in both basal and stimulated cAMP generation in the aged group[36,81,88] is consistent with several previous reports, all of which have shown functional impairment in some aspect of the adenylyl cyclase complex with age.[89] The increases in NE in the aged group are also consistent with previous results.[89] Feldman et al.[83] found and proposed an explanation for the altered responsivity within the macromolecular complex. They found that the proportion of β-adrenergic receptors capable of forming high affinity states in response to agonist exposure, (i.e., those purportedly interacting with G proteins) is reduced in lymphocytes from older subjects. High affinity states in the aged did not change with physiological challenge while those in young decreased. In contrast, Mader and Davis[87] reported short-term changes in β-adrenergic number/cell upon standing after a period of recumbency. Age-related changes in lymphocyte β-adrenergic receptor responsiveness would not result from down-regulation of receptor number/cell but rather from an increased number of receptors.[85]

A similar situation may occur in aged cardiac membranes where there is a well-documented decrease of response of cardiac myocytes to β-adrenergic agonists,[47] but alterations in β-adrenergic receptor parameters have not been demonstrated.[90] The reduction in β-adrenergic-stimulated adenylate cyclase activity[91,92] suggests an age-related disruption in the function of the macromolecular complex. However, to date the mechanisms of altered inotropic and chronotropic responsiveness have not been elucidated. Narayanan and Derby[93] found impairment in formation of the agonist-induced high affinity β-adrenergic binding site in cardiac membranes of old rats. We have not been able to replicate their finding using pindolol derivatives (Flammer, Dax, and Gregerman, unpublished observations), but we demonstrated partial impairment in myocardial membranes from 24-month-old rats compared with membranes from 6-month-old rats, using concentrations of highly liposoluble ligand [³H]-dihydroalprenolol.

These data strongly suggest that macromolecular complexes are altered during aging. The possible role of membrane composition with altered concentrations of protein components (besides the receptor) require elucidation of both resting and stimulated states of cell function.

B. Receptor Subtypes and Aging

Receptor subtypes may be defined as receptors that respond to the same natural neurotransmitters, but differ with respect to structure, [7,51,94] pharmacology,[95-97] and possibly by the second messenger system to which they are coupled.[11] Usually, subtypes are distinguished pharmacologically by assessing relative affinities for ligands which have specificity for particular subtypes. As more specific ligands have been developed, the number of subtypes within receptor types have increased. For example, with respect to adrenergic receptors α and β, subtypes were distinguished by their relative affinities for the natural catecholamines epinephrine and norepinephrine, and later for the synthetic β-adrenergic agonist isoproterenol. Gradually, a roster of increasingly specific ligands have been developed as potential therapeutic substances and enabled the identification of "subtypes of subtypes".[94,95,97-100] The subtypes may also be distinguished by different molecular structure.[7,51] *In vivo* some tissues appear to possess predominantly one subtype of receptor while others possess a number of subtypes (which presumably will recognize a neurotransmitter simultaneously). Physiological interactions of subtypes at a molecular level have been little explored and age-related studies are rare.

Dopamine receptors on target cells are pharmacologically and functionally of D1 and D2 subtypes In both human and animals, CNS dopamine receptors decline with aging. In some areas the decline may be marked and consistent, for example in the neostriatum.[101,102] Morgan et al.[101] demonstrated that in human caudate nucleus and putamen, the number/cell of D1 subtype receptors increases between 40 and 70 years, while in the caudate nucleus, D2 receptors decrease and show a highly significant correlation with age. Age-related change in affinity was not observed. These investigators have proposed that D1 binding sites increase to compensate for the age-related loss of D2 sites; the latter may in part be due to a gradual loss of neurons which express the D2 receptor[103] or possibly to reduced biosynthetic capacity of dopaminergic neurons with aging.[104-106] *In vivo* tomographic studies in humans across the adult lifespan suggest an overall decline in the dopaminergic sites in human brain.[107] It would appear that overall there is a deficit in CNS dopaminergic functions with aging, but the functional contributions of each subtype have not been elucidated.[108]

The pharmacology of the adrenergic receptor subtypes is particularly well developed. In contrast, their relations to aging processes are not. In a review by Scarpace and Abrass,[109] where studies of aging-related alterations in CNS adrenergic receptors are summarized, it is pointed out that few workers have studied α-adrenergic receptors.

The few studies performed indicate that $α_1$-adrenergic receptors are not decreasing with age.[74,110] In old humans, high affinity platelet $α_2$-adrenergic receptor number/cell decreases, contributing to the reduction in receptor-mediated inhibition of adenylyl cyclase.[111] The decrease in high affinity platelet $α_2$-adrenergic receptor number/cell in the older subject group is consistent with agonist-induced desensitization secondary to their increased levels of plasma NE. Nevertheless, findings suggest that there may be other factors in addition to a decrease in high affinity receptor number/cell which contribute to decreased receptor-mediated inhibition of adenylyl cyclase in older humans. These results could be interpreted as consistent with a functional uncoupling of the platelet $α_2$-adrenergic receptor-adenylyl cyclase complex in older humans.

Receptor subtype alterations during aging could be important in the maintenance of homeostasis or retention of function. It may be that if there is a selective alteration in one subtype, another could compensate. Such compensations may constitute normal adaptive mechanisms. Pharmacological tools for studying subtypes are currently available, particularly for catecholaminergic receptors, and should be used fruitfully in aging studies to investigate the relative functional contribution of the receptor subtypes to mechanisms of aging.

C. Interactions Between Receptors of Different Neurotransmitters During Aging

Abundant evidence suggests that interactions in receptor systems of target cells are altered with aging. These interactions may occur between seemingly unrelated transmitter systems. For example, an anorexia of old age exists which may be best explained by alteration in interactions between cholecystokinin and opiate-regulated processes and probably with other systems.[112] Allosteric modulation of ion channels may be altered: for example, between

GABA receptors and benzodiazepine receptors[113] or between ion channels in general. Prolactin administration may modulate dopamine-mediated behavior and receptors in an age-differentiated manner.[114]

Important interactions among receptors, G proteins, and second messengers stimulated by different transmitters are of great physiological relevance.[11,115,116] These interactions may be initiated by actions of quite different transmitters. While age-related alterations may depend on separately mediated transmitter actions (as above), they may also occur because of alterations in interactions. These may be dictated by more general aging-related alterations in membranes, regulatory hormones, or protein synthesis.

Altered membrane composition may affect different receptors or membrane-associated enzymes differentially.[58,117] Alternatively, more general effects such as Ca^{2+}-flux regulation may be altered,[46] as a consequence of membrane alterations. To date, manipulation of membrane composition and/or fluidity and the effects on receptor-mediated systems during aging have not been investigated extensively. Preliminary studies suggest that important mechanisms may be elucidated.[65,118] However, whether different receptor-mediated functions are differentially affected with aging remains to be investigated.

Another level of regulation of interactions of target cell membrane receptor mediated response may be the intracellular responses to the steroid and thyroid receptors. Steroid regulation may change dramatically with aging in some target cells, e.g., by altering the rates of protein synthesis (including receptor molecule synthesis) which may be impaired during aging.[119-122] In these studies, after administering irreversible receptor blockers to rats of different ages, the rate of reappearance of the appropriate receptors was found to be slower in older animals.

Legitimate criticisms of these methods, including differential partitioning of the liposoluble blockers, have been raised.[123] However, this type of experiment could also be used profitably to investigate receptor interactions and their regulation by the above-cited regulators.

VI. INTRACELLULAR TRANSDUCTION CHANGES WITH AGING

The signal transduction mechanisms are beginning to be investigated in relation to the aging process.[75,110,116] This signifies that our knowledge is still sparse, but much is to be gained from the better understanding of the altered target cell response with aging.

G protein-coupled receptors, the largest and the most versatile class of surface signal transducing proteins known, elicit biological functions which include, among others, hormone action, neurotransmission, chemotaxis, and perception of light, smell, and taste.[124]

Short peptide sequences from the receptors can activate the G proteins *in vitro*, hence the receptor structure must somehow constrain or shield these peptides in the inactive conformation. The amino acid susbtitutions in the mutant receptors must thereby hinder this constraining function and allow receptors to relax into the active conformation.[125] This structural change must somehow mimic the allosteric transition which under physiological circumstances is evoked or stabilized by agonists. Very similar effects were observed with comparable mutations of three different receptors: the β_2-adrenoreceptor which activates G_s, the α_1-adrenoreceptor which activates G_q, and the α_2-adrenoreceptor which activates G_i. Aging-related receptor characteristics are critical as they may have substantial consequences for the interpretation of primary changes. With persistent stimulation by agonists, G protein-coupled receptor/effector systems demonstrate diminished responsiveness, referred to as desensitization.[17]

The GRKs enzymes phosphorylate only the active agonist bound forms of the receptors, thus providing a tight coupling between activation and desensitization. Expression of the constitutively active mutant α_2-adrenoreceptor with ARK1 in HEK293 cells is associated with significantly higher levels of agonist-independent receptor phosphorylation than observed with wild-type receptors.[125] This further strengthens the notion that the constitutively active mutant receptors in some way mimic the agonist-bound conformation of the receptors.

A potentially important physiological ramification of the constitutive activity of such receptors is that the ability of different receptor subtypes for the same ligand to spontaneously isomerize to the active state might well differ. Such receptor subtypes would vary substantially in their properties, thus making them best suited for one or another physiological context.

Studies in this field are not available for aging. However, the findings of alterations in receptor structure which can lead to constitutive activation could profoundly modify our understanding of the altered cell response target with aging. Speculatively, aging may be related either to a constitutive inactivation of certain receptors, such as in the case of adrenergic receptors,[85] or to a constitutive activation such as in the case of certain receptors on peripheral blood cells (FMLP or CD3).[79,126] Inasmuch as one of the hallmarks of aging is altered regulation in response to external stimuli, it would seem reasonable to expect that there might be altered patterns of protein phosphorylation with age,[76,127] such as in the case of GRKs.

With the recognition of the importance of G proteins in normal signal transduction came the recognition that G protein dysfunction could lead to impaired signal transduction, and the expectation that certain human diseases involving impaired signal transduction could be due to defects at the level of the G proteins themselves. This seems to be the case in some cardiac diseases.[128]

Adenylyl cyclase, the effector that generates cAMP, is dually regulated by stimulatory (G_s) and inhibitory (G_i) G proteins. Abnormal cAMP formation, as seen in aging, can be theoretically caused by reciprocal defects of either G protein. Thus, increased cAMP formation may result from constitutive G_s activation or from loss of G_i function. Decreased ability to stimulate cAMP formation may be due to reduced G_s function or constitutive G_i activation. The implication is that loss of function of one G protein may lead to the same pathophysiologic result as constitutive activation of another protein.[13]

G proteins could be the site of defects in neuropsychiatric disease and senescence.[77] Chronic membrane depolarization of cultured neuroblastoma cells led to an increased levels of G_o.[129] Also, a PT-sensitive G protein has been implicated in long-term potentiation of memory in the hippocampus.[130] These studies raise the possibility that altered G proteins could underly changes in neuronal function that occur with aging.[115,116]

Studies on peripheral cells, primarily leukocytes, suggest that age-related reduction in β-adrenergic responsiveness in man may be due to a defect in coupling of receptor to effector.[83] Many responses to catecholamines and related agonists have been reported to decrease during aging and in aging-related diseases due to possible impairments in the coupling/uncoupling of G proteins from receptors. These impaired receptor-G protein coupling systems include muscarinic cholinergic systems in the heart and brain,[131-133] dopaminergic system in the brain,[134,135] and α- and β-adrenergic systems in a variety of cells including liver,[75,83,110] lymphocytes, and polymorphonuclear granulocytes (PMNLs).[36,85,88]

Recently, Miyamoto et al.[110] suggested that altered coupling of G proteins to parotid $α_1$-adrenergic receptor is at least partially responsible for decreased secretion during aging in rats. They demonstrated that epinephrine-stimulated $^{45}Ca^{2+}$ mobilization is reduced by nearly half between 6 and 24 months of age. In the same cell preparations, epinephrine-stimulated Ins $(1,4,5)P_3$ production is concomitantly reduced. Moreover, when G proteins were stimulated directly with GTPγS or NaF, differences in Ins $(1,4,5)P_3$ production did not occur with aging. In other experimental settings (PMNLs) we could not confirm these latter results.[37] Previous studies had not revealed aging-related loss of $α_1$-adrenergic receptor or changes in the ability of epinephrine to interact with these molecules.[74] However, since Miyamoto et al.[110] were unable to detect age diffferences in the quantity or function of any postreceptor signal transduction component, they examined the coupling of receptors to G proteins. It is conceivable that reduced α_1-adrenergic receptor-stimulated Ins $(1,4,5)P_3$ production in parotid cells of aged rats may be due to impaired uncoupling of the G protein α subunit. GTPase activity stimulation by agonist is associated with dissociation of the α subunit and is thus an index of G protein-receptor coupling and uncoupling.[110,133,136] Epinephrine was found to be much more effective in stimulating GTPase in parotid membranes from adult than old rats. These results correlate with observations made by us in lymphocytes and granulocytes stimulated by isoproterenol (Fulop, Penyige, and Seres, unpublished observations).

Alteration of receptor-G protein interaction during aging in rat parotid may be the result of an impaired dissociation of the α subunit from the G protein-receptor complex as evidenced by:

1. Inability of GppNHp to shift receptors from the high to low affinity states in parotid membranes of aged rats, and
2. Impaired stimulation of α subunit GTPase activity by epinephrine in aged preparations.[110]

However, these alterations may lie at the level of receptor, G proteins, and/or other membrane components, and precise elucidation of the mechanisms responsible for the observed defects will require both molecular genetic analysis of G proteins and receptors structure as well as an understanding of the relationship of other membrane components to the function of these regulatory proteins.

Recently, researchers on aging have also become interested in the measurement of the second messengers beyond the formation of receptor-G-protein macromolecular complex. The results are rather contradictory, but some trends are emerging. A decrease in specific inositol phosphate release was reported after stimulation of cortical alpha$_1$-adrenergic receptors, cortical muscarinic receptors, and striatal muscarinic receptors.[137] Besides age-related effects on agonist-stimulated inositol trisphosphate release,[138] carbachol stimulated $(1,3,4,5)IP_4$ formation was reduced in cerebral cortex slices of old rats.[139,140]

Aging-related changes in receptor stimulated inositol phosphate release may be dependent upon the receptor effector coupling or a change in the stoichiometry of the receptor-G protein-phospholipase C interaction. There is considerable support for the latter contention since this was also found in other cell systems such as myocytes,[141] lymphocytes, and granulocytes.[37,78,79,116] Uncoupling of the receptor-G protein-phospholipase C interaction could be caused by aging-related changes in the membrane properties (e.g., membrane fluidity), as described before, and/or the results of two other possible factors:

1. Reduction in receptor concentrations, and/or
2. Deficits early in the signal tranduction process.[142,143]

The number/cell of IP_3 receptors is decreased in the cerebellum, but not in the cerebral cortex of old rats. Furthermore the amount of Ca^{2+} released from microsomes by IP_3 decreases with age in rat brain[144] and parotid cells,[110] and resting levels of cytosolic Ca^{2+} are decreased in fibroblasts from aged humans[145] while increased in other cell types (e.g., PMNLs).[126] Impaired Ca^{2+} function appears also to be a generalized manifestation of senescence occurring both in the CNS and in the periphery.[126,143,146] Calcium/calmodulin dependent protein kinase is activated by the elevated cytosolic calcium concentration as a result of the action of IP_3 and PKC activated by DAG, the second messenger which is released simultaneously with IP_3. PKC is modified during aging in various cerebral areas, in platelets, and in lymphocytes as a result of alterations in either enzyme activity or substrate availability.[147,148]

TABLE 2   [^{3}H]-Prazosin Binding to Receptors in Livers From GRC-WISTAR Rats of Different Ages. Results Are Expressed as Mean ± SEM; n Represents the Number of Animals in Each Age Group. Statistical Differences Were Determined by ANOVA With Post Hoc Testing for Significance by Duncan's New Multiple-Range Test

Age (months)	n	B_{max} (fmol/mg)	K_d (pM)
6	6	111 ± 13	20.3 ± 1.4
12	6	132 ± 16	27.3 ± 0.6[b,c]
18	6	124 ± 4	25.2 ± 3.0[a]
24	5	125 ± 20	19.0 ± 0.9

[a] Differs from 24 months, $p < 0.05$.

[b] Differs from 24 months, $p < 0.01$.

[c] Differs from 6 months, $p < 0.05$.

VII. AGE-RELATED ALTERATIONS IN RAT LIVER ADRENERGIC RESPONSES: A MODEL FOR ALTERED TARGET CELL RESPONSE IN AGING

Glycogenolysis in liver, following maturity, is modulated by β-adrenergic receptors. Both the alpha- and β-adrenergic systems are important and their relative importance seems to change with age,[149] with consistant alterations in various strains of rats,[35,149,150] and among laboratories.[35,149,150]

Epinephrine-stimulated adenylyl cyclase activity in liver particulates prepared from rats consistent increase with age.[35,149,150] Investigation of β-adrenergic receptor number/cell has demonstrated a consistent elevation in senescent animals across species of rat[35,149,150] and among laboratories.[35,149,150] An immediate conclusion from these results is that the increase in adenylyl cyclase activity is due to an increase in β-adrenergic receptor number/cell secondary to some age-related factor. However, when we correlated adenylyl cyclase activity with β-adrenergic receptor number/cell in a group of Wistar rats from different ages and with a median life span of 24 months, there was a direct, linear relationship up to about 18 months of age, but in older rats this correlation did not hold. Rather, the less the adenylyl cyclase activity, the greater was the trend for increased β-adrenergic binding capacity.[35]

Thus, it appeared that there was an inability for the receptor signal to induce the same adenylyl cyclase response as in a younger rat with liver coupling defect. This was not reflected in the ability of the β-receptor to form a ternary complex with the G_s protein because the high affinity state of the receptor could be induced by an agonist, isoproterenol, equally well in receptors of liver membranes from rats of any age.[35] Furthermore there was no age-related change in the alpha$_1$-receptor number/cell (Table 2). One might have expected a decrease in alpha$_1$-receptor number/cell although these receptors are not coupled with the inhibitory limb of catecholamine-stimulated adenylyl cyclase responses that are predominant regulators of adrenergic-mediated glycogenolysis. It did not appear that changes in the G protein or adenylyl cyclase catalytic unit accounted for these age-related alterations; stimulation of these elements with nonreceptor-mediated ligands, such as NaF, GppNHp, which activates the G_s

protein, or the diterpene, forskolin, which activates the catalytic unit and the G protein, did not demonstrate age-related alterations. Despite these changes in the membrane adrenergic receptor-coupled system of senescent rats, the β-adrenergic-stimulated glycogenolytic response is maintained or elevated in hepatocytes.[150]

β-Adrenergic receptor increases in liver membranes during senescence in Fisher 344 rats[149] and also in Fisher 344 rats which were barrier reared.[150] In these studies, aging-related differences in catalytic unit activity stimulated by nonreceptor-mediated stimulators such as NaF or forskolin were demonstrated.

Another important feature of our studies in rat liver[35] is that the glucagon-stimulated system was investigated in parallel with the adrenergic system. The responses of two receptors can be studied within the same membrane, using the same type of coupling mechanism, and under the same conditions. Aging-related increase in glucagon-mediated adenylyl cyclase activity was not observed.

These studies with aging in liver, thus, begin to satisfy the criteria formulated by Bloom:[56] adrenergic receptors were studied as a macromolecular complex, the adrenergic receptor subtypes were considered, and another transmitter whose interactions may be important was investigated in parallel. Coupling alterations observed in liver of senescent animals may relate to the decreased fluidity of their plasma membranes.[35] Age-associated differences in the microviscosity of liver membranes have been observed.[117] The increase in β-adrenergic receptors does not occur in food-restricted rats.[151] Food restriction is a maneuver that retards many age-related alterations,[152] but to date has not been demonstrated to retard age-related membrane alterations.

VIII. SUMMARY AND CONCLUSIONS

There is ample documentation of alterations with aging in target cell responses. A uniform hypothesis for the mechanisms of these alterations has not yet been demonstrated although some trends are emerging. Methodology for investigating the mechanisms of these alterations is readily available and highly sophisticated. Molecular mechanisms may be elucidated now by employing these methodologies if studies are directed towards questioning why alterations occur, rather than further documentation of the alterations. In addition, more rigorous definition of the studied model systems is needed and their relation to aging must be clarified. Nevertheless, the documentation studies have been highly productive in investigating systems such as lymphocytes, cardiac myocytes, and hepatocytes, which are highly amenable to manipulation. Future studies could lead not only to uncovering the mechanisms of altered responses with aging, but to understanding important clinical and therapeutic issues of the aged.

ACKNOWLEDGMENTS

John Partilla performed the β-adrenergic binding experiments in rat liver reported in Table 2. His helpful comments, with those of James Hoseph, Ph.D. and Hugh Taylor, M.D. are gratefully acknowledged. Ildiko Seres participated in the experiments performed on lymphocytes and granulocytes and her work is highly appreciated and acknowledged. Mrs. Sylvianne Fumas participated in the preparation of the manuscript with her usual efficiency and insight.

REFERENCES

1. Gawler, D., Milligan, G., Spiegel, A.M., Unson, C.G. and Houslay, M.D. Abolition of the expression of inhibitory guanine nucleotide regulatory protein Gi activity in diabetes. *Nature,* 327, 229, 1987.

2. Heinsimer, J.A. and Lefkowitz, R.J. The impact of aging on adrenergic receptor function: Clinical and biochemical aspects. *J. Am. Ger. Soc.,* 33, 184, 1985.

3. Lefkowitz, R.J., Caron, M.G. and Stiles, G.L. Mechanisms of membrane-receptor regulation. Biochemical, physiological, and clinical insights derived from studies of the adrenergic receptors, *N. Engl. J. Med.,* 310, 1570, 1984.

4. Chabre, O. Conklin, B.R., Brandon, S., Bourne, H.R. and Limbird, L.E. Coupling of the 2A-adrenergic receptor to multiple G proteins. A simple approach for estimating receptor-G-protein coupling efficiency in a transient expression system. *J. Biol. Chem.,* 269, 5730, 1994.

5. Jackson, T. Structure and function of G-protein coupled receptors, in *Intracellular Messengers.* Taylor, C.W. Ed. Pergamon Press. London. 1993, Chapter 1.

6. Olete, J. and Allende, J.E. Structure and function of G proteins. in *Intracellular Messengers.* Taylor, C.W. Ed. Pergamon Press. London. 1993, Chapter 2.

7. Dixon, R.A., Kobilka, B.K., Strader, D.J., Benovic, J.L., Dohlman, H.G., Frielle, T., Bolanowski, M.A., Bennett, C.D., Rands, E., Diehl, R.E., Mumford, R.A., Slater, E.E., Sigal, I.S., Caron, M.G., Lefkowitz, R.J. and Strader, C.D. Cloning of the gene and cDNA for mammalian β-adrenergic receptor and homology with rhodopsin. *Nature,* 321, 75, 1986.

8. Lefkowitz, R.J, Cotecchia, S., Kielsberg, M.A., Pitcher, J., Koch, W.J., Inglese, J. and Caron, M.G. Adrenergic receptors: recent insights into their mechanism of activation and desensitisation. In Advances in second messenger and phosphoprotein research. Vol. 28. *Cell Signalling. Biology and Medicine of Signal Transduction.* Brown, B.L. and Dobson, P.R.N. Eds. Raven Press, New York, 1993, Chapter 1.

9. Dohlman, H.G., Thorner, J., Caron, M.G. and Lefkowitz, R.J. Model systems for the study of seven-transmembrane-segment receptors. *Annu. Rev. Biochem.,* 60, 653, 1991.

10. Strader, C.D., Sigal, I.S. and Dixon, R.A. Structural basis of beta-adrenergic receptor function. *FASEB J.,* 3, 1825, 1989.

11. Role, L. and Schwartz, J.H. Centrefold: Cross-talk between signal transduction pathways. *TINS,* 12, 1989.

12. Spiegel, A.M., Shenker, A. and Weinstein, L.S. Receptor-effector coupling by G proteins: implications for normal and abnormal signal transduction. *Endocrine Rev.*, 13, 536, 1992.

13. Spiegel, A.M., Weinstein, L.S., Shenker, A., Hernouet, S. and Merendino, J.J. G-proteins: from basic to clinical studies in advances in second messenger and phosphoprotein research. Vol. 28. *Cell Signalling. Biology and Medicine of Signal Transduction.* Brown, B.L. and Dobson, P.R.N. Eds. Raven Press, New York, 1993, Chapter 5.

14. Gilman, A.G. G proteins: transducers of receptor-generated signals. *Annu. Rev. Biochem.*, 56, 615, 1987.

15. Pitcher, J.A., Inglese, J., Higgins, J.B., Arriza, J.L., Casey, P.J., Kim, C., Benovic, J.L., Kwatra, M.M., Caron, M.G. and Lefkowitz, R.J. Role of beta gamma subunits of G proteins in targeting the beta-adrenergic receptor kinase to membrane-bound receptors. *Science,* 257, 1264, 1992.

16. Hausdorf, W.P. Caron, M.G. and Lefkowitz, R.J. Turning off the signal: desensitisation of beta-adrenergic receptor function. *FASEB J.*, 4, 2881, 1990.

17. Inglese, J., Freedman, N.J., Koch, W.J. and Lefkowitz, R.J. Structure and mechanism of the G protein coupled receptor kinases. *J. Biol. Chem.,* 268, 23735, 1993.

18. White, M.F. and Kahn, C.R. The insulin signalling system. *J. Biol. Chem.,* 269, 1, 1994.

19. Filburn, C.R. Cyclic nucleotide metabolism and action during senescence. In *Endocrine and Neuroendocrine Mechanisms of Aging,* Eds. R.C. Adelman and G.S. Roth, CRC Press, Boca Raton, FL. 1982, 25.

20. Berridge, M.J. Inositol trisphosphate and calcium signalling. *Nature,* 361, 315, 1993.

21. O'Boyle, K.M. and Waddington, J.L. Loss of rat striatal dopamine receptors with ageing is selective for D-2 but not D-1 sites: association with increased non-specific binding of the D-1 ligand [3H]piflutixol. *Eur. J. Pharmacol.,* 105, 171, 1984.

22. Thakur, M.K. Molecular mechanism of steroid hormone action during aging. A review. *Mech. Ageing Dev.,* 45, 93, 1988.

23. Bolla, R.I. Current concepts. II. Hormonal regulation of molecular events during aging. *Life Sci.,* 31, 615, 1982.

24. Roth, G.S. Altered estrogen action in the senescent rat uterus. A model for steroid resistance during aging. In *Aging, Reproduction and the Climacteric,* Eds. L. Mastroianni and C.A. Paulsen, Plenum Press. New York, 1986, 97.

25. Milligan, G. Agonist regulation of cellular G protein levels and distribution: mechanism and functional implications. *Trends in Pharmacological Sciences,* 14, 413, 1993.

26. Campbell, P.T., Hnatowitch, M., O'Dowd, B.F., Caron, M.G., Lefkowitz, R.J. and Hausdorft, W.P. Mutations of the human beta 2-adrenergic receptor that impair coupling to Gs interfere with receptor down-regulation but not sequestration, *Mol. Pharmacol.,* 39, 192, 1991.

27. Adelman, R.C. Age-dependent effects in enzyme induction — a biochemical expression of aging. *Exp. Gerontol.,* 6, 75, 1971.

28. Balin, A.K. and Allen, R.G. Mechanisms of biologic aging. *Dermatol. Clin.,* 4, 347, 1986.

29. Mooradian, A.D., Morley, J.E. and Korenman, S.G. Endocrinology in aging. Disease-A-Month, 34, 393, 1988.

30. Roth, G.S. Mechanisms of altered hormone and neurotransmitter action during aging. The role of impaired calcium mobilization. *Ann. New York Acad. Sci.,* Neuroimmunomodulation: Interventions in aging and cancer. First Stromboli Conference on Aging and Cancer, 521, 170, 1988.

31. Shock, N.W. The physiology of aging. *Sci. Am.,* 206, 100, 1962.

32. Costa, P.T., Jr. and Andres, R. Patterns of age changes. In *Clinical Geriatrics,* Ed., I. Rossman, J.B. Lippincott. New York, 1986.

33. Dax, E.M. Age-related changes in membrane receptor interactions. In *Endocrine and Metabolism Clinics of North America : Endocrinology and Aging,* Vol. 16, Ed., B. Sactor, W.B. Saunders, Philadelphia, 1988.

34. Dax, E.M. and Sugden, D. Age-associated changes in pineal adrenergic receptors and melatonin synthesizing enzymes in the Wistar rat. *J. Neurochem.,* 50, 468, 1988.

35. Dax, E.M., Partilla, J.S., Piñeyro, M.A. and Gregerman, R.I. Beta-adrenergic receptors, glucagon receptors, and their relationship to adenylate cyclase in rat liver during aging. *Endocrinology,* 120, 1534, 1987.

36. Fulop, T. Jr., Foris, G., Worum, I. and Leovey, A. Age-dependent alterations of Fc gamma receptor-mediated effector functions of human polymorphonuclear leucocytes. *Clin. Exp. Immunol.,* 61, 425, 1985.

37. Fulop, T. Jr., Varga, Z., Csongor, J., Foris, G. and Leovey A. Age-related impairment of phosphatidylinositol breakdown of polymorphonuclear granulocytes. *FEBS Lett.,* 245, 249, 1989.

38. Dax, E.M. Receptors and associated membrane events in aging. In *Rev. Biol. Res. Aging,* Vol. 2, Ed., M. Rothstein, Allen R. Liss, New York, 1985, 315.

39. Florini, J.R. (Minireview): Limitations of interpretation of age-related changes in hormone levels: illustration by effects of thyroid hormones on cardiac and skeletal muscle. *J. Gerontol.,* 44, B107, 1989.

40. Gregerman, R.I. Mechanisms of age-related alterations of hormone secretion and action. An overview of 30 years of progress. *Exp. Gerontol.,* 21, 345, 1986.

41. Greenberg, L.H. and Weiss, B. Beta-adrenergic receptors in aged rat brain. Reduced number and capacity of pineal gland to develop supersensitivity. *Science,* 201, 61, 1978.

42. Rowe, J.W. and Kahn, R.L. Human aging: usual and successful. *Science,* 237, 143, 1987.

43. Funder, J.W. Receptors, hummingbirds and refrigerators. *News Physiol. Sci.,* 2, 231, 1987.

44. Worum, I., Fulop, T., Jr., Csongor, J., Foris, G. and Leovey, A. Interrelation between body composition and endocrine system in healthy elderly people. *Mech. Ageing Dev.,* 28, 430, 1984.

45. Cooper, R.L., Goldman, J.M. and Rehnberg, G.L. Neuroendocrine control of reproductive function in the aging female rodent. *JAGS,* 34, 735, 1986.

46. Gibson, G.E. and Peterson, C. (Review): Calcium and the aging nervous system. *Neurobiol. Aging,* 8, 329, 1987.

47. Lakatta, E.G. Diminished beta-adrenergic modulation of cardiovascular function in advanced age. *Cardiol. Clin.,* 4, 185, 1986.

48. Lakatua, D.J., Nicolau, G.Y., Bogdan, C., Petrescu, E., Sackett-Lundeen, L.L., Irvine, P.W. and Haus, E. Circadian endocrine time structure in humans above 80 years of age. *J. Gerontol.,* 39, 648, 1984.

49. Miller, J.A. and Zahniser, N.R. Quantitative autoradiographic analysis of ^{125}I-pindolol binding in Fischer 344 rat brain: changes in β-adrenergic receptor density with aging. *Neurobiol. Aging,* 9, 267, 1988.

50. Kuhar, M.J. Receptor localization with the microscope. In *Neurotransmitter Receptor Binding,* Ed., H.I. Yamamura et al., Raven Press, New York, 1985, 153.

51. Hartig, P.R. Molecular biology of 5-HT receptors. *Trends in Pharmacological Sciences,* 10, 64, 1989.

52. Barnes, R.F., Raskind, M., Gumbrecht, G. and Halter, J.B. The effects of age on the plasma catecholamine response to mental stress in man. *J. Clin. Endocrinol. Metab.,* 54, 64, 1982.

53. Brodde, O.E., Prywarra, A., Daul, A., Anlauf, M. and Bock, K.D. Correlation between lymphocyte β$_2$-adrenoceptor density and mean arterial blood pressure: elevated Beta-adrenoceptors in essential hypertension. *J. Cardiovasc. Pharmacol.,* 6, 678, 1984.

54. Brodde, O.E., Anlauf, M., Graben, N. and Bock, K.D. Age-dependent decrease of alpha$_2$-adrenergic receptor number in human platelets. *Eur. J. Pharmacol.,* 81, 345, 1982.

55. Rowe, J.W. and Troen, B.R. Sympathetic nervous system and aging in man. *Endocr. Rev.,* 1, 167, 1980.

56. Bloom, F.E. Noradrenergic receptor function and aging: beyond the binding. *Neurobiol. Aging,* 9, 59, 1988.

57. Fulop, T., Jr., Utsuyama, M. and Hirokawa, K. Determination of IL-2 receptor number of Con A stimulated human lymphocytes with aging. *J. Clin. Lab. Immunol.,* 34, 31, 1991.

58. Houslay, M.D. and Gordon, L.M. The activity of adenylate cyclase is regulated by the nature of its lipid environment. In *Current Topics in Membranes and Transport,* Vol. 18, Membrane Receptors, Eds., A. Kleinzeller and B.R. Martin, Academic Press, New York, 1983, 179.

59. Murphy, M.G. Membrane fatty acids, lipid peroxidation and adenylate cyclase activity in cultured neural cells. *Biochem. Biophys. Res. Comm.,* 132, 757, 1985.

60. Neelands, P.J. and Clandinin, M.T. Diet fat influences plasma-membrane lipid composition and glucagon-stimulated adenylate cyclase activity. *Biochem. J.,* 212, 573, 1983.

61. Awad, A.B. and Clay, S.W. Age dependent alterations in lipids and function of rat heart sarcolemma. *Mech. Ageing Dev.,* 19, 333, 1982.

62. Cohen, B.M. and Zubenko, G.S. Aging and the biophysical properties of cell membranes. *Life Sci.,* 37, 1403, 1985.

63. Zs.-Nagy, I. The role of membrane structure and function in cellular aging: a review. *Mech. Ageing Dev.,* 9, 237, 1979.

64. Alvarez, E., Ruiz-Gutierrez, V., Santa Maria, C. and Machado, A. Age-dependent modification of lipid composition and lipid structural order parameter of rat peritoneal macrophage membranes. *Mech. Ageing. Dev.,* 71, 1, 1993.

65. Hershkowitz, M., Heron, D., Samuel, D. and Shinitzky, M. The modulation of protein phosphorylation and receptor binding in synaptic membranes by changes in lipid fluidity: implications for ageing. *Prog. Brain Res.,* 56, 419, 1982.

66. Schroeder, F. Role of membrane lipid asymmetry in aging. *Neurobiol. Aging,* 5,323, 1984.

67. Nohl, H. and Kramer, R. Molecular basis of age-dependent changes in the activity of adenine nucleotide translocase. *Mech. Ageing Dev.,* 14, 137, 1980.

68. Hegner, D. Age-dependence of molecular and functional changes in biological membrane properties. *Mech. Ageing Dev.,* 14, 101, 1980.

69. Chiricolo, M., Minelli, L., Licastro, F., Tabacchi, P., Zannotti, M. and Franceschi, C., Alterations of the capping phenomenon on lymphocytes from aged and Down's syndrome subjects. *Gerontology,* 30, 145, 1984.

70. Briggs, M.M. and Lefkowitz, R.J. Parallel modulation of catecholamine activation of adenylate cyclase and formation of the high affinity agonist receptor complex in turkey erythrocytes membranes by temperature and cis-vaccenic acid., *Biochemistry,* 19, 4461, 1980.

71. Miyamoto, A., Araiso, T., Koyama, T. and Ohshika, M. Membrane viscosity correlates with alpha 1-adrenergic signal transduction of the aged rat cerebral cortex. *J. Neurochem.,* 55, 70, 1990.

72. Fraeyman, N., Vanscheeuwijck, P., De Wolf, M. and Quatacker, J. Influence of aging on fluidity and coupling between beta-receptors and G-proteins in rat lung membranes. *Life Sci.,* 53, 153, 1993.

73. Ishikawa, Y., Gee, M.V., Ambudkar, I.S., Bodner, L., Baum, B.J. and Roth, G.S. Age-related impairment in rat parotid cell alpha 1-adrenergic action at the level of inositol trisphosphate responsiveness. *Biochem. Biophys. Acta,* 968, 203, 1988.

74. Ishikawa, Y, Gee, M.V., Baum, B.J. and Roth, G.S. Decreased signal transduction in rat parotid cell aggregates during aging is not due to loss of alpha 1-adrenergic receptors. *Exp. Gerontol.,* 24, 25, 1989.

75. Ishigami, A. and Roth, G.S. Age-related changes in DNA synthesis stimulated by epinephrine and isoproterenol in primary cultured rat hepatocytes. *J. Cell. Physiol.,* 158, 231, 1994.

76. Lanius, R.A., Pasqualotto, B.A. and Shaw, C.A. Age-dependent expression, phosphorylation and function of neurotransmitter receptors: pharmacological implications. *Trends In Pharmacological Sciences,* 14, 403, 1993.

77. Fulop, T., Jr., Barabas, G., Varga, Z., Csongor, J., Seres, I., Szucs, S., Szikszay, E. and Penyige, A. Alteration of transmembrane signalling with aging. Identification of G proteins in lymphocytes and granulocytes. *Cell. Signal.,* 5, 593, 1993.

78. Lipschitz, D.A. Udupa, K.D. and Indelicato, S.R. Effect of age on second messenger generation in neutrophils. *Blood,* 78, 1347, 1991.

79. Varga, Z., Bressani, N., Zaia, A.M., Bene, L., Fulop, T., Jr., Leovey, A., Fabris, N. and Damjanovich, S. Cell surface markers, inositol phosphate levels and membrane potential of lymphocytes from young and old human patients. *Immunol. Lett.,* 23, 275, 1990.

80. Roberts, T. and Steinberg, G.M. Effects of aging on adrenergic receptors. Introduction, *Fed. Proc.,* 45, 40, 1986.

81. Abrass, I.B. and Scarpace, P.J. Human lymphocyte beta-adrenergic receptors are unaltered with age. *J. Gerontol.,* 36, 298, 1981.

82. Brodde, O.E. Endogenous and exogenous regulation of human alpha- and beta-adrenergic receptors. *J. Recep. Res.,* 3, 151, 1983.

83. Feldman, R.D., Limbird, L.E., Nadeau, J., Robertson, D. and Wood, A.J. Alterations in leukocyte β-receptor affinity with aging. A potential explanation for altered β-adrenergic sensitivity in the elderly. *N. Engl. J. Med.,* 310, 815, 1984.

84. Landmann, R., Bittiger, H. and Buhler, F.R. High affinity beta-2-adrenergic receptors in mononuclear leucocytes: similar density in young and old normal subjects. *Life Sci.,* 29, 1761, 1981.

85. Gietzen, D.W., Goodman, T.A., Weiter, P.G., Graf, K., Fregeau, D.R., Magliozzi, J.R., Doran, A.R. and Maddock, R.J. Beta-receptor density in human lymphocytes membranes: changes with aging? *J. Gerontol.,* 46, B130, 1991.

86. Krall, J.F., Connelly, M., Weisbart, R. and Tuck, M.L. Age-related elevation of plasma catecholamine concentration and reduced responsiveness of lymphocyte adenylate cyclase. *J. Clin. Endo. Metab.,* 52, 863, 1981.

87. Mader, S.L. and Davis, P.B. Effect of age on acute regulation of beta-adrenergic responses in mononuclear leukocytes. *J. Gerontol.,* 44, M168, 1989.

88. Fulop, T., Jr., Foris, G. and Leovey, A. Age-related changes in cAMP and cGMP levels during phagocytosis in human polymorphonuclear leukocytes. *Mech. Ageing Dev.,* 27, 233, 1984.

89. O'Hara, N., Daul, A.E., Fesel, R., Siekmann, U. and Brodde, O.E. Different mechanisms underlying reduced beta 2-adrenoceptor responsiveness in lymphocytes from neonates and old subjects. *Mech. Ageing Dev.,* 31, 115, 1985.

90. Scarpace, P.J. Decreased β-adrenergic responsiveness during senescence. *Fed. Proc.,* 45, 51, 1986.

91. O'Connor, S.W., Scarpace, P.J. and Abrass, I.B. Age-associated decrease of adenylate cyclase activity in rat myocardium. *Mech. Ageing Dev.,* 16, 91, 1981.

92. O'Connor, S.W., Scarpace, P.J. and Abrass, I.B. Age-associated decrease in the catalytic unit activity of rat myocardial adenylate cyclase. *Mech. Ageing Dev.,* 21, 357, 1983.

93. Narayanan, N. and Derby, J. Alterations in the properties of beta-adrenergic receptors of myocardial membranes in aging: impairments in agonist-receptor interactions and guanine nucleotide regulation accompany diminished catecholamine-responsiveness of adenylate cyclase. *Mech. Ageing Dev.,* 19, 127, 1982.

94. Kobilka, B.K., Matsui, H., Kobilka, T.S., Yang-Feng, T.L., Francke, U., Caron, M.G., Lefkowitz, R.J. and Regan, J.W. Cloning, sequencing, and expression of the gene coding for the human platelet alpha$_2$-adrenergic receptor. *Science,* 238, 650, 1987.

95. Hieble, J.P., DeMarinis, R.M. and Matthews, W.D. Evidence for and against hetereogeneity of alpha 1-adrenoceptors. *Life Sci.,* 38, 1339, 1986.

96. Lai, H., Bowden, D.M. and Horita, A. Age-related decreases in dopamine receptors in the caudate nucleus and putamen of the Rhesus monkey (Macaca mulatta). *Neurobiol. Aging,* 8, 45, 1987.

97. Petrash, A.C. and Bylund, D.B. Alpha 2-adrenergic receptor subtypes indicated by [3H]yohimbine binding in human brain. *Life Sci.,* 38, 2129, 1986.

98. Bylund, D.B. Heterogeneity of alpha 2-adrenergic receptors. *Pharmacol. Biochem. Behav.,* 22, 835, 1985.

99. Johnson, R.D. and Minneman, K.P. Differentiation of alpha 1-adrenergic receptors linked to phosphatidylinositol turnover and cyclic AMP accumulation in rat brain. *Mol. Pharmacol.,* 31, 239, 1987.

100. Morrow, A.L. and Creese, I. Characterization of alpha 1-adrenergic receptor subtypes in rat brain: a reevaluation of [3H]WB 4101 and [3H]prazosin binding. *Mol. Pharmacol.,* 29, 321, 1986.

101. Morgan, D.G., Marcusson, J.O., Nyberg, P., Wester, P., Winblad, B., Gordon, M.N. and Finch, C.E. Divergent charges in D-1 and D-2 dopamine binding sites in human brain during aging. *Neurobiol. Aging,* 8, 195, 1987.

102. De Keyser, J., Ebinger, G. and Vauquelin, G. Age-related changes in the human negrostriatal dopaminergic system. *Ann. Neurol.,* 27, 157, 1990.

103. Bugiani, O., Salvarani, S., Perdelli, F., Mancardi, G.L. and Leonardi, A. Nerve cell loss with aging in the putamen. *Eur. Neurol.,* 17, 286, 1978.

104. Chaconas, G. and Finch, C.E. The effect of aging on RNA-DNA ratios in brain regions of the C57BL-6J male mouse. *J. Neurochem.,* 21, 1469, 1973.

105. Shaskan, E.G. Brain regional spermidine and spermine levels in relation to RNA and DNA in aging rat brain. *J. Neurochem.,* 28, 509, 1977.

106. Amenta, F., Zaccheo, D. and Collier, W.L. Neurotransmitters, neuroreceptors and aging. *Mech. Ageing Dev.,* 61, 249, 1991.

107. Wong, D.F., Wagner, H.N.,Jr., Dannals, R.F., Links, J.M., Frost, J.J., Ravert, H.T., Wilson, A.A., Rosenbaum, A.E., Gjedde, A., Douglass, K.H., Petronis, J.D., Folstein, M.F., Tuong, J.K., Burns, H.D. and Kuhar, M.J. Effects of age on dopamine and serotonin receptors measured by positron tomography in the living human brain. *Science,* 226, 1393, 1984.

108. Govoni, S., Rius, R.A., Battaini, F. and Trabucchi, M. Reduced cAMP-dependent phosphorylation in striatum and nucleus accumbens of aged rats: evidence of an altered functioning of D1 dopaminoceptive neurons. *J. Gerontol.,* 43, B93, 1988.

109. Scarpace, P.J. and Abrass, I.B. Alpha- and beta-adrenergic receptor function in the brain during senescence. *Neurobiol. Aging,* 9, 53, 1988.

110. Miyamoto, A., Villalobos-Molina, R. Kowatch, M.A. and Roth, G.S. Altered coupling of alpha 1-adrenergic receptor-G protein in rat parotid during aging. *Am. J. Physiol.,* 262, C1181, 1992.

111. Supiano, M.A. and Hogikyan, R.V. High affinity platelet alpha 2-adrenergic receptor density is decreased in older humans. *J. Gerontol.,* 48, B173, 1993.

112. Morley, J.E. and Silver, A.J. Anorexia in the elderly. *Neurobiol. Aging,* 9, 9-16, 1988.

113. Kochman, R.L. and Sepulveda, C.K. Aging does not alter the sensitivity of benzodiazepine receptors to GABA modulation. *Neurobiol. Aging,* 7, 363, 1986.

114. Joseph, J.A., Roth, G.S. and Lippa, A.S. Reduction of motor behavioral deficits in senescent animals via chronic prolactin administration. I. Rotational behavior. *Neurobiol. Aging,* 7, 31, 1986.

115. Spiegel, A.M. Receptor-effector coupling by G-proteins: implications for neuronal plasticity. *Progress Brain Research,* 86, 269, 1990.

116. Fulop, T., Jr. and Seres, I. Age-related changes in signal transduction. Implications for neuronal transmission and potential for drug intervention. *Drugs and Aging,* 5, 366, 1994.

117. Nokubo, M. Physical-chemical and biochemical differences in liver plasma membranes in aging F-344 rats. *J. Gerontol.,* 40, 409, 1985.

118. Cimino, M., Vantini, G., Algeri, S., Curatola, G., Pezzoli, C. and Stramentinoli, G. Age-related modification of dopaminergic and beta-adrenergic receptor system: restoration to normal activity by modifying membrane fluidity with S-adenosylmethionine. *Life Sci.,* 34, 2029, 1984.

119. Battaglia, G., Norman, A.B. and Creese, I. Age-related differential recovery rates of rat striatal D-1 dopamine receptors following irreversible inactivation. *Eur. J. Pharmacol.,* 145, 281, 1988.

120. Henry, J.M. and Roth, G.S. Modulation of rat striatal membrane fluidity: effects on age related differences in dopamine receptor concentrations. *Life Sci.,* 39, 1223, 1986.

121. Pitha, J., Hughes, B.A., Kusiak, J.W., Dax, E.M. and Baker, S.P. Regeneration of β-adrenergic receptors in senescent rats: a study using an irreversible binding antagonist. *Proc. Natl. Acad. Sci. U.S.A.,* 79, 4424, 1982.

122. Zhou, L.W., Weiss, B., Freilich, J.S. and Greenberg, L.H. Impaired recovery of alpha 1- and alpha 2-adrenergic receptors in brain tissue of aged rats. *J. Gerontol.,* 39, 538, 1984.

123. Insel, P.A. How should one study brain adrenergic receptors in aging? *Neurobiol. Aging,* 9, 64, 1988.

124. Conklin, B.R. and Bourne, H.R. Structural elements of G alpha subunits that interact with Gβy, receptors, and effectors. *Cell,* 73, 631, 1993.

125. Lefkowitz, R.J., Cotecchia, S., Samama, P. and Costa, T. Constitutive activity of receptors coupled to guanine nucleotide regulatory proteins. *Trends in Pharmacological Sciences,* 14, 303, 1993.

126. Varga, Z., Kovacs, E.M., Paragh, G., Jacob, M.P., Robert, L. and Fulop, T., Jr. Effect of elastin peptides and N-formyl-methianyl-leucyl phenylamine on cytosolic free calcium in polymorpho-nuclear leukocytes of healthy middle-aged and elderly subjects. *Clin. Biochem.,* 21, 127, 1988.

127. Ambrecht, H.J., Nemani, R.K. and Wongsurawat, N. Protein phosphorylation: changes with age and age-related diseases. *J. Am. Ger. Soc.,* 41, 873, 1993.

128. Cai, J.J., Yu, H. and Lee, H.C. Developmental changes of protein kinase C and Gs alpha in hypertrophic cardiomyopathic hamster hearts. *J. Lab. Clin. Med.,* 122, 533, 1993.

129. Luetje, C.W. and Nathanson, N.M. Chronic membrane depolarization regulates the level of guanine nucleotide binding protein Go alpha in cultured neuronal cells. *J. Neurochem.,* 50, 1775, 1988.

130. Goh, J.W. and Pennefather, P.S. A pertussis toxin sensitive G protein in hippocampal long term potentiation. *Science,* 244, 980, 1989.

131. Anson, R.M., Cutler, R., Joseph, J.A., Yamagami, K. and Roth, G.S. The effect of aging on muscarinic receptor G-protein coupling in the rat hippocampus and striatum. *Brain Res.,* 598, 302, 1992.

132. Baker, S.P., Marchand, S., O'Neil, E., Nelson, C.A. and Posner, P. Age-related changes in cardiac muscarinic receptors: decreased ability of the receptor to form a high affinity agonist binding state. *J. Gerontol.,* 40, 141, 1986.

133. Yamagami, K., Joseph, J.A. and Roth, G.S. Decrement of muscarinic receptor-stimulated low Km GTPase in striatum and hippocampus from the aged rat. *Brain Res.,* 576, 327, 1992.

134. Nomura, Y., Makihata, J. and Segawa, T. Activation of adenylate cyclase by dopamine, GTP, NaF and forskolin in striatal membranes of neonatal, adult and senescent rats. *Eur. J. Pharmacol.,* 106, 437, 1984.

135. Severson, J.A. and Randall, P.K. D2 dopamine receptors in aging mouse striatum: determination of high- and low-affinity agonist binding sites. *J. Pharmacol. Exp. Ther.,* 233, 361, 1985.

136. Dolphin, A.C. Nucleotide binding proteins in signal transduction and disease. *Trends Neurosci.,* 10, 53, 1987.

137. Mundy, W., Tandon, P., Ali, S., and Tilson, H. Age-related changes in receptor-mediated phosphoinositide hydrolysis in various region of rat brain. *Life Sci.,* 49, PL97, 1991.

138. Joseph, J.A., Kowatch, M.A., Maki, T. and Roth, C.S. Selective cross-activation/inhibition of second messenger systems and the reduction of age-related deficits in the muscarinic control of dopamine release from periperfused rat striata. *Brain Res.,* 537, 40, 1990.

139. Haba, K., Ogawa, N., Kawata, M., and Mori, A. A method for parallel determination of choline acetyltransferase and muscarinic cholinergic: application in aged-rat brain. *Neurochem. Res.,* 13, 951, 1988.

140. Pontzer, N.J., Chandler, J., Stevens, B.R., and Crews, F.T. Receptors phosphoinositol hydrolysis and plasticity of nerve cells, Progress *Brain Res.,* 86, 221, 1990.

141. Moscona- Amir, E., Henis, Y.I. and Sokolovsky, M. Aging of rat heart myocytes disrupts muscarinic receptor coupling that leads to inhibition of cAMP accumulation and alters the pathway of muscarinic stimulated phosphoinositide hydrolysis. *Biochemistry,* 28, 7130, 1989.

142. Springer, J.E., Tayrien, M.W. and Loy, R. Regional analysis of age-related change in the cholinergic system of the hippocampal formation and basal forebrain of the rat. *Brain Res.,* 407, 180, 1987.

143. Joseph, J.A., Dalton, T.K., Hunt, W.A. and Roth, G.S. Alterations in muscarinic control of striatal dopamine autoreceptors in senescence: a deficit at the ligand-muscarinic receptor interface? *Brain Res.,* 454, 149, 1988.

144. Burnett, D.M., Daniell, L.C. and Zahniser, N.R. Decreased efficacy of inositol 1,4,5-trisphosphate to elicit calcium mobilization from cerebrocortical microsomes of aged rats. *Mol. Pharmacol.*, 37, 566, 1990.

145. Peterson, C., Ratan, R.R., Shelanski, M.L. and Goldman, J.E. Cytosolic free calcium and cell spreading decrease in fibroblasts from aged and Alzheimer donors. *Proc. Natl. Acad. Sci. U.S.A.*, 83, 7999, 1986.

146. Fulop, T. Jr. Signal transduction changes in granulocytes and lymphocytes with ageing. *Immunol. Lett.*, 40, 259, 1994.

147. Magnoni, M.S., Govoni, S., Battaini, F. and Trabucchi, M. The aging brain: protein phosphorylation as a target of changes in neuronal function. *Life Sci.*, 48, 373, 1991.

148. Matsushima, H., Shimohama, S., Yamaoka, Y., Kimura, J., Taniguchi, T., Hagiwara, M. and Hidaka, H. Alteration of human platelet protein kinase C with normal aging. *Mech. Ageing Dev.*, 69, 129, 1993.

149. Graham, S.M., Herring, P.A. and Arinze, I.J. Age-associated alterations in hepatic β-adrenergic receptor/ adenylate cyclase complex. *Am. J. Physiol. (Endocrinol. Metab.)*, 253, E277, 1987.

150. Katz, M.S. Food restriction modulates β-adrenergic-sensitive adenylate cyclase in rat liver during aging. *Am. J. Physiol.*, 254, E54, 1988.

151. Dax, E.M., Ingram, D.K., Partilla, J.S. and Gregerman, R.I. Food restriction prevents an age-associated increase in rat liver beta-adrenergic receptors. *J. Gerontol.*, 44, B72, 1989.

152. Masoro, E.J. Food restriction in rodents: an evaluation of its role in the study of aging. *J. Gerontol.*, 43, B59, 1988.

153. Joyce J.N., Loeschen, S.K., Sapp, D.W. and Marschall, J.F. Age-related regional loss of caudate-putamen dopamine receptors revealed by quantitative autoradiography. *Brain Res.*, 378, 158, 1986.

154. Collier, W.L., Iacopino, L. and Amenta, F. Changes of [3H]spiroperidol binding in the renal artery of aged rabbits. *Mech. Ageing Dev.*, 28, 41, 1984.

155. Strong, R., Waymire, J.C., Samojarski, T. and Gottesfeld, Z. Regional analysis of neostriatal cholinergic and dopaminergic receptor binding and tyrosine hydroxilase activity as a function of aging. *Neurochem. Res.*, 9, 1641, 1984.

156. Severson, J.A. and Randall, P.K. D-2 dopamine receptors in aging mouse striatum: determination of high and low affinity agonist binding sites. *J. Pharmacol. Exp. Ther.*, 233, 361, 1985.

157. O'Boyle, K.M. and Waddington, J.L. A re-evaluation of changes in rat striatal dopamine receptors during development and aging. *Neurobiol. Aging*, 7, 265, 1986.

158. Kohno, A., Cinader, B. and Seeman, P. Age-related changes of adrenoreceptors in spleen lymphocytes and cerebral cortex of NZB/BIN mice. *Immunol. Lett.*, 14, 75, 1986.

159. De Blasi, A., Fratelli, M., Wielosz, M. and Lipartiti, M. Regulation of beta adrenergic receptors on rat mononuclear leukocytes by stress: receptor redistribution and down-regulation are altered with aging. *J. Pharmacol. Exp. Ther.*, 240, 228, 1987.

160. Hamilton, C.A., Jones, C.R., Mishra, N., Barr, S. and Reid, J.L. A comparison of alpha2-adrenoreceptor regulation in brain and platelets. *Brain Res.*, 347, 350, 1985.

161. Malbon, C.C. Liver cell adenylate cyclase and β-adrenergic receptors. Increased β-adrenergic receptor number and responsiveness in the hypothyroid rat. *J. Biol. Chem.*, 255, 8692, 1980.

20

Aging and Defense Mechanisms: The Immune System

Françoise Homo-Delarche, Rodolfo Goya, Jean-François Bach, and Mireille Dardenne

CONTENTS

0-8493-2446-7/95/$0.00+$.50

I. INTRODUCTION

As emphasized by Makinodan and Kay, "aging is characterized by a decline in the ability of individuals to adapt to environmental stress. This is exemplified by an inability to maintain homeostasis."[1] Of the various physiological processes which maintain homeostasis in the body, that of the immune system appears to be one of the most vulnerable, given the susceptibility to infection in the elderly. As judged by epidemiologic and animal model studies, aging induces profound alterations in the immune system, but very often these alterations are not sufficient to provoke clinically potent manifestations. Nevertheless, old individuals are more susceptible to certain infections than the general population.[2-8] Tuberculosis is more frequent in the elderly over than under 70 years of age. Viral infections, particularly of the lungs, also appear more frequent and more severe than in young adults. Response to vaccines is often reduced, but this may depend upon the individual and the vaccine.[8] Thus, many aged subjects do not mount a protective immune response against influenza or hepatitis B vaccines, whereas this is rarely seen in young healthy subjects. Other clinical manifestations may be related to the aging of the immune system. This has been suggested for the increased incidence of malignancy, the greater propensity toward autoimmune, degenerative, and possibly certain neurodegenerative disorders.[9] Autoantibodies commonly found in old individuals do not usually induce autoimmune diseases, but may contribute to the etiology of arteriosclerosis by means of immune complex deposition.[10] Such immune complexes are indeed found with abnormal frequency in the blood of aged subjects. Several authors have reported a significant correlation between the risk of death and the presence of some immunological abnormalities in old patients, such as autoantibodies[1,11] and T cell deficiency[11] or depressed delayed-type hypersensitivity reactivity.[12]

Although numerous studies have been devoted to the immune function of aging humans or animals for at least two decades, increased research in this field has been prompted in recent years by the imperatives of geriatric demographics with the hope of developing therapeutic strategies capable of potentiating the immune functions of elderly individuals. One might thus hope to increase their resistance against numerous diseases in which defects of the immune system are thought to play a role.

Analysis of the numerous data reported in the literature on the immunobiology of aging is hampered by variations in the definition of the term "aged", the medical status of the elderly individual, or the strains of mice used, and, finally, the type of assay performed. This review will attempt to present a comprehensive rather than exhaustive overview of the immunological alterations which accompany the aging process, with emphasis on the connections with the endocrine glands, essentially because of the complexity of the mechanisms involved in cellular and humoral immunity.

II. AN OVERVIEW OF THE IMMUNE SYSTEM

The aim of the immune system is the maintenance of homeostasis. It plays a major role in protecting the host against infectious agents (bacteria, viruses, parasites), neoplastic transformation, or implantation of allogeneic grafts. Alterations in functions of the immune system are frequently seen either as defects (immunodeficiencies) or as excesses (allergy and autoimmunity). Any molecule of sufficient size and diversity can induce an immune response. Then, it acts as an antigen and may provoke either a humoral immune response, producing antibodies, or a cellular immune response, involving lymphocytes. Antigen-specific immunity is often complemented and sometimes replaced by nonspecific immunity, essentially maintained by macrophages.[9,13-18]

Nonspecific immunity refers to a broad variety of host defense mechanisms including phagocytic cells (polymorphonuclear and macrophages), natural killer (NK) cells, certain antimicrobial (i.e., lysozymes) and antiviral (i.e., interferon) products, as well as the complement and kinin systems. In addition to phagocytosis, macrophages possess bactericidal and tumoricidal capacities. These functions can be enhanced following cytokine-mediated activation. Macrophages and monocytes are also of primary importance in specific immunity: they serve as accessory cells for the initial activation of lymphocytes. They are able to phagocytose and metabolize antigens and to present the "processed" antigen on their membrane to the lymphocytes in association with specific "self" markers of the major histocompatibility (gene) complex (MHC). Natural killer (NK) cells, which are cytotoxic without absolute specificity for a unique antigen-bearing cell, selectively destroy transformed cells. These cells are considered to play an important role in the general surveillance against tumor growth and perhaps viruses.

Specific immunity is associated with the establishment of immunological memory involving both cell-mediated and humoral immunity that allows the host to respond amnestically following a second contact with the antigen.

All lymphocytes are thought to arise from a common lymphoid stem cell. T lymphocytes differentiate and mature in the thymus gland. They play an effector role in cell-mediated immunity (CMI), which comprises resistance to viral infection, immunity to intracellular pathogens, allograft rejection (immunity against virus-induced tumors), and also serve as regulatory cells in CMI and humoral immunity. B lymphocytes are derived from the bursa of Fabricius in birds and from a still undefined lymphoid tissue in mammals. They are primarily involved in antibody production.

T cells comprise a large proportion of lymphocytes, (100% in the thymus, 50% in blood and lymph nodes, and 35% in the spleen). There is no clear morphological distinction between B and T cells. Nevertheless T cells are characterized by the nature of their antigen receptor and by the presence on their membrane of several specific markers. The T cell antigen receptor is a glycoprotein having a molecular weight of approximately 80 kDa and composed of two chains of slightly differing lengths. Two types are distinguished according to their constitutive chains, α/β or γ/δ.[19]

The a and b chain of the TCR are linked by disulfide bonds and consist of external variable (V) portions that interact with the MHC molecule presenting an antigenic peptide and an internal constant (C) domain. Similar to immunoglobulin (Ig) molecules, the V region domains are encoded by V region and junctional (J) region germline genes that are rearranged in T cells. In addition, diversity (D) region genes exist for the β-chain.[20,21]

The complex formed by an antigenic peptide in association with appropriate MHC molecules on an antigen-presenting cell together with the TCR α/β on a T cell determines the initiation and progression of an immune response.

Antigen recognition by the T cell receptor also requires the presence of accessory molecules which participate by transmitting the signal delivered by the antigen (CD3 molecule) or by increasing the strength of antigen-receptor binding (adhesins, CD4, CD8, LFA-1, and CD2).

The T cell repertoire of an individual is determined by positive and negative selection mechanisms that take place in the thymus and the periphery, aimed at deleting or inactivating potentially autoreactive clones.[22,23]

Following contact with an appropriate signal, usually antigen (but also nonspecific mitogens, such as phytohemagglutinin (PHA), concanavalin A (ConA), or pokeweed mitogen (PWM)), immunocompetent lymphocytes undergo activation, resulting in the polyclonal expansion of T lymphocyte populations. Sensitized T lymphocytes may be divided into different subpopulations, responsible for either regulatory, memory, or effector functions.

Subpopulations of T cells can be cytotoxic to target cells carrying the antigen to which they are sensitized. They can produce soluble mediators, cytokines, that are pharmacologically active. They can also have an immunoregulatory function, increasing or limiting (helper and suppressor effects) the level of immune, humoral, and cellular responses. Using differentiation markers, two major subpopulations can be distinguished: the CD4 subpopulation which includes T helper (Th) cells, and the CD8 subpopulation which includes cytotoxic and suppressor cells. In addition, CD4+ T cells can be separated into two subsets based upon the repertoire of cytokines produced following stimulation: Th1 cells that make predominantly interleukin-2 (IL-2), tumor necrosis factor (TNF) and interferon (IFN)-γ, and Th2 cells that make predominantly IL-4, IL-5, IL-6, and IL-10. The former are best at activating macrophages, whereas the latter preferentially activate B cells.[24]

Sensitized B lymphocytes either differentiate into plasma cells that secrete antibodies or perform memory cell functions. For the development of humoral immunity (antibody-mediated), most immune responses require cooperation between T and B cells. Some immunogens, which mostly consist of molecules with repetitive polymeric structures (such as bacterial pneumococcal, polysaccharides, staphylococcal protein A, lipopolysaccharides (LPS), and tuberculin-purified protein derivative (PPD), stimulate antibody response by B cells in the presence of minimal helper T cell activity. They are called thymus-independent antigens.

Immune responses are subjected to the influence of a complex network of immunoregulatory circuits regulated by both lymphoid and nonlymphoid cells via the production of various factors, namely cytokines. Cytokines are soluble, monomorphic (glyco)proteins released by living cells of the host in a highly regulated fashion, acting via specific cell surface receptors in picomolar to nanomolar concentrations to regulate host cell function. They not only participate in the quantitative and qualitative regulation of the immune response and intervene in the orchestration of the complex processes of hematopoiesis, wound healing, and inflammation, but are also involved in the normal physiology of nonimmunological and nonhematopoietic organ systems. Cytokines participate in the control of all immunologically relevant events, whether they concern the activation, differentiation, maturation, proliferation, apoptosis, or acquisition of effector functions of lymphocyte precursors, B, T, NK, or accessory cells. For example, under antigenic (or mitogenic) stimulation, macrophages produce interleukin 1 (IL-1).[16,25,26] Lymphocytes stimulated by an antigen or a mitogen produce, in the presence of IL-1, IL-2. IL-2 induces the proliferation of T lymphocytes which express IL-2 receptors, stimulates the production of other soluble factors such as γ-IFN, enhances B cell differentiation, and increases natural killer activity. Moreover, macrophages and T lymphocytes have been shown, among other cells, to synthesize colony-stimulating factors (CSFs) which control the production, the differentiation, and the functions of granulocytes, monocytes, and macrophages.

Finally, immune responses, either cellular or humoral, are subjected to a finely tuned positive or negative regulation. Positive regulation allows below-threshold doses of antigens to induce an immune response and negative regulation down-regulates excessive immune response. Tolerance is a state of antigen-specific central unresponsiveness. Three general tolerance mechanisms have been proposed: clonal deletion, clonal anergy, and T cell-mediated immunosuppression. Clonal deletion involves the physical elimination of cells and is achieved, at least in part, by induced programmed cell death (apoptosis). Clonal anergy, which is reversible, involves the induction of cellular unresponsiveness due to the failure to receive second or costimulatory signals necessary for cellular activation. Both processes require ligation of the T cell receptor (TCR) of the tolerized T cell, which ultimately leads to deletion or inactivation of the ligated cell. In contrast, immunosuppression is mediated by antigen specific T suppressor (Ts) cells, which inhibit immune responses by other cells.[27-29]

The mechanisms of immunoregulation and tolerance involve the participation of helper and/or suppressor cells and/or idiotypic regulation, based on Jerne's network theory.[30,31] This theory is based on the ability of the variable domains of the specific antibody molecules to be recognized (through their idiotypes) by the immune system. The interaction of idiotypes with their complementary anti-idiotypes is thought to maintain a state of dynamic equilibrium. The concept of the idiotypic network was originally limited to B cells and their antibodies, but should presently be extended to T cells. One should note here that the effect of anti-idiotypic antibodies may either be stimulatory or suppressive.[30]

III. ALTERATIONS OF CELLULAR IMMUNE RESPONSE IN AGING

Aged-related decline in immune functions has been extensively assessed in humans and rodents. Converging arguments indicate that a large part of this decline is due to T cell failure, which is thought to be primarily caused by early deterioration of thymic function.

A. Thymic Involution: Morphological and Functional Aspects

The thymus plays a fundamental role in the maturation and differentiation of T lymphocytes. Inside the thymus, T cells proliferate and progressively acquire the characteristics of mature T cells: rearrangements of genes encoding for the T cell receptor, and expression of differentiation antigens — notably the CD4 and CD8 molecules. This transformation is associated with the acquisition of the repertoire of antigen-self receptors necessary for the cognitive functions of T cells.[32-35] The aging process affects various thymic functions acting both at the level of thymocytes (the thymic lymphocytes) as well as at the nonlymphoid cells of the thymic microenvironment (essentially epithelial cells and phagocytes).

1. Morphological and Functional Alterations

In the mouse, thymus weight increases rapidly after birth, attaining its maximum size at puberty, and decreasing progressively with advancing age. This involution is associated with depletion of cortical areas and cystic changes in the epithelial cells as well as infiltration by macrophages, plasma, and mast cells. In man, thymus involution starts in the second decade, but the macroscopic appearance of the gland does not change greatly because the parenchyma is gradually replaced by fat tissue.[14,36-40] The aging process also influences the ability of thymic adherent cells to produce still unidentified factors that are able to modulate the antigen/ mitogen responses of thymocytes.[41] The thymus gland produces polypeptide hormones. Some of these thymic hormones are well characterized, such as thymopoietin, thymosin $\alpha1$, and thymulin (a zinc-containing nonapeptide, formerly called "facteur thymique sérique" or FTS).[42,43] The physiological age-dependent decline of thymulin serum levels has been extensively described.[44,45] In man, the serum thymulin level is maximal at birth, remains constant until the age of 15 to 20 years, and then declines progressively. This pattern is not restricted to thymulin, since the circulating levels of other well-defined thymic hormones such as thymopoietin and thymosin $\alpha1$ also decrease as a function of age.[36,39,42,43] The age-associated decline in circulating thymulin is also found in mice where it has been shown to parallel the involution of thymus weight. It is due to decreased synthesis rather than to peripheral destruction, since the number of thymulin-containing cells (assessed by indirect immunofluorescence using antithymulin monoclonal antibodies) diminishes at the same rate as blood levels.[46] This parallel is also observed in autoimmune mouse strains in which, however, the decrease occurs prematurely both in serum and thymus.[46] This observation is in keeping with the fact that neonatal thymectomy greatly accelerates the onset of autoimmunity in several animal models.[47-51] Neonatal and adult thymectomies hasten the onset of the immune deficiency of aging.[52] However, the accelerating effects of adult thymectomy are not immediate (several months in the mouse, unknown duration in man) and are complicated by the fact that immature peripheral T cells may mature in the absence of thymus.[53,54] It is also interesting that thymic hormone deficiencies have also been described in Down's syndrome, which presents the features of accelerated aging.[44,55]

2. Environmental Factors

The hypothesis that the thymus represents a biological clock for aging has already been suggested by several authors, but one should realize that this theory is weakened by the sensitivity of the thymus to extrinsic environmental factors,[56] such as infections or diets and neuroendocrine hormonal changes. One should note, however, that while it has been demonstrated that zinc-deficient mice or individuals have reduced thymulin levels which can be restored to normal by *in vitro* $ZnCl_2$ addition,[57] *in vitro* reactivation of thymulin activity of aging individuals has never been observed in our laboratory, in contrast to the results published by Fabris et al.[58] Evaluation of thymulin blood levels is complicated by the presence in sera from aging mice or individuals of low molecular noncompetitor inhibitory substances whose concentrations increase during aging.[58,59] These inhibitors should not be confused with high molecular weight inhibitors observed in autoimmune mice, demonstrated to be natural antithymulin antibodies.[60]

Alterations of parameters of immunity in aged mice were therefore studied consecutively by grafting young thymuses, alone or in association with other sources of lymphoid cells, (spleen or bone marrow cells), as well as by administering various thymic hormone preparations. These studies will be discussed below in more detail.

Grafting thymuses from old mice into young adult thymectomized recipients lacking circulating thymulin partially restores the circulating thymulin level. Conversely, grafting newborn thymuses is less efficient in restoring thymulin serum levels in old recipients than in young adult thymectomized recipients.[61] The data corroborate the presence of thymulin inhibitors in aging mice. It is not known, however, whether the inhibition is due to the existence of serum inhibitors in old but not in young sera and/or modulation of thymulin secretion by hormonal changes related to aging.

One of the major factors regulating thymus function is the hypothalamo-pituitary axis.[62] The regulatory control of the neuroendocrine system on the thymus has been studied by Fabris et al.[63] These authors showed that the short-lived hypopituitary dwarf mice, which lack acidophilic cells in the anterior pituitary and are deficient in growth hormone (GH), but also in prolactin (PRL) and thyroxine production, present an early involution of the thymus, which already shows "old" histological features at three months of age and other immunological defects including impaired cell-mediated immunity and early death from "wasting disease". Interestingly, the abnormal condition of these prematurely aging mice can be corrected by either GH or thyroxin treatment, but only in the presence of the thymus. More recently, Murphy et al.[64] demonstrated that dwarf mice display a deficiency in T cell progenitors, particularly CD4/CD8 double positive thymocytes which can be corrected by treatment of these mice with recombinant human GH, whereas PRL administration results in a significant increase in the number and function of antigen-specific peripheral T cells in the immunized dwarf.

In fact, a number of experimental and clinical data have now shown that various hormones, such as GH, prolactin, insulin, and thyroid hormones, positively influence the growth and function of the thymus and particularly its endocrine activity as measured by thymulin levels.[65-69] Conversely, hypophysectomy, experimental diabetes, and thyroidectomy cause a rapid decrease in thymulin plasma levels, which is corrected by hormone replacement therapy.[66,70,71]

The Buffalo/Mna rat offers an interesting model in which the thymus does not involute, but continues to grow with aging causing death at around 20 months by thoracic compression. The immune functions are well maintained in middle age as well as in old age. Hypophysectomy performed at 4 weeks of age prevents thymic overgrowth, once again underlining the close relationship existing between the thymus and the hypothalamo-pituitary axis.[72]

Removal of the adrenals or the gonads in mice, which induces an increase in thymic weight and cellularity,[73] has been the source of contradictory results with regard to thymulin levels.[71,74]

Recent experimental evidence supports the hypothesis that the physiological decline of the neuroendocrine function with aging may contribute to thymic involution. Indeed, different hormonal manipulations are able to restore thymic histology and/or thymic endocrine function in old rodents, in particular, by treatment of old animals with thyroxine,[66,71] GH,[69] or both,[70] with luteinizing hormone-releasing hormone (LH-RH) agonists which induce a chemical castration,[75] or by transplanting GH- and PRL-producing GH3 tumor cells.[76] Such hormonal treatments, which induce recovery of thymic functions in aging rats and mice, may also allow restoration of peripheral immune function.[71,76]

B. T and NK Cell Functions

1. Cell-Mediated Immunity

It is generally accepted that T cell-mediated activities decline with aging. However, it should be emphasized that contradictory results are found in the vast literature describing cellular immune functions in aging humans and animals.[1,8,77] In elderly individuals, many investigators have observed decreases in *in vivo* skin-delayed hypersensitivity responses to common antigens.[1,8,77] However, this does not appear to be an universal finding.[77,78] The reasons for these discrepancies have been analyzed elsewhere.[8,77] It has been stressed that a set of at least six antigens should be used to define anergy in the elderly. Less divergent results have been obtained on primary delayed skin reactions in response to *de novo* antigen sensitization, such as dinitrochlorobenzene, showing a clear decline with age.[1] Studies performed in mice *in vivo* have shown that several T cell-dependent functions were impaired with age. An *in vivo* age-dependent diminution in graft vs. host reaction (GVH) as well as a decrease in the resistance to challenge with syngeneic or allogeneic tumor cells have been reported.[1] Most *in vitro* experiments have revealed decreases in the proliferative T cell response of aging humans and rodents to nonspecific mitogens and allogeneic target cells.[1,8,79] This diminution appears to be more striking in mice regardless of their life span, although the magnitude and rate of decline varies with the strain examined.[80,81]

2. Cytotoxic Cells

Functional alterations of cytotoxic lymphoid and NK cells, which represent putative defense mechanisms against virus-infected and tumor cells, also occur with aging. There is general agreement that the ability to generate cytotoxic T lymphocytes and NK cells diminishes with age in animal models of senescence.[81-87] Moreover, it has been shown that old rats subjected to isolation stress present a decrease in splenic and peripheral blood NK activities compared to old control rats, concomitantly with an increased level of NK activity in bone marrow.[87] This is in contrast with the relatively unchanged activity of NK cells in different tissues from stressed young rats compared to age-matched controls. One explanation for these data is the migration of NK cells from spleen and peripheral blood to other sites, such as bone marrow. Conflicting data have been reported in humans revealing either unchanged, depressed, or even increased NK cell activity in older patients.[77,88-91]

3. T-Cell Numbers

Several possibilities may account for the age-related decline in T cell immune functions: (1) a reduction in the number of responder cells; (2) a shift in the balance among T lymphocyte regulatory and effector subsets; (3) a qualitative defect in T responder cells and/or an alteration in the production of cytokines; and (4) various combinations of these three hypotheses. Once more, it should be stressed that contradictory results have been reported regarding immune cell numbers, phenotypes, and functions in senescence.

In humans, the number of total lymphocytes, including T and B lymphocytes, has either been found unchanged or lowered by about 15 to 20%.[8,92-99] The use of monoclonal antibodies has shown that the diminution observed was primarily due to a reduction in the number of T cells, while B cell and monocyte numbers do not change appreciably. In mice and rats, the number of Thy-1+ cells decreases with age in thymus, peripheral blood, spleen, and lymphatics.[100-104] However, particularly in humans, it should be emphasized that the study of a given cell type in only one compartment is not representative of the total number of cells in the body.

4. T-Cell Subset Phenotypes

The use of monoclonal antibodies has enabled the evaluation of the pool size of the various T cell subsets. A striking increase in the number of null cells (defined as non-T, non-B, nonmonocytic cells, but CD16+Leu7+) has been found in an immunogerontological study, following the Senieur protocol (healthy and uncompromised aged individuals).[105-107] Several hypotheses have been put forward to explain this increased null cell number: positive selection, the healthiest have the highest number of null cells; the higher demand for NK cells, due to the increased occurrence of viral infections or malignant transformation, represents the majority of these null cells; an increase in NK cell number compensates for the defective T cell system, including the decreased functional activity of the individual NK cell; a primary defect of regulation or proliferation; and lastly, an age-related change in cellular compartmentalization with a migration of NK cells towards the intracellular space.[106]

With regard to subpopulations of T lymphocytes, the numbers of immature T cells have been shown to be increased in the elderly human thymus and peripheral blood,[37,108,109] and in mouse thymus and spleen.[52,110] In humans, the data reported on T cells with helper and suppressor markers have been contradictory.[8,111] In man, studies show that both subpopulations decrease to about the same extent with age,[111] but CD4+ T cells have been previously reported to be either enhanced or unchanged, while CD8+ T cells have been shown to be increased, decreased, or constant.[8] In mice, CD8+T suppressor/cytotoxic cells (Thy1+, L3T4-, Ly2+) are diminished in the thymus,[110] but increased in the spleen.[103] In contrast, lower splenic T helper cell levels (Thy1+, L3T4+, Lyt2-) are found in aged rather than in young mice.[100,102,103]

5. T-Cell Subset Functions

The study of the effect of aging on helper and suppressor T cell activities has resulted in conflicting sets of data.[8,47,111] Both functions have been shown to be increased, decreased, and unchanged. As already emphasized, this may be due to differences in cell assay and/or methodology, as well as to the selection of patients or mouse strains. An example of the decrease in T helper activity is the defect of T cells to produce or to respond to IL-2 found in most studies, both in humans and mice.[112-118] One should note, however, that recent studies in man have revealed a heterogeneity of IL-2 production[119] and that contradictory results have been obtained in rats.[120,121] It will be important to clarify this issue which is central to the understanding of the immunobiology of aging in view of the physiological importance of IL-2. Recent experiments on IL-2 mRNA expression in rat splenocytes or human peripheral blood lymphocytes have shown that the age-related decline in the ability of lymphocytes to produce IL-2 could be secondary to a decrease in their ability to express IL-2 mRNA.[122,123] Conflicting data have also been obtained with regard to response to exogenous IL-2, both in elderly humans and aged animals. In some studies an intact response has been found,[115,116,118] whereas other studies showed a defective response.[109,111] Some authors reported a decreased number of IL-2 receptors per cell[112,120,124,125] or a reduced frequency of cells expressing detectable IL-2 receptors, as measured by cytofluorometry using antibodies directed against the IL-2 receptor.[117,126,127] A possible explanation for this T cell unresponsiveness may be the inhibitory effect of endogenously produced prostaglandin E_2 (PGE_2), which has the capacity to inhibit the response of human lymphocytes to mitogens.[128] A prostaglandin-producing suppressor cell has been described which can be blocked *in vitro* and *in vivo* by the cyclooxygenase inhibitor, indomethacin, with resultant enhancement of both cellular and humoral immune responses.[128] In addition, lymphoid cells from healthy men and women over age 70 are significantly more sensitive to PGE_2 inhibition in mitogen-stimulated cultures. Moreover, the more sensitive the healthy elderly subject's lymphocytes were to PGE_2, the lower was the initial PHA response.[129,130] The increased sensitivity to PGE_2 found in some subjects was reversed *in vitro* by indomethacin. The cells most probably involved in prostaglandin production are of the monocyte-macrophage lineage. The activity of adherent cells has been suggested to be modified with aging, with regard to IL-2 production,[118] possibly via IL-1 secretion (see below). Moreover, PGE_2 production is increased with age in mice[131] and it is known that PGE_2 interferes with both IL-2 production and IL-2 receptor expression.[132]

The production of another lymphokine of importance in immunoregulation and resistance to viral infections, IFN-γ, has been reported to be normal, decreased, or increased in the elderly.[133] In another study, the synthesis and secretion of both IFN-γ and IFN-α showed an age-associated decline.[134] It thus remains to be determined whether the deficiencies in the production of these lymphokines lead to the increased susceptibility of the elderly to reactivation of varicella zoster virus or to life-threatening viral infection.

6. Subcellular Alterations

The evidence for age-dependent qualitative T cell changes has been reviewed by several authors.[111,135,136] At the membrane level, a decrease in the surface amount of Thy-1 antigen expression has been reported for old mouse cells, presenting an abnormal fluorescent pattern consisting of patchy or incomplete rings.[137] We may also recall here the already mentioned decrease in IL-2 receptor expression as well as the increase in PGE_2 sensitivity. Lower numbers of glucocorticoid and β-adrenergic receptors have also been reported in old lymphoid cells[138,139] as well as abnormalities of β-receptor redistribution and down-regulation of its expression, which normally occur under stress conditions in young rat mononuclear cells.[140] Lastly, elderly humans with intact β-adrenergic receptors present a defect in the catalytic activity of adenylate cyclase.[141] On the other hand, the expression of new or altered antigens has been observed indirectly on the surface of lymphocytes from old mice.[142,143] For example, spleen cells from young mice can proliferate in response to cells from old syngeneic mice and young mice can synthesize cytotoxic antibodies when injected with cells from old syngeneic mice.[143] Moreover, capping of T cell differentiation antigens,[144] polymerization of actin,[145] and membrane fluidity of T cells[146] are abnormal. A study suggests that many of these age-related changes occurring in the T cell membrane could be due to their increased susceptibility to lipid peroxidation.[146] Alternatively, one may incriminate an inability to transduce the signal supplied by extracellular ligands into the intracellular signals represented by Ca^{2+} and protein kinase C activators.[119] At the cytoplasmic level, aberrations in mitochondrial structures have been described which could explain the increased sensitivity of old cells to Ca^{2+} loss.[111] Imbalance of nucleotide effectors has also been noted in aging lymphocytes.[147] As recently suggested by Tollefsbol and Cohen,[136] the impairment of protein synthesis and/or degradation may be linked to the reduced induction of various enzymes involved in mitogenesis or to numerous other factors involved in cell function which are dependent upon protein synthesis. Changes at the T cell nuclear levels, either qualitative or functional, have been reviewed by Makinodan et al.[111]

IV. ALTERATIONS IN HUMORAL IMMUNE RESPONSE WITH AGING

The observation that infections caused by certain encapsulated bacteria such as *Streptococcus pneumoniae*, group B *Streptococcus*, and *Escherichia coli* K1 occur more frequently in aged humans[8] could reflect changes in humoral immunity during senescence. Indeed, it is now well documented that the humoral immune response declines with age in both humans and animals. *In vivo* and *in vitro* studies in mice have indicated that the decline in the humoral immune response is essentially due to an intrinsic defect of immunocompetent cells[148] rather than to extrinsic factors, i.e., changes in the environment or the "milieu" in which lymphoid cells live.[149]

A. Changes in Humoral Components and Humoral Response

Although the serum concentration of immunoglobulins remains constant with age, the distribution of immunoglobulin classes changes.[150,151] The serum levels of IgG and IgA are increased in the elderly, while the IgM concentration is decreased or unchanged.[8,151,152] In a longitudinal study, an association was shown between the death rate of aged individuals and decreased IgG levels.[152] Some authors have also found abnormally high IgE levels.[8,78] The levels of circulating natural allo- and xenoantibodies decline with aging, whereas those of autoantibodies to thyroglobulin, nuclear proteins, DNA, and rheumatoid factor tend to increase.[111] One may also note higher amounts of circulating immune complexes.[8,153] Lastly, the presence of "benign" homogeneous immunoglobulins (without B cell malignancy) is often seen in aging mice and humans, where it is referred to as idiopathic paraproteinemia (IP) or benign monoclonal gammapathy.[111,154-157] The frequency of IP is increased by neonatal and adult thymectomy.[157]

Most primary and secondary immune responses are impaired in aging humans and animals.[8,111] Decreased antibody response to hepatitis B virus has been demonstrated in old subjects,[158] and to influenza vaccines in both aged humans and mice.[2,159] Serum antibody titers against tetanus toxoid are significantly lower in the aged human than in the adult after booster immunization, with a concomitant decrease of *in vitro* specific IgG antibody synthesis by PWM-stimulated peripheral blood lymphocytes.[160] Defective responses to *pneumococcal polysaccharides* and *streptococcus pneumoniae* were also altered during aging.[161-164] Additionally, in mice, numerous reports have also shown reduced *in vivo* and/or *in vitro* antibody responses to several antigens.[38,111,165-169] To summarize, a general age-dependent decrease exists in the humoral response to specific antigens involving both T cell-dependent or T cell-independent antigens, but more the former than the latter. One should realize, however, that this is a general survey and that there are major individual variations.

Increased production of auto-anti-idiotypic (auto-anti-Id) antibodies as well as a high auto-anti-Id response has been described in aged animals.[150,170,171] This increase in auto-anti-Id has been shown for both thymic-independent and thymic-dependent responses.[172-174]

Humoral immunity involves factors other than immunoglobulins, such as complement, which plays an important role in opsonization. In contrast to those of immunoglobulins, complement levels as well as functional activity do not appear to be altered by aging.[78]

B. B-Cell Changes

1. B-Cell Numbers

The total number of circulating B lymphocytes remains relatively stable or only decreases slightly with age in humans and mice.[111,175,176] Conversely, in CBA mice, the number of B cells in the lymph nodes and Peyer's patches decreases with age, with a proportional increase in the bone marrow.[177,178] In other strains and hybrids, however, the number of B cells tends to increase in spleens and lymph nodes[80] or to remain constant.[179]

2. B-Cell Functions

As shown in a comparative study bearing on eight mouse strains and hybrids, the B cell mitogenic response to LPS can decrease, remain unchanged, or increase with aging, depending upon the strain tested.[80] A more recent investigation has shown that aged mice display a reduced response to Fc fragment stimulation with regard to proliferation and polyclonal antibody synthesis.[180] In rats, a decline in the response to LPS was evident at 20 months.[181] In humans, no age-related change in response to B cell mitogens has been generally observed.[111]

3. Regulatory T Cells

The cellular mechanisms underlying impaired humoral immunity in aging are extremely complex. They were first related to an impairment of the regulatory T cell function, with defective T helper activity or enhanced T suppressor activity or both.[8,182] In some cases, however, decreased suppressor activity was also documented.[183] Defective cellular interactions as well as induction of suppressive anti-idiotypic regulation could also play a role.[171]

Various populations of suppressor cells have been described including mainly T cells, but also B cells, macrophages, and nonmacrophage adherent cells.[133,170,181,183-188] Increased suppression leading to an impaired humoral immune response has been demonstrated both in *in vivo* and in *in vitro* systems; it was designated as "specific" when involving lymphoid cells and "nonspecific" when involving adherent cells such as macrophages. In aged humans, it has thus been shown that T helper and B cell functions are normal, while one could demonstrate a suppressive effect mediated through prostaglandins: the addition of indomethacin to this system completely reversed the suppression.[133,185] Aged human monocytes do not produce more prostaglandins than young ones, but aged human lymphocytes present a higher sensitivity than young ones to the suppressive effect of PGE_2.[129,130]

Another type of mechanism for decreased humoral response mediated by deficient T cells has recently been described in humans. The ability of T cells from young and elderly humans to cap membrane CD3 determinants, to proliferate in response to anti-CD3 antibody, and to produce B cell growth factors were investigated. Results showed that T cells from 50 to 80% of elderly subjects presented reductions in ligand-induced CD3-mediated proliferative events, in addition to decreased production of soluble B cell-growth factors.[189] These abnormalities in CD3-mediated signals could explain the reduced IL-2 production and reduced T helper activity observed in aging.

4. B-Cell Membrane Antigens

Senescent B cells lose their abilities to function and to respond normally.[8,74,171] This abnormality is represented, for example, by a decline in Fc-receptor-mediated regulation in mice,[180] concomitant with changes in cellular Fc receptors.[190,191] There is also a decreased density of surface B antigens, Ia and FcR, as well as μ, γ, and α immunoglobulin chains in rats.[192-194] Lastly, while resting B lymphocytes contain the cellular constituents required for normal RNA and protein synthesis in rodents, they do not respond normally to activating stimuli.[171]

5. Conclusions

Finally, it is difficult to discriminate between a primary B cell defect and a regulatory T cell abnormality which may coexist.[8,172,183] Recent investigations have shown that T cells from unprimed aged mice can down-regulate naive nonstimulated B cells and that this does not cause the elimination of these B cells ("clonal deletion"), but rather a modification of their function ("clonal anergy").[183] This may be related to the fact that T cells from aged mice, through their life-long interactions with environmental antigens, have accumulated the capacity to recognize idiotypes expressed on their own B cells, and that this recognition may lead to the down-regulation of B cell responsiveness by the production of auto-anti-idiotypic antibodies, as discussed above.

V. MONONUCLEAR PHAGOCYTIC AND POLYMORPHONUCLEAR CHANGES IN AGING

Macrophage functions have been extensively studied in aged mice and rats.[195] These studies generally showed no changes in chemotaxis, phagocytosis, or intracellular killing,[195] although one comparative study reported different patterns in three different mouse strains, with an increase in the number of nonspecific esterase-stained peritoneal cells notably in C57BL/6 mice.[196] Other reports revealed alterations in macrophage functions, such as the prevention of intracellular growth of *Toxoplasma gondii* and proliferation of tumoral cells[197] or decreased nonspecific tumor cell cytotoxicity.[8] In humans, conflicting data have also been reported.[198-200]

It was long thought that the ability of macrophages to regulate the immune reaction to mitogens and antigens, particularly at the antigen presentation level, was unaltered with age.[8,201,202] However, more recent reports indicate some age-related changes at this level. These data suggest a decreased capacity of macrophages to release IL-1 and/or of lymphoid cells to bind IL-1.[203] These abnormalities could contribute to the age-dependent decrease in IL-2 production by $Lyt1^+$ helper cells. Moreover, as already mentioned, mononuclear phagocytes produce prostaglandins, which are able to stimulate a subpopulation of suppressor T cells.[130] Although adherent aged human circulating mononuclear cells do not produce more PGE_2 than young ones,[185] a significant increase in PGE_2 production has been demonstrated in spleen cells of aged mice.[131] We may also recall here that senescent human lymphocytes appear to be highly sensitive to the PGE_2-induced suppressive effects.[128,129] Taken together, these results would indicate that: (1) endogenously produced prostaglandins are able to down-regulate IL-1 production;[204] (2) PGE_2 has a direct inhibitory effect on an early step of T cell activation, resulting in reduced IL-2 production, IL-2 receptor expression, responsiveness to exogenous IL-2 and finally, decreased proliferation.[132]

Another study has examined the role of macrophages in impaired FcR-mediated regulation and shown that, in young and old syngeneic mice, the mobile macrophage population involved was derived originally from bone marrow and eventually populates the spleen, bone marrow, and peritoneum of aged mice.[191]

Thus, macrophages may contribute to the altered immune response of old mice by either modifying the production of mediators or the sensitivity of lymphoid cells to these mediators and/or by affecting cell trafficking.

Polymorphonuclear neutrophil (PMN) constitute a first barrier against infective organisms. Since bacterial pneumoniae are relatively frequent in the elderly, alterations in PMN number and/or function cannot be excluded. Granulocytopenia is rarely found in aging.[8] Experiments concerning PMN adherence, chemotaxis, phagocytosis, and bactericidal activities have revealed intact or impaired functions for chemotaxis and phagocytosis, depending upon the investigators.[8,199,205-209] Moreover, a reduction in the generation of superoxide radicals has generally been observed.[205,207] However, no association between PMN defects and increased incidence of bacterial infections could be detected.[208]

VI. CHANGES IN HEMATOPOIETIC STEM CELLS WITH AGING

T and B lymphocytes originate from the proliferation and differentiation of bone marrow stem cells. It is important to determine whether the immunologic defects that occur with age may reflect a decrease in the number and/or functions of these stem cells or are not intrinsic to these stem cells but result from the deleterious internal environment of the aged individual: two nonexclusive possibilities.

With regard to the number of stem cells able to generate colonies in the spleen of lethally irradiated animals (referred to as spleen colony forming units (CFU-s)), an age dependent decrease is observed in some, but not all strains of mice.[80,210-212] However, since the number of nucleated cells in the bone marrow tends to increase with age,[80,210-212] the total number of marrow CFU-s does not change significantly in the strains showing decreased CFU-s concentrations. Hayflick's theory of aging, according to which cells have a genetically programmed finite life span,[56] was initially supported by experiments based on *in vitro* passages or *in vivo* (serial) adoptive transfers of bone marrow cells. However, more recent data have brought no evidence indicating that stem cell function declines with age.[213-215] Indeed, when comparing the abilities of young and old animal bone marrow stem cells to repopulate the recipient, it appears that old bone marrow cells are as active or even more active than bone marrow cells from young animals.[215,216]

With regard to the functional capacities of bone marrow cells after transfer into irradiated young recipients, no difference is observed between bone marrow from young and old animals, when assessing: (1) the levels of endogenous plaque forming cells (PFC) to a number of antigens;[217] (2) the specific PFC responses following LPS stimulation;[217] (3) the frequencies of antigen-specific cells;[179] and (4) the idiotype repertoire expressed with DNP-Ficoll antibodies.[172] However, it should be stressed that some experimental conditions limit the capacity of aged bone marrow cells to behave like young bone marrow cells: (1) bone marrow cells from antilymphocyte serum-treated mice do not interact optimally with young syngeneic thymocytes in short-term experiments;[218] (2) aged stem cells cannot be successfully transferred like young ones into thymectomized animals,[214,218] showing the importance of the thymic microenvironment to maintain their potential; and (3) spleen cells from old mice inhibit the maturation of young bone marrow cells when they are simultaneously transferred into an irradiated recipient.[148]

Recently, the age-related changes in the potential capacity of bone marrow cells to repopulate the thymus and hence to generate T cells have been studied in mice.[219] Bone marrow chimeras were produced between various combinations of young and old mice using either C57BL/6 mice only or combinations of C57BL/6 and B10 Thy 1.1 mice. The weight of the thymus, the number of thymocytes, and splenic T cells of donor origin were assessed at different times after bone marrow transplantation. It was observed that the old bone marrow was less efficient than the young in its capacity to repopulate the thymus and splenic T cell compartment. Moreover, some age-related changes appeared to occur in thymocyte progenitors. These results confirm previous studies showing an age-related decline in marrow T cell progenitors[220-221] and an accumulation of "null" bone marrow cells with age.[221]

Age-related changes in lymphopoiesis are not restricted to bone marrow lymphoid precursor cells — the environment may also play a role. Thus, injection of young bone marrow restores the T cell mitogen response and the antibody forming cell response against sheep red blood cells (SRBC) in the presence of a thymus graft in lethally irradiated old mice. Importantly, old bone marrow cells restore these immune responses in young recipients as well as young bone marrow cells, whereas old bone marrow cells do not do so in old recipients.[222] These experiments suggest that old bone marrow contains precursors that provide suppressive humoral or cellular signals when present in an old environment, but not in a young environment. Another study compared the anti-SRBC-PFC and the mitogenic and allo-cytotoxic T lymphocyte (CTL) responses in irradiated old mice, reconstituted with young bone marrow cells and newborn thymic lobes.[219] When immunologic activities were assessed 11 months later, it was found that the young cells only were incompetent with regard to their PFC response. More recently, similar studies performed without a source of young T cells showed that the antigen-specific B cell repertoire expressed by stem cells of both young and old animals is adversely affected by the old environment.[223]

The nature and molecular bases of the defect of bone marrow cell differentiation and/or proliferation observed with age remain to be determined. One cannot exclude that the thymus or T cells are involved, for example, via the production of cytokines. T cells have a major regulation of hematopoiesis, particularly on the regulation of erythropoiesis at the stem cell as well as the precursor cell levels.[224] Adult thymectomy prevents hematopoietic stem cell (CFU-s) proliferation induced by thymus-dependent but not by thymus-independent antigens. The thymic hormone, thymulin, is able to restore CFU-s response to thymus-dependent antigens in these mice.[225] The production of a cytokine, IL-3, or multi-CSF, that plays an important role in the maturation of several bone marrow cell lines as well as in the biological activities of some cells of the lymphoid lineage, has been found to be reduced with age.[226,227] Finally, there is some evidence that old animals may not be able to maintain homeostasis of the lympho-hematopoietic tissue when subjected to viral infections or psychologic stress.[228,229]

VII. THE IMPACT OF AGING ON IMMUNE-NEUROENDOCRINE INTEGRATION

In recent years a substantial body of information has accumulated showing that the immune and neuroendocrine systems share an extensive number of intercellular messengers (cytokines, hormones, and neurotransmitters) as well as their corresponding receptors.[230] The emerging view is that the immune system is functionally linked to the nervous and endocrine systems, thus constituting an integrated homeostatic network.[231,232] Within this network, the neuroendocrine system monitors and controls the physical and chemical variables of the internal milieu. On its part, the immune system perceives, through antigenic recognition, an internal image of the macromolecular and cellular components of the body and reacts to alterations of this image. It can therefore be said that the immune system participates of the "biological" homeostasis of the organism.

During early life the thymus gland appears to be essential for a proper maturation of the neuroendocrine system as suggested by the multiple endocrine alterations caused by neonatal thymectomy or congenital absence of the thymus in rodents and humans.[233] It is now known that the endocrine thymus produces a number of immunoregulatory substances, some of which are also active on nervous and endocrine circuits.[234,235] Recent *in vivo* studies have shown that in old rodents there is, in addition to a reduced activity of the endocrine thymus,[69,70] a significant desensitization of the neuroendocrine system to thymic signals. Thus, it has been reported that thymosin fraction five (TF5) and homeostatic thymus hormone (HTH), two partially purified thymic preparations, have thyrotropin (TSH)-inhibiting activity in young but not in old rats.[236,237] Furthermore, intravenous administration of HTH was also able to reduce plasma GH and increase corticosterone levels in both young and old rats, although these responses were much weaker in the old animals.

In young adult rodents, antigenic challenge induces a clear increase in circulating corticosterone levels.[238,239] This increase seems to play a role in the modulation of the immune response. Thus, adrenalectomy in rats abolishes the phenomenon of sequential antigenic competition — which is defined as the blockade of an immune response against one antigen by the administration of a second, unrelated antigen a few days before the first one.[239] It is believed that the corticosterone surge during the immune response contributes to prevent an exaggerated or nonspecific production of antibodies. Interestingly, by 12 months of age, mice lose the ability to increase their circulating levels of corticosterone during the immune response, an occurrence that is accompanied by a parallel loss of their ability to show sequential antigenic competition. It seems, therefore, reasonable to hypothesize that aging brings about a progressive disruption in immune-neuroendocrine integration which in turn could play a significant role in age-associated immunopathologies, particularly autoimmunity. Support for the latter possibility comes from studies with autoimmune animal models in which a deficient ACTH and corticosterone response to antigenic challenge has been demonstrated.[240-242]

VIII. RESTORATION AND PREVENTION OF AGE-RELATED ALTERATIONS OF THE IMMUNE SYSTEM

A number of attempts have been made to delay the onset, lower the rate, or even restore the immune functions in old animals. Such an improvement in the immune response would hopefully decrease the incidence of infections and neoplastic diseases in the elderly. These attempts comprise cell grafting, diet and immunotherapy with thymic hormones, cytokines, or other immunomodulators.

A. Cell Grafting

As already mentioned, thymus fragments or dissociated thymocytes, spleen, lymph nodes, and bone marrow cells have been grafted alone or in combination into genetically compatible, lethally irradiated old recipients, with different degrees of immunologic restoration.[61,148,213,214,218,219]

B. Diet

Many reports have pointed out the relationship existing between nutrition and immunocompetence in the elderly. Calories and protein intake, as well as dietary content in some vitamins and trace elements influence hematopoietic and/or immune functions.[77,111,243,244] For example, low protein intake in mice with a normal life span can retard the aging rate by preserving their immunologic functions which, in turn, minimizes autoimmune diseases.[111,243,245] Moreover, the life span of short-lived, autoimmune mice can be modified by the fat/protein intake ratio as well as by the type of lipids ingested.[111,246,247] More recently, it has been shown that oral administration of two amino acids — lysine and arginine — restores in old mouse mitogen responsiveness as well as the expression of T cell markers and the production of the thymic hormone thymulin.[248] The mechanism of this restoration was explained by direct amino acid supplementation or by an indirect effect, via an action of arginine on the neuroendocrine network, since arginine is known to increase GH secretion, which in turn may indirectly influence the immune system.

In addition, another study from the same group reported that a zinc-arginine combination was more effective than the treatment with arginine alone mainly on the reactivation of thymic endocrine activity and the NK activity, particularly under boosting condition by IL-2 and IFN.[249]

The role of zinc itself has been extensively investigated. First, it has been clearly shown that a mild zinc deficiency in humans induces a reduction in serum thymulin and IL-2 activity,[250] and that zinc-deficient mice or individuals have reduced thymulin levels with concomitant appearance of inactive zinc-unbound thymulin molecules.[44,59,250] Second, several studies have evidenced that zinc intake was much more reduced in aging individuals than the intake of other trace elements.[58,250,251] Moreover, the absorption of zinc is also altered in elderly, leading to relatively low zinc concentrations in the blood[251,252] or in granulocytes or lymphocytes.[250]

These observations of age-associated alterations in zinc turnover have led to the investigation of the effect that a zinc supplementation may have on the decline of immune functions. Experiments performed in rodents by applying dietary zinc supplementation during the whole life demonstrated that in these conditions many of the age-related immune modifications, including decreased thymic hormone production, reduced T helper activity, and depressed NK cytotoxicity, could be prevented by such treatment.[249] Other studies showed that a moderate dietary zinc supplementation in aging mice was able to restore some parameters of the thymic pattern observed in young mice, including normal architecture, cellularity, and hormonal function[252] or to reconstitute peripheral T cell functions,[58] whereas a physiological amount of zinc supplementation in an elderly population allowed either partial restoration of nutritional and thymic status or improvement of thymulin and IL-1 production, and an increase in response to skin-test antigens.[250,251]

The mechanism of action of zinc is probably multifaceted, due to its widespread action on different enzymes and hormones involved in various steps of immune response. Zinc is required for conferring biological activity to thymulin, a zinc-containing thymic metallopeptide. However, it is also able to regulate the activity of enzymes involved in lymphocyte proliferation and to play a role in the genetic expression of various proteins. Thus, a direct role of zinc in lymphocyte proliferation and genetic expression of IL-1 or IL-2 receptors cannot be ruled out.

Finally, enhancement of immune parameters can also be obtained *in vitro* and *in vivo* by vitamin C [253,254] and vitamin E (by inhibition of free radicals) or by vitamin and trace element supplementation, as recently evidenced by Chandra, suggesting that an optimal intake of all essential micronutrients in a physiological amount could result in an improvement of immune response and a reduction of the frequency of infection in old age.[255]

C. Immunotherapy by Thymic Hormones and Other Agents

Since involution of the thymus and decrease in thymic hormone levels preceding the loss of immunologic vigor have been observed in the elderly, a number of investigators have tried to use thymic hormones and extracts to prevent immunologic aging. First, the thymus extract (THF) was found to enhance the T cell-dependent graft vs. host (GVH) response *in vitro* of spleen cells from old but not young mice.[256] Similarly, *in vivo* administration of thymulin was shown to restore the response to PHA in thymectomized mice[257] and *in vitro* treatment increased mitogen-induced proliferation as well as IL-2 production by splenocytes of Nu/Nu mice,[258] two experimental models of complete thymic insufficiency. In old mice, *in vivo* thymulin treatment was shown to increase lymphocyte-mediated cytotoxicity,[61] and to provide, like thymopoietin, a partial reactivation of the primary humoral immune response. In contrast, multiple treatments with thymulin or thymopoietin failed to restore the resistance to line Ib leukemia or responses to T cell mitogens in thymectomized C58 mice.[259] *In vivo* administration of a thymic extract thymostimulin (TP-I) was able to increase the antitrinitrophenyl (TNP) antibody response to TNP-HRB and TNP-ficoll, suggesting that TP-I was effective in restoring helper cell activity.[260] In contrast, in humans, *in vivo* administration of TP-I failed to restore skin reactivity responses to *Candida*.[261] Thymostimulin, also increased *in vitro* mitogen-induced proliferation of old guinea pig peripheral blood lymphocytes and restored *in vivo* the mitogenic responses of peripheral blood cells and splenocytes as well as helper T cell functions.[262] Thymopentin (TP-5), the active peptide isolated from thymopoietin, has been studied *in vivo* in both normal and uncompromised elderly subjects. In normal aged subjects, TP-5 significantly enhanced T cell proliferation induced by PHA, anti-CD3, anti-CD2, and anti-CD8 monoclonal antibodies,[263] while in immunocompromised old patients it improved cutaneous delayed hypersensitivity, mitogenic responses, and IL-2 production.[264] In the last group of patients, TP-5 had no effect on either PWM-induced immunoglobulin synthesis or on lymphocyte subsets. Finally, the effects of thymosin α1 were extensively studied in mice and humans. In mice, thymosin α1 restored *in vitro* the proliferative response of lymph node cells from ovalbumin-primed aging mice, whereas when administered *in vivo* before carrier priming, it enhanced helper T cell activity.[265] *In vivo* administration of thymosin α1 to both young and old mice augmented antitetanus toxoid antibody production, without showing any effect on antipneumococcal antibody production.[266] It was further demonstrated that injection of thymosin α1 in old mice increased the splenic frequency of T cell precursors, leading to increased IL-2 production and expression of IL-2 receptors.[267] In middle-aged monkeys, the *in vivo* administration of thymosin α1 enhanced mitogen-induced proliferation and NK cell function, while it had no effect on the antibody response to tetanus toxoid vaccine.[268] Lastly, in humans, thymosin α1 was shown to augment *in vitro* the antibody response to influenza vaccine in the majority of old subjects,[269] as well as to increase the influenza vaccine response from 25 to 60% in elderly individuals in a phase III clinical trial.

The effects of thymic factors on the restoration of the immune response in old individuals are probably due to a direct action on T cell proliferation and differentiation. However, they could also be due to an indirect action on the neuroendocrine system. Indeed, thymosin peptides have recently been shown to stimulate the release of various neuropeptides, such as ACTH, LH-RH, LH, GH, PRL, and β-endorphin,[234] some of which have a stimulatory effect on thymic functions as well as peripheral immune parameters.

Attempts to enhance immune responses, particularly lymphocyte proliferation, by the addition of IL-2 to the lymphocytes of aged individuals provided conflicting data. In vitro IL-2 treatment reversed the low cytotoxic activity of old immunized lymphocytes, whereas *in vivo* IL-2 supplementation did not increase the protection mediated by old immunized T cells, but rather increased the suppression.[270]

Various immunomodulatory agents have been shown to enhance immune responses of aging animals and humans. For example, a single injection of isoprinosine into aging hamsters temporarily improved mitogen-induced stimulation, NK activity, and monocyte chemotaxis. In the elderly with chronic diseases, *in vitro* treatment with isoprinosine significantly enhanced mitogen-induced proliferation.[271] Similarly, long-term administration of levamisole restored helper as well as suppressor T cell functions in the anti-SRBC antibody response in aged mice.[272] Levamisole itself was not active *in vitro*, but exerted its effect through *in vivo* metabolites. Other agents, such as tufsin, immunocytal, and a nontoxic monophosphoryl lipid A have been shown, respectively, to increase immune cytotoxicity in aged mice, enhance purified protein derivative (PPD) tuberculin reactivity in the elderly, and restore antibody formation in old mice.[273-275]

IX. CONCLUSIONS

In conclusion, it appears that the impact of aging on the immune response is highly variable. Some individuals are able to maintain homeostasis, while others can not. Such differences may be related to environmental factors encountered during life, such as stress, therapeutic regimens, and diets. Practically, both cellular- and humoral-mediated immune responses may be altered with age. This may take place at the cellular level and regulatory, effector, and antibody-producing cells may be affected. Multiple underlying mechanisms are probably involved, such as the production of and/or response to cytokines, anti-idiotypic antibodies, or lipid mediators, particularly prostaglandins. Several immunomodulatory agents or diets may improve immune response in aged animals or humans and it would be of great interest to explore whether or not such treatments correlate with clinical improvement.

ACKNOWLEDGMENTS

The authors wish to thank Catherine Slama, Hélène Feuillet, Serge Sczulczewski, Ghislaine Lavialle, and Doreen Broneer for their help in the preparation of the manuscript.

REFERENCES

1. Makinodan, T. and Kay, M. M. B., Age influence on the immune system, *Adv. Immunol.*, 29, 287, 1980.
2. Phair, J. P., Aging and infection: a review, *J. Chronic Dis.*, 32, 535, 1979.
3. Gardner, I. D., The effect of aging on susceptibility to infection, *Rev. Infect. Diseases*, 2, 801, 1980.
4. Berk, S. L. and Smith, J. K., Infectious diseases in the elderly, *Med. Clin. North Am.*, 67, 273, 1983.
5. Schneider, E. L., Infectious diseases in the elderly, *Ann. Int. Med.*, 98, 395, 1983.
6. Yoshikawa, T. T., Aging and infectious diseases: state of the art, *Gerontology*, 30, 275, 1984.
7. Garibaldi, R. A. and Nurse, B. A., Infections in the elderly, *Am. J. Med.*, 81, 53, 1986.
8. Saltzman, R. L. and Peterson, P. K., Immunodeficiency of the elderly, *Rev. Infect. Diseases*, 9, 1127, 1987.
9. Trofatter, K. F., Immune response and aging, *Clin. Obst. Gyn.*, 29, 384, 1986.
10. Clarkson, T. B. and Alexander, N. J., Long-term vasectomy: effects on the occurence and extent of atherosclerosis in rhesus monkeys, *J. Clin. Invest.*, 65, 15, 1980.
11. Hallgren, H. M., Buckley, C. E., Gilbertsen, V. A. and Yunis, E.J., Lymphocyte phytohemagglutinin responsiveness, immunoglobulins and autoantibodies in aging humans, *J. Immunol.*, 111, 1101, 1973.
12. Roberts-Thomson, I. C., Whittingham, S., Youngchaiyud, U. and Mackay, I. R., Ageing, immune response and mortality, *Lancet*, 2, 368, 1974.
13. MacDonald, H. R., Lees, R. K., Sordat, B., Zaech, P., Maryanski, J. L. and Bron, C., Age-associated increase in expression of the T cell surface markers Thy-1, Lyt-1 and Lyt-2 in congenitally athymic (nu/nu) mice: analysis by flow microfluorometry, *J. Immunol.*, 126, 865, 1981.
14. Hirokawa, K., Autoimmunity and aging, *Concepts Immunopathol.*, 1, 251, 1985.
15. Cooper, M. D., Current concepts. B lymphocytes: Normal development and function, *New Engl. J. Med.*, 317, 1452, 1987.
16. Dinarello, C. A. and Mier, J. W., Lymphokines, *N. Engl. J. Med.*, 317, 940, 1987.
17. Royer, H. D. and Reinherz, E. L., T lymphocytes: ontogeny, function and relevance to clinical disorders, *New Engl. J. Med.*, 317, 1136, 1987.
18. Johnson, R. B., Jr., Current concepts: immunology. Monocytes and macrophages, *N. Engl. J. Med.*, 318, 747, 1988.
19. Marrack, P. and Kappler, J., The T cell receptor, *Science*, 238, 1073, 1987.
20. Davis, M. M. and Bjorkman P. J., T-cell antigen receptor genes and T-cell recognition, *Nature*, 334, 395, 1988.
21. Moss, P. A. H., Rosenberg, W. M. and Bell, J. I., The human T cell receptor in health and disease, *Annu. Rev. Immunol.*, 10, 71, 1992.
22. von Boehmer, H., Developmental biology of T cells in T-cell receptor transgenic mice, *Annu. Rev. Immunol.*, 8, 531, 1990.
23. Miller J. F. and Morahan, G., Peripheral T cell tolerance, *Annu. Rev. Immunol.*, 10, 51, 1992.
24. Swain, S. L., Bradley, L. M., Croft, M., Tonkonogy, S., Atkins, G., Weinberg, A. D., Duncan, D. D., Hedrick, S. M., Dutton, R. W. and Huston, G., Helper T-cell subsets: phenotype, function and the role of lymphokines in regulating their development, *Immunol. Rev.*, 123, 115, 1991.
25. Arai, K. I., Lee, F., Miyajima, A., Miyatake, S. and Yokota, T., Cytokines: coordinators of immune and inflammatory responses, *Ann. Rev. Biochem.*, 59, 783, 1990.
26. Kroemer, G., Moreno de Alboran, I., Gonzalo, J. A. and Martinez, C., Immunoregulation by cytokines, *Crit. Rev. Immunol.*, 13, 163, 1993.
27. Lederberg, J., Genes and antibodies, *Science*, 129, 1649, 1959.
28. Bretscher, P. and Cohn, M., A theory of self-nonself discrimination, *Science*, 169, 1042, 1970.
29. Gershon, R. K. and Kondo, K., Infectious immunological tolerance, *Immunology*, 21, 903, 1971.
30. Farid, N. D. and Lo, T. C., Antiidiotypic antibodies as probes for receptor stucture and function, *Endocrine Rev.*, 6, 1, 1985.
31. Jerne, N. K., Towards a network theory of the immune system, *Annal. Immunol. (Inst. Past.)*, 125 C, 373, 1974.
32. Reinherz, E. L. and Schlossman, S.F., Current concepts in immunology. Regulation of the immune response-inducer and suppressor T-lymphocyte subsets in human beings, *N. Engl. J. Med.*, 303, 370, 1980.
33. Scollay, R., Intrathymic events in the differentiation of T lymphocytes: a continuing enigma, *Immunol. Today*, 4, 282, 1983.
34. Rothenberg, E. and Lugo, J. P., Differentiation and cell division in the mammalian thymus, *Developmental Biol.*, 112, 1, 1985.
35. Ritter, M. A., Rozing, J. and Schuurman, H. J., The true function of the thymus?, *Immunol. Today*, 9, 189, 1988.
36. Simpson, J. G., Gray, E. S. and Beck, J. S., Age involution in the normal human adult thymus, *Clin. Exp. Immunol.*, 19, 261, 1975.
37. Singh, J. and Singh, A. K., Age-related changes in human thymus, *Clin. Exp. Immunol.*, 37, 507, 1979.

38. Kay, M. M., Immunological aspects of ageing: early changes in thymic activity, *Mech. Ageing Dev.*, 28, 193, 1984.

39. Weksler, M. E. and Siskind, G. W., The cellular basis of immune senescence, *Monogr. Devl. Biol.*, 17, 110, 1984.

40. Steinmann, G. G., Changes in the human thymus during ageing, *Current Top. Pathol.*, 75, 43, 1986.

41. Sato, K., Chang, M. P. and Makinodan, T., Influence of age on the ability of thymic adherent cells to produce factors in vitro which modulate immune responses of thymocytes, *Cell. Immunol.*, 87, 473, 1984.

42. Bach, J. F., Thymulin (FTS-Zn), *Clin. Immunol. Allergy*, 3, 133, 1983.

43. Zatz, M. A. and Goldstein, A. L., Thymosins, lymphokines, and the immunology of aging, *Gerontology*, 31, 263, 1985.

44. Fabris, N., Mocchegiani, E., Amadio, L., Zannotti, M., Licastro, F. and Franceschi, C., Thymic hormone deficiency in normal ageing and Down's syndrome: is there a primary failure of the thymus?, *Lancet*, 1, 983, 1984.

45. Dardenne, M., Bach, M. A. and Bach, J. F., Thymic hormones and aging. in *Immunology and Ageing*, Fabris, N., Ed., Martinius Nijhoff, Boston, 1982, 139.

46. Savino, W., Dardenne, M. and Bach, J.F., Thymic hormone containing cells. II. Evolution of cells containing the serum thymic factor (FTS or thymulin) in normal and autoimmune mice, as revealed by anti-FTS monoclonal antibodies. Relationship with Ia bearing cells, *Clin. Exp. Immunol.*, 52, 1, 1983.

47. Wick, G., Kite, J. H., Jr. and Witebsky, E., Spontaneous thyroiditis in the obese strain of chickens. IV. The effect of thymectomy and thymobursectomy on the development of the disease, *J. Immunol.*, 104, 54, 1970.

48. Roubinian, J. R., Papoian, R. and Talal, N., Effects of neonatal thymectomy and splenectomy on survival and regulation of autoantibody formation in NZB/NZW F1 mice, *J. Immunol.*, 118, 1524, 1977.

49. Steinberg, A. D., Roths, J. B., Murphy, E. D., Steinberg, R. T. and Raveche, E. S., Effects of thymectomy or androgen administration upon the autoimmune disease of MLR/Mp-lpr/lpr mice, *J. Immunol.*, 125, 871, 1980.

50. Smith, H. R., Chused, T. M., Smathers, P. A. and Steinberg, A. D., Evidence for thymic regulation of autoimmunity in BXSB mice: acceleration of disease by neonatal thymectomy, *J. Immunol.*, 130, 1200, 1983.

51. Hang, L., Theophilopoulos, A. N., Balderas, R. S., Francis, S. J. and Dixon, F.J., The effect of thymectomy on lupus-prone mice, *J. Immunol.*, 132, 1809, 1984.

52. Dutartre, P. and Pascal, M., Thymectomy at weaning. An accelerated aging model for the mouse immune system, *Mech. Ageing Dev.*, 59, 275, 1991.

53. Mackay, I. R., Ageing and immunological function in man, *Gerontologia*, 18, 285, 1972.

54. MacDonald, H. R., Phenotypic and functional characteristics of "T-like" cells in nude mice, *Exp. Cell. Biol.*, 52, 2, 1984.

55. Franceschi, C., Licastro, F., Chiricolo, M., Bonetti, F., Zannotti, M., Fabris, N., Mocchegiani, E., Fantini, M. P., Paolucci, P. and Masi, M., Deficiency of autologous mixed lymphocyte reactions and serum thymic factor level in Down's syndrome, *J. Immunol.*, 126, 2161, 1981.

56. Hayflick, L., The aging process: current theories, *Drug-Nutrients Interactions*, 4, 13, 1985.

57. Dardenne, M., Savino, W., Wade, S., Kaiserlian, D., Lemonnier, D. and Bach J. F., In vivo and in vitro studies of thymulin in marginally zinc-deficient mice, *Eur. J. Immunol.*, 14, 454, 1984.

58. Fabris, N., Mocchegiani, E., Muzzioli, M. and Provinciali, M., The role of zinc in neuroendocrine-immune interactions during aging, *Ann. N.Y. Acad. Sci.*, 621, 314, 1991.

59. Dardenne, M., Savino, W., Gastinel, L. N. and Bach, J. F., Thymulin, zinc and ageing, in EURAGE Symposium on *Lymphoid Cell Functions in Ageing*; de Weck, A. L., Ed., Rijswijk, 1984, 187.

60. Dardenne, M., Savino, W. and Bach, J. F., Autoimmune mice develop antibodies to thymic hormone. Production of anti-thymulin monoclonal autoantibodies from diabetic (db/db) and B/W mice, *J. Immunol.*, 133, 740, 1984.

61. Bach M. A. and Beaurain, G., Respective influence of extrinsic and intrinsic factors on the age-related decrease of thymic secretion, *J. Immunol.*, 122, 2505, 1979.

62. Cooper, E. L., Immune systems and neuroendocrines, *Ill. Med. J.*, 171, 223, 1987.

63. Fabris, N., Pierpaoli, W. and Sorkin, E., Lymphocytes, hormones and ageing, *Nature*, 240, 557, 1972.

64. Murphy, W. J., Durum, S. K. and Longo, D. L., Differentiation effects of growth hormone and prolactin on murine T cell development and function, *J. Exp. Med.*, 178, 231, 1993.

65. Dardenne, M., Savino, W., Gagnerault, M. C., Itoh, T. and Bach, J. F. Neuroendocrine control of thymic hormonal production. I. Prolactin stimulates in vivo and in vitro the production of thymulin by human and murine thymic epithelial cells, *Endocrinology*, 125, 3, 1989.

66. Fabris, N., Muzzioli, M. and Mocchegiani, E., Recovery of age-dependent immunological deterioration in Balb/c mice by short-term treatment with L-thyroxine, *Mech. Ageing. Dev.*, 18, 327, 1982.

67. Nagy, E., Berczi, I. and Friesen, H. G., Regulation of immunity in rats by lactogenic and growth hormones, *Acta Endocrinol.*, 102, 351, 1983.

68. Savino, W., Wolf, B., Aratan-Spire, S. and Dardenne, M., Thymic hormone containing cells. IV. Fluctuations in the thyroid hormone levels in vivo can modulate the secretion of thymulin by the epithelial cells of young mouse thymus, *Clin. Exp. Immunol.*, 55, 629, 1984.

69. Goya, R. G., Gagnerault, M. C., Leite-de-Moraes, M. C., Savino, W. and Dardenne, M., In vivo effects of growth hormone on thymus function in aging mice, *Brain, Behav. Immunity*, 6, 341, 1992.

70. Goya, R. G., Gagnerault, M. C., Sosa, Y. E., Bevilacqua, J. A. and Dardenne, M., Effects of growth hormone and thyroxine on thymulin secretion in aging rats, *Neuroendocrinology*, 58, 338, 1993.

71. Fabris, N. and Mocchegiani, E., Endocrine control of thymic serum factor production in young-adult and old mice, *Cell. Immunol.*, 91, 325, 1985.

72. Harrison, D. E., Archer, R. and Astle, C. M., The effect of hypophysectomy on thymic aging in mice, *J. Immunol.*, 129, 2673, 1982.

73. Grossman, C. J., Regulation of the immune system by sex steroids, *Endocrine. Rev.*, 5, 435, 1984.

74. Dardenne, M., Savino, W., Duval, D., Kaiserlian, D., Hassid, J. and Bach, J. F., Thymic hormone-containing cells. VII. Adrenals and gonads control the in vivo secretion of thymulin and its plasmatic inhibitor, *J. Immunol.*, 136, 1303, 1986.

75. Greenstein, B. D., Fitzpatrick, F. T. A., Kendall, M. D. and Wheeler, M. J., Regeneration of the thymus in old male rats treated with a stable analog of LHRH, *J. Endocr.*, 112, 345, 1987.

76. Kelley, K. W., Brief, S., Westly, H. J., Novakofski, J., Bechtel, P. J., Simon, J. and Walker, E. B., GH3 pituitary adenoma cells can reverse thymic aging in rats, *Proc. Natl. Acad. Sci. U.S.A.*, 83, 5663, 1986.

77. Delafuente, J. C., Immunosenescence. Clinical and pharmacologic considerations, *Med. Clin. North Am.*, 69, 475, 1985.

78. Phair, J. P., Kauffman, C. A., Bjornson, A., Gallagher, J., Adams, L. and Hess, E. V., Host defenses in the aged: evaluation of components of the inflammatory and immune responses, *J. Infect. Dis.*, 138, 67, 1978.

79. Kay, M. M., An overview of immune aging, *Mech. Ageing Dev.*, 9, 39, 1979.

80. Kay, M. M., Mendoza, J., Diven, J., Denton, T., Union, N. and Lajiness, M., Age-related changes in the immune system of mice of eight medium and long-lived strains and hybrids. I. Organ, cellular and activity changes, *Mech. Ageing Dev.*, 11, 295, 1979.

81. Goodman, S. A. and Makinodan, T., Effect of age on cell-mediated immunity in long-lived mice, *Clin. Exp. Immunol.*, 19, 533, 1975.

82. Herberman, R. B., Nunn, M. E. and Lavrin, D. H., Natural cytotoxic reactivity of mouse lymphoid cells against syngeneic and allogeneic tumors. I. Distribution of reactivity and specificity, *Int. J. Cancer*, 16, 216, 1975.

83. Kiessling, R., Klein, E., Pross, H. and Wigzell, H., Natural killer cells in the mouse. II. Cytotoxic cells with specificity for mouse Moloney leukemia cells. Characteristics of the killer cells, *Eur. J. Immunol.*, 5, 117, 1975.

84. Weindruch, R., Devens, B. H., Raff, H. V. and Walford, R. L., Influence of dietary restriction and aging on natural killer cell activity in mice, *J. Immunol.*, 130, 993, 1983.

85. Albright, J. W. and Albright, J. F., Age-associated impairment of murine natural killer activity, *Proc. Natl. Acad. Sci. U.S.A.*, 80, 6371, 1983.

86. Albright, J. W. and Albright, J. F., Age-associated decline in natural killer (NK) activity reflects primarily a defect in function of NK cells, *Mech. Ageing Dev.*, 31, 295, 1985.

87. Ghoneum, M., Gill, G., Assanah, P. and Stevens, W., Susceptibility of natural killer cell activity of old rats to stress, *Immunology*, 60, 461, 1987.

88. Fernandes, G. and Gupta, S., Natural killing and antibody-dependent cytotoxicity by lymphocyte subpopulations in young and aging humans, *J. Clin. Immunol.*, 3, 141, 1981.

89. Nagel, J. E., Collins, G. D. and Adler, W.H., Spontaneous or natural killer cytotoxicity of K562 erythroleukemic cells in normal patients, *Cancer Res.*, 41, 2284, 1981.

90. Penschow, J. and Mackay, I. R., NK and K cell activity of human blood: differences according to sex, age and disease, *Ann. Rheum. Dis.*, 39, 82, 1980.

91. Tsukamaya, D., Breitenbucher, R., Steinberg, S., Allen, J., Nelson, R., Gekker, G., Keane, W. and Peterson, P., Polymorphonuclear leukocyte, T-lymphocyte, and natural killer cell activities in elderly nursing home residents, *Eur. J. Clin. Microbiol.*, 5, 468, 1986.

92. Diaz-Jauanen, E., Strickland, R. G. and Williams, R. C., Studies of human lymphocytes in the newborn and the aged, *Am. J. Med.*, 58, 620, 1975.

93. Kishimoto, S., Tomino, S., Inomata, K., Kotegawa, S., Saito, T., Kuroki, M., Mitsuya, H. and Hisamitsu, S. Age-related changes in the subsets and functions of human T lymphocytes, *J. Immunol.*, 121, 1773, 1978.

94. Nagel, J. E., Chrest, F. J. and Adler, W. H., Enumeration of T lymphocyte subsets by monoclonal antibodies in young and aged humans, *J. Immunol.*, 127, 2086, 1981.

95. O'Leary, J. J., Jackola, D. R., Hallgren, H. M., Abbasnezhad, M. J. and Yasmineh, W. G., Evidence for a less differentiated subpopulation of lymphocytes in people of advanced age, *Mech. Ageing Dev.*, 21, 109, 1983.

96. Weksler, M. E. and Hütteroth, T. H., Impaired lymphocyte function in aged humans, *J. Clin. Invest.*, 53, 99, 1974.

97. Yamakido, M., Yanagida, J., Ishioka, S., Matsuzaka, S., Hozawa, S., Akiyama, M., Kobuke, K., Inamizu, T. and Nishimoto, Y., Detection of lymphocyte subsets by monoclonal antibodies in aged and young humans, *Hirosh, J. Med. Sci.*, 34, 87, 1985.

98. Murasko, D. M. and Goonewardene, I. M., T-cell function in aging: mechanisms of decline, *Ann. Rev. Gerontol. Geriatr.*, 10, 71, 1990.

99. Ben-Yehuda, A. and Weksler, M. E., Immune senescence: mechanisms and clinical implications, *Cancer Invest.*, 10, 525, 1992.

100. el Demellawy, M. and el Ridi, R., Age-associated decrease in proportion and antigen expression of CD8+/CD4+ thymocytes in BALB/c mice, *Mech. Ageing Dev.*, 62, 307, 1992.

101. Haaijman, J. J., Ure, J. M. and Micklem, H. S., Mouse T and B lymphocyte subpopulations: changes with age, in *Immunology and Ageing*, Fabris, N., Ed., Martinus Nijhoff, The Hague, 1982, 86.

102. Vissinga, C.S., Dirven, C. J. A. M., Steinmeyer, F. A., Benner, R. and Boersma, W. J., Deterioration of cellular immunity during aging. The relationship between age-dependent impairment of delayed-type hypersensitivity reactivity, interleukin-2 production capacity, and frequency of Thy-1+, Lyt-2- cells in C57BL/Ka and CBA/Rij mice, *Cell Immunol.*, 108, 323, 1987.

103. Dutartre, P., Annat, J. and Pascal, M., Flow cytometric analysis of membrane receptors evolution during mouse aging, *Periodicum. Biologorum.*, 89, 131 (abstract), 1987.

104. Ebersole, J. L., Steffen, M. J. and Pappo, J., Secretory immune responses in ageing rats. II. Phenotype distribution of lymphocytes in secretory and lymphoid tissues, *Immunology*, 64, 289, 1988.

105. Ligthart, G. J., Schuit, H. R. E., and Hijmans, W., Subpopulations of mononuclear cells in ageing: expansion of the null cell compartment and decrease in the number of T and B cells in human blood, *Immunology*, 55, 15, 1985.

106. Lighart, G.J., Van Vlokhoven, P.C., Schuit, H. R. E., Hijmans, W., The expanded null cell compartment in ageing: increase in the number of natural killer cells and changes in T-cell and NK-cell subsets in human blood, *Immunology*, 59, 353, 1986.

107. Krishnaraj, R. and Blandford, G., Age-associated alterations in the human natural killer cells. 2. Increased frequency of selective NK subsets, *Cell. Immunol.*, 114, 137, 1988.

108. Moody, C. E., Innes, J. B., Staiano-Coi, L., Incefy, G. S., Thaler, H. T. and Weksler, M. E., Lymphocyte transformation induced by autologous cells. XI. The effect of age on the autologous mixed lymphocyte reaction, *J. Immunol.*, 44, 431, 1981.

109. Pahwa, S. G., Pahwa, R.N. and Good, R.A., Decreased in vitro humoral immune responses in aged humans, *J. Clin. Invest.*, 67, 1094, 1981.

110. Yoshikai, Y., Matsuzaki, G., Kishihara, K., Yokokura, T. and Nomoto, K., Age-associated increase in the expression of T-cell antigen receptor γ-chain in conventional and germ-free mice, *Infect. Immun.*, 56, 2069, 1988.

111. Makinodan, T., Lubinski, J. and Fong, T. C., Cellular, biochemical, and molecular basis of T cell senescence, *Arch. Pathol. Lab. Med.*, 111, 910, 1987.

112. Gillis, S., Kozak, R., Durante, M. and Weskler, M. E., Immunological studies of aging. Decreased production of and response to T cell growth factor by lymphocytes from aged humans, *J. Clin. Invest.*, 67, 937, 1981.

113. Miller, R. A. and Stutman, O., Decline, in aging mice, of the anti-2,4,6-trinitrophenyl (TNP) cytotoxic Tcell response attributable to loss of Lyt-2-, interleukin 2-producing helper cell function, *Eur. J. Immunol.*, 11, 751, 1981.

114. Thoman, M. L. and Weigle, W. O., Cell-mediated immunity in aged mice: an underlying lesion in IL-2 synthesis, *J. Immunol.*, 128, 2358, 1982.

115. Thoman, M. L. and Weigle, W.O., Lymphokines and aging: interleukin-2 production and activity in aged animals, *J. Immunol.*, 127, 2102, 1981.

116. Kennes, B., Brohée, D. and Nève, P., Lymphocyte activation in human ageing. V. Acquisition of response to T cell growth factor and production of growth factors by mitogen-stimulated lymphocytes, *Mech. Ageing Dev.*, 23, 103, 1983.

117. Vie, H. and Miller, R.A., Decline, with age, in the proportion of mouse T cells that express IL-2 receptors after mitogen stimulation, *Mech. Ageing Dev,* 33, 313, 1986.

118. Chang, M. P., Makinodan, T., Peterson, W. J. and Strehler, B. L., Role of T cells and adherent cells in age-related decline in murine interleukin 2 production, *J. Immunol.*, 129, 2426, 1982.

119. Barcellini,W., Borghi, M. O., Sguotti, C., Palmieri, R., Frasca, D., Meroni, P. L., Doria, G. and Zanussi, C., Heterogeneity of immune responsiveness in healthy elderly subjects, *Clin. Immunol. Immunopathol.*, 47, 142, 1988.

120. Gilman, S. C., Rosenberg, J. S. and Feldman, J. D., T lymphocytes of young and aged rats. II. Functional defects and the role of interleukin-2, *J. Immunol.*, 128, 644, 1982.

121. Gilman, S. C., Lymphokines in immunological aging, *Lymphokine Res.*, 3, 119, 1984.

122. Wu, W., Pahlavani, M., Cheung, H. T. and Richardson, A., The effect of aging on the expression of interleukin 2 messenger ribonucleic acid, *Cell. Immunol.*, 100, 224, 1986.

123. Nagel, J. E., Chopra, R. K., Chrest, F. J., McCoy, M. T., Schneider, E. L., Holbrook, N. J. and Adler, W. H., Decreased proliferation, interleukin 2 synthesis, and interleukin 2 receptor expression are accompanied by decreased mRNA expression in phytohemagglutinin-stimulated cells from elderly donors, *J. Clin. Invest.*, 81, 1096, 1988.

124. Negoro, S., Hara, H., Miyata, S., Saiki, O., Tanaka, T., Yoshizaki, K., Igarashi, T. and Kishimoto, S., Mechanisms of age-related decline in antigen-specific T cell proliferative response: IL-2 receptor expression and recombinant IL-2-induced proliferative response of purified TAC-positive T cells, *Mech. Ageing Dev.*, 36, 223, 1986.

125. Proust, J. J., Kittur, D. S., Buchholz, M. A. and Nordin, A. A., Restricted expression of mitogen-induced high affinity IL-2 receptors in aging mice, *J. Immunol.* 141, 4209, 1988.

126. Nagel, J. E., Chopra, R K., Powers, D. C. and Adler, W. H., Effect of age on the human high affinity interleukin 2 receptor of phytohaemagglutinin stimulated peripheral blood lymphocytes, *Clin. Exp. Immunol.*, 75, 286, 1989.

127. Orson, F. M., Saadeh, C. K., Lewis, D. E. and Nelson, D. L., Interleukin 2 receptor expression by T cells in human aging, *Cell. Immunol.*, 124, 278, 1989.

128. Goodwin, J. S., Changes in lymphocyte sensitivity to prostaglandin E, histamine, hydrocortisone, and X irradiation with age: studies in a healthy elderly population, *Clin. Immunol. Immunopathol.*, 25, 243, 1982.

129. Goodwin, J. S. and Messner, R. P., Sensitivity of lymphocytes to prostaglandin E2 increases in subjects over age 70, *J. Invest.*, 64, 434, 1979.

130. Goodwin, J. S. and Ceuppens, J., Regulation of the immune response by prostaglandins, *J. Clin. Immunol.*, 3, 295, 1983.

131. Rosenstein, M. M. and Strausser, H. R., Macrophage-induced T cell mitogen suppression with age, *J. Reticuloendothel. Soc.*, 27, 159, 1980.

132. Vercammen, C. and Ceuppens, J. L., Prostaglandin E2 inhibits human T-cell proliferation after crosslinking of the CD3-Ti complex by directly affecting T cells at an early step of the activation process, *Cell. Immunol.*, 104, 24, 1987.

133. Antonaci, S., Jirillo, E., Lucivero, G., Gallitelli, M., Garofalo, R. and Bonomo, L., Humoral immune response in aged humans: suppressor effect of monocytes on spontaneous plaque forming cell generation, *Clin. Exp. Immunol.*, 52, 387, 1983.

134. Abb, J., Abb, H. and Deinhardt, F., Age-related decline of human alpha and interferon gamma production, *Blut*, 48, 285, 1984.

135. Doggett, D. L., Chang, M. P., Manikodan, T. and Strehler, B. L., Cellular and molecular aspects of immune system aging, *Mol. Cell. Biochem.*, 37, 137, 1981.

136. Tollefsbol, T.O. and Cohen, H.J., Expression of intracellular biochemical defects of lymphocytes in aging: proposal of a general aging mechanism which is not cell specific, *Exp. Gerontol.*, 21, 129, 1986.

137. Brennan, P. C. and Jaroslow, B. N., Age-associated decline in theta antigen on spleen thymus-derived lymphocytes of B6CF1 mice, *Cell. Immunol.*, 15, 51, 1975.

138. Schocken, D. D. and Roth, G. S., Reduced β-adregenic receptor concentrations in ageing man, *Nature*, 267, 856, 1977.

139. Petrovic, J. S. and Markovic, R. Z., Changes in cortisol binding to soluble receptor proteins in rat liver and thymus during development and ageing, *Dev. Biol.*, 45, 176, 1975.

140. De Blasi, A., Fratelli, M., Wielosz, M. and Lipartiti, M., Regulation of beta adrenergic receptors on rat mononuclear leukocytes by stress: receptor redistribution and down-regulation are altered with aging, *J. Pharmac. Exp. Ther.*, 240, 228, 1987.

141. Abrass, I. B. and Scarpace, P. J., Catalytic unit of adenylate cyclase: reduced activity in aged-human lymphocytes, *J. Clin. End. Metab.*, 55, 1026, 1982.

142. Gozes, Y., Umiel, T., Meshorer, A. and Trainin, N., Syngeneic GvH induced in popliteal lymph nodes by spleen cells of old C57BL/6 mice, *J. Immunol.*, 121, 2199, 1978.

143. Callard, R. E., Basten, A. and Blanden, R. V., Loss of immune competence with age may be due to a qualitative abnormality in lymphocyte membranes, *Nature*, 281, 218, 1979.

144. Gilman, S. C., Woda, B. A. and Feldman, J. D., T lymphocytes of young and aged rats. I. Distribution, density and capping of T antigens, *J. Immunol.*, 127, 149, 1981.

145. Cheung, H. T., Rehwaldt, C. A., Twu, J. S., Liao, N. S. and Richardson, A., Aging and lymphocyte cytoskeleton: age-related decline in the state of actin polymerization in T lymphocytes from Fischer F 344 rats, *J. Immunol.*, 138, 32, 1987.

146. Hendricks, L. C. and Heidrick, M. L., Susceptibility to lipid peroxidation and accumulation of fluorescent products with age is greater in T-cells than B-cells, *Free Rad. Biol. Med.*, 5, 145, 1988.

147. Tam, C. F. and Walford, R. L., Alterations in cyclic nucleotides and cyclase-specific activities in T lymphocytes of aging normal humans and patients with Down's syndrome, *J. Immunol.*, 125, 1665, 1980.

148. Price, G. B. and Makinodan, T., Immunologic deficiencies in senescence. I. Characterization of intrinsic deficiencies, *J. Immunol.*, 108, 403, 1972.

149. Price, G. B. and Makinodan, T., Immunologic deficiencies in senescence. II. Characterization of extrinsic deficiencies, *J. Immunol.*, 108, 413, 1972.

150. Klinman, N. R., Antibody-specific immunoregulation and the immunodeficiency of aging, *J. Exp. Med.*, 154, 547, 1981.

151. Weksler, M. E., Senescence of the immune system, *Med. Clin. North. Am.*, 67, 263, 1983.

152. Buckley, C. E., Buckley, E. G. and Dorsey, F. C., Longitudinal changes in serum immunoglobulin levels in older humans, *Fed. Proc.*, 33, 2036, 1974.

153. Goodwin, J. S., Searles, R. P. and Tung, K. S., Immunological responses of healthy elderly population, *Clin. Exp. Immunol.*, 48, 403, 1982.

154. Radl, J. and Hollander, C. F., Homogeneous immunoglobulins in sera of mice during aging, *J. Immunol.*, 112, 2271, 1974.

155. Radl, J., Hollander, C. F., van der Berg, P. and De Glopper, E., Idiopathic paraproteinemia. I. Studies in an animal model — the ageing C57BL/KaLwRij mouse, *Clin. Exp. Immunol.*, 33, 395,1978.

156. Radl, J., De Glopper, E. D. , Schuit, H. R. and Zurcher, C., Idiopathic paraproteinemia. II. Transplantation of the paraprotein-producing clone from old to young C57BL/KaLwRij mice, *J. Immunol.*, 122, 609, 1979.

157. Radl, J., Idiopathic paraproteinemia. A consequence of an age-related deficiency in the T immune system. Three-stage development — a hypothesis, *Clin. Immunol. Imunopathol.*, 14, 251, 1979.

158. Denis, F., Mounier, M., Hessel, L., Michel, J. P., Gualde, N., Dubois, F., Barin, F. and Goudeau, A., Hepatitis-B vaccination in the elderly, *J. Infect. Diseases*, 149, 1019, 1984.

159. Effros, R. B. and Walford, R. L., Diminished T-cell response to influenza virus in aged mice, *Immunology*, 49, 387, 1983.

160. Kishimoto, S., Tomino, S., Mitsuya, H., Fujiwara, H., and Tsuda, H., Age-related decline in the in vitro and in vivo syntheses of anti-tetanus toxoid antibody in humans, *J. Immunol.*, 125, 2347, 1980.

161. Shapiro, E. D. and Clemens, J. D., A controlled evaluation of the protective efficacy of pneumococcal vaccine for patients at high risk of serious pneumoccoccal infections, *Ann. Int. Med.*, 101, 325, 1984.

162. Ammann, A. J., Schiffman, G. and Austrian, R., The antibody responses to pneumococcal capsular polysaccharides in aged individuals, *Proc. Soc. Exp. Biol. Med.*, 164, 312, 1980.

163. Ruben, F. L. and Uhrin, M., Specific immunoglobulin-class antibody responses in the elderly before and after 14-valent pneumococcal vaccine, *J. Infect. Diseases*, 151, 845, 1985.

164. Musher, D. M., Chapman, A. J., Goree, A., Jonsson, S., Briles, D. and Baughn, R.E., Natural and vaccine-related immunity to Streptococcus pneumoniae, *J. Infect. Diseases*, 154, 245, 1986.

165. Segre, M. and Segre, D., Humoral immunity in aged mice. I. Age-related decline in the secondary response to DNP of spleen cells propagated in diffusion chambers, *J. Immunol.*, 116, 731, 1976.

166. Goidl, E. A., Innes, J. B. and Weksler, M. E., Immunological studies of aging. II. Loss of IgG and high avidity plaque-forming cells and increased suppressor cell activity in aging mice, *J. Exp. Med.*, 144, 1037, 1976.

167. Weksler, M. E., Innes, J. B. and Goldstein, G., Immunological studies of ageing. IV. The contribution of thymic involution to the immune defiencies of aging mice and reversal with thymopoietin 32-36, *J. Exp. Med.*, 148, 996, 1978.

168. Callard, R. E. and Basten, A., Immune function in aged mice. IV. Loss of T cell and B cell function in thymus-dependent antibody responses, *Eur. J. Immunol.*, 8, 552, 1978.

169. Miller, R. A., Aging and immune function, *Int. Rev. Cytol.*, 124, 187, 1991.

170. Goidl, E. A., Thorbecke, G. J., Weksler, M. E. and Siskind, G.W., Production of auto-anti-idiotypic antibody during the normal immune response: changes in the auto-anti-idiotypic response and the idiotype repertoire associated with aging, *Proc. Natl. Acad. Sci. U.S.A.*, 77, 6788, 1980.

171. Wade, A.W. and Szewczuk, M. R., Aging, idiotype repertoire shifts, and compartmentalization of the mucosal-associated lymphoid system, *Adv. Immunol.*, 36, 143, 1984.

172. Goidl, E. A., Schrater, A. F., Thorbecke, G. J. and Siskind, G. W., Production of auto-anti-idiotypic antibody during the normal immune response. IV. Studies of the primary and secondary responses to thymus-dependent and -independent antigens, *Eur. J. Immunol.*, 10, 810, 1980.

173. Goidl, E. A., Choy, J. W., Gibbons, J. J., Weksler, M. E., Thorbecke, G. J. and Siskind, G. W., Production of auto-antiidiotypic antibody during the normal immune response. VII. Analysis of the cellular basis for the increased auto-anti-idiotype antibody production by aged mice, *J. Exp. Med.*, 157, 1635, 1980.

174. Szewczuk, M. R. and Campbell, R. J., Loss of immune competence with age may be due to auto-anti-idiotypic antibody regulation, *Nature*, 286, 164, 1980.

175. Schulze, D. H. and Goidl, E. A., Age-associated changes in antibody-forming cells (B cells), *Proc. Soc. Exp. Biol. Med.*, 196, 253, 1991.

176. Otte, R. G., Wormsley, S. and Hollingsworth, J. W., Cytofluorographic analysis of pokeweed mitogen-stimulated human peripheral blood cells in culture: age-related characteristics, *J. Am. Ger. Soc.*, 31, 49, 1983.

177. Haaijman, J. J. and Hijmans, W., Influence of age on the immunological activity and capacity of the CBA mouse, *Mech. Ageing Dev.*, 7, 375, 1978.

178. Benner, R. and Haaijman, J. J., Aging of the lymphoid system at the organ level. With special reference to the bone marrow as site of antibody production, *Dev. Comp. Immunol.*, 4, 591, 1980.

179. Zharhary, D., T cell involvement in the decrease of antigen-responsive B cells in aged mice, *Eur. J. Immunol.*, 16, 1175, 1986.

180. Thoman, M. L., Morgan, E. L. and Weigle, W. O., Role of Fc receptors in lymphocyte activation: deficiency in T- and B-lymphocytes from aged animals, *Mol. Immunol.*, 19, 1239, 1982.

181. Cheung, H. T., Vovolka, J. and Terry, D. S., Age- and maturation-dependent changes in the immune system of Fisher F344 rats, *J. Reticuloendothel. Soc.*, 30, 563, 1981.

182. Segre, D. and Segre, M., Humoral immunity in aged mice. II. Increased suppressor T cell activity in immunologically deficient old mice, *J. Immunol.*, 116, 735, 1976.

183. Zharhary, D. and Klinman, N. R., Antigen responsiveness of the mature and generative B cell populations of aged mice, *J. Exp. Med.*, 157, 1300, 1983.

184. DeKruyff, R. H., Kim, Y. T., Siskind, G. W. and Weksler, M. E., Age-related changes in the in vitro immune response: increased suppressor activity in immature and aged mice, *J. Immunol.*, 125, 142, 1980.

185. Delfraissy, J. F., Galanaud, P., Wallon, C., Balavoine, J. F. and Dormont, J., Abolished in vitro antibody response in elderly: exclusive involvement of prostaglandin-induced T suppressor cells, *Clin. Immunol. Immunopathol.*, 24, 377, 1982.

186. Doria, G., Mancini, C. and Adorini, L., Immunoregulation in senescence: increased inducibility of antigen-specific suppressor T cells and loss of cell sensitivity to immunosuppression in aging mice, *Proc. Natl. Acad. Sci. U.S.A.*, 79, 3803, 1982.

187. Globerson, A., Abel, L., Barzilay, M. and Zan-Bar, I., Immunoregulatory cells in aging mice. I. Concanavalin A-induced and naturally occurring suppressor cells, *Mech. Ageing Dev.*, 19, 293, 1982.

188. Antel, J. P., Oger, J. J. , Wrabetz, L. G., Arnason, B. G. and Hopper, J. E., Mechanisms responsible for reduced in vitro immunoglobulin secretion in aged humans, *Mech. Ageing Dev.*, 23, 11, 1983.

189. Whisler, R. L. and Newhouse, Y. G., Function of T cells from elderly humans: reductions of membrane events and proliferative responses mediated via T3 determinants and diminished elaboration of soluble T-cell factors for B-cell growth, *Cell. Immunol.*, 99, 422, 1986.

190. Weiner, H. L., Moorhead, J. W. and Claman, H. N., Anti-immunoglobulin stimulation of murine lymphocytes. I. Age-dependency of the proliferative response, *J. Immunol.*, 116, 1656, 1976.

191. Scribner, D. J. and Moorhead, J. W., Anti-immunoglobulin stimulation of murine lymphocytes. VII. Identification of an age-dependent changes in accessory cell function, *J. Immunol.*, 128, 1377, 1982.

192. Woda, B. A. and Feldman, J. D., Density of surface immunoglobulin and capping on rat B lymphocytes. I. Changes with aging, *J. Exp. Med.*, 149, 416, 1979.

193. Woda, B. A., Yguerabide, J. and Feldman, J. D., Mobility and density of AgB, "Ia", and Fc receptors on the surface of lymphocytes from young and old rats, *J. Immunol.*, 123, 2161, 1979.

194. Rosenberg, J. S., Gilman, S. C. and Feldman, J. D., Activation of rat B lymphocytes. II. Functional and structural changes in "aged" rat B lymphocytes, *J. Immunol.*, 128, 656, 1982.

195. Brouwer, A. and Knook, D. L., The reticuloendothelial system and aging: a review; *Mech. Ageing Dev.*, 21, 205, 1983.

196. Wustrow, T. P., Denny, T. N., Fernandes, G. and Good, R. A., Changes in macrophages and their functions with aging in C57BL/6J, AKR/J, and SJL/J mice, *Cell. Immunol.*, 69, 227, 1982.

197. Gardner, I. D. and Remington, J. S., Aging and the immune response. II. Lymphocyte responsiveness and macrophage activation in Toxoplasma gondii-infected mice, *J. Immunol.*, 120, 944, 1978.

198. Gardner, I. D., Lim, S. T. K. and Lawton, J. W., Monocyte function in ageing humans, *Mech. Ageing Dev.*, 16, 223, 1981.

199. Antonaci, S., Jirillo, E., Ventura, M. T., Garofalo, A. R. and Bonomo, L., Non-specific immunity in aging: deficiency of monocyte and polymorphonuclear cell-mediated functions, *Mech. Ageing Dev.*, 24, 367, 1984.

200. Olmos, J. M., de Dios, B., Garcia, J. D., Sanchez, J. J. and Jimenez, A., Monocyte function in the elderly, *Allerg. et Immunopath.*, 14, 369, 1986.

201. Callard, R. E., Immune function in aged mice. III. Role of macrophages and effect of 2-mercaptoethanol in the response of spleen cells from old mice to phytohemagglutinin, lipopolysaccharide and allogeneic cells, *Eur. J. Immunol.*, 8, 697, 1978.

202. Rosenberg, J. S., Gilman, S. C. and Feldman, J. D., Effects of aging on cell cooperation and lymphocyte responsiveness to cytokines, *J. Immunol.*, 130, 1754, 1983.

203. Bruley-Rosset, M. and Vergnon, I., Interleukin-1 synthesis and activity in aged mice, *Mech. Ageing Dev.*, 24, 247, 1984.

204. Kunkel, S. L., Chensue, S. W. and Phan, S. H., Prostaglandins as endogenous mediators of interleukin 1 production, *J. Immunol.*, 136, 186, 1986.

205. Van Epps, D. E., Goodwin, J. S. and Murphy, S., Age-dependent variations in polymorphonuclear leukocyte chemiluminescence, *Infect. Immunity*, 22, 57, 1978.

206. Charpentier, B., Fournier, C., Fries, D., Mathieu, D., Noury, J. and Bach, J. F., Immunological studies in human ageing. I. In vitro functions of T cells and polymorphs, *J. Clin. Lab. Immunol.*, 5, 87, 1981.

207. Nagel, J. E., Pyle, R. S., Chrest, F. J. and Adler, W. H., Oxidative metabolism and bactericidal capacity of polymorphonuclear leukocytes from normal young and aged adults, *J. Gerontol.*, 37, 529, 1982.

208. Laharrague, P., Corberand, J., Fillola, G., Nguyen, F., Fontanilles, A.M, Gleizes, B., Gyrard, E. and Jean, C., Impairment of polymorphonuclear functions in hospitalized geriatric patients, *Gerontology*, 29, 325, 1983.

209. Fülöp, T., Jr., Foris, G., Worum, I, Paragh, G. and Leövey, A., Age related variations of some polymorphonuclear leukocyte functions, *Mech. Ageing Dev.*, 29, 1, 1985.

210. Chen, M. G., Age-related changes in hematopoietic stem cell populations of a long-lived hybrid mouse, *J. Cell. Physiol.*, 78, 225, 1971.

211. Davis, M. L., Upton, A. C. and Satterfield, L. C., Growth and senescence of the bone marrow stem cell pool in RFM/Un mice, *Proc. Soc. Exp. Biol. Med.*, 137, 1452, 1971.

212. Silini, G. and Andreozzi, U., Haematological changes in the ageing mouse, *Exp. Geront.*, 9, 99, 1974.

213. Hirokawa, K., Kubo, S., Utsuyama, M., Kurashima, C., and Sado, T., Age-related change in the potential of bone marrow cells to repopulate the thymus and splenic T cells in mice. *Cell. Immunol.*, 100, 443, 1986.

214. Harrison, D. E. and Astle, C. M., Loss of stem cell repopulation ability upon transplantation. Effects of donor age, cell number and transplantation procedure, *J. Exp. Med.*, 156, 1767, 1982.

215. Harrison, D. E., Long-term erythropoietic repopulating ability of old, young and fetal stem cells, *J. Exp. Med.*, 157, 1496, 1983.

216. Weksler, M. E., The immune and the aging process in man, *Proc. Soc. Exp. Biol. Mech.*, 165, 200, 1980.

217. Gorczynski, R. M., Chang, M. P., Kennedy, M., MacRae, S., Benzing, K. and Price, G. B., Alterations in lymphocyte recognition repertoire during ageing. I. Analysis of changes in immune response potential of B lymphocytes from non-immunized mice, and the role of accessory cells in the expression of that potential, *Immunopharmacol.*, 7, 179, 1984.

218. Farrar, J. J., Loughman, B. E. and Nordin, A. A., Lymphopoietic potential of bone marrow cells from aged mice: comparison of the cellular constituents of bone marrow from young and aged mice, *J. Immunol.*, 112, 1244, 1974.

219. Hirokawa, K., Sato, K. and Makinodan, T., Restoration of impaired immune functions in aging animals. V. Long-term immunopotentiating effects of combined young bone marrow and newborn thymus grafts, *Clin. Immunol. Immunopath.*, 22, 297, 1982.

220. Tyan, M. L., Age-related decrease in mouse T cell progenitors, *J. Immunol.*, 118, 846, 1977.

221. Twomey, J. J., Luchi, R. J. and Kouttab, N. M., Null cell senescence and its potential significance to the immunobiology of aging, *J. Clin. Invest.*, 70, 201, 1982.

222. Astle, C. M. and Harrison, D. E., Effects of marrow donor and recipient age on immune responses, *J. Immunol.*, 132, 673, 1984.

223. Gorczynski, R. M., Diversity in the lymphocyte recognition repertoire is altered during ageing, *Biomed. Pharmacotherapy*, 41, 124, 1987.

224. Lepault, F., Fache, M. P. and Frindel, E., Role of the thymus in CFU-S differentiation and proliferation, *Leukemia Res.*, 5, 379, 1981.

225. Lepault, F., Dardenne, M. and Frindel, E., Restoration by serum thymic factor of colony-forming unit (CFU-S) entry into DNA synthesis in thymectomized mice after T-dependent antigen treatment, *Eur. J. Immunol.*, 9, 661, 1979.

226. Chang, M. P., Utsuyama, M., Hirokawa, K. and Makinodan, T., Decline in the production of interleukin-3 with age in mice, *Cell. Immunol.*, 115, 1, 1988.

227. Li, D. D., Chien, Y. K., Gu, M. Z., Richardson, A. and Cheung, H. T., The age-related decline in interleukin 3 expression in mice, *Life Sci.*, 43, 1215, 1988.

228. Kay, M. M., Parainfluenza infection of aged mice results in autoimmune disease, *Clin. Immunol. Immunopathol.*, 12, 301, 1979.

229. Williams, L. H., Udupa, K. B. and Lipschitz, D. A., Evaluation of age on hematopoiesis in the C57BL/6 mouse, *Exp. Hematol.*, 14, 827, 1986.

230. Blalock, J. E., Harbour-McMenamin, D. and Smith, E. M., Peptide hormones shared by the neuroendocrine and immunologic systems, *J. Immunol.*, 135, 8585, 1985.

231. Goya, R. G., The immune-neuroendocrine homeostatic network and aging, *Gerontology*, 37, 208, 1991.

232. Homo-Delarche, F. and Dardenne, M., The neuroendocrine-immune axis, *Seminars in Immunopathol.*, 14, 221, 1993.

233. Michael, S. D., Taguchi, O. and Nishizuka, Y., Effect of neonatal thymectomy on ovarian development and plasma LH, FSH, GH, and PRL in the mouse, *Biol. Reprod.*, 22, 343, 1980.

234. Hall, N. R., McGillis, J. P., Spangelo, B. L. and Goldstein, A. L., Evidence that thymosins and other biologic response modifiers can function as neuroactive immunotransmitters, *J. Immunol.*, Suppl. 135, 806, 1985.

235. Hall, N. R., O'Grady, M. P. and Farah, J. M.,Thymic hormones and immune function mediation via neuroendocrine circuits, in *Thymic Hormones and Immune Function Mediation Via Neuroendocrine Circuits*, Academic Press, New York, 1991, 515.

236. Goya, R. G., Takahashi, S., Quigley, K. L., Sosa, Y. E., Goldstein, A. L. and Meites, J., Immune-neuroendocrine interactions during aging: age-dependent thyrotropin-inhibiting activity of thymosin peptides, *Mech. Ageing Dev.*, 41, 219, 1987.

237. Goya, R. G., Sosa, Y. E., Quigley, K. L., Gottschall, P. E., Goldstein, A. L. and Meites, J., Differential activity of thymosin peptides (thymosin fraction five) on plasma thyrotropin in female rats of different ages, *Neuroendocrinology*, 47, 379, 1988.

238. Besedovsky, H., Sorkin, E., Keller, M. and Muller, J., Changes in blood hormone levels during the immune response, *Proc. Soc. Exp. Biol. Med.*, 150, 466, 1975.

239. Besedovsky, H. O., Del Rey, A. and Sorkin, E., Antigenic competition between horse and sheep red blood cells as a hormone-dependent phenomenon, *Clin. Exp. Immunol.*, 37, 106, 1979.

240. Schauenstein, K., Fassler, R., Dietrich, H., Schwarz, S., Kromer, G. and Wick, G., Disturbed immune-endocrine communication in autoimmune disease. Lack of corticosterone response to immune signals in obese strain chickens with spontaneous autoimmune thyroiditis, *J. Immunol.*, 139, 1830, 1987.

241. Sternberg, E. M., Hill, J. M., Chrousos, G. P., Kamilaris, T., Listwak S. J., Gold, P. W. and Wilder, R. L., Inflammatory mediator-induced hypothalamic-pituitary-adrenal axis activation is defective in streptococcal cell wall arthritis-susceptible Lewis rats, *Proc. Natl. Acad. Sci. U.S.A.*, 86, 2374, 1989.

242. Sternberg, E. M., Chrousos, G. P., Wilder, R. L. and Gold, P. W. The stress response and the regulation of inflammatory disease, *Ann. Int. Med.*, 117, 854, 1992.

243. Weindruch, R. H., Kristie, J. A., Cheney, K. E. and Walford, R. L., Influence of controlled dietary restriction on immunologic function in aging, *Fed. Proc.*, 38, 2007, 1979.

244. Lipschitz, D. A., Nutrition, aging, and the immuno-hematopoietic system, *Clin. Geriatric Med.*, 3, 319, 1987.

245. Homsy, J., Morrow, W. J. and Levy, J. A., Nutrition and autoimmunity: a review, *Clin. Exp. Immunol.*, 65, 473, 1986.

246. Smith A. D., Conroy, D. M. and Belin, J., Membrane lipid modification and immune function, *Proc. of the Nutrition Society*, 44, 201, 1985.

247. Robinson, D. R., Prickett, J. D., Polisson, R., Steinberg, A. D. and Levine, L., The protective effect of dietary fish oil on murine lupus, *Prostaglandins*, 30, 51, 1985.

248. Fabris, N. and Mocchegiani, E., Arginine-containing compounds and thymic endocrine activity, *Thymus*, 19, S21, 1992.

249. Mocchegiani, E., Muzzioli, M., Santarelli, L. and Fabris, N., Restoring effect of oral supplementation of zinc and arginine on thymic endocrine activity and peripheral immune functions in aged, *Arch. Gerontol. Geriat.*, S3, 267, 1992.

250. Prasad, A. S., Meftah, S., Abdallah, J., Kaplan, J., Brewer, G. J., Bach, J. F. and Dardenne, M., Serum thymulin in human zinc deficiency, *J. Clin. Invest.*, 82, 1202, 1988.

251. Boukaïba, N., Flament, C., Acher, S., Chappuis, P., Piau, A., Fusselier, M., Dardenne, M. and Lemonnier, D., A physiological amount of zinc supplementation: effects on nutritional, lipid, and thymic status in an elderly population, *Am. J. Clin. Nutri.*, 57, 566, 1993.

252. Dardenne, M., Boukaïba, N., Gagnerault, M. C., Homo-Delarche, F., Chappuis, P., Lemonnier, D. and Savino, W., Restoration of the thymus in aging mice by in vivo zinc supplementation, *Clin. Immunol. Immunopathol.*, 66, 127, 1993.

253. Delafuente, J. C., Prendergast, J. M. and Modigh, A., Immunologic modulation by vitamin C in the elderly, *Int. J. Immunopharmac.*, 8, 205, 1986.

254. Kennes, B., Dumont, I., Brohee, D., Hubert, C. and Neve, P., Effect of vitamin C supplements on cell-mediated immunity in old people, *Gerontology*, 29, 305–310, 1983.

255. Chandra, R. K., Effect of vitamin and trace-element supplementation on immune responses and infection in elderly subjects, *Lancet*, 340, 1124, 1992.

256. Friedman, D., Keiser, V. and Globerson, A., Reactivation of immunocompetence in spleen cells of aged mice, *Nature*, 251, 545, 1974.

257. Bash, J. A., Dardenne, M., Bach, J. F. and Waksman, B. H., In vitro responses of rat lymphocytes following adult thymectomy. III. Prevention by thymic factor of increased suppressor activity in the spleen, *Cell Immunol.*, 26, 308, 1976.

258. Palacios, R., Fernandez, C. and Sideras, P., Development and continuous growth in culture of interleukin 2-producer lymphocytes from athymic nu/nu mice, *Eur. J. Immunol.*, 12, 777, 1982.

259. Martinez, D., Field, A. K., Schwam, H., Tytell, A. A. and Hilleman, M. R., Failure of thymopoietin, ubiquitin and synthetic serum thymic factor to restore immunocompetence in T-cell deficient mice, *Proc. Soc. Exp. Biol. Med.*, 159, 195, 1978.

260. D'Agostaro, G., Frasca, D., Garivini, M. and Doria, G., Immunorestoration of old mice by injection of thymus extract : enhancement of T cell-T cell cooperation in the in vitro antibody response, *Cell Immunol.,* 53, 207, 1980.

261. Quinti, I., Pandolfi, F., Fiorilli, M., Zolla, S., Moro, M. L., and Aiuti, F., T-dependent immunity in aged humans. I. Evaluation of T-cell subpopulations before and after short term administration of a thymic extract, *J. Gerontology*, 36, 674, 1981.

262. Falchetti, R., Cafiero, C. and Caprino, L., Impaired T-cell functions in aged guinea-pigs restored by thymostimulin, *Int. J. Immunopharmac.,* 4, 181, 1982.

263. Barcellini, W., Meroni, P. L. , Borghi, M. O., Frasca, D., Perego, R. Doria, G. and Zanussi, C., In vivo immunopotentiating activity of thymopentin in aging humans: modulation of IL-2 receptor expression, *Clin. Immunol. Immunopathol.,* 48, 140, 1988.

264. Meroni, P. L., Barcellini, W., Frasca, D., Sguotti, C., Borghi, M. O., De Bartolo, G., Doria, G. and Zanussi, C., In vivo immunopotentiating activity of thymopentin in aging humans: increase of IL-2 production, *Clin. Immunol. Immunopathol.*, 42, 151, 1987.

265. Frasca, D., Adorini, L. and Doria, G., Enhanced frequency of mitogen-responsive T cell precursors in old mice injected with thymosin $\alpha 1$, *Eur. J. Immunol.*, 17, 727, 1987.

266. Ershler, W. B., Hebert, J. C., Blow, A. J., Granter, S. R. and Lynch, J., Effect of thymosin $\alpha 1$ on specific antibody response and susceptibility to infection in young and aged mice, *Int. J. Immunopharmac.*, 7, 465, 1985.

267. Frasca, D., Adorini, L., Mancini, C. and Doria, G., Reconstitution of T cell functions in aging mice by thymosin alpha1, *Immunopharmacol.,* 11, 155, 1986.

268. Ershler, W. B., Coe, C. L., Laughlin, N., Klopp, R. G., Gravenstein, S., Roecker, E. B. and Schultz, K. T., Aging and immunity in non-human primates. II. Lymphocyte response in thymosin-treated middle-aged monkeys, *J. Gerontology*, 43, B142; 1988.

269. Ershler, W. B., Moore, A. L. and Socinski, M. A, Influenza and aging : age-related changes and the effects of thymosin on the antibody response to influenza vaccine, *J. Clin. Immunol.*, 4, 445, 1984.

270. Bruley-Rosset, M. and Payelle, B., Deficient tumor-specific immunity in old mice: in vivo mediation by suppressor cells, and correction of the defect by interleukin 2 supplementation in vitro but not in vivo, *Eur. J. Immunol.,* 17, 307, 1987.

271. Delafuente, J. C. and Panush, R. S. Pharmacologic immunoenhancement in the elderly : in vitro effects of isoprinosine, *Clin. Immunol. Immunopathol.*, 47, 363, 1988.

272. Morimoto, C., Abe, T. and Homma, M., Restoration of T-cell function in aged mice with long-term administration of levamisole, *Clin. Immunol. Immunopathol.*, 12, 316, 1979.

273. Bruley-Rosset, M., Hercend, T., Rappaport, H., and Mathé, G., Immunorestorative capacity of tuftsin after long-term administration to aging mice, *Ann. N.Y. Acad Sci.*, 419, 242, 1983.

274. Tomai, M. A., Solem, L. E., Johnson, A. R. and Ribi, E., The adjuvant properties of a nontoxic monophosphoryl lipid A in hyporesponsive aging mice, *J. Biol. Response. Mod.*, 6, 99, 1987.

275. Miller, R. A., Immunodefiency of aging: restorative effects of phorbol ester combined with calcium ionophore, *J. Immunol.*, 137, 805, 1986.

PART V

Conclusions and Perspectives

21

Outlook on Neuroendocrine Aging

Paola S. Timiras

CONTENTS

I. INTRODUCTION

The phenomenological or causal implication of endocrine decrements in the aging process was born simultaneously with the emergence of endocrinology as a separate biomedical field. The physiologists Brown-Sequard and d'Arsonval reported at a meeting of the Society of Biology of Paris (1889) that potent substances they called "internal secretions" existed in animal tissues and that aging and disease resulted from their lack. Inasmuch as the "feebleness of old men" would be in part due to the decline in testicular function, administration of testicular extracts would restore their physical strength, sexual vigor, and improved mental activity. This first attempt at hormone replacement therapy was associated with a "notable augmentation of the powers of action of the nervous centers;" it established from its very beginning the relationship of "internal secretions" to the nervous system.[1]

    The fact that these attempts at rejuvenation did not fall completely into disrepute but rather opened a vast scientific future within the next few years (1890–1895) is due to imminent

0-8493-2446-7/95/$0.00+$.50
© 1995 by CRC Press Inc.

clinical and experimental breakthroughs: thyroid extracts were proven to effectively treat human and animal myxedema; adrenomedullary extracts were shown to possess strong vasopressor activity; and grafts of pancreatic tissue were able to prevent or ameliorate experimental diabetes mellitus in dogs. In the following decade, the existence of powerful extracts of specific tissues was confirmed and their active substances were given the name of "hormones" (by physiologists Bayliss and Starling). The elusive goal of "a cure for aging" was replaced by the study of the regulation of metabolism, growth, development, and cell communication by means of chemical messengers.[1]

Since these early studies, endocrinologists and neuroendocrinologists have pursued their interest in aging. As the Phoenix arises reborn from its ashes, the neuroendocrine theories of aging emerge, continually revitalized by the new cellular and molecular discoveries underlying endocrine and neural mechanisms.[2,3] In the present chapter, early and current neuroendocrine theories will be reviewed briefly with reference to the chapters where supportive data and abundant bibliographic references for these theories are presented.

The second part of this chapter proposes future research to combine both physiologic synthesis and molecular reductionism. Homeostasis and reproduction, necessary for survival of the individual and the species, depend on complex processes that include a myriad of chemical reactions catalyzed by specific molecules. The entity that bridges molecular, endocrine, and neural controls is the gene that directs self-perpetuation and homeostasis throughout the lifespan. Complementary molecular, genetic and physiologic studies are needed to elucidate the signals that trigger aging.

II. NEUROENDOCRINE THEORIES OF AGING

In preceding chapters, the neuroendocrine theories (or hypotheses) of aging have emphasized their uniqueness supported by the number of experimental and clinical observations, and by the validity of therapeutic interventions. Depending on the major structure/function involved, they have focused on signals from the hypothalamus/limbic structures, neurotransmitters, the pituitary, and the relations with the immune system; they will be so presented here.

A. The Hypothalamic "Disregulation" Hypotheses

Given the well proven, essential role of the hypothalamus and some of the limbic structures in regulating adaptation to the environment and reproduction, these hypotheses have postulated that changes in hypothalamic and limbic function may trigger the signal for aging, as they signal earlier stages of the lifespan.[2] Changes involving hypothalamic/limbic nuclei may be characterized by

- Differential timetable of aging,
- Alterations in hormonal feedbacks, and
- Shifts in sensitivity to hormonal and environmental stimuli.

1. Differential Timetable of Aging: Hypothalamic/Limbic Disregulation

The hypothalamus and limbic system are comprised of several, relatively discrete nuclei. Occasionally, a particular function can be ascribed to a specific nucleus (e.g., the suprachiasmatic nucleus for the regulation of biologic rhythms; the hippocampus for the encoding of memory). In most cases, larger areas, including more than one nucleus, are implicated in a function (e.g., regulation of sex hormones and sexual behavior by hypothalamic anterior and preoptic areas together with limbic hippocampus and amygdala). Differences in the timetable of aging of these various areas or the specific aging of a group of commanding or "pacemaker" cells may change the adult type into an old-age pattern of regulation. Differential and localized aging agrees with the concept of a regionally circumscribed rather than a global aging of the brain.[2]

2. Functional Deafferentation

Aging changes in hypothalamic morphology reveal little cell loss but a progressive damage to dendrites and synapses. Of the regulatory systems that maintain homeostasis, none receives more diversified information or affects as many functions as does the hypothalamus. With aging, neurons would become "deafferented" (separated), that is, less capable of responding to hypothalamic and extrahypothalamic stimuli. For example, in old rats and mice, changes in the arcuate nucleus of the hypothalamus resembling those found in estrogen-treated animals at a young age may result in a functional deafferentation, that is, separation of the arcuate nucleus from the medial preoptic area with consequent decrease in dopamine concentration associated with high prolactin levels and loss of LH surge. Estrogens, like corticoids, might damage hypothalamic and perhaps also limbic neurons. Reproduction in senescent female rodents (but probably not in humans), impaired by deterioration of the preoptic arcuate pathway, may be reinstated at least temporarily by a variety of substances and conditions (e.g., administration of hormones, the antioxidant vitamin E, the dopamine precursor, L-DOPA, ether inhalation or cold stress, caloric restriction) which all increase hypothalamic catecholamines that stimulate the hypothalamo-pituitary-ovarian axis (Chapters 2, 4, and 7).

3. Alterations in Feedbacks and Hypothalamic Sensitivity

Due to its central location in the brain, the hypothalamus mediates communication among cerebral structures. When portions of this "switchboard" become inoperative or excessively stimulated, feedbacks or signals (endocrine, autonomic, immune, thermoregulatory, behavioral) may be abolished or misdirected with consequent loss of complexity (as in the "chaos theory of senescence").[4,5] One example shows that the age-related neuronal death in the hippocampus results in reduced inhibition of hypothalamic CRH release associated with a rise in the hypothalamic threshold to the negative feedback by corticosteroids; such loss of an inhibitory control would lead to adrenocortical hyperactivity (as postulated by the "glucocorticoid cascade hypothesis", Chapter 14).

Aging may be associated with a shift or unequal and discordant patterns of change in the sensitivity of the hypothalamus to specific hormones. Such change may be mediated by alterations in the number and affinity of receptors (T3 receptors in the brain and liver, Chapter 5; insulin receptors in adipose cells, Chapter 10; T3 and corticosteroid receptors in neuronal and glial cells, Chapter 16; receptors for growth factors, Chapter 18; and receptors for catecholamines, Chapters 4, 17, and 19). Changes in hormonal sensitivity of target cells and tissues may also depend on changing activity of cell enzymes and susceptibility to cell death as well as capacity for cell proliferation, as they are influenced by genetic make-up and environmental influences.

Neuroendocrine profiles undergo continuous subtle changes which culminate in reprogramming at birth, puberty, adulthood, menopause, and senescence. From each reprogramming emerge different physiologic activities specific for each stage of the life cycle. Program disruption may occur spontaneously at any age but becomes more prevalent and less repairable with old age.

B. The Neurotransmitter Deficiency or Imbalance Hypotheses

As with the hormones, excess, deficits, or imbalance of neurotransmitters and changes in the responsiveness of target cells may cause profound alterations of physiologic endpoints capable of inducing aging. Initially, a relatively small group of defined neurotransmitters, then an increasing number of substances with neurotransmitter and neuromodulator properties, have been implicated in neuroendocrine regulation. Several neurotransmitters, chemically diverse (e.g., amines, amino acids, peptides, or gases), may be synthesized, released, or taken up by the same neuronal or glial cell (Chapter 16). Major functions considered here include:

- Informational role and cell-to-cell communication,
- Plasticity,
- Receptors and target cells, and
- Genetic connections.

1. Informational Role: A General Function?

Information processing in the nervous and endocrine systems involves neural and endocrine cells talking with each other or with target cells. Neurotransmitters released from the presynaptic axon, bind on the surface of the postsynaptic cell, trigger intracellular events (e.g., opening or closing of membrane channels), and initiate metabolic and functional responses. Phylogenetically, several substances (e.g., neurotransmitters, hormones, growth factors, cytokines) serve as communicators not only in complex organisms (e.g., mammals) but also in plants and unicellular organisms. They serve as "informational substances" (i.e., "as words in the vocabulary of life"). This global view of biochemical messages vitiates the criticism leveled at the neuroendocrine theories that they lack universal application because not all organisms have complex neuroendocrine systems. In all organisms there exist molecules that regulate, modulate, and convey information; their alteration with the passage of time may lead to misinformation, with consequent aging and death.

Another criticism of the neuroendocrine theories is that they lack specificity: age-associated deficits in neuroendocrine cells result from the same basic changes directed by the genome in all cells that age. Even if this were true, functional consequences of neuroendocrine aging may uniquely endanger survival because:

- The neuroendocrine system, due to its complexity, is particularly vulnerable to alterations with aging,
- Due to its regulatory role in homeostasis, alterations in this system widely affect all body functions,
- The number and efficiency of the repertoire of integrative responses available during adulthood will diminish with advancing age with consequent limitation (convergence) of strategies for adaptation and survival.

2. Synaptic and Neurotransmitter Plasticity: Benefit or Damage?

With aging, decrease in neuronal number and, especially, in dendrites and synapses is inevitably associated with changes in the corresponding neurotransmitters (Chapter 16). However, the nervous system, and particularly its neuroendocrine counterpart, are modifiable or "plastic", capable of adapting to external and internal demands and, thus, of controlling their responses. The classic view that in most mammals neurons cannot regenerate after birth is being replaced by evidence that, in fact, they are capable of regeneration when their immediate microenvironment provides favorable conditions (e.g., availability of growth factors, removal of inhibitory agents from intercellular matrix).[6] Additionally, glial cells continue to divide throughout life and to exhibit compensatory plasticity (Chapter 16).

Functionally, early experiences may induce life-long structural, behavioral, and neurologic changes, such as the beneficial effects of neonatal handling in reducing the loss of neurons in the hippocampus induced by glucocorticoids in aged animals (Chapter 14). Administration of dopamine (through its precursor L-DOPA) in diseases associated with a loss of dopaminergic neurons (e.g., Parkinson's disease) may replace dopaminergic connections and actions. Similarly, administration of drugs elevating brain catecholamines increased the lifespan of rats and mice. However, in other cases, attempts at recovery in old brains may remain unsuccessful or of inconsistent benefit (e.g., failure of restoring cholinergic transmission by administration of choline precursors or agonists or antiacetylcholinesterases after cholinergic neuronal loss in the nucleus of Meynert, characteristic of Alzheimer's dementia).

In other cases still, attempts at repair may be harmful. Accumulation of one of the microtubule assembly proteins (MAPs), tau protein (including some of its fetal forms), may contribute to the formation of paired-helical filaments and neurofibrillary tangles, characteristic of Alzheimer's disease. The demand for tau protein increases with aging to facilitate regeneration of lost dendrites and axons; production of adult and fetal forms of tau proteins would be accelerated with consequent accumulation of abnormal proteins in aging neurons and tangle formation.

3. Neurotransmitter Imbalance

The multiplicity of chemical messengers released by neural cells, and the heterogeneity of their changes in response to endogenous and exogenous stimuli, suggest that functional alterations with aging are more likely to derive from imbalance among neurotransmitters than from the global alteration of single neurotransmitters. For example, a study of rats from birth to death (in old age) show that major changes occur in catecholamines with development, and then levels remain constant throughout adulthood. With old age, serotonin concentrations remain unchanged in several brain areas (cerebral cortex, hypothalamus, cerebellum, corpus striatum) until very old age when they increase slightly, whereas levels of catecholamine progressively decrease.

Generally, it is the area of greatest concentration of a neurotransmitter that exhibits the most severe decrement with aging: this is the case of dopamine in the substantia nigra (alterations in gait and motor disturbances) and the hypothalamus (increased prolactin levels), of acetylcholine in the basal forebrain (nucleus of Meynert) (cognitive and memory deficits), and of norepinephrine in the locus ceruleus (adrenergic and hormonal deficits).

In senescence, the continuing decline in catecholamines (Chapter 4), the progressive decrease in growth hormone from the pituitary (Chapter 3) and DHEA and aldosterone from the adrenal cortex (Chapter 2), the subtle modification of thyroid function (Chapter 5), the sharp changes in gonadal hormones and gonadotropins (Chapters 7, 8, 9, and 13), the alterations in the responsiveness of tissues to insulin (Chapters 10 and 11) and to glucocorticoids (Chapters 14 and 16) contribute to a reprogramming of the hypothalamo-pituitary-endocrine relationships. The brain catecholaminergic profile, promoting growth and anabolism in young and adult ages, gives way in old age to a relatively predominant serotonergic/catabolic profile with less competence for homeostasis and high incidence of disease.[7,8]

4. Changes in Neurotransmitter Receptors and Rhythmicity

Changes in neurotransmitter, hormone, and cytokine receptors with aging are discussed in previous chapters, particularly 14 to 20.

Several neurotransmitters and hormones follow various rhythms regulated by external cues, of which the daily light/dark cycle is a most common example. In humans, as well as in other animals and plants, certain time variations (e.g., daily, weekly, monthly, yearly) are maintained in the absence of environmental periodicity and their persistence has been ascribed to the presence of endogenous synchronizers acting through neural and endocrine signals. For example, those related to specific neurotransmitters (e.g., serotonin) and hormones (e.g., melatonin) and the interactions between the two have been implicated not only in the photoperiod regulation of reproductive events, but also in the modulation of a large number of other functions (Chapter 4). Melatonin from the pineal gland controls thermoregulation, feeding and sexual behaviors, cardiovascular functions, and through its interactions with serotonin, participates in regulation of secretion of ACTH, corticosterone, β-endorphin, prolactin, renin, vasopressin, oxytocin, GH and LH, and the sleep/wake cycle.[9,10] Many of these rhythmic functions are altered with aging (Chapters 3, 4, 7, 8, and 14). Loss of complexity (chaos) in the dynamics of healthy organ and system functions (e.g., loss of complex variability in cardiovascular control, pulsatile hormone release, electroencephalographic potentials) may lead with aging to impaired ability to adapt to stress.[11]

Hormonal shifts may be triggered by changes occurring in secretion/levels of neurotransmitters. In the rat, for example, a peak in the circadian hypothalamic serotonin cycle triggers the surge of LH preceding ovulation so that, given the proper hormonal (estrogen) environment, the actual levels of serotonin are less important for inducing the LH surge than a properly timed peak in the neurotransmitter. Depression of the hypothalamic peak by neonatal administration of serotonin inhibitors or it displacement by changes in light/dark daily cycles will block LH surge and alter the length of the reproductive period by accelerating both onset of reproduction and its termination.

5. The Genetic Connection

The strong linkage of genes to lifespan is verified by the simple observation that some species live longer than others and by other convincing evidence (Chapters 1 and 15). The relationship of steroid and thyroid hormones to the viral oncogene erbA suggests, despite differences in chemistry and function, a genetic relationship (Chapter 16). Steroid (including adrenocortical and gonadal) and thyroid hormone receptors are products of a superfamily of genes. The kinship of these receptors suggests that they may all be part of regulatory proteins that have a function, over evolutionary time, to match the increasing needs (homeostasis, longer lifespan) of the more complex organisms. The cloning of steroid and thyroid hormone receptors represents a logical outcome of current efforts to understand neuroendocrine actions and the role that they may be playing in aging and longevity.

Genes hold the codes to these molecules, but what substances turn the genes on and off? And, once activated, how do their products, hormones and neurotransmitters, interact with the products of other genes?

6. Interventions: Drugs, Diet, Transplants

The proposition is that aging may depend on neuroendocrine signals, and current knowledge of neural and endocrine functions have provided a rationale for the use of a variety of interventions to treat aging-associated diseases as well as to delay aging.[5] Some of these measures are discussed throughout this book.

C. Pituitary (and Other Endocrine) Hypotheses

Contrasting observations range from:

- Involutional changes of organs and tissues induced by pituitary lack or hypofunction and resembling those of old age,
- Acceleration of aging processes and contribution to the pathology of senescence by pituitary hormones.

These changes may be caused directly by hormonal actions or indirectly by hormone-induced alterations of metabolism and food intake. In the rat, food intake is increased by thyroid and growth hormones, corticosteroids, and insulin, and decreased by thyroidectomy and hypophysectomy. Long-term undernutrition in humans and rodents is accompanied by low circulating levels of the hormones secreted by the anterior pituitary and its target endocrines. Dietary restriction by various means, especially when initiated at weaning, delays maturation (e.g. onset of reproductive function is delayed) and extends (by as much as 30 to 40%) the lifespan in rodents. Hypophysectomy represents an alternative means, although less effective, of inducing chronic underfeeding in rats. Dietary restriction may operate through complex neuroendocrine signals mediated by neurotransmitters, hypothalamic hypophysiotropic hormones, and cellular and molecular actions of hormones on tissues, especially the CNS.[4]

Changes in pituitary secretion with aging may involve alterations in the synthesis of the hormones or in their metabolism due to impaired activity of the enzymes responsible for their cleavage from larger precursor molecules (Chapter 3) or the presence of polymorphic forms with varying biologic potency (Chapters 5 and 7). Polymorphism, although present at all ages, increases in old age when it is also associated with a decline in the carbohydrate content of glycoprotein hormones. Insulin is another hormone with possibly impaired synthesis (and efficiency?) in the elderly (Chapters 10 and 11). The functional significance of these altered forms remains to be clarified.

Other hormones may play a key role in longevity. Among these, thyroid hormones by their regulatory role on basal metabolism and on brain function have been singled out as possible regulators of aging (Chapter 5). Some of the steroid hormones, mainly DHEA, may also lengthen the lifespan (Chapter 2). In view of the close interactions among endocrine glands and the complexity of endocrine, neurotransmitter, and immune signals, it may be unrealistic to ascribe aging to alterations of a single endocrine gland, even those with many actions such as the pituitary and thyroid. Aging, rather, may result from multineural and multiendocrine disturbances.

1. Progeria and Progeroid Syndromes

These syndromes are examples in which length of lifespan depends on a strong genetic component. Progeria (premature old age) and progeroid (progeria-like) syndromes resemble but do not quite duplicate the total pathophysiology of aging: each syndrome represents the acceleration of some aging characteristics, including endocrine dysfunctions. The genetic variants determine accelerations or decelerations of changes in the senescent phenotypes and these may result from or be influenced by hormonal factors. While the expression of these syndromes is obscure, among the many causes suggested, neuroendocrine dysfunction is supported by a number of symptoms such as stunted somatic growth and impaired gonadal development.

D. Neuroendocrine-Immune Interactions

The immune system, also implicated in aging, originally viewed as essentially autonomous, has an autonomy more apparent than real. It is now abundantly clear that the immune system is subject to neural and endocrine influences and exerts, in turn, a reciprocal influence on these systems.[12,13] A knowledge of these extremely complex and not fully understood interactions is based on information that is rapidly accruing and is quite convincing. A brief discussion of the relations of neuroendocrine and immune systems in body defenses and aging is presented in Chapter 20.

III. OUTLOOK

As previously discussed, aging may result from a multiplicity of factors, both genetic and environmental, rather than from a single, unifying cause. In the present uncertainty, neuro-immuno-endocrine theories of aging have an important role to play. Which of these theories is the correct one and, indeed, whether changes with advancing age in neural, immune, and endocrine functions are the cause or consequence of aging remains to be verified. Yet, the pursuit of the study of these theories is important for it will provide, as it has already done in the past, future breakthroughs in our understanding and treatment of the aging process.

The notion that biologic functions may be reduced to principles of physics and chemistry has culminated in the view held by many molecular biologists that the organism is a simple sum of its molecular and cellular parts. However, it is apparent that unique complexities arise at each level of organization which cannot be simply explained or predicted by the knowledge of the components parts of an organism. Although it may be possible to catalog any molecule in the cell and any cell in an organ, this information fails to explain adequately the complex interactions among molecules in a cell, cells in an organ, and organs in a multisystem organism. Structure and function of each body component must be integrated by physiologic coordination (homeostasis) as regulated by the nervous, endocrine, and immunologic systems. Both reductionism (illustrated by molecular biology) and synthesis (illustrated by physiology) should be viewed as complementary and not as competitive methods of studying biologic activities.

In this general framework, the concept of "pacemaker" or command cells situated in specific brain areas and expressing themselves through genetic, neural, hormonal, and immune signals provides a useful model for devising experiments for the control of aging, its induction, prevention, and modulation. Identification of the responsible signals at the cellular and molecular levels has provided a better understanding of the aging process and further progress with this methodology is expected. The rapid advances in gene modification make it possible to envision modification of synthesis of proteins that regulate adaptation (in somatic cells perishing with the individual) and units of inheritance that regulate reproduction (and survive the death of the individual).

Current experimentation, combining molecular, cellular, and biomedical methodology, is poised to advance research and foster discoveries in aging studies. From the many potentially effective areas of research that have been discussed throughout this book, some may be regarded as especially worthy of continuing investigation:

- The study of cell proliferation, differentiation, and death — hormones, local growth factors, cytokines, extracellular matrix components, and cell-cell interactions contribute to inhibit or activate the expression of growth stimulatory factors or induce growth suppressor genes and gene products;
- The study of binding of chemical signals on target cell receptors — secondary messengers induced by tyrosine kinase cell surface receptors activate intracellular transduction pathways and ultimately affect nuclear transcription with induction/repression of particular sets of target genes;
- The study of changes with aging in target cells (involving receptors, energy metabolism, ionic content and transport) — with consequent differential responsiveness to their microenviroment and differential responsiveness to replacement therapy with endocrine and local hormones, neurotransmitters, and cytokines.

Other important aspects of research are concerned with:

- The biotechnologic synthesis of valuable new products that can be utilized for replacement therapy and treatment (following the successful synthesis of human growth hormone, insulin, erythropoietin, interferons, and others);
- The interactions between neuroendocrine and immune agents and other factors such as medications, leisure drugs, constituents of the diet;
- The use of transgenic animals as well as tissue culture techniques to investigate a wide range of cell functions (e.g., gene expression, production of membrane and cytoplasmic proteins) acting directly and specifically on target cells.

Information obtained from experimental studies must be integrated with clinical aspects of aging in humans to improve the physiologic competence (homeostasis) and adaptation of the individual. Therefore the success of medicine in the future will depend on:

- The ability of health professionals to adapt biotechnologic advances to the prevention and treatment of disabilities and diseases at all ages but particularly in old age,
- An educated use of these techniques to avoid unnecessary and inappropriate high technology in older persons.

Although shifting economic conditions and changing societal needs are issues that have not been dealt with in this book, human health cannot be separated from the environment. To insure a long and healthy life, improvements in economic, social, as well as ethical circumstances must continue to evolve and change together with scientific, biologic, and medical progress in order to sustain a coalition of efforts towards wellness and longevity.

REFERENCES

1. Timiras, P. S., Neuroendocrinology of aging: retrospective, current and prospective views, in, *Neuroendocrinology of Aging,* Meites, J., Ed., Plenum Press, New York, 1983, 5.
2. Timiras, P. S., Ed., *Physiological Basis of Aging and Geriatrics,* 2nd ed., CRC Press, Boca Raton, FL, 1994.
3. Finch, C. E., *Longevity, Senescence, and the Genome,* University of Chicago Press, Chicago, 1990.
4. Everritt, A. V. and Walton, J. R., Eds., *Regulation of Neuroendocrine Aging,* (Interdisciplinary Topics in Gerontology, Vol. 24), Karger, Basel, 1988.
5. Frolkis, V. V. and Muradian, K. K., *Life Span Prolongation,* CRC Press, Boca Raton, FL, 1991.
6. Timiras, P. S., Privat, A., Giacobini, E., Lauder, J., and Vernadakis, A. Eds., *Plasticity and Regeneration of the Nervous System,* Advances in Experimental Medicine and Biology, Vol. 296, Plenum Press, New York, 1991.
7. Meites, J., Aging of the endocrine brain. Basic and clinical aspects, in *Brain Endocrinology,* 2nd ed., Motta, M., Ed., Raven Press, New York, 1991, 449.
8. Proceedings of a workshop, Parma, Italy, 1991, Psychoneuroendocrinology of aging: the brain as target organ of hormones, *Psychoneuroendocrinology,* 17, 277, 1992.
9. Van de Kar, L. D., and Brownfield, M. S., Serotonergic neurons and neuroendocrine function, *News Physiol. Sci.,* 8, 202, 1993.
10. Ebadi, M., Samejima, M., and Pfeiffer, R. F., Pineal gland in synchronizing and refining physiological events, *News Physiol. Sci.,* 8, 30, 1993.
11. Lipsitz, L. A., and Goldberger, A. L., Loss of complexity and aging. Potential applications of fractals and chaos theory to senescence, *JAMA,* 267, 1806, 1992.
12. Fabris, N., Biomarkers of aging in the neuroendocrine-immune domain. Time for a new theory of aging?, *Ann. N. Y. Acad. Sci.,* 663, 335, 1992.
13. Reichlin, S., Neuroendocrine-immune interactions, *N. Engl. J. Med.,* 329, 1246, 1993.

INDEX